Clinical Manual
of Health
Assessment

Fourth Edition

Clinical Manual of Health Assessment

Arden C. Bowers, RN, MS

Former Associate Professor,
Department of Nursing,
College of Santa Fe,
Santa Fe, New Mexico

June M. Thompson, RN, MS

Assistant Professor of Nursing,
Prairie View College of Nursing,
Texas A & M University,
Houston, Texas

With contributions by

Mindi Miller, RN, PhD

Adjunct Professor,
Department of Human Performance and Health Sciences,
Rice University,
Houston, Texas

with 670 illustrations

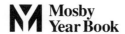

Mosby
Year Book

St. Louis Baltimore Boston Chicago London Philadelphia Sydney Toronto

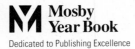
Mosby
Year Book
Dedicated to Publishing Excellence

Editor Terry Van Schaik
Developmental Editors Janet R. Livingston, Sally Adkisson
Project Manager Patricia Tannian
Production Editor Betty Hazelwood
Designer David Zielinski

Fourth edition

Previous editions copyrighted 1980, 1984, and 1988

Printed in the United States of America.

Mosby—Year Book, Inc.
11830 Westline Industrial Drive
St Louis, MO 63146

Library of Congress Cataloging-in-Publication Data

Bowers, Arden C.
    Clinical manual of health assessment / Arden C. Bowers, June M.
  Thompson; with contributions by Mindi Miller.—4th ed.
        p.   cm.
    Includes bibliographical references and index.
    1. Nursing assessment. I. Thompson, June M., 1946–.
  II. Miller, Mindi. III. Title.
    [DNLM: 1. Diagnosis. 2. Health. 3. Health Status. WB 200
B786c]
RT48.B68 1991
616.07′5—dc20
DNLM/DLC
for Library of Congress   91-31339
                                                             CIP
ISBN 0-8016-0826-0

92 93 94 95 96 GW/VH   9 8 7 6 5 4 3 2 1

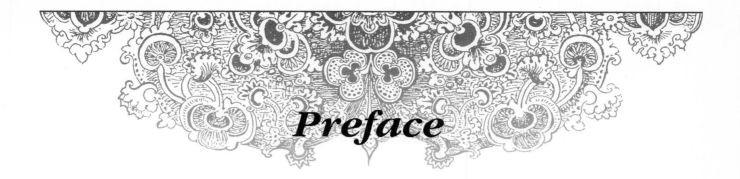

Preface

This manual is designed for use in a clinical or laboratory setting as a procedural guide for students who are learning health assessment. Each chapter offers the knowledge necessary to proceed with a given portion of assessment, the explicit skills for the student to perform, and the expected findings that result from individual assessment efforts.

New to this edition are anatomy and physiology summaries for 13 clinical chapters. This inclusion permits students to review an applicable knowledge base before proceeding with the practice component of assessment.

Integrated into each clinical chapter, separate sections on age-group considerations for newborns, children, pregnant women, and older adults enable students to perform a thorough health assessment on all clients. These sections include some deviations from normal findings so that the student can be alert to common health problems specific to clients of each age group. Some information is repeated in the age-related sections so that the student can locate specific data for immediate clinical reference. Although this approach is somewhat redundant, it allows each section to stand alone.

The chapter on functional assessment includes a generic tool for assessing the capability of healthy and disabled clients of all ages to function satisfactorily within their given environments. This chapter addresses the aging population, the heightened awareness of problems faced by disabled people, and the trend toward self-care in the home and other alternatives to hospitalization. Functional assessment is meant to complement the traditional assessment approach.

The manual is divided into four areas: the total health data base chapter; 14 clinical chapters that present specific systems or body regions for study; the integration chapter, which offers a detailed outline of the entire health assessment process; and the functional assessment chapter. Each chapter can be used as a single unit of study. The 14 clinical chapters follow a consistent format, comprising the following sections:

1. *Vocabulary.* A list of defined terms associated with the system or region of study.
2. *Anatomy and physiology.* A review of anatomy and physiology that provides background needed to perform body-system assessment.
3. *Cognitive objectives.* An outline of defined learning needs.
4. *Clinical outline.* An outline of clinical entities that must be assessed.
5. *History.* An in-depth systemic or regional history that investigates common problems, complaints, and client risk potential.
6. *Clinical guidelines.* A procedural outline that includes examiner behaviors and clinical entities to be assessed, expected normal findings, and common deviations from normal findings. Throughout the manual this section is supported with illustrations.
7. *Clinical tips and strategies.* Notes and helpful hints for the beginning student regarding examination techniques and client behaviors.
8. *Sample recording: normal findings.* An example of a written description of normal findings.
9. *History and clinical strategies.* A discussion of approaches and additional history data for each age group: the newborn, the child, the childbearing woman, and the older adult.
10. *Clinical variations.* A detailed outline of the examination procedure, anticipated normal findings, and commonly identified deviations for each age group: the newborn, the child, the childbearing woman, and the older adult.
11. *Study questions.* A quiz section that demonstrates the student's understanding of manual material and monitors progress. Answers are provided at the end of the book.
12. *Suggested readings.* Additional readings complement the information in each chapter.

The assessment procedures are elaborate and detailed. The format of the book guides the student through cognitive application, a sequence of skill maneuvers, and detailed descriptors of common findings within normal limits and of findings that extend beyond normal. The illustrations, photographs, and careful description of findings assist students in being accountable for the results of their assessment efforts. However, this text does not attempt to lead students to diagnoses. Giving meaning to the findings requires clinical practice, preceptorship, and further study.

v

We have found that the clinical guidelines are extremely useful in the laboratory setting. We suggest to our students that they read aloud and discuss procedures while following along with a fellow student. The students are asked to describe the procedure, their rationale for their behaviors, and the characteristics of the findings as they progress. They frequently complete a practice session by writing out their actual findings for one another to critique.

To assist instructors further in assessing student progress, we have included a test bank with this edition. The test questions relate to the Cognitive Objectives, found at the beginning of each chapter in the book.

This manual is designed to provide the student with an orderly, thorough method of collecting and categorizing accurate and well-defined data in preparation for subsequent professional care.

Arden C. Bowers
June M. Thompson

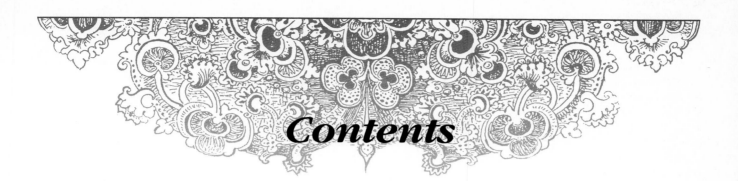

Contents

Introduction

Assessment of an individual begins with careful, deliberate, and concrete observations of the whole person. Textbooks traditionally divide the remainder of the examination process into parts composed of body systems or regions. This division is convenient for the learner, who functions cognitively and clinically in logically sequenced segments, gradually coordinating the segments to form a total process of assessment.

This manual proceeds in a logical fashion. The whole person is assessed, from a personal viewpoint, through the use of the health history chapter (Chapter 1). Simultaneously, the examiner must be aware of the information provided in the chapter on general and mental status assessment (Chapter 2). The examiner begins collecting objective data as soon as the client is encountered and throughout the history-taking session. Dress, mannerisms, general body movement, and behavior are observed and noted as contributions to the final summary. Thereafter the student can proceed through the remaining clinical chapters, segment by segment, gradually using and synthesizing knowledge until all the parts are fitted together. The final chapter offers a detailed outline for fitting examiner behavior and clinical findings into a coordinated procedure and total summary.

We have used this manual in the laboratory setting for several years and have noted that predictable levels of learning are exhibited by the student. These phases must be acknowledged by both learner and teacher in designing and evaluating student progress.

A knowledge base is essential to the learner before psychomotor skills can be practiced. Anatomy and physiology supply the rationale for performing an examination and for the presence of normal findings. A cognitive introduction to the use of instruments and the practices of observation, palpation, auscultation, and percussion prepares the student for laboratory performance. Interviewing skills and analytical thinking are necessary prerequisites for acquiring an accurate and effective data base.

Much of the laboratory time is devoted to the mechanical aspects of the examination. Students need to concentrate on how to position the client (usually a fellow student) and how to maneuver their own bodies during the examination. They need to practice the skills of percussion, auscultation, and palpation. The use of equipment and the sequence of maneuvers are frequently the focus of attention before any cognitive application can occur.

Some body systems require a great deal of psychomotor skill. For example, use of the ophthalmoscope is difficult, and much time is consumed in manipulating the instrument and the client's and examiner's bodies. We have found that deep palpation of the abdomen is a new experience for many students and that tactile awareness is an acquired skill. Giving *meaning* to the findings that result from the process of examination may not occur until after several practice sessions.

When the learner is comfortable with the physical maneuvers, attention can then be given to the findings and their significance. Learners must be encouraged to describe findings in concrete terms rather than to simply label a part as "normal" or "OK." Normal findings have variations, with many gray areas between normal and abnormal. Examiners must be precise about what they have found and be able to clearly convey descriptions to others. We have found that beginning students have a difficult time accounting for their findings. They benefit greatly by verbally describing their findings as they examine and by writing up the results of the examination in each laboratory session.

Simulated abnormal findings can be taught in a laboratory. For example, audiovisual equipment can demonstrate skin lesions or abnormal heart sounds. However, the real application of performing a full assessment and sorting the resultant data does not usually occur until the student practices in a clinical setting with a preceptor. It is our belief that knowing the significance of findings and responding to them with direct intervention or referral to others is a lifelong learning process.

The chapter on functional assessment requires a different framework for approach and analysis on the part of the student. Functional assessment bypasses body systems. It explores the capacity of an individual to manipulate his environment to his satisfaction. The client's "satisfaction" is dependent on his biological, psychosocial, and spiritual state, as well as the biological, psychosocial, and spiritual resources in his environment.

To analyze and intervene using functional information obtained from the client, the practitioner must be knowledgeable about nursing diagnoses and rehabilitation concepts.

We certainly acknowledge that human beings are more than the sum of their parts. They are dynamic entities interacting with the environment to attain or maintain a state of maximum well-being. As the student begins to pool information about a person, the development of a problem list, a client profile, a risk profile, and a functional profile should occur.

The therapeutic application of the information in that final summary requires further professional knowledge beyond the scope and intent of this book. Recognizing client strengths, setting priorities with the client for seeking solutions to problems, and taking into account all the environmental variables that alter the client's state of well-being involve additional professional preparation.

This manual is designed to provide the student with an orderly, thorough method of collecting and categorizing accurate and well-defined data in preparation for subsequent professional care.

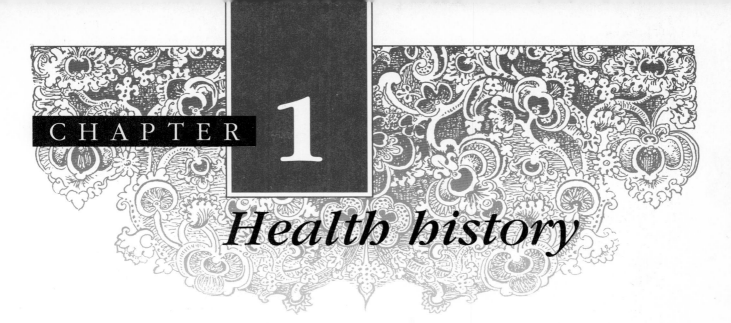

CHAPTER 1

Health history

VOCABULARY

active listening State of selective attention and alertness that encompasses the skill of observation so that verbal and nonverbal cues are registered and clarified in an interaction; involves data absorption, retention, and exchange for clarification of meaning.

assessment Process of gathering and analyzing subjective and objective client data for summarization of a client's status.

data base Collection or store of information

subjective Portion of the client data that is supplied by the client; the client's perceptions of himself.

objective Portion of the client data that is perceived by the examiner through physical examination or obtained from other external sources (such as laboratory studies).

empathic response State of mind that enables one to view another as that person views himself; coupled with interviewing skills that enable an examiner to verbally or nonverbally respond to a client statement without coloring or altering the client's intended meaning.

silence A deliberate examiner response (sometimes very difficult for the examiner) to a client statement; allows time for client reflection.

facilitative behaviors Examiner behaviors (verbal or nonverbal) that encourage the client to continue.

EXAMPLES: Leaning forward, nodding head, maintaining eye contact, or saying, "Um-hum," "Yes," "Please go on," etc.

reflection Repetition of key words from the client's last statement to encourage elaboration.

EXAMPLE: The client says, "I feel as though I'm going to explode." The examiner responds, "Explode?"

interpretive reflection Rearrangement or rewording of the client's statement.

EXAMPLE: The client says, "When you have that much pain, you just want to give up." The examiner responds, "You feel frustrated and helpless."

exacerbation Increase in intensity of signs or symptoms.

hypothesis Formation of an idea that relates available information to a probable cause. (*Note:* In the context of research, *hypothesis* has a broader meaning.)

incidence The number of times an event occurs.

precipitating factor Event or entity that hastens the onset of another event.

EXAMPLE: Chronic overeating is a precipitating factor for obesity.

predisposing factor (risk factor) Event or entity that contributes to the cause of another event.

EXAMPLE: A family history of obesity increases the risk for obesity.

problem list Compilation of findings that appear at the end of the data base; may be diagnoses (medical or nursing), clusters of interrelated findings, or isolated findings that the examiner wishes to pursue but cannot label or attach to other findings.

EXAMPLE: *diagnoses*—herpes simplex, knowledge deficit; *clusters*—polydipsia, polyuria, polyphagia; *finding*—lower back pain.

questions

closed Question posed in such a way that the respondent is directed toward a brief answer or a "yes" or "no"; does not encourage the respondent to elaborate.

EXAMPLE: "Has your back pain improved since the last visit?"

open A broadly stated question that encourages a free-flowing, open response.

EXAMPLE: "How has your back been feeling since your last visit?"

directive General term for a question or series of questions that leads the client in the questioner's channel of thinking. (*Note:* Most of the questions in the review of systems are directive.)

EXAMPLES: "Have you ever noticed blurred vision? Double vision?" "Do you see spots or floaters?"

probing Form of directive questioning that enables the examiner to pursue a line of thinking to prove or disprove a hypothesis.

leading A question worded in such a way that it suggests the answer to the respondent.

EXAMPLE: "Do you find that your chest pain radiates to your left arm or shoulder?" versus "Does your chest pain ever move around or locate in another area?"

remission Disappearance or diminishment of signs or symptoms.

sign Objective finding; one perceived by the examiner.

significant negative Absence of a finding that is often significant in clarifying the client's status.

EXAMPLE: A client with diagnosed congestive heart failure shows no sign of ankle edema. (This is significant and should be reported as negative, or not present, because it clarifies the client's physical status for the reader.)

suspended judgment State of mind that permits the examiner to pose questions without allowing the answers to convey a meaning that would alter the completion or direction of the ensuing questions; suspended meaning allows both the examiner and the client to maintain an open state of inquiry versus pursuing a narrowed line of questioning to support the meaning of a given answer.

symptom Subjective indicator or sensation perceived by the client.

PRINCIPLES AND CONCEPTS

A health history is a compilation of client information (data) gathered through a systematic interview for the purpose of identifying and serving client needs. The mode and content of the interview and the ensuing data base will vary. The format presented in this text is known as the *long form*. It covers everything that an examiner could want to know about a client. Practitioners who use this format can spend from 1 to 3 hours collecting, compiling, and collating client data. The long form is known also as the *exhaustive method* for problem solving because its framework incorporates nonjudgmental descriptors of every aspect of the human condition. It does not urge the user to hypothesize about symptoms or to veer from the format to pursue an idea or a suspected diagnosis. The long form discourages straying from pure data collection and encourages the examiner to remain in a state of suspended judgment until all the facts have been gathered for sifting and analysis.

In clinical situations in which time and space are limited, the student may find the exhaustive method to be impractical. Seasoned preceptors may use a questioning mode, which quickly launches into specific probing questions. For example, if a client has presenting symptoms of weight loss, thirst, polyuria, and excessive hunger, the experienced examiner might immediately ask about a family history of diabetes, vaginal irritation, and skin infections. The exhaustive style would pursue a detailed symptom analysis (see box, p. 11) to clarify each symptom; family history and review of specific systems would come later. Each approach has advantages, depending on the (1) intent of the interview, (2) condition of the client, (3) knowledge base and experience of the examiner, (4) constraints of the clinical setting, and (5) expectations of the client.

Intent of the Interview

Medical inquiry has traditionally focused on exploration of *effects* (symptoms), which leads to *cause* (diagnosis), which leads to *cure*. The intent is to spend a minimum amount of time lingering on the effects and to quickly check hunches (hypotheses) about causes (suspected diseases), which leads to prescriptions for treatment. Reaching the stage of checking hunches can sometimes be accomplished quickly if the symptoms are localized (e.g., earache). If the client has broad or vague presenting symptoms (e.g., fatigue or weight loss), the examiner remains longer in a state of suspended judgment to clarify such factors as onset and duration, before asking probing, directive questions. The physician will branch off into an area of questioning to prove or disprove a hypothesis. If probing in this fashion disproves the hunch, the physician returns to nonjudgmental inquiry to get more information until another hypothesis forms, which leads to further probing.

Nursing inquiry frequently elicits more information about the effects. The nurse is interested in how the client functions within his environment. Pathological factors are relevant, but nurses recognize that causes may stem from such conditions as environmental influences, family relationships, or the client's coping skills. Nurses tend to inquire more closely and broadly about effects and to remain in suspended judgment for a longer time to gather this information.

Boundaries between traditional medical and nursing modes are no longer distinct. Physicians, especially those in primary care settings, are being taught and urged to gather a broad data base and to give more attention to the client effects. Nurses have extended into some of the medical functions and are posing questions in the traditional medical mode to uncover disease. Many professional people are becoming more holistically oriented. The holistic philosophy demands that the examiner acquire complete information about each client because the philosophy holds that illness cannot be separated from wellness and both are entrenched in the client's environment and life-style.

Some practitioners have a completely nondirective approach, which is often used in a psychological interview. The client is asked the reason for the visit and is encouraged to give information in whatever order and pace he devises. Probing and confrontation are deliberately delayed to give the client total freedom of expression.

Regardless of approach, it is extremely important that the examiner understand the *purpose* of the interview.

The history format is intended to be flexible and to be used as a vehicle for effective, efficient information gathering.

Condition of the Client

Urgency dictates expediency. A client with severe pain should not be subjected to a prolonged history. Biographical data may be delayed to pursue the chief complaint, followed by a symptom analysis and selected system review. This approach enables the examiner to hypothesize quickly and identify the cause, which leads to prompt alleviation of pain. A client with depression might be given more time to freely divulge feelings and surrounding circumstances without interference from the examiner. An elderly client with multiple symptoms, a long history of illness and hospitalizations, and numerous problems at home would benefit from a full data base (exhaustive) approach.

Knowledge Base and Experience of the Examiner

To hypothesize about causes, one must have a store of knowledge to draw from, since human perceptions are narrowed by lack of knowledge and experience. A beginner cannot invent directive questions that lead to diagnosis. Therefore students are urged to prolong the state of suspended judgment and to get full details about clients. The process of hypothesizing channels one's thinking and perceptions into a specific area and shuts out extraneous information. Lack of knowledge blurs the difference between what is extraneous and what is significant. Students should have experience with gathering a full data base. In this way they learn the value of each component of the history, and they give themselves and the client more time to sift through the facts to arrive at a series of findings.

Constraints of the Clinical Setting

Practitioners with nondirective approaches or holistic beliefs can become frustrated (and ineffective) in a clinic setting that allocates 30 minutes for each client appointment. Time and space can dictate a philosophy and practice mode regardless of examiner intent or client condition. If cost-effectiveness calls for rapid patient turnover, the examiner must either function accordingly within that value system, change the system, or become creative in accomplishing his intent. A full data base can be gathered over time. In some instances clients can complete portions of the history at home or in the waiting room. It is pointless to record a full data base if no one is going to read it or use the information. Gathering such data also is misleading to the client if identified problems are not followed up. Students sometimes become frustrated when they cannot use a full data base in a real-life setting. Yet it is a valuable lesson

to be knowledgeable about the potential for a complete history and to have to relinquish portions of it for expediency. The student is aware of what is missing and may choose to question the value of expediency.

Expectations of the Client

A client with a painful ingrown toenail wants relief. He does not expect to discuss the condition of his neighborhood or his relationship with significant others. Because many clinics have an episodic care modality, clients have been conditioned to present tangible symptoms for diagnosis and treatment. They do not expect a 3-hour interview, even if they have multiple problems, and they may be confused or annoyed by a long interview. Other clients do expect adequate time for relaying all of their circumstances, and they benefit from such attention. Some clients expect a leisurely interview session and have difficulty with efficient conveyance of information. It is extremely important that the examiner, the client, and the health agency are clear about *why* the history is being taken. If an examiner has only 15 minutes, this information should be shared with the client at the onset. People generally become more efficient when they know that time is limited. If the interview will be lengthy, the client should be prepared and accepting of this.

With most histories both the examiner and the client benefit if the examiner is nondirective for the first 5 to 10 minutes of the interview. The client is asked the reason for the visit and allowed to freely convey information in his own fashion. This requires active listening, observing, and empathic skills on the part of the questioner. The practitioner can make observations about the client's behaviors and verbal styles, as well as gain spontaneous information from the client. This approach also establishes a condition of trust between client and professional. At the same time, the client is observing the examiner. He needs to know that he has the examiner's full attention and concern. A state of suspended judgment broadens the examiner's perceptions and increases openness for inflow of data; it allows for patient priorities to be identified. It is human nature to hypothesize and to probe. The examiner must be aware when he or she is doing this and acknowledge that directive questions are being posed. Otherwise the client can easily be steered into a thinking channel that diverts from his original one.

At some point the history taking moves into a probing style (hypothesis generation and follow-up). It may go back and forth between probing, asking nonjudgmental questions, allowing free flow of conversation, and more probing. The questioner must judge the importance of being nondirective versus redirecting the client to answer specific questions. Sometimes practitioners with nondirective styles need to learn to interrupt and retrace a line of thinking. Directive people must concentrate and develop a facilitative style to permit client expression. This practice is both an art and a science.

A model for clinical problem solving is shown in Fig. 1-1. Note that the history-taking aspect of problem solving is contained in the first four steps of the process. Step 3 denotes the shift from nonjudgmental to directive questioning. This may precede step 2 in certain situations or may not occur until the entire history has been taken.

The expanded data base outline that follows provides a method for collecting data about the client's physiological, psychological, and sociocultural health. It also includes questions about the client's past health and the health of the family. When integrated, the information becomes the client's *health data base*. The practitioner must analyze and organize the data base to formulate the following:

- A subjective data problem list (including physiological symptoms and psychological, social, or environmental

factors that concern the client and/or the examiner). This will later be combined with the physical assessment problem list to develop a total problem list in the final write-up.
- A risk profile (risk factors related to certain body systems are listed in subsequent chapters).
- A client profile (a summary, from the *client's* viewpoint, of his life-style and ability to cope with self-care).

These data will serve as a constant resource for comparison as the client's condition changes and he provides new information in future assessments.

COGNITIVE OBJECTIVES

At the end of this chapter the learner will demonstrate knowledge of the effective techniques and components of the health history by the ability to do the following:

- Apply the terms that are listed in the vocabulary section.
- Discuss the rationale and options for examiner behav-

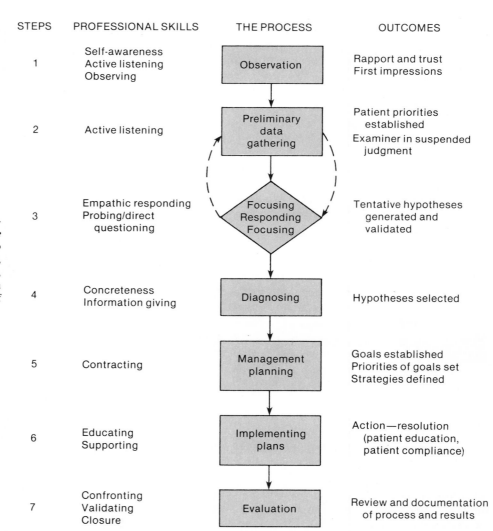

Fig. 1-1 Clinical problem solving. (Modified from *Comprehensive humanistic health care.* The Ohio State University, Grant No. 713297, Health Resources Administration, Department of Health and Human Services, Cherry McPherson, chief investigator, 1980-1983.)

STEPS	PROFESSIONAL SKILLS	THE PROCESS	OUTCOMES
1	Self-awareness Active listening Observing	Observation	Rapport and trust First impressions
2	Active listening	Preliminary data gathering	Patient priorities established Examiner in suspended judgment
3	Empathic responding Probing/direct questioning	Focusing Responding Focusing	Tentative hypotheses generated and validated
4	Concreteness Information giving	Diagnosing	Hypotheses selected
5	Contracting	Management planning	Goals established Priorities of goals set Strategies defined
6	Educating Supporting	Implementing plans	Action—resolution (patient education, patient compliance)
7	Confronting Validating Closure	Evaluation	Review and documentation of process and results

iors as they gather and analyze health data for the
following:
1. Well person (does not belong in following categories)
2. Well childbearing woman
3. Well newborn
4. Well child
5. Well older adult
- Define the 10 components of the adult data base.
- List the sections of the social history and provide at least one example of relevant information gathered in each section.
- List and define the 11 components of the analysis of a symptom.
- Recognize the characteristics of the newborn, the child, and the childbearing woman that are collected in addition to or as substitution for the adult data base.
- Recognize the characteristics of the older adult that are collected in addition to or as substitution for the adult data base.

CLINICAL OUTLINE

- At the end of this chapter the learner will conduct a systematic and accurate assessment of an individual's health status using the following format:
  1. Biographical data
  2. Reason for visit (chief complaint)
  3. Present health status (general summary and symptom analysis; also known as *history of present illness—HOPI)*
  4. Current health data
  5. Past health status
  6. Family history
  7. Review of physiological systems
  8. Psychosocial history
  9. Health maintenance efforts
  10. Environmental health status
- The learner will complete the assessment with the following:
  1. Problem list
  2. Risk profile
  3. Client profile

EXPANDED CLINICAL OUTLINE
FOR THE ADULT
Biographical Data

- Name
- Age
- Race
- Culture
- Address and telephone number
- Marital status
- Children and family in home (if not family, significant others)
- Occupation

- Means of transportation to health care facility if pertinent
- Description of home and size and type of community

Reason for Visit

One statement that describes the reason for the client's visit or the chief complaint, stated in the client's own words.

Present Health Status

- Summary of client's current major health concerns
- If illness is present, record symptom analysis (see p. 11)
  1. When client was last well
  2. Date of problem onset
  3. Character of complaint
  4. Nature of problem onset
  5. Course of problem
  6. Client's hunch of precipating factors
  7. Location of problem
  8. Relation to other body symptoms, body positions, and activity
  9. Patterns of problem
  10. Efforts of client to treat
  11. Coping ability

Current Health Data

- Current medications
  1. Type (prescription, over-the-counter drugs, vitamins, etc.)
  2. Prescribed by whom
  3. When first prescribed
  4. Amount per day
  5. Problems
- Allergies (description of agent and reactions)
  1. Drugs
  2. Foods
  3. Contact substances
  4. Environmental factors
- Last examinations (physician/clinic, findings, advice, and/or instructions)
  1. Physical
  2. Dental
  3. Vision
  4. Hearing
  5. ECG
  6. Chest radiograph
  7. Pap smear (females)
  8. Tuberculosis tine test
- Immunization status (dates or year of last immunization)
  1. Tetanus, diphtheria, pertussis
  2. Mumps
  3. Rubella
  4. Polio
  5. Influenza

Past Health Status

Although each of the following is asked separately, the examiner must summarize and record the data *chronologically:*

- Childhood illnesses: rubeola, rubella, mumps, pertussis, scarlet fever, chickenpox, strep throat
- Serious or chronic illnesses: scarlet fever, diabetes, kidney problems, hypertension, sickle cell anemia, seizure disorders, blood infections
- Serious accidents or injuries: head injuries, fractures, burns, other trauma
- Hospitalizations: description of, including reason for, location, primary care providers, duration
- Operations: what, where, when, why, by whom
- Emotional health: past problems, help sought, support persons
- Obstetrical history
  1. Complete pregnancies: number, pregnancy course, postpartum course, and condition, weight, and sex of each child
  2. Incomplete pregnancies: duration, termination, circumstances (including abortions and stillbirths)
  3. Summary of complications

Family History

Family members include the client's blood relatives, spouse, and children. Specifically the interviewer should inquire about the client's maternal and paternal grandparents, parents, aunts, uncles, spouse, and children, as well as about the general health, stress factors, and illnesses of other family members. Questions should include a survey of the following:

Alzheimer's disease	Mental illnesses
Cancer	Developmental delay
Diabetes	Alcoholism
Heart disease	Endocrine diseases
Hypertension	Sickle cell anemia
Epilepsy (or seizure disorder)	Kidney disease Unusual limitations
Emotional stresses	Other chronic problems

The most concise method to record these data is by a family tree. Fig. 1-2 is an example.

Review of Physiological Systems

The purpose of this component of the data base is to collect information about the body regions or systems and their function.

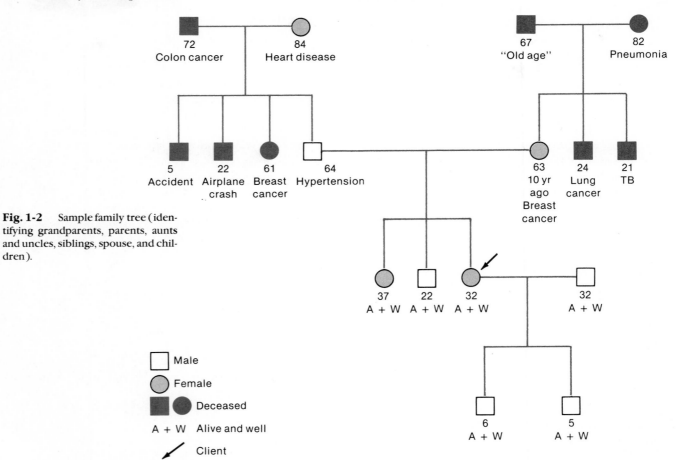

Fig. 1-2 Sample family tree (identifying grandparents, parents, aunts and uncles, siblings, spouse, and children).

- General—reflect from client's previous description of current health status
  1. Fatigue patterns
  2. Exercise and exercise tolerance
  3. History of weakness episodes, if any
  4. History of fever, sweats, if any
  5. Frequency of colds, infections, or illnesses
  6. Ability to carry out activities of daily living
- Nutritional
  1. Client's average, maximum, and minimum weights during past month; 1 year; 5 years
  2. History of weight gains or losses (time element); specific efforts to change weight
  3. Twenty-four-hour diet recall, as on p. 14 (helpful to mail the client a chart to fill in before visit)
  4. Cultural and/or religious practices regarding intake
  5. Current appetite
  6. Extreme deviations in physical activity that would affect appetite (e.g., athletic or immobilization influences)
  7. Person(s) who buys and prepares food
  8. Person(s) client normally eats with
  9. Availability of money to buy preferred food
  10. Status of ability to chew; condition of teeth or dentures
  11. Client's self-evaluation of nutritional status
- Integumentary
  1. Skin
     a. Skin disease, problems, lesions (wounds, sores, ulcers)
     b. Skin growths, tumors, masses
     c. Excessive dryness, sweating, odors
     d. Pigmentation changes or discolorations
     e. Pruritus (itching)
     f. Texture changes
     g. Temperature changes
  2. Hair
     a. Changes in amount, texture, character
     b. Alopecia (loss of hair)
     c. Use of dyes
  3. Nails
     a. Changes in appearance, texture
- Head
  1. Headache (characteristics, including frequency, type, location, duration, care for)
  2. Past significant trauma
  3. Dizziness
  4. Syncope
- Eyes
  1. Discharge (characteristics)
  2. History of infections, frequency, treatment
  3. Pruritus
  4. Lacrimation (excessive tearing)
  5. Pain in eyeball

  6. Spots (floaters)
  7. Swelling around eyes
  8. Cataracts, glaucoma
  9. Unusual sensations or twitching
  10. Vision changes (generalized or vision field)
  11. Use of corrective or prosthetic devices
  12. Diplopia (double vision)
  13. Blurring
  14. Photophobia
  15. Difficulty reading
  16. Interference with activities of daily living
- Ears
  1. Pain (characteristics)
  2. Cerumen (wax)
  3. Infection
  4. Hearing changes (describe)
  5. Use of prosthetic devices
  6. Increased sensitivity to environmental noise
  7. Vertigo
  8. Ringing and cracking
  9. Care habits
  10. Interference with activities of daily living
- Nose, nasopharynx, and paranasal sinuses
  1. Discharge (characteristics)
  2. Epistaxis
  3. Allergies
  4. Pain over sinuses
  5. Postnasal drip
  6. Sneezing
  7. General olfactory ability
- Mouth and throat
  1. Sore throats (characteristics)
  2. Tongue or mouth lesion (abscess, sore, ulcer)
  3. Bleeding gums
  4. Hoarseness
  5. Voice changes
  6. Use of prosthetic devices (dentures, bridges)
  7. Altered taste
  8. Chewing difficulty
  9. Swallowing difficulty
  10. Pattern of dental hygiene
- Neck
  1. Node enlargement
  2. Swellings, masses
  3. Tenderness
  4. Limitation of movement
  5. Stiffness
- Breasts
  1. Pain or tenderness
  2. Swelling
  3. Nipple discharge
  4. Changes in nipples
  5. Lumps, dimples
  6. Unusual characteristics
  7. Breast examination (pattern, frequency)

- Cardiovascular
  1. Cardiovascular
     a. Palpitations
     b. Heart murmur
     c. History of heart disease
     d. Hypertension
     e. Chest pain (character and frequency)
     f. Shortness of breath
     g. Orthopnea
     h. Paroxysmal nocturnal dyspnea
  2. Peripheral vascular
     a. Coldness, numbness
     b. Discoloration
     c. Peripheral edema
     d. Varicose veins
     e. Intermittent claudication
- Respiratory
  1. History of asthma
  2. Other breathing problems (when, precipitating factors)
  3. Sputum production
  4. Hemoptysis
  5. Chronic cough (characteristics)
  6. Shortness of breath (precipitating factors)
  7. Night sweats
  8. Wheezing or noise with breathing
- Hematolymphatic
  1. Lymph node swelling
  2. Excessive bleeding or easy bruising
  3. Petechiae, ecchymoses
  4. Anemia
  5. Blood transfusions
  6. Excessive fatigue
  7. Radiation exposure
- Gastrointestinal
  1. Food idiosyncrasies
  2. Change in taste
  3. Aphagoproxia or dysphagia (inability to swallow or difficulty in swallowing)
  4. Indigestion or pain (associated with eating?)
  5. Pyrosis (burning sensation in esophagus and stomach with sour eructation)
  6. Ulcer history
  7. Nausea/vomiting (time, degree, precipitating and/or associated factors)
  8. Hematemesis
  9. Jaundice
  10. Ascites
  11. Bowel habits (diarrhea/constipation)
  12. Stool characteristics
  13. Change in bowel habits
  14. Hemorrhoids (pain, bleeding, amount)
  15. Dyschezia (constipation resulting from habitual neglect in responding to stimulus to defecate)
  16. Use of digestive or evacuation aids (what, how often)

- Urinary
  1. Characteristics of urine
  2. History of renal stones
  3. Hesitancy
  4. Urinary frequency (in 24-hour period)
  5. Change in stream of urination
  6. Nocturia (excessive urination at night)
  7. History of urinary tract infection, dysuria (painful urination), urgency, flank pain
  8. Suprapubic pain
  9. Dribbling or incontinence
  10. Stress incontinence
  11. Polyuria (excessive excretion of urine)
  12. Oliguria (decrease in urinary output)
  13. Pyuria
- Genital
  1. General
     a. Lesions
     b. Discharges
     c. Odors
     d. Pain, burning, pruritus
     e. Venereal disease history
     f. Satisfaction with sexual activity
     g. Birth control methods practiced
     h. Sterility
  2. Men
     a. Prostate problems
     b. Penis and scrotum self-examination practices
  3. Women
     a. Menstrual history (age of onset, last menstrual period [LMP], duration and amount of flow, problems)
     b. Amenorrhea (absence of menses)
     c. Menorrhagia (excessive menstruation)
     d. Dysmenorrhea (painful menses), treatment method
     e. Metrorrhagia (uterine bleeding at times other than during menses)
     f. Dyspareunia (pain with intercourse)
- Musculoskeletal
  1. Muscles
     a. Twitching
     b. Cramping
     c. Pain
     d. Weakness
  2. Extremities
     a. Deformity
     b. Gait or coordination difficulties
     c. Interference with activities of daily living
     d. Walking (amount per day)
  3. Bones and joints
     a. Joint swelling
     b. Joint pain
     c. Redness
     d. Stiffness (time-of-day related)

e. Joint deformity

f. Crepitus (noise with joint movement)

g. Limitations of movement

h. Interference with ADLs (activities of daily living)

4. Back

a. History of back injury (characteristics of problems, corrective measures)

b. Interference with ADLs

- Central nervous system

1. History of central nervous system disease

2. Fainting episodes

3. Seizures

a. Characteristics

b. Medications

4. Cognitive changes

a. Inability to remember (recent vs. distant)

b. Disorientation

c. Phobias

d. Hallucinations

e. Interference with ADLs

5. Motor-gait

a. Coordinated movement

b. Ataxia, balance problems

c. Paralysis (partial vs. complete)

d. Tic, tremor, spasm

e. Interference with ADLs

6. Sensory

a. Paresthesia (patterns)

b. Tingling sensations

c. Other changes

- Endocrine

1. Diagnosis of disease states (e.g., thyroid, diabetes)

2. Changes in skin pigmentation or texture

3. Changes in or abnormal hair distribution

4. Sudden or unexplained changes in height and weight

5. Intolerance of heat or cold

6. Exophthalmos

7. Goiter

8. Hormone therapy

9. Polydipsia (increased thirst)

10. Polyphagia (increased food intake)

11. Polyuria

12. Anorexia (decreased appetite)

13. Weakness

- Allergic and immunological (optional; use if client indicates allergy history; note precipitating factors in each case.)

1. Dermatitis (inflammation or irritation of skin)

2. Eczema

3. Pruritus

4. Urticaria (hives)

5. Sneezing

6. Vasomotor rhinitis (inflammation and swelling of mucous membrane of nose, nasal discharge)

7. Conjunctivitis (inflammation of conjunctiva)

8. Interference with ADLs

9. Environmental and seasonal correlation

10. Treatment techniques

- Any other physiological problems or disease states not specifically discussed. (If present, explore in detail [e.g., fatigue, insomnia, nervousness]).

Psychosocial History

- General statement of client's feelings about self

- Feelings of satisfaction or frustration in interpersonal relationships

1. Home, occupants

2. Client's position in home relationships

3. Most significant relationship (in and out of home)

4. Community activities

5. Work or school relationships

6. Family cohesiveness patterns

- Activities of daily living

1. General description of work, leisure, and rest distribution

2. Significant hobbies or methods of relaxation

3. Family demands

4. Community activities and involvement

5. Ability to accomplish all that is desired during period of day/week

- General statement about client's ability to cope with ADLs

- Occupational history

1. Jobs held in past

2. Current employer

3. Educational preparation

4. Satisfaction with present and past employment

5. Time spent at work versus time spent at play

- Recent changes or stresses in client's life-style (e.g., divorce, moving, new job, family illness, new baby, financial stresses)

- Patterns in which client copes with situations of stress

- Response to illness

1. Client's ability to cope during own or others' illness

2. Client's family and friends' response during periods of illness

- History of psychiatric care or counseling

- Feelings of anxiety or nervousness (characteristics and coping mechanisms)

- Feelings of depression (such symptoms as insomnia, crying, fearfulness, marked irritability, or anger)

- Changes in personality, behavior, or mood

- Use of medications or other techniques during times of anxiety, stress, or depression

- Habits

1. Alcohol

a. Kinds (beer, wine, mixed drinks)

b. Frequency per week

    c. Pattern over past 5 years; 1 year
    d. Drinking companions
    e. Alcohol consumption variances (increase) when anxious or stressed
  2. Smoking
    a. Kind (pipe, cigarette, cigar)
    b. Amount per week; day
    c. Pattern over past 5 years; 1 year
    d. Enclosed with others who smoke
    e. Smoking amount variances (increase) when anxious or stressed
    f. Desire to quit smoking (methods, attempts)
  3. Coffee and tea
    a. Amount per day
    b. Pattern over past 5 years; 1 year
    c. Consumption variances (increase) when anxious or stressed
    d. Physiological effects
  4. Other
    a. Overeating or sporadic eating (e.g., always in refrigerator, soft drink abuse, cookie jar syndrome)
    b. Nail biting
    c. "Street drug" usage
    d. Nervous noneating
• Financial status
  1. Sources
  2. Adequacy
  3. Recent changes in resources and expenditures

Health Maintenance Efforts

• General statement of client's own physical fitness
• Exercise (amount, type, frequency)
• Dietary regulations; special efforts (describe in detail)
• Mental health; special efforts, such as group therapy, meditation, yoga (describe in detail)
• Cultural or religious practices
• Frequency of physical, dental, and vision health assessment

Environmental Health

• General statement of client's assessment of environmental safety and comfort
• Hazards of employment (inhalants, noise, heavy lifting, psychological stress, machinery)
• Hazards in home (concern about fire, stairs to climb, inadequate heat, open gas heaters, inadequate toilet facilities, pest control, inadequate space)
• Hazards in neighborhood (noise, water, and air pollution, inadequate police protection, heavy traffic on surrounding streets, isolation from neighbors, overcrowding)
• Community hazards (unavailability of stores, market, laundry facilities, drugstore, access to bus line)

ANALYSIS OF A SYMPTOM

In addition to the health data base, the examiner must be prepared to collect in-depth information about a symptom. The format presented on p. 11 is a data collection tool that can be used for physiological, psychological, or sociological symptoms.

Chief Complaint

A chief complaint is a one-sentence or brief statement using the client's words to describe the reason for the visit. Details about the complaint are included in the "Present Health Status," p. 5, or the symptom analysis (box on p. 11).

CLINICAL TIPS AND STRATEGIES

• **Complete data collection and analysis take practice and constant validation with an experienced practitioner:** Use *all* the steps; each is important. Write up as many histories for review by an experienced practitioner as possible; it takes practice to write successfully.
• **The examiner needs ample time:** Negotiate for time and space with your employer. Next, contract for an extended time period with your client; collecting a full data base from an individual may take an hour or more.
• **"Episodic care" may be appropriate for a simple, short-term concern:** In this case it may not be appropriate for the examiner to collect a complete data base, so a systematic and routine manner of collecting episodic care data must be developed. In the box below is a list of data that should be collected about every episodic care problem.
• **Tips on interviewing can facilitate data collection:**
  1. Pose questions without suggesting answers: "Tell me about your pain," not "Does your pain travel down your arm?"
  2. Begin questioning with the most *recent* episode (if client has experienced a number of "attacks" over

---

EPISODIC ASSESSMENT

• Chief complaint
• Analysis of the symptom or complaint (see box, p. 11, for details)
• Interrelationship of current problem to other body systems (would include a review of associated body systems; vague symptoms, such as weakness or fatigue, must be thoroughly explored by reviewing all body systems)
• Relation of current problem to past health and health maintenance

a period of time) and then move on to preceding episodes. The client is most likely to remember specific details of the most recent episode.
3. Begin questioning with the most *urgent* problem (if client presents a number of complaints that are worrying him): "What brought you to the clinic today?"

4. Chronology is the anchor of the history; request calendar dates and clock times.
5. Use simple language (e.g., instead of saying *void*, use *urinate* or *pass your water*).
6. Pose one question at a time.
7. Keep the client politely on track: "Before we go on to that, I would like to hear more about. . . . "

SYMPTOM ANALYSIS

1. **Last time client was entirely well**
   a. Patient may confuse onset of symptom with the first time he was *concerned* about it.
   b. Major symptom may have been preceded by other less alarming ones (e.g., fatigue) that the client will not recall unless questioned.
2. **Date of current problem onset**
   a. Ask client to name specific date and time if possible.
   b. Inquire about the setting at the time of onset to help establish chronology (time of day; month).
   c. Ask client how he was feeling before symptom onset.
3. **Character (description of the qualities of the problem)**
   a. Move back to quoting the client: What is the pain like? "Like being stabbed?" "Squeezed in a vise?"
   b. Determine severity (does it interfere with ADLs?).
4. **Nature of problem onset**
   a. Ask if the onset was slow? Abrupt? Noticeable to others?
   b. Use quotes if possible.
5. **Client's hunch of precipitating factors**
   a. Determine aggravating or alleviating factors.
   b. Word questions to avoid influencing answers, for example, *angina*: "What effect does walking have?" or *vertigo*: "What happens if you move your head?"
6. **Course of problem (determine if client continued with normal activity during episode)**
   a. Consistent
   b. Intermittent
   c. Duration
7. **Location of problem**
   a. Pinpoint
   b. Generalized, vague
   c. Radiation patterns
8. **Effect on other systems and activities**
   a. Symptoms, signs
   b. Body functions or positions
   c. Activities (body movement, exercise)
   d. Appetite
9. **Patterns**
   The client may exhibit a symptom that has been occurring intermittently over time. Most previous questions have elicited data about the quantity and quality of *one* episode. This section concerns multiple episodes, identifies patterns, and provides an overview of chronology.
   a. *Timing.* Relate incidences to number of times per hour; day; week; month; inquire about client's well-being during the intervals.
   b. *Duration and quality variations.* May indicate a stepping up or increase in intensity over time. ("Has it been getting any better? Worse? Staying the same?")
   c. *Exacerbations or remission.* Try to associate with other symptoms, activities, or precipitating factors.
10. **Efforts to treat**
    a. Home remedies (what and when)
    b. Body positions (e.g., bed rest)
    c. Over-the-counter medications
    d. Prescription medications and physician visits (give details)
11. **In-depth exploration of client's life-style and coping ability as related to the symptom**
    a. Pose questions to discover an association between daily activities and the symptom.
       (1) What mandatory activities make the symptom worse? For example, if stair climbing causes chest pain, does the client have to use stairs at home or at work?
       (2) What activities are altered or curtailed because of the symptom? For example, if the client complains of nocturnal urination, how much sleep is lost? Is fatigue a problem? Is it possible to sleep during the day?
       (3) Do altered activities pose a threat to the client? If client complains of diminished vision or glare, is driving hazardous? Is reading part of job?
    b. Pose questions that indicate an association between client's ability to deal with current life-style and the symptom. For example, if a mother complains of marked fatigue, does this interfere with child-rearing activities or management of the home?
    c. A general question such as, "What does this problem *mean* to you?" might help to summarize the previous questions. It also permits the client to voice an emotional response to changes or problems. It may help the examiner to grasp more fully the impact or severity of the symptom.

8. Clarify the client's responses: What do these really mean to the client? Do they mean the same to you?
   a. Quasimedical terms
      (1) Tumor
      (2) Nervous breakdown
      (3) Sick-to-the-stomach
      (4) Pneumonia
      (5) Sciatica
      (6) Dizziness
      (7) Heart attack
      (8) Diarrhea
   b. Quantities (unclear)
      (1) A lot
      (2) Often
      (3) Once in a while
9. At the end of the interview, summarize (aloud) what the client has said.

- **Sometimes a client will diagnose himself:** If the examiner accepts a diagnosis from a client, he or she should record it in quotations and follow up with a summary of the symptoms that prompted diagnosis (e.g., *hemorrhoids*—involves five or six drops of bright red blood on tissue, associated with once-a-week constipation, pain localized at anus with each daily bowel movement, palpable tags at anal area).
- **The examiner should be aware of hazards of interviewing:**
  1. Nonverbal cues that indicate the examiner is rushed, bored, preoccupied, disapproving, or generally disinterested are usually sensed by the client and can greatly alter or shorten the interview.
  2. Disapproval can overtake an examiner for many reasons. For example, the client's mode of dress, life-style, language, failure to follow a previously prescribed regimen, or body appearance may trigger a conscious or unconscious response. The examiner must monitor his or her own reactions and accept the client as is.
  3. The examiner and client need a quiet, private environment with adequate chairs and writing space; if the surroundings are noisy, confusing, and intrusive, the accuracy and the quality of the data will be affected.
  4. Failing to take the time to establish a relationship and launching into "the facts" for the sake of expediency are intimidating and disconcerting. It usually takes only a minute or two to introduce oneself and conduct a general inquiry about the client's well-being.
- **Avoid the use of the terms *normal, negative, healthy,* or *well*:** Each of these terms has a different meaning to individual examiners with different levels of expertise. The beginning practitioner is encouraged to use descriptive terminology to define significant findings or significant negatives to describe "normal" states.
- **Use an outline of the history format:** The beginning examiner cannot memorize all the data categories and should carry a pocket guide to use as a reference.
- **Use a clipboard or a small notebook for taking notes:** The examiner will need a portable, hard surface to write on. This will permit seating comfort and maintenance of eye contact.
- **Note:** The client often does not present a tidy package of symptoms for analysis at the onset of the interview. Symptoms will be uncovered as the examiner pursues information in the review of systems. The examiner *must* stop and analyze these problems as thoroughly as those presented initially.

SAMPLE ADULT DATA BASE WRITE-UP

Once the data base is collected, it must be organized, synthesized, and documented. Following is a sample data base write-up. Refer to "The Newborn" (p. 15), "The Child" (p. 17), "The Childbearing Woman" (p. 22), and "The Older Adult" (p. 24) to make the appropriate changes.

Biographical data

Cynthia M. Stoner; 32 years old; white; female; married; two sons, ages 6 and 7; 3792 Hedge Creek Lane, Maysville, Ohio; lives in single-family dwelling owned by family; home described as three-bedroom, "comfortable," in midst of rural community.

Reason for visit

Time for Pap smear; "lower abdominal discomfort off and on;" desire to lose weight.

Present health status

Health during past 5 years has been good; during past year has noted 15-pound weight gain and periods of not feeling "up to par"; complains of being "tired" much of the time; no fatigue pattern identified; currently most significant concern is lower abdominal discomfort.

Initial problem onset 8 months ago; since then increased episodes and severity; increased discomfort before menses,

SAMPLE ADULT DATA BASE WRITE-UP—cont'd

with increased flatus and full bladder; discomfort described as nonradiating, sharp, and stabbing; pinpoint location in LLQ; client perceives problem associated with uterus or left ovary; coping methods: client aware of discomfort but problem not interfering with activities of daily living.

Current health data

1. Current medications
   a. None prescribed
   b. No over-the-counter drugs
2. Allergies
   a. Seasonal and environmental: pollen, dust, grass; no treatment
   b. Denies food, drug, contact allergies
3. Last examinations
   a. Physical, Pap smear, chest x-ray: September 1989
   b. Dental: June 1990
   c. Vision: October 1989
   d. Hearing: high school
   e. ECG: 1983
   f. Tuberculosis tine test: 1988
4. Immunizations
   a. Polio: 1982
   b. Diphtheria, tetanus: 1988
   c. Influenza, mumps, rubella, pertussis: none

Past health status

1959-1969 Childhood diseases: measles, mumps, chicken-pox
1968 Tonsillectomy: Marion, Ohio, Dr. Harris
1971 Appendectomy: Marion, Ohio, Dr. Spencer
1972 Hospitalized for hepatitis
1974 Fracture of left tibia from riding accident; uncomplicated
1980 Surgery: benign left breast cyst removed, Delaware, Ohio, Dr. Southwood
1982 Pregnancy: delivered healthy 7 lb, 2 oz boy; vaginal delivery, uncomplicated
1983 Pregnancy: delivered healthy 7 lb, 9 oz boy; vaginal delivery; complications—high blood pressure, fluid retention, hospitalized 3 weeks before induced delivery; recovered to healthy state within 2 weeks after delivery
1983 Tubal ligation, Delaware, Ohio, Dr. Southwood

Family history

See Fig. 1-2.

Review of physiological systems

1. General: Client considers herself in "good health" but has periods of fatigue with physical and emotional stress. Feels rested after sleep periods. Client states she would feel better if she could lose 20 pounds and exercise more regularly.
2. Nutritional
   Current weight: 142 lb; height: 5 feet, 4 in

Weight past year: 138 to 140 lb
Weight past 5 years: 120 to 138 lb
   Client considers the accompanying dietary recall to be typical. She states, "I know better than to eat all that junk." Dietary efforts have been sporadic; major methods involved skipping meals (breakfast and lunch) and protein (meat and salad) diets; no efforts in past 8 months.
   Client considers current appetite "too good." She enjoys eating and eats more when nervous or worried. Client does grocery shopping. States she buys foods that her children and husband like. Money or transportation not a problem.
3. Integumentary
   a. Skin: denies lesions, masses, discolorations. Some pruritus during winter; clears with lotion.
   b. Hair: denies texture changes and loss; uses color rinse monthly to maintain lightened color; no scalp irritation reported from the rinse.
   c. Nails: states she has always had brittle nails.
4. Head: periodic headaches in occipital area and back of neck usually follow tension period and are relieved by aspirin and rest (no more than four aspirin tablets/week consumed).
5. Eyes: denies infections and discharge from eyes; seasonal periorbital swelling associated with pollen allergy. Denies visual changes, diplopia, blurring, photophobia, pain in eyeball, and excessive tearing. Client wears glasses for reading (past 3 years).
6. Ears: complains of chronic hearing problem (multiple ear infections as child); states hearing difficulty does not interfere with activities of daily living: "just certain sounds are not clear." Denies pain, infections, and vertigo; frequent complaints of ringing and cracking in ears. Cares for ears with cotton-tipped swabs.
7. Nose, nasopharynx, and paranasal sinuses: denies epistaxis, sinus problems, postnasal drip, and olfactory deficit; seasonal sneezing and discharge associated with allergies.
8. Mouth and throat: denies sore throats, lesions, gum irritation, chewing and swallowing difficulties, hoarseness, and voice changes. Brushes teeth two times a day and uses dental floss.
9. Neck: denies tenderness or range-of-motion difficulties.
10. Breast: breast tenderness before menses; breasts "feel lumpy"; "small amount of yellow" bilateral nipple discharge present since birth of second child. Examines own breasts each month after menstrual period. Breast biopsy with cyst removed in 1980. Client considers breasts to be "cystic, lumpy."
11. Cardiovascular: denies chest pain, shortness of breath, and palpitations. No known history of heart murmurs, heart disease, or hypertension. Feet always feel cold. Denies discoloration and peripheral edema.
12. Respiratory: denies breathing difficulties, chronic cough, and shortness of breath.

Continued.

SAMPLE ADULT DATA BASE WRITE-UP—cont'd

13. Hematolymphatic: describes periods of fatigue related to stress or excessive work. Denies lymphatic swelling, excessive bleeding, and bruising. Never tested for anemia.
14. Gastrointestinal: denies eating and digestion problems. Periodic pyrosis usually follows rapid food ingestion or occurs during stressful period. Denies hematemesis, jaundice, and ascites. Bowel movement once each day. Stools are soft and brown. Denies difficulty with diarrhea and constipation. No known hemorrhoids.
15. Urinary: describes urine as yellow and clear. Voiding frequency four or five times in 24 hours. Denies voiding difficulties, dysuria, urgency, and flank pain. Infrequent nocturia. Denies polyuria and oliguria. Complains of frequent episodes of stress incontinence since birth of second child. Condition becoming no worse but does present problem during laughing, running, or lifting heavy objects.
16. Genital: LMP, 6-14-90. Periods normally 28 to 30 days apart, regular intervals, heavy flow with clotting and cramps in first 24 hours. Cramps controlled by aspirin. LLQ pain increases just before menses. Denies genital lesions, discharges, and VD history. Sexually active; satisfied with sexual activity.

17. Musculoskeletal extremities: denies muscular weakness, twitching, and pain; gait difficulties and extremity deformities; joint swelling, pain, stiffness, and crepitus; history of back injury problems.
18. Central nervous system: denies changes in cognitive function, coordination, and sensory defects.
19. Endocrine: denies endocrine disease, history of skin changes, polydipsia, polyuria, polyphagia, anorexia, and weakness.
20. Allergic: describes allergy problems as seasonal (August to October). Treatment consists of symptomatic relief by a "cortisone shot" and an unidentified prescription. During allergic season client reports sneezing, vasomotor rhinitis, conjunctivitis; no interference with activities of daily living.

Psychosocial history

Client states she feels good about herself most of the time. She experiences episodes of depression and fatigue and expresses a feeling that she should "do more" with her life.

Client expresses feelings of satisfaction with family members and friends. She considers her husband her best friend but also speaks of two other very close female friends. She counts on her friends to help her "talk through" stress periods. Considers family very close; communication channels are open.

Client's energies revolve around maintaining home, raising two small sons, and working part-time (12 hours/week) at a local flower shop. Denies membership in clubs or church. Spends weekends just relaxing with family. Feels stressed and at times "angry" when husband's business keeps him away on weekends. Client states that much of her time is spent meeting the needs of others. States she would like more time for herself.

As soon as children are older, client hopes to return to college to complete degree in horticulture (5 terms to go). Client loves work at flower shop and would like to either take a college course or two or work a few more hours at the flower shop. Husband supports career goals but for now believes client's job is at home with the children (seems to be a stress point).

Husband just accepted job promotion. Now travels approximately 12 days of the month. This seems to cause direct stress and creates child care problems during client's working hours.

Client denies previous psychiatric counseling or feelings of anxiety or nervousness that she could not cope with. Methods of coping most frequently are (1) easy and sometimes inappropriate expression of anger, (2) increased sleeping, and (3) eating. To relax, client enjoys reading, playing with children, and going out with husband.

Client denies use of drugs or medications.

Alcohol: 3 or 4 glasses of wine a week

Smoking: none

Twenty-four-hour dietary recall

FOOD EATEN	AMOUNT	CALORIES
Breakfast		
Toast with peanut butter and butter	1 slice	214
Coffee with cream	8 oz	30
Orange juice	4 oz	100
		344
Lunch		
Hamburger sandwich	1	250
Salad with ranch dressing	6 oz	105
Coffee with cream	8 oz	30
		385
Dinner		
Swiss steak	3 oz	300
Baked potato	1	230
Green beans	4 oz	27
Bread	2 slices	228
Water		
		785
Snacks		
Iced cupcake	1	200
Carbonated beverage	8 oz	105
		305
TOTAL		1819

SAMPLE ADULT DATA BASE WRITE-UP—cont'd

Coffee: 4 or 5 cups a day; no increase over the past 5 years. Increased consumption with stress (6 to 8 cups/day).

Overeating: increased with stress; eats most when alone and after children go to bed.

Financial status: client feels they could do more as a family if there were more money but states there are no serious financial problems.

Health maintenance efforts

No specific health maintenance efforts. Health care patterns inconsistent, as stated.

Environmental health

Client believes her home and neighborhood environment are safe and without hazards. Client is exposed to fertilizer fumes at flower shop, but ventilation is adequate.

Subjective problem list

1. Periods of fatigue
2. LLQ pain: cyclical with menses: does not interfere with activities of daily living; increased severity and frequency past 8 months
3. Stress incontinence past 5 years; not increased in severity
4. Seasonal allergies: symptomatically treated; do not interfere with activities of daily living
5. Feet cold "most of time"
6. Long-standing hearing difficulty (since childhood); does not interfere with activities of daily living
7. Overweight for height and build; 22 lb weight gain in past 5 years; 4 lb in past year

8. Poor dietary habits
9. Needs Pap smear
10. Feels trapped at times by home and child-raising responsibilities; husband travels approximately 12 days a month

(Final problem list is developed, and priorities are established after physical assessment.)

Risk profile

1. Family cancer history
   Maternal: mother, breast cancer; uncle, lung cancer
   Paternal: aunt, breast cancer; grandfather, colon cancer
   Client: cystic breasts; already has had one cyst removed (1980); client examines breasts regularly
2. Weight: Steady weight gain since 1982; attempts at regular dieting and exercise programs have failed
3. Irregular health maintenance program: health care visits, diet, exercise
4. At times client does not feel self-fulfilled; believes she is always meeting needs of others and neglecting self

Client profile

Client views herself as a healthy and resourceful 32-year-old woman. Physiologically she is bothered by (1) LLQ discomfort, (2) overweight state, and (3) periodic fatigue.

Psychologically and sociologically, stresses viewed by client are (1) husband traveling too often, (2) feeling burdened periodically by family and household responsibilities, (3) desiring to return to college or become more actively involved in outside activities, and (4) fearing breast cancer. In summary, client views coping skills as adequate to meet present stresses.

 The Newborn

TOTAL HEALTH DATA BASE

The neonatal period is the first 30 days of life. Data collected on day 30 will differ from data obtained shortly after birth. Data related to 1-month-old infants will be addressed in the sections on "The Child," beginning on page 17. The gestational age and well-being of an infant will influence the information needed for the data base; therefore at-risk newborns should receive additional assessment by neonatal experts.

General guidelines should be followed when assessing any newborn's physical condition and adjustment from intrauterine to extrauterine life. Maternal history is an important aspect of the total health data base of the newborn.

Biographical Data

- Name: mother's name and infant's name and sex; multiple births may be listed as infant A or B, etc., until the infants are given names
- Age: gestational age, and date and time of birth
- Birth weight in pounds, ounces, grams
- Race
- Parents' culture
- Socioeconomic factors of family
- Address and telephone number of parents or family
- Siblings and family in home
- Parents' means of transportation for follow-up infant examinations

• Description of parents' home, and size and type of community

Birth Data

For pediatric and older clients, health data are collected at the time of a health care visit. For the newborn, the total health data base relates to the childbirth history and early assessment.

Present Health Status

• Obstetric factors pertinent to the newborn's health
• Present infant condition, including gestational assessment data, and neurological assessment data

Current Health Data

• Medications: vitamin K, standard eye care, other medications ordered, such as antibiotics
• Tests performed, such as cultures

Past Health Status

See numbers 1 to 3 in the *Past Health Status* section for "The Child," p. 18.

Family History

Any incidence of sibling problems during the newborn period should be reviewed.

Review of Physiological Systems

• Overall assessment
  1. Vital signs
  2. Weight
  3. Measurements: length, head and chest circumference
• Assessment tests
  1. Apgar scores
  2. Gestational age assessment
  3. Behavioral and neurological tests
• Integumentary
  1. Vernix, lanugo, meconium staining
  2. Texture, color
  3. Hair and nail (characteristics)
• Head and neck
  1. Head and face shape, circumference, symmetry
  2. Sutures, fontanels
  3. Neck mobility, length
• Nose and mouth
  1. Mouth shape, structure, symmetry
  2. Nose structure, symmetry, function
• Ears and auditory
  1. Symmetry, shape, position
  2. Eardrum, fluid (characteristics)
  3. Startle reflex to loud noises
• Eyes and visual system

  1. External eye symmetry, size, position; ocular movements
  2. Pupil size, scleral condition, red reflex
• Thorax and lungs
  1. Clavicles, ribs, xiphoid
  2. Chest symmetry, size, shape
  3. Respiratory and heart rates
  4. Crying characteristics and skin color
• Cardiovascular
  1. Heart position, rate, sounds
  2. Pulse rate, capillary refill
• Breasts
  1. Areola size, discharge
• Gastrointestinal, abdomen, and rectum
  1. Abdominal symmetry, shape, bowel sounds
  2. Liver, spleen, kidney position
  3. Umbilicus characteristics: two arteries, one vein; drying
  4. Patent anus, meconium within 24 hours of birth
• Male genitourinary
  1. Testes, scrotum, urethra position, size, symmetry
  2. Urine color; voiding frequency
• Female genitourinary
  1. Labia minora and majora, clitoris, vulva, vagina size, position, discharge
  2. Urine color; voiding frequency
• Musculoskeletal
  1. Spine position, symmetry
  2. Limb symmetry, range of motion
  3. Gluteal folds, hips abduct without difficulty
• Neurological
  1. Responses to touch, noise
  2. Symmetry in movement
  3. Position, muscle tone of head, extremities

Psychosocial History

Parent-infant attachment should be observed. Parenting patterns are assessed and documented.

Health Maintenance Efforts

See section on "The Child," p. 22.
• Follow-up clinic appointments should be scheduled. If the mother and infant are discharged before testing for phenylketonuria, an appointment for testing must be assured. Future bilirubin testing, if needed, must be planned.
• Support systems for breast-feeding, home phototherapy, or other needed services should be intact before discharge.

Environmental Health

See section on "The Child," p. 22.
• Parents should make use of an infant car seat.
• Infant furniture and supplies should be tested for safety.

3. Blue spells
4. Excessive crying
- Growth and development
Unlike the developmental data collected under current health status, this section includes a survey of significant developmental milestones.
  1. General statement as to how this child compares with siblings
  2. Parent's opinion of whether child's growth and development have been normal
  3. Notation of age of events: rolled over, sat up, walked, first tooth, first words, toilet trained
- State age and complications of each: chickenpox, rubella, measles, mumps, whooping cough, hay fever
- State age and complications of each serious or chronic illness: meningitis or encephalitis, pneumonia or chronic lung problems, rheumatic fever, asthma, hay fever, scarlet fever, diabetes, kidney problems, hypertension, sickle cell anemia, seizure disorders, blood infections, etc.
- State age and extent of each serious injury: head injuries, fractures, burns, traumas, poisonings, etc.
- Hospitalizations: list reason, location, primary care providers, duration, and how child reacted to hospitalization
- Operations: what, where, when, why, by whom
- Emotional health: past behavior problems, help sought, support persons, how child reacted to stress

Family History

Family members include the client's blood relatives. Specifically the interviewer should inquire about the client's maternal and paternal grandparents, parents, aunts, uncles, and siblings. The interviewer should inquire about the general health, stress factors, and illnesses of family members. Questions should include a survey of the following:

Cancer	Hypertension
Diabetes	Sickle cell anemia
Heart problems	Blindness
Developmental delay	Endocrine disorders
Learning problems	Kidney diseases
Cystic fibrosis	Birth defects
Asthma	Infant deaths
Other allergies	Other chronic problems
Seizure disorders	

Review of Physiological Systems

- General
  1. Frequency of colds, infections, or illnesses
  2. Frequency of fevers, sweats
  3. Fatigue patterns
  4. Energetic or overactive patterns
- Nutritional
  1. Recent weight gain or loss (describe)

2. Appetite
3. Twenty-four-hour diet recall, including types, amount of food eaten (formula, breast milk, meat, fruits, vegetables, cereals, juices, eggs, sweets, milk, snacks), and frequency (e.g., number of times a day or week)
4. Child feeding self
5. Where child eats
6. Who child eats with
7. Parent's perception of child's nutritional status (note problems)
8. Vitamin supplements
9. Junk food consumption (amount and kinds)
- Integumentary
  1. Skin
     a. Chronic rashes
     b. Easy bruising or petechiae
     c. Easy bleeding
     d. Acne (treatment pattern)
     e. Excessive sweating
     f. Skin diseases, problems, or lesions
     g. Pruritus
     h. Pigmentation changes, discolorations, mottling
     i. Excessive dryness
     j. Skin growths or tumors
  2. Hair
     a. Changes in amount, texture, characteristics
     b. Infections, lice
     c. Alopecia
  3. Nails
     a. Changes in appearance
     b. Cyanosis
     c. Texture
- Head
  1. Headache (characteristics, including frequency, type, location, duration, care for)
  2. Past significant trauma
  3. Dizziness
  4. Syncope
- Eyes
  1. Strabismus
  2. Discharge
  3. Complaint of vision changes
  4. Reading difficulty
  5. Sits close to television
  6. History of infections
  7. Pruritus
  8. Excessive tearing
  9. Pain in eyeball
  10. Swelling around eyes
  11. Cataracts
  12. Unusual sensations or twitching
  13. Excessive blinking
  14. Eye injury history
  15. Wears glasses

3. Bones and joints
   a. Joint swelling
   b. Joint pain
   c. Redness, stiffness
   d. Joint deformity
   e. Fracture or dislocation history
4. Back
   a. History of back injury
   b. Curvature of spine
   c. Characteristics of problems and corrective measures
- Central nervous system
  1. General
     a. Unusual episodic behaviors
     b. History of central nervous system diseases
     c. Birth injury
  2. Seizure: febrile versus afebrile
  3. Speech
     a. Stuttering
     b. Speech misarticulations
     c. Language delay
  4. Cognitive changes
     a. Hallucinations
     b. Passing out episodes
     c. Staring spells
     d. Learning difficulties
  5. Motor-gait
     a. Coordination
     b. Developmental clumsiness
     c. Balance problems
     d. Tic
     e. Tremor, spasms
  6. Sensory
     a. Pain pattern
     b. Tingling sensations
- Endocrine
  1. Diagnosis of disease states (e.g., thyroid, diabetes)
  2. Changes in skin texture (e.g., increased or decreased dryness or perspiration)
  3. Pigmentation
  4. Abnormal hair distribution
  5. Sudden or unexplained changes in height and weight
  6. Intolerance to heat or cold
  7. Exophthalmos
  8. Goiter
  9. Polydipsia
  10. Polyphagia
  11. Polyuria
  12. Anorexia
  13. Weakness
  14. Precocious puberty
- Allergic and immunological
  1. Dermatitis
  2. Eczema

3. Pruritus
4. Urticaria
5. Sneezing
6. Vasomotor rhinitis
7. Conjunctivitis (inflammation of conjunctiva)
8. Interference with ADLs
9. Environmental and seasonal causes
10. Treatment techniques

Psychosocial History

- General status
  1. General statement of child's feelings about self
  2. Parents' observations of child's feeling of self
- Caretakers and family
  1. Who lives in child's home
  2. Primary care provider for child
  3. Child's position in home environment
  4. Relationships among members
- Friends
  1. Child's relationships with friends, classmates, siblings
  2. Age of playmates—older, younger, same age
  3. Ability to make friends easily
- Activities of daily living
  1. General
     a. General description of typical day
     b. Sleep patterns and naps: sound sleeper or fretful, numbers of hours per 24 hours, nightmares, other nighttime activity (e.g., wakes up at night), parents' response
     c. Kinds of play: amount of active and quiet play per 24 hours, television time per 24 hours
     d. Significant hobbies or methods of relaxation (for older child)
  2. Family
     a. Activities of families as unit
     b. Methods of discipline within family
     c. Effectiveness of discipline
     d. Who disciplines child
     e. Child's reaction to discipline
     f. Parents or providers: type of employment, type of child care provided if both parents work
     g. Availability of emotional support for mother for her care of child and opportunity to be away from child
  3. School
     a. Present grade in school or level of nursery care
     b. School performance
     c. Behavior problems
     d. Grades skipped
     e. Learning problems; special classes required, if any
     f. Attitude about school
     g. Rate of absenteeism

for labor, delivery, child rearing
- Means of transportation if pertinent
- Description of home, and size and type of community

Reason for Visit

Prenatal visits should be clearly delineated. Telephone calls or unscheduled visits, such as coming to the clinic with symptoms of urinary tract infection, premature labor, or other problems, should be noted.

Present Health Status

Data specific to a childbearing woman include her present nutritional status, motherhood coping abilities, and general physical well-being. Allergies and sensitivities should be noted.

Current Health Data

Information should be gathered that relates to the woman's current health and pregnancy status. Note the client's and her partner's blood type. The pregnant woman's date of delivery should be determined, as well as any current conditions suggesting health risks for her or her fetus.

Past Health Status

A pregnant woman's gravida (number of previous pregnancies), parity (number of children born alive), abortions (both spontaneous "miscarriages" and "therapeutic" pregnancy interruptions), and information about her live or deceased offspring should be noted. The conditions and outcomes of previous pregnancies should be recorded. Data about previous labor patterns should be explored. Patients who have recently delivered should be assessed for involution patterns.

Family History

A pregnant woman's history should include the childbearing history of her mother and sister(s). Questions should be asked about any family history of diabetes, renal disease, or hereditary disorders.

Review of Physiological Systems

An assessment of physiological systems includes data obtained during a general adult examination, plus findings pertinent to pregnancy or after delivery.
- Overall assessment
  1. Vital signs
  2. Weight
  3. Urine tests for protein, ketones
- Fetal assessment tests
  1. Presumptive and probable signs of pregnancy
  2. Measurement of fundal height
- Integumentary
  1. Skin marks, lines, varicosities
  2. Sweat gland production
- Head and neck
  1. Thyroid gland (may be enlarged)
- Nose and mouth
  1. Nose bleeding
  2. Nasal stuffiness
  3. Gum bleeding
- Ears and auditory
  1. Slight hearing loss
- Eyes and visual
  1. Visual changes
- Thorax and lungs
  1. Increased respiratory rate
  2. Changes in thoracic cage
- Cardiovascular
  1. Increased heart rate
  2. Changes in blood pressure
  3. Supine hypotension syndrome, positive roll-over test
- Breasts
  1. Enlargement, engorgement
  2. Tingling feeling
  3. Development of colostrum, milk
- Gastrointestinal, abdomen, and rectum
  1. First trimester nausea
  2. Heartburn, esophageal reflux
  3. Bowel habits, hemorrhoids
- Genitourinary
  1. Vaginal, cervical, uterine changes
  2. Renal changes
  3. Postdelivery involution
- Musculoskeletal
  1. Posture changes
  2. Shifted gait

Psychosocial History

Adjustment to parenthood should be assessed. Emotional stability data should be collected, which would include, for example, the incidence of excessive crying, social withdrawal, or decisions related to infant care.

Health Maintenance Efforts

Physical fitness and activities directed toward childbearing should be assessed. Prenatal, vision, and dental appointments should be made and kept. Dietary planning should be noted.

Environmental Health

Environmental factors are particularly important during childbearing because of the risks of teratogens. Exposure to toxins should be assessed and preventive steps taken.

HISTORY AND CLINICAL STRATEGIES

A profile of the client and family should be delineated. It is helpful to have the family visit routinely, so that the physical and psychosocial health of the family can be assessed. A new mother may feel left out when attention is directed toward her infant. Concentration on the needs of the entire family is important.

 The Older Adult

TOTAL HEALTH DATA BASE

Geriatric clients are not different from other adults. There is no specific age when concerns related to the aging process warrant additional screening questions to complete an accurate data base.

The following questions and concerns are directed toward elderly adults. Many of the questions concern problems of disability, chronic illness, or normal changes that take place with aging. There are many older people who do not have chronic illnesses, disabilities, or marked aging changes that affect their daily lives. The practitioner can use the following format when it seems to be appropriate.

Biographical Data

- Name
- Age
- Race
- Culture
- Address and telephone number
- Marital status
- Children and family in home
- Occupation/retirement status
- Means of transportation to health care facility if pertinent
- Description of home, and size and type of community

Reason for Visit

Some elderly clients present a multitude of problems. Some complaints are long-standing (e.g., stiff joints, hypertension, dry skin, chronic constipation), and others are more acute. Certain problems are not easily identified and, with skilled questioning, emerge as the assessment progresses (e.g., depression, weight loss, weakness, difficulty caring for self at home).

Other clients tend to minimize pain or other symptoms. Older individuals may not manifest fever associated with infection to the extent that younger clients do. Some elderly individuals complain less of pain (e.g., cholecystitis, angina) or seem to experience less pain. New symptoms may be attributed to "getting old" and therefore are not reported as significant.

It takes time and patience to identify the *priorities* of the client's concerns (which may be different from the examiner's priorities). It often takes time and patience to establish the actual reason for the visit.

The final statement describing the reason(s) should be brief, stated in the client's own words, and limited to the *client's* immediate concerns. The final problem list, risk profile, and client profile can absorb (identify) the multiplicity of concerns that are not directly related to the chief complaint.

Present Health Status

- Summary of client's current major health concerns
- If illness is present, record of symptom analysis (box, p. 11)
  1. When client was last well
  2. Date of problem onset
  3. Character of complaint
  4. Nature of problem onset
  5. Course of problem
  6. Client's hunch of precipitating factors
  7. Location of problem
  8. Relation to
     a. Other body symptoms
     b. Body positions
     c. Activity
  9. Patterns of problem
  10. Efforts of client to treat
  11. Coping ability

Current Health Data

- Current medications (include prescriptions, over-the-counter drugs, vitamins, home remedies)
  1. Name of drug
  2. Prescribed when and by whom
  3. When first prescribed
  4. Amount prescribed per day
  5. Amount taken per day
  6. Problems with compliance: complicated or inconvenient dosage schedule, large number and variety of drugs prescribed, visual difficulty (unable to read label), unpleasant side effects, inability to afford drugs, difficulty swallowing or administering, inability to get to pharmacy, client fearful of addiction, client considers drug ineffective, client overdosing to relieve symptoms. If the client is taking a large number of prescribed drugs (often prescribed by different physicians), request that all medications be brought in for review. Clients are often unaware of the names or the purposes of all their drugs.
- Allergies (describe agent and reactions)
  1. Drugs
  2. Foods
  3. Contact substances
  4. Environmental factors
- Last examination (note physician/clinic, findings, advice, and/or instructions)

1. Physical
2. Dental
3. Vision
4. Hearing
5. ECG
6. Chest radiograph
7. Pap smear (women)
8. Mammography
9. Proctoscopy
10. Tonometry
11. Tuberculosis tine test
- Immunization status (note dates or year of last immunization)
  1. Tetanus, diphtheria
  2. Mumps
  3. Rubella
  4. Polio
  5. Influenza

Past Health Status

- Childhood illnesses: rubeola, rubella, mumps, pertussis, scarlet fever, chickenpox, strep throat
- Serious or chronic illnesses: Parkinson disease, diabetes, hypertension, arthritis, bone diseases, cardiovascular disease, stroke, respiratory disease, kidney or urinary problems, nervous or seizure disorders, blood diseases or infections, gastrointestinal dysfunction, gynecological disorders, cancer, thyroid problems, diseases of eyes or ears
  If client offers a diagnosis that is not confirmed by health records, note it in quotes.
- Serious accidents or injuries: head injuries, fractures, burns, other trauma
- Hospitalizations: elaborate upon, listing reason, location, primary care providers, duration
- Operations: what, where, when, why, by whom
- Emotional health: past problems, help sought, support persons
- Obstetrical history
  1. Complete pregnancies: number, pregnancy course, postpartum course, and condition, weight, and sex of each child
  2. Incomplete pregnancies: duration, termination, circumstances, including abortions and stillbirths
  3. Summary of complications

An elderly individual's health history may be lengthy, complicated, and time consuming to amass and organize. If the individual has no difficulty with vision or writing skills, it is helpful to have this portion completed at home in advance of the assessment.

Family History

Family members include the client's blood relatives, spouse, and children. Specifically the interviewer should inquire about the client's maternal and paternal grand-parents, parents, aunts, uncles, spouse, and children, as well as the general health, stress factors, and illnesses of family members. Questions should include a survey of the following:

Alzheimer's disease	Developmental delay
Cancer	Alcoholism
Diabetes	Endocrine diseases
Heart disease	Sickle cell anemia
Hypertension	Kidney disease
Epilepsy (or seizure disorder)	Unusual limitations
Emotional stresses	Other chronic problems
Mental illness	

The most concise method to record these data is by a family tree. With the geriatric client an elaborate family history may be less meaningful as a predictor of potential medical problems, since many familial diseases are contracted at an earlier age. Cancer and diabetes are exceptions. However, the family tree serves as a reference for knowing what experiences (perhaps fears) the client has had with diseases, disabilities, and causes of death.

Review of Physiological Systems

- General—reflect from client's previous description of current health status
  1. Fatigue patterns
  2. Exercise and exercise tolerance
  3. History of weakness episodes, if any
  4. History of fevers, sweats, if any
  5. Frequency of colds, infections, or illnesses
  6. Activities of daily living assessment (optional package; to be used if client has multiple complaints or disabilities, such as visual loss, limited energy, motor skill deficits, mental difficulties, arthritic changes); see box on next page. When the multiplicity of diseases, symptoms, and side effects strikes an individual, the general health status is sometimes best assessed in terms of the *impact of disability* on one's daily life. This tool is particularly helpful if the client is living alone or with an elderly companion or spouse.
- Nutritional
  1. Client's average, maximum, and minimum weights during past month; 1 year; 5 years
  2. History of weight gains or losses (time element); specific efforts to change weight—if dieting, describe efforts and type of diet used.
  3. If client is on special diet, describe
  4. Current appetite patterns—food type preferences (e.g., sweets, fruits, convenience foods), amounts consumed at one time, hunger more marked at certain times of day or night, loss or gain in appetite recently or over past year
  5. Food consumption patterns (e.g., three meals a day, smaller meals five or six times a day, eating

ACTIVITIES OF DAILY LIVING (ADL) ASSESSMENT

A. Self-care
   1. Dressing, undressing, clothing
      a. Keeping clothes in good repair (mending)
      b. Accessing clothes
      c. Getting into and out of underwear (bra, girdle, underpants, pantyhose, stockings, garter belt)
      d. Putting on and removing pants
      e. Getting arms in sleeves
      f. Managing zippers, buttons, snaps (especially in back), ties
      g. Putting on socks, shoes, tying laces
      h. Applying prostheses (e.g., glasses, hearing aids)
   2. Grooming and hygiene
      a. Washing, drying, brushing hair
      b. Brushing teeth
      c. Cleaning and putting in dentures
      d. Shaving
      e. Caring for nails (feet and hands)
      f. Applying makeup
      g. Preparing bath water and testing temperature
      h. Getting into and out of tub, shower
      i. Reaching and cleaning all body parts
   3. Elimination
      a. Position altered for urination or sitting on toilet
      b. Ability to wipe self
      c. Lowering onto and rising from toilet
B. Mobility
   1. Difficulty climbing or descending stairs (Is bedroom/bathroom on upper level? How many stairs/flights to apartment or house?)
   2. Sitting up and rising from bed
   3. Lowering to or rising from chair
   4. Walking (short and long distances); describe necessity for walking
   5. Opening doors
   6. Reaching items in cupboards
   7. Necessity for lifting (and any difficulty)
C. Communication
   1. Dialing telephone
   2. Reading numbers
   3. Hearing over telephone
      4. Answering door
      5. Immediate access to neighbors, help
D. Eating (see *nutritional* section, which begins on p. 25, for details about appetite, weight, food consumption)
   1. Access to market
   2. Preparing food (opening cans and packages, using stove, reaching dishes, pots, utensils)
   3. Handling knife, fork, spoon (cutting meat)
   4. Getting food to mouth
   5. Chewing, swallowing
E. Housekeeping, laundry, house upkeep
   1. Making bed
   2. Sweeping, mopping floors
   3. Dusting
   4. Washing dishes
   5. Cleaning tub, bathroom
   6. Picking up clutter (to client's satisfaction)
   7. Taking out trash, garbage
   8. Use of basement (stairs, cleaning)
   9. Laundry facilities (in home or near residence, washtub, clothesline)
   10. Yard care (garden, bushes, grass)
   11. Other home-maintenance concerns (e.g., access to fuse box, storm windows, furnace filters, painting)
F. Medications
   1. Large number of prescriptions (may be many)
   2. Ability to remember
   3. Ability to see labels/directions
   4. Medications kept in one area
G. Access to community
   1. Busline
   2. Walking
   3. Driving (self or service from others)
   4. Church, dry cleaning, drugstore, bank, health care facility, dentist, other community agencies
H. Other
   1. Caring for spouse/relative/companion
   2. Financial management (able to write checks, make payments, cash checks)
   3. Care of pet(s)

---

at night). Eating pattern variances from day to day. Who client eats with, if anyone. A 24-hour recall may not be indicative of client's real eating pattern, which may vary greatly from day to day.

6. Specific foods and amounts consumed; a 24-hour recall, if appropriate, or foods consumed over a week or a month
7. Fluid intake (24-hour estimate)
8. Person who buys and prepares food
9. If someone else prepares and buys food, client's satisfaction with this; ability to maintain special diet
10. If client buys own food, ask about access to market, walking (clarify distance), bus, driving, taxi, frequency of trips to market
11. If client prepares food in own home, ability to cope with any preparation problems (e.g., fatigue, eating alone, decreased vision, refrigerator, stove, water in rural area)
12. Problem with chewing (dentures fit or loose,

teeth loose or painful, edentulous)
13. Problem with swallowing, choking
14. Ability to afford the food desired and needed
15. Client's summary of own nutritional status
- Integumentary
  1. Skin
     a. Skin disease or skin problems or lesions (wounds, sores, ulcers)
     b. Growths, tumors, masses
     c. Excessive dryness, sweating, odors
     d. Pigmentation changes or discolorations
     e. Pruritus, scratching
     f. Texture changes
     g. Temperature changes
     h. Increased or excessive bruises, excoriations (especially in skinfolds), redness, or trauma marks
     i. Healing pattern of bruises, cuts, etc. (time element)
     j. Decreased sensation to pain, heat
     k. Increased sensation to pain, heat, cold, itching
     l. Chronic sun exposure; sensitivity
  2. Hair
     a. Thinning, falling out, dulling
     b. Texture changes
     c. Brittleness, breaking
     d. Use of dyes, permanents
  3. Nails
     a. Brittleness, peeling, breaking
     b. Changes in appearance, texture
     c. Toenails: thickening, difficulty cutting
- Head
  1. Headache (do full symptom analysis)
  2. Past significant trauma
  3. Dizziness (associated with body position or change—sitting up, standing, or head/neck movement)
  4. Syncope
- Eyes
  1. History of glaucoma
  2. Cataracts, infections (frequency, treatment)
  3. Discharge characteristics
  4. Itching
  5. Lacrimation (excessive tearing)
  6. Loss (or decrease) of tears
  7. Pain in eyeball
  8. Swelling around eyes
  9. Spots, floaters
  10. Unusual visual effects (e.g., light flashes, halos or rainbows around lights)
  11. General vision changes
  12. Loss of lateral vision (narrowing fields, tunnel vision)
  13. Double vision
  14. Sensitivity to glare

15. Difficulty with night vision
16. Difficulty distinguishing colors (e.g., traffic lights)
17. Photophobia
18. Blurring
19. Difficulty reading
20. Use of corrective or prosthetic devices (bifocals)
21. Unusual sensations, twitching
22. If bifocals, any problems with adjusting to far vision (e.g., stepping up on a curb)
23. Interference with activities of daily living caused by vision changes
- Ears
  1. Pain (pattern, position related)
  2. Cerumen
  3. Infection
  4. Vertigo
  5. Ringing and cracking
  6. Care habits
  7. Hearing changes
  8. Use of prosthetic devices
  9. Increased sensitivity to environmental noise
  10. Interference with activities of daily living
  11. Does conversation (of others) sound garbled or distorted?
  12. Client's perception of effectiveness of hearing aid, if used; person who prescribed it; when; how much it is used by client
- Nose, nasopharynx, paranasal sinuses
  1. Discharge (characteristics)
  2. Epistaxis
  3. Allergies
  4. Pain over sinuses
  5. Postnasal drip
  6. Sneezing
  7. Dry nasal passages/crusting
  8. Painful nose breathing
  9. Mouth breathing
  10. General olfactory ability
- Mouth and throat
  1. Sore throats
  2. Sore mouth
  3. Dry mouth
  4. Lesions (sores, ulcers, bumps on tongue, mouth, gums)
  5. Bleeding gums
  6. Burning mouth, palate, tongue
  7. Toothache
  8. Loose teeth
  9. Missing teeth
  10. Altered taste
  11. Chewing difficulty
  12. Swallowing difficulty
  13. Prosthetic devices (dentures, bridges)
  14. If client has dentures:

a. Wearing habits (e.g., for meals only, for appearance only, always, seldom, or never wears)

b. Wearing problems (e.g., rubbing or tenderness, looseness, clicking noises, talking difficulty, whistling dentures)

c. Cleaning habits and problems

15. Sores at corner of mouth (associated with edentulous patients or ill-fitting dentures)

16. Bad breath

17. Bad taste in mouth

18. Hoarseness

19. Voice changes

20. Pattern of dental hygiene

- Neck
  1. Node enlargement
  2. Swelling, masses
  3. Tenderness
  4. Limitation of movement
  5. Stiffness

- Breasts
  1. Pain or tenderness
  2. Swelling
  3. Nipple discharge
  4. Changes in nipples
  5. Lumps, dimples
  6. Unusual characteristics
  7. Irritated skin under pendulous breasts, rubbing bra
  8. Breast examination pattern, frequency

- Cardiovascular
  1. Cardiovascular—chest pain may be reduced, even absent, in elderly; dyspnea on exertion may be a primary symptom.
     a. Chest pain (do full symptom analysis)
     b. Dyspnea on exertion (specify *amount* of exertion, e.g., three stairs vs. one flight with 2-minute rest at landing; walking one block vs. walking from bed to bath)
     c. Palpitations
     d. Unusual breathing patterns (e.g., Cheyne-Stokes)
     e. Orthopnea
     f. Paroxysmal nocturnal dyspnea
     g. Episodes of confusion
  2. Peripheral vascular
     a. Coldness
     b. Loss of sensation to pain, touch
     c. Exaggerated response to cold (pain)
     d. Pain associated with exercise
     e. Color changes (especially feet and ankles: bluish-red or ruddy, mottling, pallor, associated with position)
     f. Swelling (specify time of day; do full symptom analysis)
     g. Varicosities

h. Constrictive clothing (e.g., girdles, garters, or stockings rolled at knees)

3. Heart and hypertension medications: toxicity symptoms

   The examiner need not pose questions about all these symptoms but should be alert to symptom groupings or patterns of drug reactions. Many clients take digitalis preparations, diuretics, and/or antihypertensive medications. The box below shows the major side effects and chief symptoms associated with toxicity.

- Respiratory
  1. History of wheezing, bronchitis, other breathing problems
  2. Painful breathing (on deep or regular inspirations)
  3. Smoking (detailed questions covered under habits)
  4. Chronic cough (do full symptom analysis—specify time of day or night that cough is bothersome)
  5. Sputum production (amount, color, time element)
  6. Hemoptysis
  7. Night sweats
  8. Exertional capacity (report present status and any recent change)
     a. Shortness of breath (SOB) with heavy, sustained work (e.g., lifting, digging, snow shoveling)
     b. SOB with sudden high-speed exercise (e.g., jogging, brisk walking, bicycling)
     c. SOB with exertion at slower pace (e.g., slow walk around the block, light housekeeping)
     d. SOB with slight exertion (e.g., rising from chair, walking from one room to another)
  9. Less active or immobilized recently or in past year for reasons other than respiratory (e.g., foot problems, fractured hip, arthritic pain)

MEDICATIONS: TOXICITY SYMPTOMS

Digitalis	Diuretics	Antihypertensives
Anorexia	Fatigue	Lethargy
Nausea, vomiting, diarrhea	Weakness	Mood disturbances
Headache	Muscle cramps	Sedation
Drowsiness	Gastrointestinal	Postural syncope
Vision changes (yellow, brown, green vision, halos around lights)	distress	Dizziness
	Confusion	Nausea
		Diarrhea
Dysrhythmias (all varieties)		Fluid retention
Confusion		Drug rash

- Hematolymphatic
  1. Lymph node swelling
  2. Excessive bleeding or easy bruising
  3. Petechiae, ecchymoses
  4. Anemia
  5. Blood transfusions
  6. Excessive fatigue
  7. Radiation exposure
- Gastrointestinal
  1. Abdominal pain (heartburn, indigestion, pain in lower abdomen; specify if pain is associated with eating, before or after; do full symptom analysis)
  2. Excessive belching (sour taste, associated with pain)
  3. Anorexia
  4. Nausea, vomiting
  5. Food idiosyncrasies (long-standing or recent)
  6. Bloating
  7. Flatulence
  8. Rumbling bowel
  9. Diarrhea
  10. Swollen abdomen
  11. Jaundice
  12. Hemorrhoids (pain, bleeding, amount)
  13. Bowel habits (frequency, defecation difficulty, straining)
  14. Change in bowel habits
  15. Description of stool (color, size, consistency)
  16. Constipation (describe client's concern in detail, including use of digestive or evacuation aids)
- Urinary
  1. Characteristics of urine; note changes (color, odor, clarity)
  2. Voiding pattern (in 24-hour period), number of times client is up at night, any recent change in pattern
  3. Characteristics of urine
  4. Urination pattern/problems (retention, incomplete emptying, straining to void, change in force of stream—requires man to stand closer to toilet—hesitancy, dribbling, incontinence with stress, sneezing, coughing)
  5. Painful urination
  6. Urgency, frequency
  7. Oliguria
  8. Polyuria
  9. Pyuria
  10. Hematuria
  11. Flank, groin, low back, or suprapubic pain
- Genital
  1. General
     a. Lesions
     b. Discharges
     c. Odors
     d. Pain, burning, pruritus
     e. Veneral disease history
     f. Sexually active—if so, satisfaction with sexual activity
  2. Men
     a. History of prostate trouble
     b. Scrotal lumps, masses, surface changes
     c. If uncircumcised, difficulty retracting foreskin
     d. Scrotum self-examination practices
     e. Does client have full erection, can he maintain erection to his satisfaction, complete ejaculation?
     f. Pain preceding, during, or following erection
  3. Women
     a. Menopause history (onset, course, LMP, associated problems, residual problems, any bleeding since LMP)
     b. Any severe problems with menstrual history
     c. Soreness or tenderness of vagina
     d. Pressure sensation within vagina
     e. Dyspareunia
- Musculoskeletal—history of injuries, fractures, dislocation, whiplash
  1. Muscles
     a. Twitching
     b. Cramping
     c. Weakness or pain with use (location of weakness; activity, such as stair climbing, altered by weakness)
     d. Manual dexterity problems
     e. Other interferences with ADLs
  2. Extremities
     a. Deformity or coordination difficulties
     b. Problems with shoes (fit, rubbing)
     c. Restless legs
     d. Transient paresthesia—need to move legs at night
  3. Gait
     a. Any alterations noted by client (e.g., weakness, balance, difficulty with steps, fear of falling)
     b. Walking aids (cane, walker, special shoes; client's perception of effectiveness of aids; any difficulty maneuvering aid)
  4. Bones and joints
     a. Joint swelling, pain, redness, deformity
     b. Stiffness (pronounced at certain times of day, associated with or after activity or inactivity)
     c. Limited movement (specify location, which joint)
     d. Crepitus
     e. Interference with ADLs
  5. Back
     a. Pain (do full symptom analysis)
     b. Stiffness

c. Corrective measures (use of bed board, special mattress, prosthetic devices)
d. Interference with activities of daily living
e. Client's assessment of effectiveness of prosthetic devices; any difficulty applying

- Central nervous system—history of any disease
  1. Seizure (characteristics, medications for)
  2. Speech
     a. Unusual speech patterns
     b. Aphasia
     c. Dysarthria (stammering)
  3. Cognitive changes
     a. Inability to remember (recent vs. remote)
     b. Disorientation
     c. Phobias
     d. Hallucinations
     e. Passing out episodes
     f. Inteference with activities of daily living
  4. Motor-gait
     a. Coordinated movement
     b. Ataxia, balance problems
     c. Paralysis (partial vs. complete)
     d. Tic
     e. Tremor, spasm
     f. Interference with activities of daily living
  5. Sensory
     a. Tingling sensations
     b. Areas of paresthesia (patterns)
     c. Other changes
- Endocrine
  1. Diagnosis of disease states (e.g., thyroid, diabetes)
  2. Changes in skin pigmentation or texture
  3. Changes in or abnormal hair distribution
  4. Sudden or unexplained changes in height and weight
  5. Intolerance of heat or cold
  6. Exophthalmos
  7. Goiter
  8. Hormone therapy
  9. Polydipsia
  10. Polyphagia
  11. Polyuria
  12. Anorexia
  13. Weakness
- Allergic and immunological (optional; use if client indicates allergic history; note precipitating factors in each case.)
  1. Dermatitis
  2. Eczema
  3. Pruritus
  4. Urticaria
  5. Sneezing
  6. Vasomotor rhinitis

7. Conjunctivitis
8. Interference with activities of daily living
9. Environmental and seasonal changes
10. Treatment techniques

- Any other physiological problems or disease states not specifically discussed that client has; explore in detail.

Psychosocial History

- General statement of client's feeling about self
- Relatives and friends, in home, or nearby (sexual needs, affection, support). If individual lives alone: (a) to what extent is being alone tolerated; (b) does client have sufficient and satisfactory access to family and friends; and (c) does client have a pet? If client lives with family: (a) are relationships satisfactory (with spouse, children, grandchildren); (b) does client participate in activities (meals, recreation) with family; and (c) does client participate in family decisions; is there conflict?
- Environment: is it adequately warm, sufficiently and conveniently spacious, sufficiently private, comfortable, safe, and affordable?
- Time/energy: too much or too little time to carry out daily life; does client have sufficient energy to meet needs?
- Activities of daily living (see p. 26 for details)
  1. General description of work, leisure, and rest distribution
  2. Significant hobbies or methods of relaxation
  3. Family demands
  4. Community activities and involvement (e.g., church, club)
  5. Transportation
     a. Automobile: estimate amount of driving; does client consider himself safe (last driving test); financial problems with gas, upkeep, insurance
     b. Bus: easy access; availability to necessary and desired destinations; problems getting onto bus, tolerating wait
     c. Taxi: estimate amount used (financial burden)
     d. Driving services from others: availability, convenience
     e. Walking: problems with distance, carrying packages, using curbs and stairs, bad weather, fear of traffic
  6. Occupational/volunteer history
     a. Major jobs held in past
     b. Current employment
     c. Volunteer and community activities
     d. Satisfaction with present activities
  7. Work/retirement concerns
     a. Reduced/fixed income
     b. Moving or selling home
     c. Role change/time adjustment

d. Problems in relationship with spouse because of retirement
- General statement about client's ability to cope with activities of daily living
- Recent changes or stresses in life-style: illness of self or family member; death of spouse, close friend, or family member; retirement, moving, financial changes
- Patterns in which client copes with stress: use of resources; worry pattern
- Any history of psychiatric care or counseling
- Feelings of anxiety or nervousness: describe characteristics and coping mechanisms
- Feelings of depression (consider such symptoms as insomnia, crying, fearfulness, marked irritability, or anger; review medication intake)
- Changes in personality, behavior, mood
- Specific feelings of satisfaction or frustration: aging changes, setting goals and meeting them, work activities, use of leisure time, mental capacity, intellectual capacity, aspirations
- Use of drugs or other techniques during times of anxiety or stress
- Response to illness
  1. Does the client cope satisfactorily during times of own or others' illness?
  2. Do the client's family and friends respond satisfactorily during periods of illness?
- Physical well-being; particular fears and concerns about death/disability
- Habits
  1. Alcohol
     a. Kinds (beer, wine, mixed drinks)
     b. Frequency per week
     c. Pattern over past 5 years; 1 year
     d. Drinking companions?
     e. Drinks when anxious?
  2. Smoking
     a. Kind (pipe, cigarette, cigar)
     b. Amount per week; day
     c. Pattern over past 5 years; 1 year
     d. Enclosed with others who smoke?
     e. Smokes when anxious?
     f. Desire to quit smoking? (method of attempts)
  3. Coffee and tea
     a. Amount per day
     b. Pattern over past 5 years; 1 year
     c. Drinks more coffee when anxious?
     d. Physiological effects
  4. Sleep
     a. Any alteration in sleep pattern recently or in past year?
     b. Sleep needs being met (fatigue)
     c. Concerns about interruptions at night (e.g., pain, SOB, nocturia, light sleeping, insomnia—

specify difficulty falling asleep, staying asleep, awakening too early in morning)
     d. Excessive napping during day
     e. Inability to stay awake
     f. Describe *all* client efforts to regulate sleep (e.g., drugs, prescriptions, alcohol, warm milk, reading)
  5. Other
     a. Overeating, sporadic eating
     b. Nail biting
     c. Withdrawal (e.g., sleeping)
- Financial status
  1. Sources
  2. Adequacy
  3. Recent changes in resources/expenditures

Health Maintenance Efforts

- General statement of client's physical fitness
- Exercise: amount, type, frequency
- Dietary regulations: special efforts (describe in detail)
- Mental health: special efforts, such as group therapy, meditation, yoga
- Cultural or religious practices
- How often client seeks:
  1. Physical health assessment
  2. Dental health assessment
  3. Vision health assessment

Environmental Health

- General statement of client's assessment of environmental safety and comfort; if client's community considered safe
- Hazards of employment: inhalant, noise, heavy lifting, psychological stress, machinery
- Hazards in the home: concern about fire, stairs to climb, inadequate heat, open gas heaters, inadequate toilet facilities, pest control, inadequate space
- Hazards in neighborhood: noise, water pollution, air pollution, inadequate police protection, heavy traffic on surrounding streets, isolation from neighbors, overcrowding
- Community hazards: unavailability of grocery stores, laundry facilities, drugstore; bus line access
- Safety assessment (optional; to be used if client is disabled or has difficulty with activities of daily living. This section suggests some major hazards.)
  1. Gait and balance problems
     a. Slippery or irregular surfaces (floors, icy sidewalks, rug edges, small rugs, risers on stairs not fastened down)
     b. Obstructions or clutter (on stairs, extension cords)
     c. Steep, dark stairs (cellar)
     d. Stairs without handrails

e. Inadequate space for maneuvering walker, cane, wheelchair
f. Slippery bathtub (oil in bath water)
g. Shoes without support, untied laces
h. Climbing: use of ladders to paint, make home repairs, replace light bulb, etc.
i. Excessively long clothing
j. Walking in heavy traffic areas

2. Decreased vision
   a. Insufficient illumination in home (dark hallways, stairways, no night light)
   b. Glare from polished floors, excess lighting
   c. Missing the bottom step
   d. Bifocals (client has difficulty with far vision, descending stairs, curb)
   e. Medication errors

3. Decreased sensitivity to pain and heat
   a. Hot bath water
   b. Heating pads, hot water bottles

4. Other
   a. Fire hazards: loose sleeves over stove burner, frayed electric cords, open heaters, stove burners left on, smoking (especially in bed)
   b. Driving and traffic accidents: slow reaction time, decreased vision, difficulty turning head with upper torso (arthritis), walking too slow for traffic signals

HISTORY AND CLINICAL STRATEGIES

- Many older people don't seem to "fit" into traditional clinics. If there is a tight appointment schedule, the examiner and client have time for little other than assessing immediate, acute problems.
  1. Older clients often have a long story to tell (especially medical history)
  2. Their reaction time may be slower; it takes longer for them to reflect and respond to questions.
  3. Many of them have had unpleasant experiences being hurried or pressured (in department stores, heavy traffic, etc.); they may enter the health care facility with a reluctance to take up the examiner's time.
  4. It takes *time* to develop trust with clients so that they will be willing to share their concerns.

- If clinic (or employer) policies cannot be altered to meet geriatric client needs, some alternatives might be helpful.
  1. Gather and organize all available history data from other sources before interviewing the client.
  2. Ask the client to complete the medical history at home (if no vision or writing problems exist).
  3. Spread out the data base collection over several appointments.
  4. Supplement clinic visits with a home visit.
  5. Set aside 1 day a week or month for prolonged appointments to collect initial data base from new clients.
  6. Insist that time be made available! Otherwise, the client's needs are not being fully assessed.

- Assess limitations of hearing and sight early in the interview: visual and hearing losses can distort information exchange. The examiner may believe the client is confused; the client may merely have difficulty hearing the examiner.

- Do not shout. This rarely helps in communicating with those who have diminished hearing; it often further distorts conversation.

- Directly face the client for a full view of the face; speak slowly and distinctly.

- Refer to "Clinical Tips and Strategies," p. 12, for further suggestions.

 Study Questions

A series of statements about the total health data base follows; mark each statement as either "T" for true or "F" for false.

1. _____ The history format is intended to be flexible.
2. _____ During preliminary data gathering, patient priorities are established.
3. _____ The chief complaint should be stated in the client's own words.
4. _____ A family tree should be used to describe relationships only among immediate family members living together.
5. _____ When posing questions, do not suggest answers.
6. _____ An immunization history is part of a patient's current health data.
7. _____ Childbearing women should be assessed for exposure to teratogens.
8. _____ Maternal history is not part of the newborn's health data.
9. _____ Depending on their ages, a child's health history may be separated from that of his parents.
10. _____ Assessment of elderly patients' activities of daily living is an optional part of their health data.

SUGGESTED READINGS
General

Barsky AJ and others: Evaluating the interview in primary care medicine, *Soc Sci Med (Med Psychol Med Sociol)* 14A(6):653, 1980.

Bates B: *A guide to physical examination,* ed 4, Philadelphia, 1987, JB Lippincott, p 1.

Ber R, Alroy G: The teaching of history-taking and diagnostic thinking: description of a method, *Med Educ* 15:97, 1981.

Diekelmann N: *Primary health care of the well adult,* New York, 1977, McGraw-Hill.

Engle GL, Morgan WL: *Interviewing the patient,* London, 1973, WB Saunders.

Gordon M: *Nursing diagnosis: process and application,* ed 2, New York, 1987, McGraw-Hill.

Malasanos L, Barkauskas V, Stoltenberg AK: *Health assessment,* ed 4, St Louis, 1990, Mosby−Year Book.

Platt FW, McMath JC: Clinical hypocompetence: the interview, *Ann Intern Med* 91(6):898, 1979.

Prior JA, Silberstein JS, Stang JM: *Physical diagnosis: the history and examination of the patient,* ed 6, St Louis, 1981, Mosby−Year Book.

Seidel HM, Ball JW, Dains JE, Benedict GW: *Mosby's guide to physical examination,* ed 2, St Louis, 1991, Mosby−Year Book.

The newborn

Auvenshine MA, Enriquez MG: *Maternity nursing: dimensions of change,* Belmont, Calif, 1985, Wadsworth.

Beischer NA, MacKay EV: *Obstetrics and the newborn: an illustrated textbook,* ed 2, Philadelphia, 1986, WB Saunders.

Bobak LM, Jensen MD: *Essentials of maternity nursing,* ed 3, St Louis, 1987, Mosby−Year Book.

Judd JM: Assessing the newborn from head to toe, *Nurs '85* 15(12):34, 1985.

Kiernan BS, Scoloveno MA: Assessment of the neonate, *Top Clin Nurs* 8(1):1, 1986.

The organization for Obstetrical, Gynecological, and Neonatal Nurses (NAACOG): *Physical assessment of the neonate,* OGN nursing practice resource, Washington, DC, Oct 1986, The Association.

Pillitteri A: *Maternal-newborn nursing: care of the growing family,* ed 3, Boston, 1985, Little, Brown.

Scanlon JW and others: *A system of newborn physical examination,* Baltimore, 1979, University Park Press.

Scharping EM: Physiological measurements of the newborn, *Matern Child Nurs J* 8:70, 1983.

Seidel HM, Ball JW, Dains JE, Benedict GW: *Mosby's guide to physical examination,* ed 2, St Louis, 1991, Mosby−Year Book.

Whaley LF, Wong DL: *Nursing care of infants and children,* ed 4, St Louis, 1991, Mosby−Year Book.

The child

De Angelis C: *Basic pediatrics for the primary health care provider,* ed 2, Boston, 1984, Little, Brown.

Malasanos L, Barkauskas V, Stoltenberg-Allen K: *Health assessment,* ed 4, St Louis, 1990, Mosby−Year Book.

Pillitteri A: *Nursing care of the growing family: a child health text,* Boston, 1977, Little, Brown.

Powell ML: *Assessment and management of developmental changes and problems in children,* ed 2, St Louis, 1981, Mosby−Year Book.

Seidel HM, Ball JW, Dains JE, Benedict GW: *Mosby's guide to physical examination,* ed 2, St Louis, 1991, Mosby−Year Book.

Whaley LF, Wong DL: *Essentials of pediatric nursing,* ed 3, St Louis, 1989, Mosby−Year Book.

The childbearing woman

Auvenshine MA, Enriquez MG: *Maternity nursing: dimensions of change,* Belmont, Calif, 1985, Wadsworth.

Beischer NA, MacKay EV: *Obstetrics and the newborn: an illustrated textbook,* ed 2, Philadelphia, 1986, WB Saunders.

Bobak IM, Jensen MD: *Essentials of maternity nursing,* ed 3, St Louis, 1991, Mosby−Year Book.

Gilbert ES, Harmon JS: *High-risk pregnancy and delivery: nursing perspectives,* St Louis, 1986, Mosby−Year Book.

The Organization for Obstetrical, Gynecological, and Neonatal Nurses (NAACOG): *Antenatal assessment. I. Maternal profile.* Update Series.

Pillitteri A: *Maternal-newborn nursing: care of the growing family,* ed 3, Boston, 1985, Little, Brown.

Pritchard JA, MacDonald PC: *Williams' obstetrics,* ed 17, New York, 1985, Appleton-Century-Crofts.

Seidel HM, Ball JW, Dains JE, Benedict GW: *Mosby's guide to physical examination,* ed 2, St Louis, 1991, Mosby−Year Book.

Update Series, Continuing Professional Education Center, (CPEC), Princeton, NJ.

Whitley N: *A manual of clinical obstetrics,* Philadelphia, 1985, JB Lippincott.

The older adult

Burnside IM, editor: *Nursing and the aged,* ed 2, New York, 1981, McGraw-Hill.

Ebersole P, Hess P: *Toward healthy aging: human needs and nursing,* ed 3, St Louis, 1990, Mosby−Year Book.

Kerzner LJ, Greb L, Steel K: History-taking forms and the care of geriatric patients, *J Med Educ* 57(5):376, 1982.

Matteson M, McConnell ES: *Gerontological nursing: concepts and practice,* Philadelphia, 1988, WB Saunders.

Meneilly GS, Minaker KL: Obtaining the geriatric history, *Contemp OB/GYN,* Sept. 1986, p 177.

Tideiksaar R, Kay AD: What causes falls? A logical diagnostic procedure, *Geriatrics* 41(12):32, 1986.

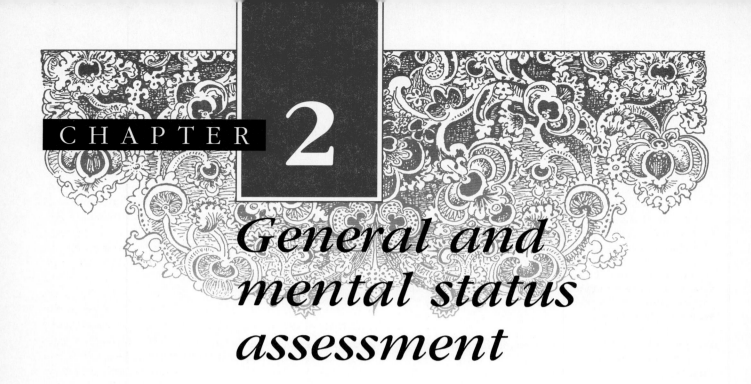

2

General and mental status assessment

VOCABULARY

affect Observable behaviors indicating an individual's feelings or emotions.

apathy Lack of emotional expression; indifference to stimuli or surroundings.

blocking Interruption in a train of thought, loss of an idea, or repression of a feeling or idea from conscious awareness; can be a normal behavior or, in extreme form, indicative of abnormality.

coherency Conversation and behavior that convey thoughts, feelings, ideas, and perceptions in a logical and relevant manner.

compulsive behavior A repetitive act that usually originates from an obsession; extreme anxiety emerges if the act is not completed.

confabulation The fabrication of events or sequential experiences often recounted to cover up memory gaps.

delusion Persistent belief or perception that is illogical or improbable.

dementia A broad term that indicates impairment of intellectual functioning, memory, and judgment.

depersonalization Sense of being out of touch with one's environment; loss of a sense of reality and association with personal events.

dysarthria Speech disorder involving difficulty with articulation and pronunciation of specific sounds; results from loss of control over muscles of speech.

dysphasia Speech disorder involving difficulty with use of language and words to convey meaning to others; often associated with cerebral vascular accidents.

dysphonia Difficulty in controlling laryngeal speech sounds; can be a normal event, such as male vocal changes occurring at puberty.

euphoria Sense of elation or well-being; can be a normal feeling or exaggerated to the extent of distorting reality.

hallucination Sensory perception that does not arise from an external stimulus; can be auditory, visual, tactile, gustatory, or olfactory.

illusion Perceptual distortion of an external stimulus.

EXAMPLE: Mirage in a desert.

labile emotions Unpredictable, rapid shifting of expression of feelings.

neologism Newly invented word or phrase that has meaning understood only by the person who coins it; often accompanies psychotic states.

neurosis Ineffective or troubled coping mechanism stemming from anxiety or emotional conflict.

obsession Persistent thought or idea that preoccupies the mind; not always realistic and may result in compulsive behavior.

paranoia Sense of being persecuted or victimized; suspicious of others.

phobia Uncontrollable, often unreasonable, and intense fear of a specific object or event.

psychosis Any major mental disorder characterized by greatly distorted perceptions and severe disorganization of personality.

schizoid Exhibiting behaviors or having characteristics that resemble schizophrenia.

schizophrenia Any one of a large group of psychotic disorders characterized by marked distortion of reality and disorganization of personality characteristics.

sensorium Status of level of consciousness and orientation to surroundings.

PRINCIPLES AND CONCEPTS

When a practitioner initially observes a client (perhaps from across the room), the practitioner is presented with a steady stream of data. Some of this information may not be processed at a conscious level. The examiner may quickly decide that the client looks "ill," "depressed," "alert," or "pleasant." Many of those observations cannot be classified under body systems, but they are vitally important and must be reported in concrete terms. The word *ill* does not convey a clear message to the reader. The following description does:

Skin is ashen, cool to touch, and moist. The client is slumped in a chair, and body and extremities appear limp. Client does not establish eye contact and responds to all questions in a monotone "yes" or "no."

Observation skills are enhanced through practice and a concentrated awareness of incoming perceptions. Every element of the examiner's behavior and capacity for observation should be deliberate and focused on the client. A simple handshake indicates the client's ability to extend the arm, to firmly grip the hand, to respond with a smile or facial expression acknowledging an introduction, and to establish and maintain eye contact. It also permits the examiner to feel the coolness or warmth and dryness or moisture of the palm. Stammering, hand wringing, sighing respirations, and speaking loudly are examples of hundreds of cues that the examiner can observe and report without such judgmental descriptors as "normal," "abnormal," or "well-adjusted." Judgment occurs later, when the examiner puts together the client's version of self, the examiner's observations, and physical findings.

The purpose of this chapter is to clarify and organize specific, observable behaviors that are valid indications of the client's general state, as well as his emotional and mental well-being.

Cognitive Functions

A client's orientation to time, person, and place is usually made apparent in the first few minutes of the interview. Client statements about concerns that brought him to the interview usually include references to self, acknowledgment of being present in the setting, and time-related events leading up to the present. Note that "normal" people can lose track of time or forget the day's date when they are anxious or stressed. People who live in an isolated environment—away from media, other people, or associations with time-related stimuli (e.g., clocks, calendars, a job to report to, or bills to pay at a certain time)—may find time irrelevant and elusive. Failure to report the present month, season, or year usually extends beyond moderate anxiety or isolation.

It should also be remembered that individuals who have been transported to a hospital, clinic, or other strange environments may have difficulty grasping where they are. A sense of self or self in relation to others (e.g., inability to identify one's child) is usually the last phase of orientation that is lost. Chemical substance ingestion, psychotic states, and advanced brain or physical deterioration can all be contributors to disorientations.

An individual's attention span can be disrupted when he is anxious, depressed, in pain, or affected by chemical substance ingestion; a decrease in attention span can be an early indicator of mental or emotional dysfunction. A full attention span is present when one can follow and complete a train of thought. This usually can be ascertained as conversation with the client proceeds in the interview. Shifting the subject in midsentence and failure to recall a question just posed are two examples of inability to maintain concentration. If the examiner notices that one or both of these behaviors are occurring, he or she should ask simpler, shorter questions that call for brief and simple answers to acquire necessary information. A lengthy history should be curtailed.

Recent memory loss is a failure to recall something that occurred within minutes or a few hours before the present. Remote memory loss is a failure to remember an event that took place days, weeks, or even years ago. Recent memory loss is much more common and is usually apparent as the continuity of an interview begins to break down. The client cannot connect a stated complaint with a series of events because he has forgotten the stated complaint. The client may repeat the same sentence or story several times; telling it each time as though it has never been stated. Sometimes clients are aware that their memories falter, and the anxiety about this only exaggerates the effects. Others, as they grow older, fear a loss of memory, and the fear becomes a reality as their anxiety interferes with their capacity to recall. Recent memory may diminish with some but not all elders. Some clients are skilled at masking memory loss. They are aware of it and are embarrassed. They provide a diversion through social conversation, humor, and changing the subject to avoid exposing a memory gap. Alzheimer disease is the most common cause of recent memory dysfunction. Remote memory loss is usually detected when the client cannot recall the more distant past (e.g., past hospitalizations, an anniversary date, or other important life events). Remote memory loss is associated with advanced organic dementia and some schizophrenic states.

Judgment enables one to conduct a life that is satisfactory in one's own thinking, as well as in the thinking of those who live and deal with that person (e.g., family, employers, neighbors, friends). "Good" judgment enables one to (1) plan ahead, (2) assess what is and make use of it, (3) weigh a situation and consider all the factors to reach a decision, and (4) consider options and the effects on self and others. "Normal" judgment covers a wide range of behaviors, includng sensible, eccentric, and impetuous. "Normal" judgment can be temporarily impaired with added stressors or anxiety states. It can be seriously or permanently impaired with alcoholism, psychotic states, substance abuse, mental retardation, manic states, and brain deterioration. In history taking, the examiner might suspect a judgment malfunction if the client reports a long series of crises over an extended period. Posing questions about hypothetical situations and asking for client-devised solutions will identify severe problems (see p. 39).

The underlying intelligence of a client is noted as he proceeds with the interview; talks about himself, his problems, and his relationship with others; and reflects with the examiner about the causes and consequences of his present condition. Basic intelligence is conveyed through one's access to basic information and everyday activities (e.g., completion of elementary or high school, ability to drive an automobile and acquire a license, and capacity to acquire and maintain a job.) The level of one's vocabulary might indicate a lack of education or a mental dysfunction. An extreme paucity of wordage should be noted; other very simple words can be used to request the client's definition to identify severe problems (see p. 39). The capacity to engage in abstract reasoning and to identify similarities (see p. 39 for example questions) are also ways to determine basic intelligence.

Emotional Status

Anxiety and depression are common emotional states that most people experience at some time in their life. Clients who present themselves in a health care setting are very likely to exhibit some of these behaviors as a "normal" response to being in an unfamiliar arena, perhaps with a concern that something is wrong with them. Anxiety or depression may also be present to such an extent that either state could be deemed "abnormal." Following is a list of behaviors and complaints that can serve as general indicators of levels or degrees of these states. Again, the judgment that a given set of observations is "normal" or "abnormal" should be withheld until all data is gathered and analyzed. The following characteristics may be observed in the mildly to moderately anxious client and in the client who is moderately to severely anxious.

Mild to moderate anxiety

- Can focus on conversation and respond appropriately
- Demonstrates increased alertness and eye contact

- Shows signs of muscle tension (leans forward, listens intensely) and is fidgety and restless
- Frequently wets lips with tongue
- Has higher voice pitch, asks rapid-fire questions and gives rapid-fire responses
- Has increased respirations and moderately increased perspiration

Moderate to severe anxiety

- Has very limited or no ability to focus on conversation
- May either appear frozen/immobilized or have extreme muscle tension with jerky, erratic movements
- Frequently wets lips or clenches jaw and breathes through teeth
- Has higher pitch with rapid, rambling mode of speech, or speaking capacity may be shut down
- Has increased respirations, pants, or is breathless; has clammy skin, may feel cold and appear pale
- Complains of palpitations, dizziness, chills, urinary frequency, diarrhea, chest pain, and/or abdominal pain

Depressive Behaviors: Signs and Symptoms

Signs and symptoms of depressive behavior are listed as follows. It should be noted that none of these manifestations are indicative of either mild or severe depression. Severity is indicated by the intensity and duration of the behaviors and symptoms and the extent to which these entities disrupt the client's life.

- Diminished body movements
- Slowed movements
- Slouched posture
- Subdued voice, low pitch and volume, monotone
- Decreased eye contact
- Absent or diminished smile or constant, unchanging smile
- Sighing respirations
- Tearfulness
- Indecisive responses: either cannot make a decision or not sufficiently engaged to make a decision
- Reports appetite change (anorexia, weight loss, increased appetite, weight gain)
- Reports lack of energy
- Reports loss of interest in daily activities
- Reports insomnia (unable to fall asleep, awakens in the middle of the night, or awakens very early in the morning)
- Reports that early morning is always the most difficult time of the day
- Reports constipation
- Reports nagging muscular pains, backache, or vague symptoms

(The statement from the client that he has thought about suicide is *always serious* and becomes increasingly urgent if the client (1) has a history of suicide attempts, (2) has no access to a personal support system,

(3) has entertained or devised a method for self-destruction, and (4) is in a high-risk category for suicide (see p. 38).

Clients may present a variety of affects (observable behaviors indicating feelings or emotions) that noticeably alter the interview and should be carefully observed. Labile emotions are conveyed as rapid and dramatic shifts of behaviors, swinging from weeping to elation. Some individuals may exhibit an inappropriate euphoria—accompanied by rapid-fire conversation, flight of ideas (abrupt shifts in topics), denial of illness or adversity, or delusions—with intervals of irritability and defensiveness. A blunted or flat affect—frequently associated with some medication side-effects, depression, and schizophrenic disorders—is manifested through limited facial expressions, flattened or noncommittal responses, reduced physical movement, and inability to initiate conversation. Bizarre or inappropriate affects include euphoria, seductive behaviors, unpredictable shifts of conversation, contradictory statements, and hyperactive physical activity.

Moods are experienced internally, and even though the examiner can observe affect, an inquiry about "how does it feel?" can reveal how the client perceives self and lives on a day-to-day basis. The sadness of depression may be so consuming that the client can barely function, or it may occur only at certain times of the day, month, or year. Both anxiety and depression are bound with stressors—either the presence or creation of them or the client's capacity to resolve or cope with them. Any affective disturbance should be observed and followed with questions about how it feels, how one perceives self, and how one copes with one's life.

Thought Process and Content

Coherency is a broad term indicating an individual's ability to convey thoughts, feelings, intentions, and perceptions in a logical and rational manner. Coherency can be interrupted by a variety of disorders, including schizophrenic states, severe depression or anxiety, impaired verbal communication, and organic brain syndromes. Use of bizzare words; rapid and unpredictable shifts of topics; severe withdrawal or halted, limited language; blocking; and constant repetition of words are examples of thought process interruptions. The individual is easily distracted, or preoccupied, and words and sentences are fragmented. Incoherency can be observed as a mild deterrent to relevant flow of conversation, or it can be an extreme set of behaviors, including the utterance of jibberish or unintelligible sounds.

Thought content disruptions are persistent, irrational thoughts, ideas, or beliefs that invade the continuity of one's thoughts and actions. Individuals with phobias, obsessions, or compulsive behaviors will report that their daily lives are disrupted by fears (which may escalate to terror) of certain activities, objects, or entities. They may describe a constant preoccupation with a need to perform an activity repeatedly or a fixation on avoidance of something (e.g., fear of germs and a preoccupation with cleaning, or fear of open spaces, heights, or enclosures). Delusions occur in many different forms and degrees of severity and frequently interfere with personal relationships. Jealousy, ideas of persecution, and grandiose schemes or sense of self are examples. Delusions may exist to the point that an individual is out of touch with reality, or they may be confined to specific situations. Extreme anxiety or schizophrenia may cause one to feel removed from his environment or unable to maintain a sense of identity. Severe perceptual distortions may be presented in the form of hallucinations or illusions.

COGNITIVE OBJECTIVES

At the end of this chapter the learner will demonstrate knowledge of assessment of the client's general and mental status by the ability to do the following:
- Apply the terms that are listed in the vocabulary section.
- Identify major components of the general assessment.
- Point out some common behaviors associated with mild to moderate anxiety.
- Identify some common behaviors associated with moderate to severe anxiety.
- Distinguish some common behaviors associated with depression.
- Identify methods by which an examiner can validate the suspicion that a client is disoriented.
- Point out characteristics of behaviors associated with hallucinations.
- Identify some disorders that can disrupt thought content.
- Identify selected newborn, child, childbearing woman, and older adult variations of behavior associated with general and mental status.

CLINICAL OUTLINE

At the end of this chapter the learner will perform a systematic assessment of the general and mental status of the client, demonstrating the ability to do the following:
- Describe specific behaviors related to observation of the client:
  1. Initial response to examiner
  2. Body appearance
  3. Posture
  4. Body movements

5. Gait
6. Facial expression
7. Vocal tones
8. Speech patterns: pace, clarity, word and sentence delivery, volume, accent, or foreign language
9. Apparel
10. Grooming/hygiene
11. Odors
12. General mannerisms
- Describe specific behaviors indicating the client's cognitive functions:
  1. Orientation to person, place, time
  2. Attention span and concentration ability
  3. Memory—recent and remote
  4. Ability to make judgments
  5. Abstract reasoning ⎫
  6. Underlying intelligence ⎬ Optional history
     a. Access to basic ⎪ questions
        information
     b. Vocabulary
     c. Similarities
  7. Ability to read and write ⎭
- Describe specific behaviors indicating the client's emotional status.
- Describe specific behaviors that show the client's ability to sustain a clear thinking process: coherency, thought content, clarity of perceptions.
- Summarize results of the assessment with a written description of findings.

HISTORY

Most of the information needed for the assessment of the "normal" client's mental status can be obtained through the use of the general questions in the "Psychosocial History" (Chapter 1, p. 10). Basically, these questions ask the client: How do you feel about yourself? Are you living in a relatively low-stress environment? Are your coping abilities adequate to meet the stressors that you encounter in your daily living?

The answers to these questions can become more apparent by observing the client's general behavior (described subsequently). If the client's self-assessment and the examiner's assessment are congruent and if the results indicate that the client is coping adequately to meet personal needs, further questioning is not necessary. However, if there is an incongruity between what the client states and the behavior displayed, if behavior disturbances are noted, or if activities of daily living are interrupted, the following detailed questions are helpful.
- Anxiety or depressive states
  1. Do you have difficulty falling asleep, staying asleep, or being wakeful early in the morning?
  2. Describe your general mood in the morning.

3. Have you noticed any marked changes in appetite or eating habits?
4. Have you recently lost or gained weight?
5. Do you have periods of despondency or nervousness to the extent that you feel unable to cope? If so, how do you treat yourself? Is it effective?
6. Do you ever have crying spells?
7. Have there been any marked changes in your sexual habits or desires?
8. Have you noticed any change in the amount of energy you have to accomplish daily functions?
9. Do you have any difficulty making decisions?
10. Have you noticed any increase in irritability? Restlessness? Listlessness?
11. Do you ever feel as though you do not care about anything?
12. Do you spend much of your time alone? (Estimate number of waking hours per day, per week.)
13. Who are your significant friends, that is, individuals you trust and who are available when you need them?
14. If you had a crisis in the middle of the night, is there a resource you could seek; someone whom you know would be available?
15. History of psychiatric counseling and use of medications have been explored in the original data base, but they should be carefully reviewed.
16. Have you ever thought of hurting yourself or ending your life? (If so, describe past methods and any specific plans for future attempts.)
17. Presence of suicide risk factors should be determined.
    a. Teenage and early adulthood years
    b. Older adulthood (over 60 years)
    c. Previous attempts of suicide
    d. Expression of wish to die (risk increases if tangible plans are intact for killing self)
    e. Failing or terminal health state
    f. Marked or abrupt disengagement from friends, family, support system
    g. Recent, major disruption of life, such as loss of job or money, or loss of loved one
    h. Teenager coping with family disruption, or loss of boyfriend/girlfriend
    i. Teenager with sudden drop in grades or loss of interest in school, friends, or appearance
- Orientation
  1. Person: Can you give me your full name, address, and telephone number? Do you recall what my name is? Can you give me the full name of your closest relative?
  2. Place: Do you recall the name of this health agency?

What part of town do you live in? What is the name of this town? This country?

3. Time: Do you recall what day it is? Month? Year?

- Attention span/concentration

This can best be tested by giving the client a series of directions to follow, a sequence of behaviors. For example, "I would like you to reach into your purse, pull out your billfold, find an identification card, and show it to me. Then I would like you to empty your change purse on the table and put all the dimes and nickels in one stack and the quarters and pennies in another stack." Assuming there is no hearing, vision, or motor dysfunction, the client can be observed (and timed) going through the sequence of behaviors. If immobilized, the client can repeat a short story that you have related or describe a personal story. The examiner should be alert for (1) a total shift in direction of subject matter or sequence of behavior midway through the process or (2) conversation or sequenced behavior dwindling to silence or inactivity before being completed.

- Memory
  1. Recent: What did you have for breakfast this morning? What time did you arrive at the agency today? What time was your appointment? Ask client to repeat a series of three to six numbers.
  2. Remote: Can best be tested by having the client describe medical history, high school graduation, first job, when married, etc. (Provided the examiner is able to verify the information).

- Ability to make judgments (offering solutions to hypothetical situations)
  1. What would you do if you saw a man picking someone's pocket right in front of you?
  2. What would you do if the newspaper deliverer came to the door to collect and you discovered you had no available change?

- Abstract reasoning

Ask the client to explain what the following proverbs mean:
  1. A bird in the hand is worth two in the bush.
  2. Not to decide is to decide.
  3. Every cloud has a silver lining.

- Emotional status alerations (previous questions related to anxiety and depression are relevant in this area)
  1. Inquire again about stressors (e.g., money, intimate relationship, death or illness in family or friends, employment problems).
  2. How are you feeling right now?
  3. Do you consider your present feelings to be a problem in your daily life? If so, do you feel the problem is temporary or curable?

4. Describe a typical day at home (and/or at school, work), and tell which times or experiences are easiest for you and which are difficult.

5. Do you think you need help with your problem?

- If underlying intelligence appears to be minimal, the following questions or tests will be helpful.
  1. Client's access to basic information. In what direction does the sun set? How many months are in a year? What month follows July? In what state is Philadelphia?
  2. Client's vocabulary level. Ask the client to define a list of words. The list should begin with simple words and progress to more difficult ones, for example, chair, trouble, tender, posture, maximum.
  3. Ability to see similarities. Ask the client to describe how the following words are alike: a carrot and a potato, a dog and a cat, a lantern and a candle, a rose and perfume, an automobile and a train, etc.
  4. Ability to read and write. Ask the client to write his name and address on a sheet of paper. Ask the client to read newsprint (also a test for near vision). *Note:* Inability to read and write is not always a measure of intelligence, but is useful information for a practitioner when devising a care plan.

- Thought content disruptions
  1. Do you have certain thoughts or feelings that consistently return or disrupt your thinking? Are you able to control them?
  2. Do you ever lose control of your thoughts?
  3. Is your thinking the same as, as good as, or better than it was 5 years ago?
  4. Do you ever have trouble making decisions about everyday events?
  5. Do you have any dreadful or uncontrollable fears that keep returning?
  6. Do you ever have the feeling that something dreadful is going to happen?
  7. Do you feel that you have enemies or that someone is trying to harm you, discredit you, or control you?
  8. Do you feel that you are being watched or followed?
  9. Do you ever feel guilty about your behavior or your feelings?
  10. Do you ever have the feeling that you are losing touch with what is happening around you?

- Perception distortion
  1. Do you ever hear voices or strange noises?
  2. Do you ever see visions, lights, or people that others cannot see?
  3. Do you ever experience strange odors or tastes?
  4. Have you ever experienced strange sensations (warm, cold, or pressure) on your skin?

Text continues on p. 45.

CLINICAL GUIDELINES

	EVALUATION	
ASSESSMENT PROCEDURE	**NORMAL FINDINGS**	**DEVIATIONS FROM NORMAL**
1. Observe the whole client and the client's interaction with the environment for: a. Client's initial response to examiner 　(1) Examiner introduces self, clarifies client's name, offers hand in greeting, and sits down to be at eye level with client	Client responds with smile or facial expression acknowledging examiner's presence; establishes eye contact; offers own name; extends hand in greeting	Client does not attain or maintain eye contact; does not acknowledge presence of examiner with facial expression, body gesture, or extension of hand Client may jump up, interrupt, or talk through examiner May be tearful or grimacing with pain
(2) Examiner explains own role to client and begins interview with broad, open question	Client attentive, nodding head, maintaining eye contact, leaning toward examiner	Client looking away, eyes closed, eyes wandering around room; body pulled back in chair or leaning forward, exhibiting tense posture
2. Make more specific observations regarding: a. Body appearance (Height and weight measured with scale and results compared with standards [Tables 2-1 and 2-2])	Height not unusual	Excessively tall or short

TABLE 2-1 Weights* for men (according to frame, ages 25-59) for greatest longevity †

HEIGHT (IN SHOES)‡		SMALL FRAME	MEDIUM FRAME	LARGE FRAME
FEET	INCHES			
5	2	128-134	131-141	138-150
5	3	130-136	133-143	140-153
5	4	132-138	135-145	142-156
5	5	134-140	137-148	144-160
5	6	136-142	139-151	146-164
5	7	138-145	142-154	149-168
5	8	140-148	145-157	152-172
5	9	142-151	148-160	155-176
5	10	144-154	151-163	158-180
5	11	146-157	154-166	161-184
6	0	149-160	157-170	164-188
6	1	152-164	160-174	168-192
6	2	155-168	164-178	172-197
6	3	158-172	167-182	176-202
6	4	162-176	171-187	181-207

Courtesy Metropolitan Life Insurance Company, copyright 1983.
* Weights in pounds (in indoor clothing weighing 5 pounds).
† Metropolitan no longer labels these weights "ideal" or "desirable" because these adjectives mean different things to different people.
‡ Shoes with 1-inch heels.

TABLE 2-2 Weights* for women (according to frame, ages 25-59) for greatest longevity †

HEIGHT (IN SHOES)‡		SMALL FRAME	MEDIUM FRAME	LARGE FRAME
FEET	INCHES			
4	10	102-111	109-121	118-131
4	11	103-113	111-123	120-134
5	0	104-115	113-126	122-137
5	1	106-118	115-129	125-140
5	2	108-121	118-132	128-143
5	3	111-124	121-135	131-147
5	4	114-127	124-138	134-151
5	5	117-130	127-141	137-155
5	6	120-133	130-144	140-159
5	7	123-136	133-147	143-163
5	8	126-139	136-150	146-167
5	9	129-142	139-153	149-170
5	10	132-145	142-156	152-173
5	11	135-148	145-159	155-176
6	0	138-151	148-162	158-179

Courtesy Metropolitan Life Insurance Company, copyright 1983.
* Weights in pounds (in indoor clothing weighing 3 pounds).
† Metropolitan no longer labels these weights "ideal" or "desirable" because these adjectives mean different things to different people.
‡ Shoes with 1-inch heels.

	EVALUATION	
ASSESSMENT PROCEDURE	**NORMAL FINDINGS**	**DEVIATIONS FROM NORMAL**
	Body appears symmetrical in terms of size and placement of parts	Unilateral wasting or hypertrophy; asymmetrical body alignment
	Body fat is sparse or moderate and evenly distributed	Wasted, cachectic appearance; obesity, odd fat cushion distribution (e.g., confined to abdomen, hips, or buttocks)
	Body parts present and in proportion	Arms or legs exceptionally short; extremities missing
	Arm span equals height; distance between crown and pubis nearly equal to distance between pubis and soles of feet	Arm span exceeds body height
	Skin color evenly distributed; skin smooth	Sallow, pale, flushed; patchy discoloration of skin; marked wrinkling (localized or general)
	Muscle well or moderately developed or defined	Muscle wasting (localized or general)
	Hair evenly distributed over scalp, present in brows, lashes; moderate to light distribution over extremities, torso	Hirsutism; absence of scalp or body hair or excessive thinning
b. Posture	Shoulders back and relaxed; arms resting at sides or on chair; feet resting on floor; body relaxed in chair or on examining table	Asymmetrical posture (e.g., guarding or contractures); tense posture; client at edge of chair, curled up in bed; back/neck rigid (client must move torso to view side); Rigid posture with extremities held in flexion (Fig. 2-1); slumped in chair

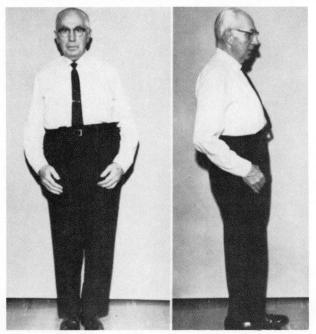

Fig. 2-1 Parkinson disease may be manifested in a series of different behaviors. Note staring, fixed facial expression, and posture rigidity with arms held close to sides in semiflexed position. (From Prior JA, Silberstein JS, Stang JM: *Physical diagnosis: the history and examination of the patient*, ed 6, St Louis, 1981, Mosby—Year Book.)

Continued.

ASSESSMENT PROCEDURE	EVALUATION	
	NORMAL FINDINGS	DEVIATIONS FROM NORMAL
c. Body movements	Movements deliberate, smooth, and coordinated; client sits motionless for brief periods, alternating with body position shifts and gestures	Jerky, fidgety, constant movement; tremors (localized or general)
	Client can sit up in bed, swing legs to side; able to rise to standing position from sitting position with smooth even movements	Movements very slow or very fast; client fails to move certain parts (e.g., may be splinting or guarding a painful area); hemiplegia or paraplegia; total absence or paucity of movement of arms, torso, or legs; movement uncoordinated (e.g., client slips when trying to rise; falls into chair rather than easing into it)
d. Gait	Steps even and smooth	Client watches feet while moving
	Heel-strike, midstance, push-off, and swing phases easily executed	Stumbles, shuffles, staggers, limps (midstance phase shortened with painful leg or foot); steps uneven; one leg not functioning; lurching or propulsive, spastic or scissors gait
e. Facial expression	Eye contact maintained much of time	No eye contact; staring fixedly (*Note:* A fixed gaze may indicate an effort to lip-read.)
	Smile alternating with serious or thoughtful expressions appropriate to conversation	Face immobile, expressionless; constant smile; grimacing (pain associated)
		Face puffy, flushed, pale; excessive perspiration on forehead, upper lip
		Dark circles under eyes (may be normal)
	Facial features symmetrical	Asymmetrical features (Fig. 2-2)
		Tearful expression
		Brow constantly furrowed
		Eyes darting around or constantly wandering about room
		Tics, tremors, lip biting or licking
		Squinting (inability to see)

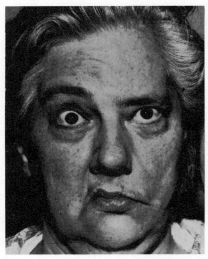

Fig. 2-2 Asymmetrical features. Note that flaccid left side of face flattens nasolabial fold, deepens line at left corner of mouth, shows marked discrepancy of eyebrow levels, and diminishes lines on left side of forehead. (From Prior JA, Silberstein JS, Stang JM: *Physical diagnosis: the history and examination of the patient,* ed 6, St Louis, 1981, Mosby–Year Book.)

	EVALUATION	
ASSESSMENT PROCEDURE	**NORMAL FINDINGS**	**DEVIATIONS FROM NORMAL**
f. Vocal tones	Moderate in pitch and volume; voice clear, firm, and audible; plentiful and varied inflections of tone in conversation	Very high pitched, loud, weak, inaudible, hoarse, monotone (*Note:* Depression, drug usage, and Parkinson disease are common causes.)
g. Speech		
(1) Pace	Moderate pace; may slow down with difficult or serious topic; may accelerate with excitement	Constantly rapid or very slow
(2) Clarity	Words easily understood. Enunciation of vowels and consonants clear	Slurred, garbled speech. Client misses particular consonants at beginning of words or mispronounces vowels
(3) Word and sentence pattern	Style of verbal response may be brief or loquacious; client pauses to think	Paucity of words (e.g., confined to yes/no responses); constant stream of words; words or sentences reflect loss of train of thought; stammering; interjection of numerous pauses (e.g., uhs, ums)
(4) Accent or foreign language	Accent varies according to origin	Accent very heavy (determine whether client able to use English language sufficiently to convey and receive messages)
h. Apparel	Clothing fits body	Clothing too tight, too small, too large (*Note:* May indicate recent weight loss or gain.)
	Shoes are intact and appear to fit snugly over feet	Skin bulges over top of shoes (may indicate edema or weight gain); shoes have holes or slits cut or worn in them (often done to minimize discomfort related to foot lesions, weight gain, or edema)
	Clothing clean, pressed, and "appropriate" for occasion (*Note:* Appropriate must be *broadly* defined; dress varies with age, lifestyle, financial resources, culture, climate)	Clothing dirty, rumpled; distinctly bizarre dress or combination of colors
i. Grooming/hygiene	Hair brushed, shiny	Hair disheveled, dull, broken ends
	Men: shaved or trimmed facial hair	Unshaved
	Nails clean (*Note:* Some employment leaves nails chronically dirty.)	Dirty, ragged nails
	Women: moderate or no makeup	Bizarre makeup
	Shoes fitted and clean (*Note:* Cleanliness is subjective and may or may not be an indication of normalcy.)	Shoes ill fitted, dirty
j. Odors	No odor (*Note:* Some cultures do not promote use of deodorants.)	Pungent ammonia or fetid breath odors; foul body odors
k. General mannerisms	Client may be quiet, thoughtful, somewhat passive (frightened) or active, moderately talkative, and demonstrative with body language	Tearful, angry, suspicious, questioning, evasive; constantly laughing and inappropriately joking; noticeably subdued

Continued.

CLINICAL GUIDELINES—cont'd

ASSESSMENT PROCEDURE	EVALUATION	
	NORMAL FINDINGS	DEVIATIONS FROM NORMAL
	Client shows no acute distress signs; breathing even and moderately slow; facial expression relaxed	Shows acute distress signs, such as dyspnea, pain (client splints, guards a part, limits movement), grimacing, moaning, writhing, coughing, wheezing, marked lethargy, drowsiness

3. Observe mental status regarding:
  a. Cognitive functions
    (1) Orientation to person, place, and time (Specific questions should be used only if examiner cannot assess orientation through conversation and general health interview)
	Client indicates orientation to person, place, and time through discussion of history	Client cannot deliver accurate biographical data (e.g., address, name); cannot name the agency that he is currently in; cannot identify year, month (*Note:* Many "normal" people cannot recall the day of the month!)

(2) Attention span and concentration	Client can complete entire thought process (e.g., when describing a pain, client can recall location, duration, onset, character, etc., without wandering off subject)	Client cannot complete a thought; may digress in middle of sentence
(3) Recent memory	Client accurately responds to questions about very recent events (e.g., How did you get to the clinic this morning? What did you have for breakfast?)	Client cannot recall very recent events (*Note:* Client's laugh may indicate embarrassment, may be an attempt to change subject or distract examiner.)
(4) Remote memory	Client delivers medical history accurately	Client cannot recall remote events
(5) Ability to make judgments	Client usually indicates ability to make judgments when describing personal health care practices and decisions made about maintaining or following health care routines	Client gives no indication that he can perceive a particular situation accurately and follow through with appropriate decisions
(6) Abstract reasoning (usually tested by asking client to explain proverbs)	Client offers appropriate explanation	Client cannot explain meaning
b. Emotional status, affect, mood	Client responds with smiles alternating with thoughtful or serious facial expressions appropriate to conversation; body behaviors indicate relaxation or mild to moderate anxiety	Client demonstrates behavior indicating depression or moderate to severe anxiety or indicates through general questions that activities of daily living are impeded or altered by mood, that coping capacity is inadequate
	Client describes self as well adjusted, generally happy, or appropriately concerned about present health alteration	Mood may be intense, defensive, or hostile; mood shifts may be extreme and unpredictable

	EVALUATION	
ASSESSMENT PROCEDURE	**NORMAL FINDINGS**	**DEVIATIONS FROM NORMAL**
c. Thought processes and perceptions		
(1) Coherency and relevance	Client can complete entire thought (e.g., full symptom analysis description) without losing track of ideas or digressing; answers to examiner's questions direct and appropriate	Ideas run together within sentence or stream of thought; illogical ideas associated
(2) Thought content	Consistent, logical, and free-flowing thinking demonstrated as client describes history and self	Thoughts interrupted with signs of complusive or obsessive ideas (going off on a tangent); marked doubting and indecisiveness; phobias; free-floating anxieties; ideas of persecution, delusion; feelings of unreality
(3) Perceptions	Client indicates to examiner, through descriptions of self a consistent awareness of reality; client perception of objects and surroundings consistent with those of examiner	Client has illusions; hallucinations interfere with client's flow of perceptions
	Client can accurately follow all directions; breathe deeply, sit up, walk to the other end of the room, tell about last hospitalization, etc.	Psychotic client may demonstrate preoccupation with self and little or no interest in examiner's activity
		Affect may be inappropriate, (euphoric, flat, depersonalized, erratic, or easily distracted)
		Ritualistic, repetitive posturing or gestures may be evident
		Client may have periods of complete immobility

CLINICAL TIPS AND STRATEGIES

- **The first 5 to 10 minutes of the interview belong to the client:** The examiner can begin with a very broad question, such as "What brings you to the clinic today?" This enables the client to talk freely about concerns and priorities and enables the practitioner to observe the client's verbal, nonverbal, and general behavior patterns.
- **Most clients are anxious:** Normal mild to moderate anxiety may create a number of unusual behaviors—hyperactivity, stammering, excessive perspiration, excessive giggling, or listlessness. All these behaviors are worth noting in the final summary, but the examiner should be cautious about labeling behaviors as abnormal.
- **The client is observing the examiner:** The examiner must be acutely aware of personal behavior so that feelings of concern, caring, concentration, and confidence are conveyed, as well as interest.

SAMPLE RECORDING: NORMAL FINDINGS

The client is a neatly attired, clean-shaven, 42-year old man. Facial expressions are alert, appropriate to the conversation, and coupled with frequent eye contact with examiner. Varied vocal tones are well modulated, and speech is audible and articulate. Body movements are smooth and coordinated.

General mood is one of seriousness accompanied by mild postural tension and intense listening behaviors while symptoms are discussed. Conversation indicates orientation to time, person, and place. Client is able to offer logical and reasonable contributions to the discussion of the problem and can describe past attempts at dealing with the difficulty.

The Newborn

HISTORY AND CLINICAL STRATEGIES

- The newborn should not mind being undressed or examined but will lie quietly on the examination table or the parents's lap (if not tired or cold) and will cooperatively allow the examiner to collect the appropriate assessment data.
- The examiner should collect history data before undressing the infant. During the history collection, observe the interaction between parent and child and how the child responds to the parent's techniques. Chapter 1 further describes specific information regarding parenting stresses and infant responses to stress.
- Newborns have an amazing ability to interact with their environments. Parents should get to know their infants. A parenting or infant stimulation class may help the family function more optimally.
- Infants deprived of early, positive interaction may develop such conditions as failure to thrive. Infants need consistent caretakers.
- Parental abusive behaviors toward each other or their offspring should be assessed, and appropriate referrals made.

The Child

HISTORY AND CLINICAL STRATEGIES

- The general and mental assessments of the child are patterned after those of the adult. The examiner must carefully observe the child interacting with the environment, the parents, and the examiner. Depending on the child's age and development, the examiner should observe for various normal behaviors. Following is an initial summary. Other areas are further detailed in the data base in Chapter 1 and in subsequent clinical chapters.

  The *6-month-old to 2-year-old child* is acutely aware of the environment, viewing the parent as protector and the examiner as the enemy. The examiner must evaluate the child with the assistance of the parent in eliciting various responses. During this time, observe the parent-child interaction. If the child does not cooperate, how does the parent respond? Does the child have eye contact with the examiner? Does the child separate with difficulty from the parent? It is anticipated that the child will respond most favorably if examined while sitting on the parent's lap.

  The *child from ages 2 to 4 years* is curious to find out who the examiner is and what will take place, but still clings to the parent for security. After becoming familiar with the examiner, the child should relax and enter into game playing, conversation, and free expression of giggles and smiles. The examiner should again observe parent-child interactions and the child's ability to communicate and cooperate with the examiner.

  The preschool *child from 4 to 6 years of age* will generally cooperate with the examiner and separate with ease from the parent. The examiner should evaluate the child's maturity, eye contact, attention span, and interaction with the parent.

  In general, as the child matures, developmental progression, an increased attention span, the ability to cooperate with the examiner, and decreased dependence on the parent should be observed. Any deviation from this should stimulate the examiner to develop a thorough behavior profile for the child based on the history and physical data.

- The examiner must be alert to common behavioral problems in children and common behavioral concerns of parents. Although the actual mental status examination follows the same guidelines as for the adult client, other common problems or concerns should be screened for. In each of the following situations the examiner should employ the elements of symptom analysis to develop a situational profile.

  1. Intellectual limitations of the child: the parent may feel the child is not performing to capacity.
  2. Short attention span: the parent may feel that the child is unable to maintain concentration appropriate for age.
  3. Inability to problem-solve: the parent may express concern that the child is unable to perform tasks or solve problems appropriate for age.
  4. Communication difficulties: the child may have difficulty with speech development, eye contact, or communication with parents or peers.
  5. Variability: the child's mood is unpredictable— one minute happy or organized, the next minute unhappy or disorganized.
  6. Emotional immaturity: the child may lag in development, acting impulsively without thinking through the consequences, even though there has been experience with a similar problem.
  7. Hyperactivity: the child demonstrates an inappropriate amount of activity for age; the parent may state that the child has a difficult time sitting still or following through with an activity; may demonstrate a repetitive activity, such as finger tapping.
  8. Perception difficulties: the child may demonstrate a pattern of inappropriate behaviors that might be a sign of difficulties with perception. Common difficult concepts are the differences between right and left, up and down, in and out, before and after. The child may also demonstrate an inability to complete a puzzle appropriate for age, difficulty learning to tie a shoe, or difficulty screwing or unscrewing the lid on a jar.
  9. Aloneness: the preschool or school-age child may

not interact with or play with other children.

10. Change in routine: the child may have difficulty with or react violently to a change in routine.

11. Personal contact: the infant or child may not like to be cuddled, does not extend the arms to be picked up, or does not like to be held.

- Other common stress behaviors that the examiner must note are thumb sucking, nail biting, teeth grinding, rocking, or stuttering.

- In general, the examiner must assess how the child is developing and coping with the environment. As the examiner collects developmental, psychological, and physical data, patterns or collective signs that indicate how the child is coping with the environment and how the parent is coping with the child must be observed. Areas of the text most likely to facilitate this collective analysis are the *Psychosocial History* sections for "The Child" in Chapters 1, 14, and 15.

 ## *The Childbearing Woman*

HISTORY AND CLINICAL STRATEGIES

- An overall assessment of a client and family can unveil beliefs and values about the childbearing and child-rearing experience. Appearance, actions, and speech should be analyzed to help determine physiological and psychosocial health.

- Grooming and hygiene practices are especially important during pregnancy and delivery.
  1. Tight clothing that constricts uterine growth or blood circulation should be discouraged.
  2. Support hose and support bras help prevent varicosities and strain.
  3. Cotton underwear and hygiene help prevent infection, especially *Candida,* which causes thrush.

- Hormonal shifts may cause mood swings and postpartum depression. Women with a history of stress, depression, or other emotional problems may experience more family adjustment difficulties. Physiological symptoms may be associated with a woman's mental health, so an assessment must include general and mental factors.

- The weight gain during pregnancy averages 25 to 30 pounds. Diets to lose weight are usually discouraged during pregnancy. A woman's overall height and weight should be assessed, and appropriate weight gain and dietary habits should be encouraged.

 ## *The Older Adult*

HISTORY AND CLINICAL STRATEGIES

Elderly clients can be observed and assessed in the same manner as other adult clients.

- It is helpful to remember that elderly individuals are frequently subject to a greater number and intensity of stressors than are younger people. They invariably suffer losses: loss of friends and loved ones through death, loss of occupation through retirement, and loss of a youthful body and energy. They are frequently subject to changes in living conditions, financial status, and positions of authority and impact previously ensured in work, parenting, and social environments. There is no indication that the number and intensity of stressors can predict the individual's responses; in terms of depression, withdrawal, anxiety, or grieving, however, the examiner must be alert for signals indicating a maladaptive response.

- It is estimated that 500,000 to 1 million elders suffer from physical and psychological abuse in this country (Kallman, 1987). In recent years authorities have developed profiles (or characteristics) of abused individuals to assist in the identification of these victims. Some of the common signs, symptoms, and characteristics are the following:
  1. Lives at home with adult child and/or grandchild
  2. Has cognitive impairment
  3. Exhibits physical dependency needs that make great demands on the caregiver
  4. Shows signs of fearfulness or extreme compliance when the caregiver is present
  5. Frequently denies abuse if asked
  6. Has unexplainable (and repeated) bruises, scratches, excoriations, burns, or other injuries
  7. Shows evidence of poor hygiene, malnutrition, and general neglect
  8. Is isolated from visitors and outsiders

  Abuse may be subtle and is often difficult to assess and confirm. The examiner should be well informed on the subject before assessment and intervention take place.

- The examiner should also be alert for signs of confusion. Many elderly people are confused as a result of a physical illness. Confusion may be the first indicator of an altered health state, and its onset is usually sudden. Early indications of confusion are the following:
  1. Limited attention span (losing track of thought in midsentence or indicating loss of attention through nonverbal behavior, such as breaking eye contact during a conversation)
  2. Loss of recent memory (remote memory may remain intact)
  3. Emotion lability (sudden episode of tearfulness)
  4. Decreased use of judgment (inability to think through a situation and make decisions)
  5. Confusion that is exaggerated at night (wandering or sleeplessness) and diminishes or disappears during the day

- Some physiological states that might be associated with confusion follow:

1. Infectious process
2. Cardiorespiratory disturbances
3. Metabolism disorders
4. Trauma
5. Alcohol or drug abuse
6. Neoplasms

Most often, confusion associated with altered health states is reversible. This kind of confusion is usually compounded when elderly individuals are admitted to hospitals. Loss of a familiar environment and daily routines creates complex problems.

Mild confusion can sometimes be masked in clients who have well-preserved social skills. They can participate in polite conversations and skirt issues or direct questions that they are unsure of.

Hearing loss or visual impairment can be mistaken for confusion. The examiner should assess early in the interview the client's ability to receive communications.

- Depression in the elderly can be accompanied by a thinking or memory impairment, which tends to occur most often with the very elderly depressed individual. Clients who complain of a "bad memory" should be further assessed for depression. Cognitive impairment related to depression is usually reversible if the depression is successfully treated.
- Organic brain syndrome is not a disease. The term describes brain changes that result in a variety of altered client behaviors. The onset is usually slow and can be manifested in an intermittent or progressive fashion. A stable environment and a limited number of stressors can be therapeutic. Altered behaviors associated with this syndrome vary greatly according to the individual clients. Some common behaviors are as follows:
  1. Diminished emotional responsiveness

2. Disorientation (especially to time and place)
3. Depression (often in the form of apathy or withdrawal)
4. Confabulation
5. Agitation
6. Paranoic beliefs
7. Loss of interest in appearance
8. Shortened attention span
9. Decreased intellectual skills
10. Decreased ability to make judgments

- Alzheimer disease is a progressive degeneration of the brain that results in a gradual, steady decline in cognitive and emotional functioning. The onset of symptoms may occur in late middle age but the incidence increases markedly in old age. The progression of symptoms varies widely, ranging from 1 to 15 years' duration. Signs and symptoms include the following:
  1. Memory loss (short term, initially)
  2. Restlessness, agitation
  3. Lack of spontaneity
  4. Mood swings
  5. Poor judgment in daily activities
  6. Irritability
  7. Gradual, insidious disorientation (eventually in all spheres)
  8. Eventual movement and gait disturbances
  9. Eventual incoherency
  10. Eventual coma and death
- Risk factors for Alzheimer disease include the following:
  1. A family history
  2. Being female
  3. Being over 80 years old
- The examiner must assess the client's use of drugs (over-the-counter and prescribed) and alcohol if confusion or disorientation is suspected.

Study Questions

General

1. Name eight general areas of behavior to look for while performing a general assessment, beginning with:
   a. Posture
   b.
   c.
   d.
   e.
   f.
   g.
   h.
2. A symptom that a client might exhibit if mildly anxious is:
   ☐ a. Breathlessness
   ☐ b. Dizziness
   ☐ c. Increased alertness
   ☐ d. Abdominal cramps
   ☐ e. None of the above
3. A sign of severe anxiety is:
   ☐ a. Intense listening
   ☐ b. Increased alertness
   ☐ c. Constipation
   ☐ d. Inability to clearly focus on present situation
   ☐ e. None of the above
4. Which of the following behavior(s) might be seen with depression:
   ☐ a. Slow body movements
   ☐ b. Indecisive response
   ☐ c. Constipation
   ☐ d. b and c
   ☐ e. a, b, and c
5. When an individual appears to be disoriented, the examiner can validate this suspicion by:
   ☐ a. Asking the client to name the present month or year
   ☐ b. Asking the client to describe personal feelings
   ☐ c. Asking the client to define words on a vocabulary list
   ☐ d. All of the above
   ☐ e. None of the above
6. If an individual can follow a series of brief, simple directions without prompting, the client is:
   ☐ a. Intelligent
   ☐ b. Able to control attention span
   ☐ c. Not depressed
   ☐ d. Not hallucinating
   ☐ e. None of the above

7. A client may be deemed incoherent if he:
   ☐ a. Wears bizarre clothing
   ☐ b. Expresses the wish to die
   ☐ c. Expresses feelings of self-worthlessness
   ☐ d. Exhibits rapid, unpredictable shifts of topics
   ☐ e. Is afraid of heights
8. A delusion is:
   ☐ a. Perceptual distortion of an external stimulus
   ☐ b. Persistent belief or perception that is illogical
   ☐ c. Repression of a feeling or idea from conscious awareness
   ☐ d. Impairment of intellectual functioning and memory

The Newborn

9. Infants deprived of loving interaction have a higher likelihood of developing:
   ☐ a. Eyesight defects
   ☐ b. Otitis media
   ☐ c. Failure to thrive syndrome
   ☐ d. Retractions, flaring, and grunting

The Child

10. A child who perceives the parent as a protector and the examiner as an enemy is probably:
    ☐ a. 2 to 6 months old
    ☐ b. 6 months to 2 years old
    ☐ c. 18 months to 3 years old
    ☐ d. 3 to 5 years old

The Childbearing Woman

11. Postpartum depression is usually associated with:
    ☐ a. Methargen ingestion
    ☐ b. Hormonal shifts
    ☐ c. Hereditary factors
    ☐ d. Constricting clothes

The Older Adult

12. An elderly client with cognitive impairment, malnutrition, bruising, and physical dependency needs has characteristics pertinent to the profile of:
    ☐ a. An abused person
    ☐ b. A client with Alzheimer disease
    ☐ c. A recently retired person
    ☐ d. An "elderly primipara"

SUGGESTED READINGS
General

Anxiety: programmed instruction, recognition and intervention, *Am J Nurs* 65:9, 1965.

Bates B: *A guide to physical examination,* ed 4, Philadelphia, 1987, JB Lippincott.

Braverman BG, Shook J: Spotting the borderline personality, *Am J Nurs* 87(2):200, 1987.

Malasanos L, Barkauskas V, Stoltenberg AK: *Health assessment,* ed 4, St Louis, 1990, Mosby—Year Book.

Nowack M: Initial development of an inventory to assess stress and health risk, *Am J Health Promotion* 4(3):173, 1990.

Snyder JC, Wilson MF: Elements of a psychological assessment, *Am J Nurs* 77(2):235, 1977.

Thompson JM, McFarland GK, Hirsch JE: *Mosby's Manual of Clinical Nursing,* ed 2, St Louis, 1989, Mosby—Year Book.

The newborn

Auvenshine MA, Enriquez MG: *Maternity nursing: dimensions of change,* Belmont, Calif, 1985, Wadsworth.

Bobak IM, Jensen MD: *Essentials of maternity nursing,* ed 3, St Louis, 1991, Mosby—Year Book.

Erickson ML: *Assessment and management of developmental changes in children,* St Louis, 1976, Mosby—Year Book.

Whaley LF, Wong DL: *Essentials of pediatric nursing,* ed 3, St Louis, 1989, Mosby—Year Book.

The child

DeAngelis C: *Basic pediatrics for the primary health care provider,* ed 2, Boston, 1984, Little, Brown.

Pillitteri A: *Nursing care of the growing family: a child health text,* Boston, 1977, Little, Brown.

Powell ML: *Assessment and management of developmental changes and problems in children,* ed 2, St Louis, 1981, Mosby—Year Book.

Whaley LF, Wong DL: *Essentials of pediatric nursing,* ed 3, St Louis, 1989, Mosby—Year Book.

The childbearing woman

Auvenshine MA, Enriquez MG: *Maternity nursing: dimensions of change,* Belmont, Calif, 1985, Wadsworth.

Bobak IM, Jensen MD: *Essentials of maternity nursing,* ed 3, St Louis, 1991, Mosby—Year Book.

Humenick SS: *Analysis of current assessment strategies in the health care of young children and childbearing families,* Norwalk, Conn, 1982, Appleton-Century-Crofts.

Pilitteri A: *Maternal-newborn nursing: care of the growing family,* ed 3, Boston, 1985, Little, Brown.

Pritchard JA, MacDonald PC: *Williams' obstetrics,* ed 17, New York, 1985 Appleton-Century-Crofts.

The older adult

Burnside LM: *Nursing and the aged,* ed 3, New York, 1988, McGraw-Hill.

Dychtwald, K: *Wellness and health promotion for the elderly,* Rockville, Md, 1986, Aspen Systems.

Ebersole P, Hess P: *Toward healthy aging,* ed 3, St Louis, 1990, Mosby—Year Book.

Janz M: Clues to elder abuse, *Geriatr Nurs* 11(5):220, 1990.

Kallman H: Detecting abuse in the elderly, *Med Aspects Human Sexuality* 21(3):89, 1987.

Quinn MJ, Tomita SK: *Elder abuse and neglect,* New York, 1986, Springer.

Steinberg FU, editor: *Care of the geriatric patient,* ed 6, St Louis, 1983, Mosby—Year Book.

Wolanin MO, Phillips LR: *Confusion: prevention and care,* St Louis, 1981, Mosby—Year Book.

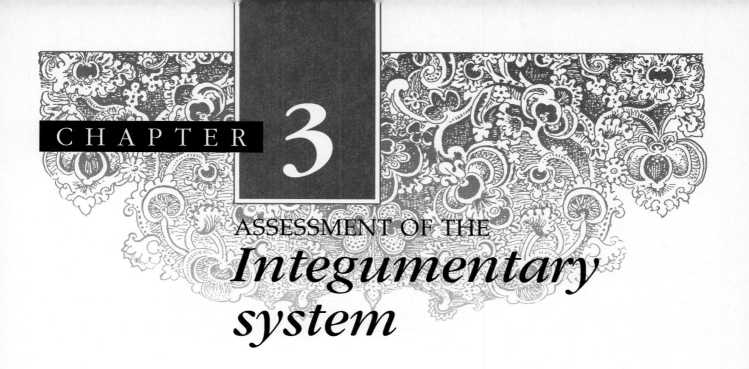

CHAPTER 3

ASSESSMENT OF THE
Integumentary system

VOCABULARY

annular Describes a lesion that forms a ring around a clear center of normal skin.

apocrine sweat glands Secretory dermal structures located in the axillae, nipples, areolae, scalp, face, and genital area; develop at puberty and respond to emotional stimulation.

atrophy Diminution of size or wasting; can also refer to loss of elastic tissue resulting in a slightly sunken epidermis that wrinkles easily when pulled to the side.

bulla Elevated, circumscribed, fluid-filled lesion greater than 1 cm in diameter.

bunion Abnormal prominence on the inner aspect of the first metatarsal head (described in Chapter 14); the skin over the prominence may be reddened, broken, and tender from pressure and friction.

callus Hyperkeratotic area caused by pressure or friction; usually not painful.

circinate Circular.

circumscribed Well defined, limited, and encircled.

confluent Describes lesions that run together.

contusion (bruise) Swelling, discoloration, and pain without a break in the skin; caused by a blow to the area.

corn Hyperkeratotic, slightly raised, circumscribed lesion caused by pressure over a bony prominence; usually on the fourth or fifth toe; painful if pressure or friction is persistent.

crust Dried serum, blood, or purulent exudate on the skin surface.

desquamation Sloughing process of the cornified layer of the epidermis; when accelerated, the process can cause peeling, scaling, and loss of the deeper layers of skin.

diffuse Spread out, widely dispersed, copious.

ecchymosis Discoloration of skin or the mucous membrane caused by leakage of blood into the subcutaneous tissue; can also be a bruise.

eccrine sweat glands Secretory dermal structures distributed over the body that secrete water and electrolytes and regulate body temperature; heat, emotional reactions, and physical exercise are the primary stimulants for secretion.

eczematous Describes a superficial inflammation characterized by scaling, thickening, crusting, weeping, and redness.

erosion Wearing away or destruction of the mucosal or epidermal surface; often develops into an ulcer.

erythematous Redness (of the skin).

excoriation Scratch or abrasion on the skin surface.

fissure Linear crack in the skin.

herpetiform Describes a cluster of vesicles resembling herpes lesions.

induration Hardening of the skin, usually caused by edema or infiltration by a neoplasm.

ischemia Diminished supply of blood to a body organ or surface; characterized by pallor, coolness, and pain.

keloid Hypertrophic scar tissue; prevalent in non-white races.

keratosis Overgrowth and thickening of the cornified epithelium.

lichenification Thickening of the skin characterized by accentuated skin markings; often the result of chronic scratching.

macule Flat, circumscribed lesion of the skin or mucous membrane; 1 cm or less in diameter.

necrosis Localized death of tissue.

nevus Congenital, pigmented area on the skin.

EXAMPLES: Mole, birthmark.

nodule Solid skin elevation that extends into the dermal layer; 1 cm or less in diameter.

papule Solid, elevated, circumscribed, superficial lesion; 1 cm or less in diameter.

paronychia Inflammation of the skinfold that adjoins the nail bed; characterized by redness, swelling, and pain; may be pustular.

patch Flat, circumscribed lesion of the skin or mucous membrane; more than 1 cm in diameter.

petechiae Tiny, flat, purple or red spots on the surface of the skin resulting from minute hemorrhages within the dermal or submucosal layers.

plaque Solid, elevated, circumscribed, superficial lesion; more than 1 cm in diameter.

pruritus Itching.

purpura Hemorrhage into the tissue, usually circumscribed; lesions may be described as petechiae, ecchymoses, or hematomas, according to size.

pustule Vesicle or bulla that contains pus.

reticular Describes a netlike pattern or structure of veins on a tissue surface.

scale Small, thin flakes of epithelial cells.

sebaceous glands Secretory dermal structures that produce sebum, an oily substance; puberty stimulates production, and the primary areas for secretion are in the face, chest, and upper part of back.

seborrhea Group of skin conditions characterized by noninflammatory, excessively dry scales or by excessive oiliness.

telangiectasia Dilation of a superficial capillary or network of small capillaries that produces fine, irregular red lines on the skin surface.

tumor Solid skin elevation extending into the dermal layer; more than 1 cm in diameter.

turgor Normal resiliency of the skin.

ulcer Circumscribed crater on the surface of the skin or mucous membrane that leaves an uncovered wound.

urticaria (hives) Pruritic wheals, often transient and allergic in origin.

vesicle Fluid-filled, elevated, superficial lesion; 1 cm or less in diameter.

wheal Elevated, solid, transient lesion; often irregularly shaped but well demarcated; an edematous response.

ANATOMY AND PHYSIOLOGY REVIEW

The skin is composed of three layers: the epidermis, the dermis, and the hypodermis (Fig. 3-1). The epidermis has an outer, cornified layer that serves as a protective barrier and regulates water loss. The underlying epidermal layers fold into the dermis and contain hair roots, apocrine sweat glands, eccrine sweat glands, and sebaceous glands. Hair and nails arise from these underlying layers and are composed primarily of keratin (produced by keratin cells, which are generated in the epidermis). Melanocytes, located in the base epidermal layer, secrete melanin, which provides pigment for the skin and hair and serves as a shield against ultraviolet radiation. The epidermis is avascular and is shed and replaced with new cells about every 30 days.

The dermis is formed of connective tissue and is highly vascular. The blood vessels dilate and constrict in response to external heat and cold and internal stimuli, such as anxiety or hemorrhage, resulting in the regulation of body temperature and blood pressure. The dermal blood nourishes the epidermis, and the dermal connective tissue provides support for the outer layer. The dermis also contains sensory fibers that react to touch, pain, and temperature. The arrangement of connective tissue enables the dermis to stretch and contract with body movement. Dermal thickness varies from 1 to 4 mm in different parts of the body.

The hypodermis is composed primarily of loose connective tissue interspersed with subcutaneous fat. These fatty cells help to retain heat and to provide a protective cushion and a storage for calories.

• • •

Alterations in the skin, hair, or nails can be responses to external stimuli (e.g., bacterial invasion, trauma, sun, or extended pressure) or internal forces (e.g., allergic response, systemic disease manifestations, diminished capillary supply, pregnancy, or aging). Lesions may be difficult to diagnose because people often treat themselves with home remedies, which may change the configuration or course of the lesion. Diagnosis is difficult also because the source of the problem may be a combination of factors.

The examiner should develop a descriptive vocabulary that clearly conveys the onset, present state, and course of manifestations and events associated with the alteration. For the beginning examiner, the vocabulary associated with disease states is much less important than the capacity to describe an entity clearly and concisely. Tables 3-1 and 3-2 illustrate and describe basic skin lesions and offer examples of common diseases or causes. *Text continues on p. 58.*

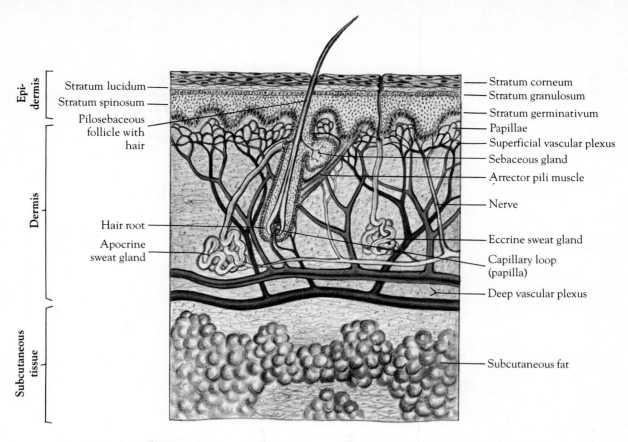

Fig. 3-1 Structures of skin. (From Thompson JM, McFarland GK, Hirsch JE, and others: *Mosby's manual of clinical nursing,* ed 2, St Louis, 1989, Mosby–Year Book.)

TABLE 3-1 **Primary skin lesions** (initial spontaneous manifestations of underlying pathological process)

LESION	DESCRIPTION	EXAMPLES
Macule	Flat, nonpalpable, circumscribed; less than 1 cm in diameter; brown, red, purple, white, or tan in color	Freckles, flat moles, rubella, rubeola
Patch	Flat, nonpalpable, irregularly shaped macule; greater than 1 cm in diameter	Vitiligo, port-wine marks

Modified from Thompson JM, McFarland GK, Hirsch JE, and others: Mosby's manual of clinical nursing, *ed 2, St Louis, 1989, Mosby–Year Book.*

Continued.

LESION		DESCRIPTION	EXAMPLES
Papule		Elevated, palpable, firm, circumscribed; less than 1 cm in diameter; brown, red, pink, tan, or bluish red in color	Warts, drug-related eruptions, pigmented nevi
Plaque		Elevated, flat topped, firm, rough, superficial papule; greater than 1 cm in diameter; may be coalesced papules	Psoriasis, seborrheic and actinic keratoses
Wheal		Elevated, irregular-shaped area of cutaneous edema; solid, transient, changing; variable diameter; pale pink in color	Urticaria, insect bites
Nodule		Elevated, firm, circumscribed, palpable; deeper in dermis than papule; 1 to 2 cm in diameter	Erythema nodosum, lipomas
Tumor		Elevated, solid; may or may not be clearly demarcated; greater than 2 cm in diameter; may or may not vary from skin color	Neoplasms

LESION	DESCRIPTION	EXAMPLES
Vesicle	Elevated, circumscribed, superficial, filled with serous fluid; less than 1 cm in diameter	Blister, varicella, herpes zoster (clustered vesicles)
Bulla	Vesicle; greater than 1 cm in diameter	Blister, pemphigus vulgaris
Pustule	Elevated, superficial; similar to vesicle, but filled with purulent fluid	Impetigo, acne, variola
Cyst	Elevated, circumscribed, palpable, encapsulated; filled with liquid or semisolid material	Sebaceous cyst
Telangiectasia	Fine, irregular red line produced by dilation of capillary	Telangiectasia in rosacea

TABLE 3-2   Secondary skin lesions (later evolution of a primary lesion or external trauma to the primary lesion)

LESION		DESCRIPTION	EXAMPLES
Scale		Heaped-up keratinized cells; flaky exfoliation; irregular; thick or thin; dry or oily; varied size; silver, white, or tan in color	Psoriasis, exfoliative dermatitis
Crust		Dried serum, blood, or purulent exudate; slightly elevated; size varies; brown, red, black, tan, or straw in color	Scab on abrasion, eczema
Lichenification		Rough, thickened epidermis, accentuated skin markings caused by rubbing or irritation; often involves flexor aspect of extremity	Chronic dermatitis
Scar		Thin to thick fibrous tissue replacing injured dermis; irregular; pink, red, or white in color; may be atrophic or hypertrophic	Healed wound or surgical incision
Keloid		Irregularly shaped, elevated, progressively enlarging scar; grows beyond boundaries of wound; caused by excessive collagen formation during healing	Keloid from ear piercing or burn scar

Modified from Thompson JM, McFarland GK, Hirsch JE, and others: Mosby's manual of clinical nursing, *ed 2, St Louis, 1989, Mosby–Year Book.*

LESION		DESCRIPTION	EXAMPLES
Excoriation		Loss of epidermis, linear or hollowed-out crusted area, dermis exposed	Abrasion, scratch
Fissure		Linear crack or break from epidermis to dermis, small, deep, red	Athlete's foot, cheilosis
Erosion		Loss of all or part of epidermis; depressed, moist, glistening; follows rupture of vesicle or bulla; larger than fissure	Varicella, variola after rupture
Ulcer		Loss of epidermis and dermis, concave, varies in size, exudative, red or reddish blue	Decubiti, stasis ulcers
Atrophy		Thinning of skin surface and loss of skin markings; skin translucent and paperlike	Striae, aged skin

COGNITIVE OBJECTIVES

At the end of this chapter the learner will demonstrate knowledge of assessment of the integument by the ability to do the following:

- Apply the terms that are listed in the vocabulary section.
- Identify relationships and primary functions of these integumentary components:
  1. Stratum corneum
  2. Epidermis
  3. Dermis
  4. Sebaceous gland
  5. Eccrine sweat gland
  6. Apocrine sweat gland
  7. Subcutaneous tissue
  8. Keratin
  9. Melanin
- Point out differentiating characteristics of 12 common primary lesions:
  1. Macule
  2. Papule
  3. Nodule
  4. Vesicle
  5. Patch
  6. Plaque
  7. Tumor
  8. Bulla
  9. Pustule
  10. Wheal
  11. Cyst
  12. Telangiectasia
- Identify client conditions or situations that increase the importance of periodic skin assessment.
- Identify pressure points for assessment of an immobilized, recumbent, or chair-bound client.
- Point out the characteristics of sequential skin alterations in response to continued pressure.
- Identify some systemic or local conditions that affect the skin, hair, and nails.
- Identify selected characteristics of the integumentary examination for the newborn, the child, the childbearing woman, and the older adult.

CLINICAL OUTLINE

At the end of this chapter the learner will perform a systematic assessment of the integumentary system, demonstrating the ability to do the following:

- Obtain a pertinent health history from a client.
- Demonstrate and describe the results of inspection and palpation of the following skin characteristics:
  1. Color
  2. Moisture
  3. Temperature
  4. Texture
  5. Thickness variations
  6. Mobility and turgor
  7. Hygiene
  8. Lesions
- Demonstrate and describe the results of inspection and palpation of nails for the following:
  1. Configuration
  2. Consistency
  3. Color
  4. Adherence to nail bed
- Demonstrate and describe the results of inspection of hair for the following:
  1. Distribution and configuration
  2. Texture
  3. Color
  4. Quantity
  5. Parasites
- Summarize results of the assessment with a written description of findings.

HISTORY

- Is there a family history of skin problems (chronic, allergic, intermittent, or acute in nature)?
- Does anyone at home (or closely associated with client) have any skin lesions, itching, or infections?
- Does the client use any home remedies or local applications of any kind on the skin?
- What is the client's assessment of the "delicacy" or "sensitivity" of the skin? Do cuts, bruises, or minor injuries heal fast enough and without complications? Does the client feel diminished or heightened skin sensitivity to discomfort?
- What are the client's sun-exposure circumstances: outdoor work or sunbathing habits?
- Facial care: What cosmetics, soaps, or cleansing agents are used? How does the client manage pimples or minor lesions (by squeezing or picking)?
- Hair care: What shampoos, rinses, coloring, or lubricating agents are used? Have there been any recent changes in hair care patterns?
- Does the client have difficulty cutting or clipping fingernails or toenails? What instruments are used?
- Itching (sometimes unaccompanied by rash or redness) should be located. Is it generalized or more intense in certain areas? Is it intermittent? More pronounced at certain times of the day (or night)? How severe is it? Does it interfere with daily activities (especially sleep)? Does the client have problems with scratching?
- Dry skin: Is it more intense in certain areas of the body or generalized? Does the client use bath oils or powder? How would the client estimate the degree of humidity at home or at work (especially in the winter)? Is the skin dryness seasonal, intermittent, constant? Is it associated with itching?
- Additional questions for any skin problem:
  1. Is the problem seasonal?
  2. Is it associated with stress?

3. Are there occupational hazards (e.g., skin contact materials, radiation, abnormal lighting)?
4. What drugs are being taken (prescribed and over the counter), especially recent prescriptions or purchases?
5. Is the problem associated with leisure activities (e.g., weekends, hiking, swimming, yard work, hobbies involving use of special materials)?
6. How is the client adjusting to the problem (e.g., use of wig or excessive cosmetics to cover up the problem, fear of rejection, fear of infecting others)?

- Multiple cuts or bruises need to be followed by careful inquiry. The examiner should consider the possibility of abuse. Posing direct or indirect questions about the source of injury will depend on the situation, the condition of the client, the relationship between practitioner and client, and information gathered previously regarding the client and the family.
- Multiple cuts or bruises might also indicate frequent falls. The underlying cause for the falls should be considered (e.g., dizziness, alcohol or drug abuse, sensorium disturbances). *Text continues on p. 66.*

CLINICAL GUIDELINES

ASSESSMENT PROCEDURE	EVALUATION	
	NORMAL FINDINGS	DEVIATIONS FROM NORMAL

1. Gather equipment
  a. Gloves
  b. Ruler to measure small lesions; Wood's lamp to examine fluorescing lesions
  c. Flashlight with transilluminator to determine if cysts or masses contain fluid
2. Be certain there is adequate light
3. Inspect and palpate the skin for:
  a. Color
    (1) General tone (best determined in areas of body not exposed to sun)
	Deep to light brown, whitish-pink to ruddy-pink, olive, and yellow overtones	Diffuse, marked hyperpigmentation
		General pallor (loss of underlying red tones in dark skin)
		Ashen-gray appearance
		Yellow tone (jaundice)
		General redness or flush (Table 3-3)

TABLE 3-3 Differences in color changes of racial groups

COLOR CHANGE	LIGHT SKIN	DARK SKIN
Cyanosis	Blue tinge, especially in palpebral conjunctiva (lower eyelid), nail bed, earlobes, lips, oral membranes, soles, and palms	Ashen-gray lips and tongue
Pallor	Loss of rosy glow in skin, especially face	Ashen-gray appearance in black skin More yellowish-brown color in brown skin
Erythema	Redness easily seen anywhere on body	Much more difficult to assess; rely on palpation for warmth or edema
Ecchymoses	Purple to yellowish-green areas; may be seen anywhere on skin	Very difficult to see unless in mouth or conjunctiva
Petechiae	Purple pinpoints most easily seen on buttocks, abdomen, and inner surfaces of the arms or legs	Usually invisible except in oral mucosa, conjunctiva of eyelids, and conjunctiva covering eyeball
Jaundice	Yellow staining seen in sclera of eyes, skin, fingernails, soles, palms, and oral mucosa	Most reliably assessed in sclera, hard palate, palms, and soles

From Whaley LF, Wong DL: Nursing care of infants and children, *ed 3, St Louis, 1987, Mosby–Year Book.*

Continued.

CLINICAL GUIDELINES—cont'd

ASSESSMENT PROCEDURE	EVALUATION	
	NORMAL FINDINGS	DEVIATIONS FROM NORMAL
(2) Uniformity	Sun-darkened areas	Localized hyperpigmentation (especially in skinfolds, nail beds, old scars)
	Areas of lighter pigmentation in dark-skinned individuals (palms, nail beds, lips) Fig. 3-2)	Pigmentation around ankles (Fig. 3-3) Patchy or localized hypopigmentation (associated with inflammation, scaling, atrophy, scarring)
	Labile pigment areas often associated with use of birth control pills or pregnancy (cheeks, forehead, axillae, linea alba, areolae, flexor surface of wrist, genital area)	
	Crinkled skin areas appear darker (knees, elbows)	
	Calloused areas appear yellow (palms, soles)	
(3) Extremities (examine at heart level)		Marked pallor or mottling of extremities (especially when elevated) Deep, dusky-red color of dependent extremities
	Dark-skinned (Mediterranean origin) individual may have lips with blue hue	Cyanosis (dusky, blue pallor), especially lips, areas around mouth, nail beds, extremities
	Vascular flush areas (cheeks, neck, upper chest, genital area) may appear red, especially with excitement or anxiety	
	Skin color masking, incurred through use of cosmetics, tanning agents	

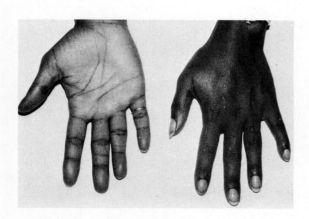

Fig. 3-2   Area of light pigmentation on black skin.

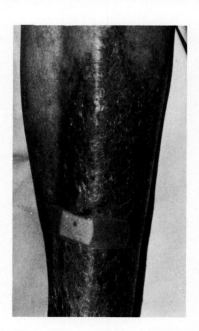

Fig. 3-3   Stasis dermatosis pigmentation.

ASSESSMENT PROCEDURE	EVALUATION	
	NORMAL FINDINGS	DEVIATIONS FROM NORMAL
b. Moisture	Dampness in skinfolds Increased perspiration associated with warm environs or activity Wet palms, scalp, forehead, axillae often associated with anxiety	Excessive dryness and flaking (Fig. 3-4) Excessive perspiration Onset of excessive oiliness May use Wood's lamp to identify fluorescing lesions; blue or green fluorescence indicates presence of fungal infection
c. Surface temperature (examiner's hand should be warm)		Excessive coolness (general or localized), especially extremities Excessive heat (general or localized)
d. Texture: stroke inner aspect of client's arms with finger pads	Smooth, even, soft	Rough, dry, coarse Velvety smooth Corns form from pressure, usually over fourth or fifth toe
e. Thickness	Wide body variation Skin of palms and soles normally much thicker than that of face or scalp; callused areas form from pressure and rubbing	Excessive thickness (generalized change in condition or localized, especially extremities)
f. Mobility and turgor: pick up skin under clavicle where there is usually no excess (Fig. 3-5)	Skin moves easily when lifted and returns to place immediately when released	Skin remains in pinched position (tenting) and returns slowly to place (Fig. 3-6)

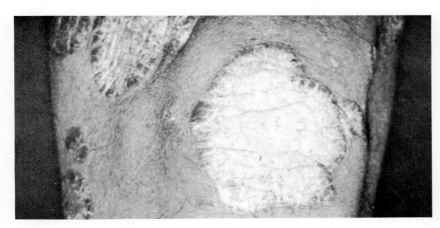

Fig. 3-4 Psoriasis of knee. (From Stewart WD, Danto JL, Maddin S: *Dermatology: diagnosis and treatment of cutaneous disorders,* ed 4, St Louis, 1978, Mosby—Year Book.)

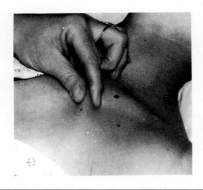

Fig. 3-5 Testing for skin turgor.

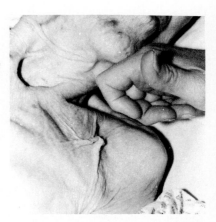

Fig. 3-6 Tenting associated with loss of skin turgor.

Continued.

CLINICAL GUIDELINES—cont'd

ASSESSMENT PROCEDURE	EVALUATION	
	NORMAL FINDINGS	DEVIATIONS FROM NORMAL
g. Hygiene	Skin clean, free of odor	Decreased mobility with edema (skin appears shiny, taut)
h. Surface alterations or lesions	Striae (stretch marks, usually silver or pink) (Fig. 3-7)	Edema present (legs, feet, fingers, eyelids)
		Crusted, dirty, marked body odor
		Macules, papules, nodules, vesicles, patches, plaque, tumors, bullae, pustules, wheals, cysts, telangiectasias (see Tables 3-1 and 3-2)
	Freckles (prominent in sun-exposed areas)	Increased vascularity
	Some birthmarks	Mixed lesions
	Some flat and raised nevi (in various shades of brown, tan, or near skin color)	
	Patchy depigmented areas (vitiligo unassociated with inflammation, scaling, or scarring) (Fig. 3-8)	
i. Trauma-induced surface alterations		Bruises, scabs, lacerations, needle marks

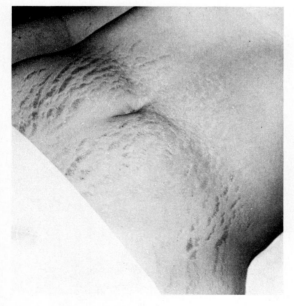

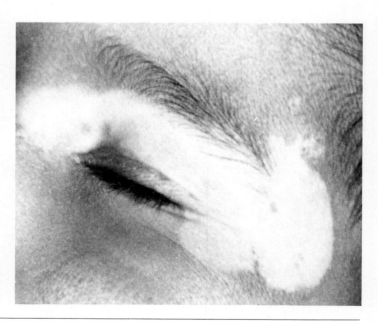

Fig. 3-7 Abdominal striae.

Fig. 3-8 Vitiligo. (From Stewart WD, Danto JL, Maddin S: *Dermatology: diagnosis and treatment of cutaneous disorders,* ed 4, St Louis, 1978, Mosby–Year Book.)

	EVALUATION	
ASSESSMENT PROCEDURE	**NORMAL FINDINGS**	**DEVIATIONS FROM NORMAL**
4. Identify and inspect all pressure-prone areas for immobilized, recumbent, or chair-bound client (Fig. 3-9) for: a. Color	Initial pallor (if there has been sustained pressure) quickly becomes red; redness (reactive hyperemia) then returns to original skin color	Prolonged blanching (ischemia) or, most often, redness (reactive hyperemia) is marked and extends over a prolonged period (area is engorged with blood)
b. Surface temperature	Localized area is same temperature as surrounding skin	Localized area is warmer than surrounding tissue
c. Surface characteristics	Skin is intact	Cell and skin damage stages: 1. Prolonged redness with unbroken skin 2. Prolonged redness (that does not blanch) with excoriation 3. Full thickness of skin is lost Serosanguineous drainage

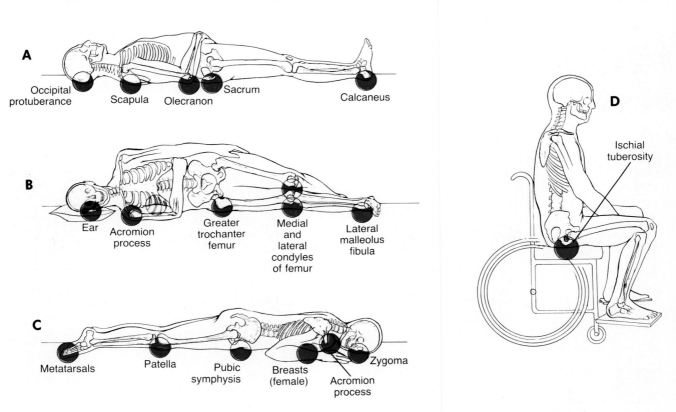

Fig. 3-9 Bony prominences vulnerable to pressure. **A,** Supine. **B,** Side lying. **C,** Prone. **D,** Sitting. (Modified from Forbes EJ, Fitzsimons VM: *The older adult: a process for wellness,* St Louis, 1981, Mosby–Year Book.)

Continued.

CLINICAL GUIDELINES—cont'd

ASSESSMENT PROCEDURE	EVALUATION	
	NORMAL FINDINGS	DEVIATIONS FROM NORMAL
		4. Invasion of deeper tissues (subcutaneous and/or muscle) Open ulcer (may be necrotic, bone may be visible) Purulent drainage (thick crust may be present)
5. Inspect and palpate the nails for: a. Configuration	Nail edges smooth and rounded Nail base angle 160 degrees Nail surface flat or slightly curved	Edges bitten, ragged Clubbing Spooning: secondary to iron deficiency anemia, syphilis, use of strong detergents; transverse depressions; nail depressions may be response to systemic diseases (e.g., syphilis, peripheral vascular disease, uncontrolled diabetes) (Figs. 3-10 and 3-11)
b. Consistency	Smooth, hard surface Uniform thickness	Excessive and/or irregular thickening, flaking
c. Color	Variations of pink Dark-skinned individual may have pigment deposits in nail beds	Yellow discoloration may indicate psoriasis or fungal infections Cyanotic Very pale Splinter hemorrhages Redness at nail bed (paronychia)
d. Adherence to nail bed	Nail base feels firm when palpated	Nail base not firm Nail base tender on palpation

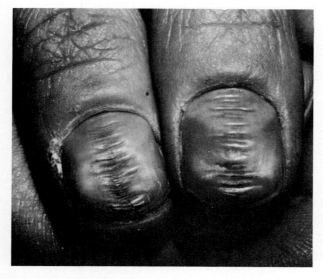

Fig. 3-10 Median nail dystrophy. (From Habif TP: *Clinical dermatology: a color guide to diagnosis and therapy,* St Louis, 1985, Mosby–Year Book.)

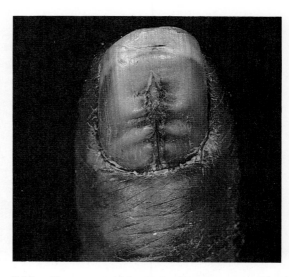

Fig. 3-11 Transverse ridging secondary to recurrent local inflammatory cutaneous disease. (From Stewart WD, Danto JL, Maddin S: *Dermatology: diagnosis and treatment of cutaneous disorders,* ed 4, St Louis, 1978, Mosby–Year Book.)

	EVALUATION	
ASSESSMENT PROCEDURE	**NORMAL FINDINGS**	**DEVIATIONS FROM NORMAL**
6. Inspect and palpate scalp and hair for:		
a. Surface characteristics	Scalp smooth	Scalp flaky; scaling, reddened, or open lesions
	Hair shiny	Hair dull
b. Distribution and configuration	"Normal" varies with individuals; hair may be present on scalp, lower face, nares, ears, axillae, anterior chest around nipples, arms, legs, back of hands and feet, back, and buttocks	Sudden or marked increase or decrease in body hair
	Female pubic configuration forms inverted triangle (Fig. 3-12) (hairline may extend up linea alba)	Alteration of pubic configuration appropriate to male or female
	Male configuration is upright triangle with hair extending up linea alba to umbilicus (Fig. 3-13)	
c. Texture	Scalp hair may be fine or coarse	Increased coarseness of body hair
	Fine hair over body	Dryness, brittleness, or coarseness of scalp hair
	Coarse hair in pubic and axillary areas	
d. Color	Wide variation from pale blond to black	
	Color may be masked or changed with rinses, dyes	
7. Inspect hair for:		
a. Quantity	"Normal" varies according to individuals	Excess body hair (hirsutism)
	Gradual symmetrical balding of scalp hair in some men	Female: hair growth intensified on upper lip, chin, cheeks, chest, and from pubic crest to umbilicus
		Excessive loss of body hair
		Scalp hair: asymmetrical or patchy balding (alopecia)
		Marked hair loss
b. Parasites		Body lice (especially in pubic and axillary areas)
		Head lice and nits in scalp

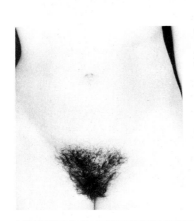

Fig. 3-12 Normal triangular configuration of female pubic hair.

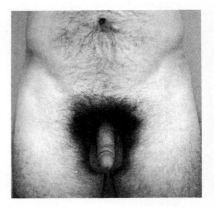

Fig. 3-13 Normal configuration of male pubic hair.

CLINICAL TIPS AND STRATEGIES

- **The entire skin surface should be inspected:** The client should be completely undressed for skin examination because of the following:
  1. Clients may be unaware of alterations in areas that are inaccessible to them (e.g., the back, under skinfolds).
  2. Older adults, persons with diabetes, and others sometimes have decreased sensitivity to pain (especially in extremities), and infected or ulcerated lesions can be missed when direct inspection is neglected.

- **Skinfolds are usually warm and moist and may harbor bacteria, parasites (e.g., scabies) and fungi:** Axillae, groins, and areas under pendulous breasts are sites often overlooked. Also, obese people have more skinfolds.

- **The bottoms of the feet and the areas between the toes should be inspected:** Even undressed clients may wish to keep their shoes and socks or stockings on, but they should be removed.
  1. Circulatory inadequacy, which occurs with many systemic disorders, may result in infections or lesions that are often painless and dangerous.
  2. Feet endure weight-bearing, pressure, and friction from ill-fitted shoes every day. The contour and alterations of normal shape should be explored through examination and inquiry about comfort.

- **Long, jagged, thick toenails should be considered a problem:** Sometimes elderly, obese, or disabled people cannot reach their feet to provide self-care. Very thick toenails may require (1) a special instrument to cut and/or (2) regular inspection and trimming by another person. Long toenails interfere with shoe fit.

- **Long, jagged, dirty fingernails also should be considered a problem:** It may mean that the client cannot provide self care. Dirty, jagged fingernails can be the cause of infections elsewhere on the body if the individual scratches.

- **Lesions or surface alterations should be described:** The following categories should be used:
  1. Distribution and location (e.g., confined to face, trunk, extremities, sun-exposed areas, or general distribution with no pattern; placement on symmetrical body parts)
  2. Surface and color characteristics (e.g., confluent, macular)
  3. Lesion dimension: use metric system; do not compare tumors or nodules with fruits or vegetables
  4. Color and condition of surrounding tissue

- **Beginning examiners often have a difficult time describing findings in a concise, accurate manner:** The vocabulary section at the beginning of this chapter is very useful. Many of the words are adjectives that briefly convey an explicit lesion pattern or arrangement. For example, "confluent vesicles" is an efficient way to state that small, fluid-filled lesions all run together. The examiner should become familiar with these terms.

- **Wearing gloves is appropriate when examining any lesion:** Washing hands is a necessity after any inspection.

 The Newborn

HISTORY AND CLINICAL STRATEGIES

Skin color should be observed when infants are resting, as well as when they are crying. Skin and hair characteristics provide gestational age data. The examiner should assess a newborn's skin as described below:

- Newborns can be undressed easily for a comprehensive integumentary examination. The practitioner must carefully examine all the folds, crevices, and wrinkles of the infant's skin, observing skin characteristics, irritations, or rashes. The infant must not be allowed to chill.

- The examiner should note integumentary characteristics present at birth that are considered deviations within normal limits, including mongolian spots, hemangiomas, café au lait spots, and lanugo.

- The examiner should note integumentary characteristics present at birth or shortly thereafter that may indicate disease, including jaundice appearing within 24 hours of birth, cyanosis in the nonchilled infant, tufts of hair over the spine or sacrum, and dermatoglyphics of the palm.

> ### SAMPLE RECORDING: NORMAL FINDINGS
>
> **Skin:** Pink, moist, soft, warm, and elastic. No lesions, discolorations, excess thickening, trauma, odor, or edema.
> **Nails:** Pink, smooth, and hard. No clubbing, biting, or thickening or tenderness on palpation.
> **Body hair:** Moderate, uniform distribution. Male pubic configuration.
> **Scalp and hair:** Moderately thick, evenly distributed brown hair. Scalp clean. No flaking, lesions, or tenderness.

CLINICAL VARIATIONS: THE NEWBORN

CHARACTERISTIC OR AREA EXAMINED	NORMAL FINDINGS	DEVIATIONS FROM NORMAL
1. Birth covering	Vernix caseosa: waxy, greasy, whitish-yellow material, especially in body creases Temperature decreased after birth (should not fall below 97° F)	Diminished vernix in postterm infants Contour distortions (may be masses, tumors, nodules)
2. Skin	Smooth, soft, opaque, thin; red when crying Eccrine and apocrine glands are nonfunctional Some desquamation on feet, hands, groin Urticaria neonatorum; erythema toxicum: transitory skin lesions; 1 to 2 mm, whitish-yellow papules, pustules, or splotchy macules Milia: sebaceous gland white cysts, 1 mm, on nose, chin, cheeks, forehead Slight swelling of extremities, eyelids, buttocks (after breech delivery)	Transparent, visible in preterm infants; cracked, leathery, desquamated, dry in postterm infants Perspiration (seen with drug withdrawal, overheating) Few or absent heel creases in preterm infants; many creases over entire plantar area in postterm infants Pinpoint hemorrhages (petechiae) (may be from delivery trauma or other pathology) Ecchymoses (may be from breech or traumatic delivery) Edema (may be from systemic problem, e.g., infant respiratory distress syndrome, hydrops fetalis, congestive heart failure)
3. Color	Pink, flushes, mottles, pales quickly Transitory blue hand, feet color (acrocyanosis) Cut-glass mottling; disappears when warmed Slight jaundice in 2 to 3 days (physiological jaundice) Half body from head to feet darker than other side (harlequin color; rare, nonpathological temporary autonomic imbalance) Dark-skinned infants: melanotic pigmentation Red, flat areas (superficial teleangiectasia); on nape of neck (storkbite); on upper lip, eyelids (flame nevi)	Beefy red, ruddy, plethoric (may be from polycythemia) Pallor (may be from anemia, blood loss) Ashen-gray cyanosis (may be from sepsis or cardiac or respiratory problems) Jaundice within first day (nonphysiological hyperbilirubinemia) Persistent mottling
4. Hair	Fine, downy hair (lanugo)	Little or no lanugo on very preterm infant; abundant on preterm infant; mostly bald on postterm infant
5. Nails	Extend beyond nail bed	Absent or deformed nails; may be fetal alcohol syndrome, anticonvulsant syndromes, or systemic diseases (e.g., renal or bone anomalies)

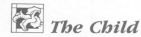 *The Child*

HISTORY AND CLINICAL STRATEGIES

- Integumentary characteristics change as the child develops, including appearance of pubic and axillary hair and acne.
- Integumentary characteristics occur as either primary or secondary lesions caused by local irritations, communicable diseases, or infectious processes, including the following*:
  1. Primary lesions
     a. *Poor skin turgor,* resulting from dehydration
     b. *Macules,* seen in scarlet fever, rubeola, and roseola infantum
     c. *Papules,* seen in ringworm, pityriasis rosea, psoriasis, or eczema
     d. *Vesicles* (or blisters), seen in poison ivy, chickenpox (varicella), and herpes zoster (shingles)
     e. *Bullae,* seen in burns or on palms and soles of children with scarlet fever
     f. *Pustules,* seen in impetigo, acne, and staphylococcal infections
     g. *Wheals,* usually associated with pruritus and seen in insect bites, hives, and urticaria
     h. *Petechiae,* usually associated with systemic disease, such as meningococcemia, bacterial endocarditis, or nonthrombocytopenic purpura; needs immediate referral
  2. Secondary lesions, which are alterations in the skin caused by another problem, such as trauma, unclean surface area, or continuous irritation
     a. *Scales,* seen in very dry skin or cradle cap
     b. *Crusts* (dried blood, scales, pus), from infected dermatitis, such as impetigo
     c. *Excoriation,* seen in scrapes after falling
     d. *Erosions* or *ulcers,* seen in infected, sloughing tissue or pressure sores
     e. *Scars,* seen in healing tissue
     f. *Lichenification,* seen over body areas where child chronically rubs or scratches

*Modified from Alexander MM, Brown MS: *Pediatric history taking and physical diagnosis for nurses,* ed 2, New York, 1979, McGraw-Hill.

- The integumentary history of the pediatric client should include all the components of the adult history. In addition, the examiner should inquire about the following situations:
  1. Specific exposure to communicable diseases
  2. Specific exposure to other children with environmentally caused skin problems, such as poison ivy or scabies
  3. If integumentary signs were present at birth or shortly thereafter, how these signs have changed or progressed since birth or the last visit
  4. If signs such as cyanosis, pallor, or jaundice are found, an expanded, detailed history
  5. Care and cleansing routines for children with such conditions as a diaper rash, dry skin, or acne
  6. Environmental contacts for children with rashes; dry, patchy skin; or areas of irritation
  7. A detailed history of young children with rashes or skin irritations regarding skin care routines, soap or lotions used, new foods eaten, new detergents or fabrics exposed to, as well as parental treatment techniques
- The pediatric client must be completely undressed for the integumentary system examination to be adequately evaluated. The age and shyness of the child will determine examination techniques.
  1. *Babies and toddlers* usually enjoy being undressed, which makes the integumentary examination easy. Special attention should be given to the fat creases, the diaper area, and the scalp.
  2. Because of the acquired modesty of *preschoolers* and *school-age children,* the integumentary examination is more difficult. It may be necessary for the examiner to integrate this examination with other components of the physical assessment, for example, to provide integumentary assessment of the abdominal area while evaluating the abdomen. The hazard of this approach is that subtle skin problems or changes may be missed. At the completion of the examination the examiner must feel confident that total integumentary evaluation has been achieved. Again, this includes all folds and crevices.
  3. Modesty is perhaps the biggest concern of *older school-age children* and *adolescents.* Examination criteria are the same as for the adult client. Special attention should be paid to acne, complexion, and rashes that can develop around the genital area.

- As the examiner evaluates the skin, signs of child abuse or neglect must not go unnoticed. Examples of problems include multiple bruises above the knees and elbows, multiple bruises at different stages of healing, or bruises reflecting belt or electrical cord marks; cigarette burns or burns with even lines of demarcation that could indicate submersion; or any injury that does not coincide with the history. For example, the parent states that her 18-month-old child fell into hot bathtub water, but the clinical observation shows a submersion burn up to the waist with an even line of termination. There is no evidence of splash burns of the hands, face, or chest. A more subtle observation of child neglect involves the parents' nontreatment of obvious integumentary problems, for example, a diaper rash that has been allowed to progress to the point of blistering, infection, and bleeding. These situations require in-depth investigation and referral.
- If a rash is identified, it is important for the examiner to determine the body surface involved, the rash migration and evolutionary pattern, and home care tried. *Text continues on p. 77.*

CLINICAL VARIATIONS: THE CHILD

CHARACTERISTIC OR AREA EXAMINED	NORMAL FINDINGS	DEVIATIONS FROM NORMAL
1. Skin color	Older children: same as adult Similar color tones	Cyanosis (suggests low oxygenation) Pallor (may be from anemia) Plethora (may be polycythemia) Increased cyanosis of lower extremities (may indicate aortic or congenital heart defect)
2. Moisture	Perspiration present in all children over 1 month of age	Perspiration in infant less than 1 month of age Excessive sweating, as seen in children with fever, hypoglycemia, hyperthyroidism, or heart disease
3. Texture	Smooth, soft, flexible Dryness and flakiness of skin in infants less than 1 month of age (shedding of vernix caseosa); may appear as white, cheesy skin Presence of *milia*: small, white papules over nose and cheeks, which are plugged sebaceous glands that may remain for 2 months	Dryness or flakiness in children over 1 month Dryness or scaling between fingers or toes (may be from ringworm) Scaling over knees, elbows, or behind ears (may be from eczema) Scaliness of palms and soles (seen with scarlet fever) Dermatoglyphics: straight, single folds seen across the upper palm of hands at base of fingers in children with Down syndrome Dryness or chafing of diaper area
4. Thickness	Varying degrees of adipose tissue, dimpling of skin over joint areas	Skin dimpling at areas other than over joints

Continued.

CLINICAL VARIATIONS: THE CHILD—cont'd

CHARACTERISTIC OR AREA EXAMINED	NORMAL FINDINGS	DEVIATIONS FROM NORMAL

5. Mobility and turgor
  a. Pinch large area of skin over lower abdomen
  b. Palpate the calf
	Skin rises with pinch but falls quickly when released
	
	Full, taut skin
		Skin remains in pinched position (Fig. 3-14)
		Loose and "extra" skin
		Edema

6. Hygiene	Skin free from odor, clean	Dirty, crusted, or excoriated areas: skinfolds, diaper area, behind ears, neck region; dirty appearance

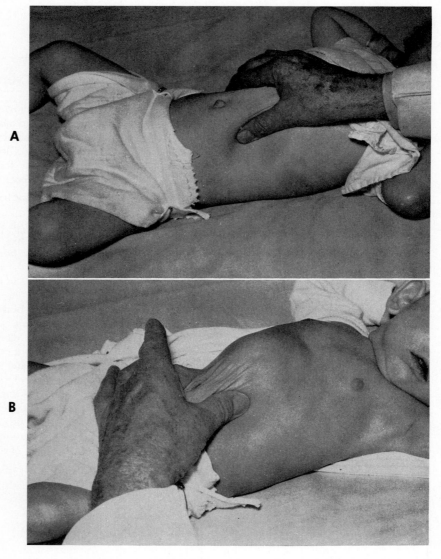

Fig. 3-14 **A,** Good tissue turgor. **B,** Poor tissue turgor. (From Prior JA, Silbertstein JS, Stang JM: *Physical diagnosis: the history and examination of the patient,* ed 6, St Louis, 1981, Mosby—Year Book.)

CHARACTERISTIC OR AREA EXAMINED	NORMAL FINDINGS	DEVIATIONS FROM NORMAL

7. Skin surface
  a. Alterations in pigmentation
	Mongolian spots*: irregularly shaped, darkened flat areas over sacral area and buttocks; usually seen in black or darkly pigmented children; may be gone by first or second year
	Note size and location
	Café au lait spots*: light, cream-colored spots found on darkened backgrounds
	Note size and location
	Hemangiomas*: increase in pigmentation with crying
	  1. *Flat capillary*
	    a. Storkbites: small red or pink spots often seen on back of neck, upper lip, or upper eyelid (Fig. 3-15); usually disappear by age 5
		Vitiligo: absence of pigmentation in areas
		
		Multiple areas of spots

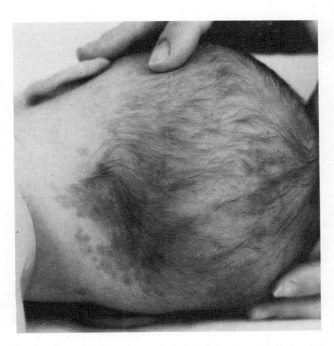

Fig. 3-15 Storkbite. (From Bobak IM, Jensen MD, Zalar MK: *Maternity and gynecologic care: the nurse and the family,* ed 4, St Louis, 1989, Mosby–Year Book. Courtesy Mead Johnson & Co.)

*These lesions are commonly seen in the pediatric client. Many practitioners consider them a "normal" deviation. Beginners in assessment should consider all pigment alterations as problems until experience enables them to recognize common deviations within normal limits.

Continued.

CLINICAL VARIATIONS: THE CHILD—cont'd

CHARACTERISTIC OR AREA EXAMINED	NORMAL FINDINGS	DEVIATIONS FROM NORMAL
	b. Port-wine stain: large, flat, bluish-purple capillary area; most frequently found on face along distribution of fifth cranial nerve (Fig. 3-16); usually does not disappear spontaneously; not accompanied by nervous system complications 2. *Raised capillary:* strawberry mark, slightly raised, reddened area with sharp demarcation line; may be 2 to 3 cm in diameter; appears at birth or within first few months and usually gone by age 5 (Fig. 3-17) Note size and location	Port-wine stains, accompanied by nervous system complications

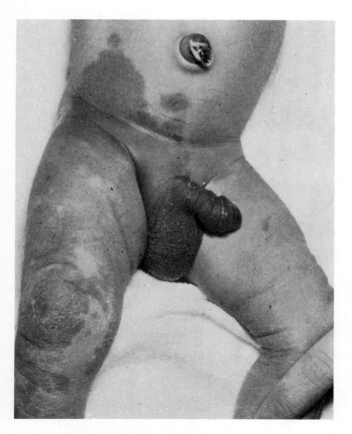

Fig. 3-16   Port-wine stain. (From Bobak IM, Jensen MD, Zalar MK: *Maternity and gynecologic care: the nurse and the family,* ed 4, St Louis, 1989, Mosby—Year Book. Courtesy Mead Johnson & Co.)

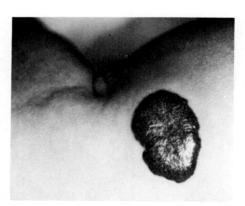

Fig. 3-17   Strawberry mark. (From Shirkey HC: *Pediatric therapy,* ed 6, St Louis, 1980, Mosby—Year Book.)

CHARACTERISTIC OR AREA EXAMINED	NORMAL FINDINGS	DEVIATIONS FROM NORMAL
	3. *Cavernous hemangioma:* reddish-blue, round masses of blood vessels; may continue to grow until child is 10 to 15 months old Note size and location Child should be reevaluated frequently	Some may require surgical removal
	4. *Nevus* (mole): may vary in size and number; brown in pigmentation Note size, location, and number Large nevi or those in irritating areas must be frequently evaluated for change	Large, hairy nevi Bathing trunk nevi
b. Common lesions	*Ecchymoses,* bruises: commonly seen below knees and elbows	*Ecchymoses,* bruises, seen elsewhere on the body, or multiple bruises seen at different stages of healing *Macules,* as seen in measles, German measles, or drug rash (Fig. 3-18) *Papules,* as seen in tinea (ringworm) or psoriasis (Fig. 3-19)

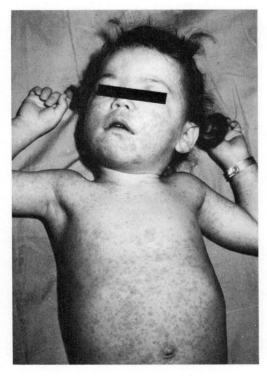

Fig. 3-18   Macule rash of measles. (From Krugman S, Katz SL: *Infectious diseases of children,* ed 7, St Louis, 1981, Mosby–Year Book.)

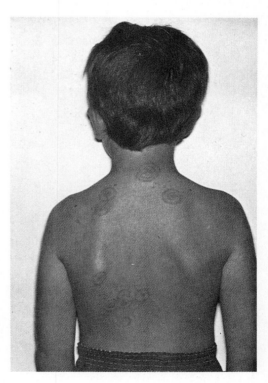

Fig. 3-19   Papules as seen in ringworm. (From Verbov J, Morley N: *Color atlas of pediatric dermatology,* Philadelphia, 1983, JB Lippincott.)

Continued.

CLINICAL VARIATIONS: THE CHILD—cont'd

CHARACTERISTIC OR AREA EXAMINED	NORMAL FINDINGS	DEVIATIONS FROM NORMAL
		Vesicles (blebs), as seen in chicken pox, herpes simplex, herpes zoster, or poison ivy (Fig. 3-20)
		Pustules, as seen in impetigo or scabies (Fig. 3-21)
		Xanthomas: small yellow plaques seen across nose of newborn
		Miliaria (prickly heat): tiny red irritation (Fig. 3-22)

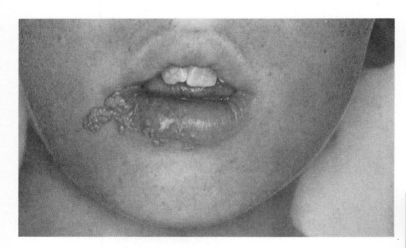

Fig. 3-20 Vesicles as seen in herpes simplex. (From Verbov J, Morley N: *Color atlas of pediatric dermatology,* Philadelphia, 1983, JB Lippincott.)

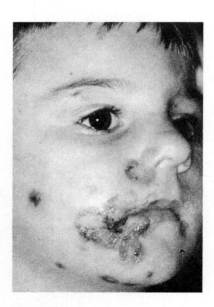

Fig. 3-21 Pustules as seen in impetigo. (From Verbov J, Morley N: *Color atlas of pediatric dermatology,* Philadelphia, 1983, JB Lippincott.)

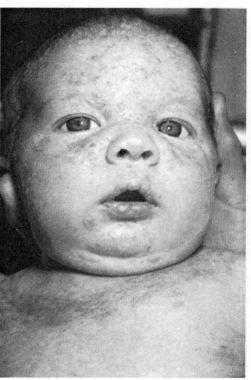

Fig. 3-22 Miliaria prickly heat rash. (From Verbov J, Morley N: *Color atlas of pediatric dermatology,* Philadelphia, 1983, JB Lippincott.)

CHARACTERISTIC OR AREA EXAMINED	NORMAL FINDINGS	DEVIATIONS FROM NORMAL
		Hives (wheals or urticaria), as seen in allergic reactions (Fig. 3-23) *Petechial rash,* or macular type of rash that does not blanch with palpation or pressure (may indicate meningococcemia, a medical emergency) *Acne,* resulting in blackheads, papules, pustules, and cysts (Fig. 3-24)

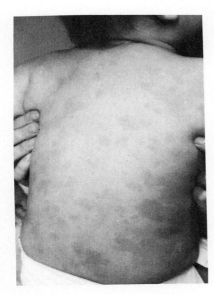

Fig. 3-23 Urticaria. (From Verbov J, Morley N: *Color atlas of pediatric dermatology,* Philadelphia, 1983, JB Lippincott.)

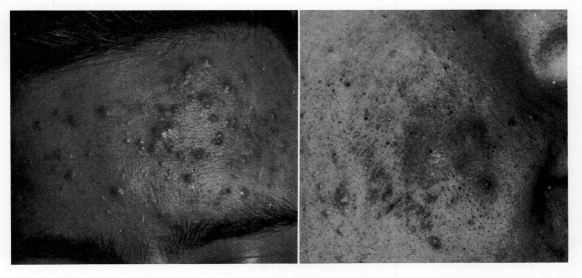

Fig. 3-24 Acne vulgaris. (From Stewart WD, Danto JL, Maddin S: *Dermatology: diagnosis and treatment of cutaneous disorders,* ed 4, St Louis, 1978, Mosby–Year Book.)

Continued.

CLINICAL VARIATIONS: THE CHILD—cont'd

CHARACTERISTIC OR AREA EXAMINED	NORMAL FINDINGS	DEVIATIONS FROM NORMAL
8. Nails		
a. Configuration	Generally longer than wider	Nail beds wider than longer; may be seen in children with Down syndrome or other congenital malformations
b. Consistency	Soft nails in infants and small children; become hardened with age	Pitting of nails, as seen with fungal diseases
c. Color	Same as adult	
d. Adherence to nail bed	Same as adult	Paronychia: commonly seen infection around nail bed (Fig. 3-25)
9. Scalp and hair		
a. Scalp	Smooth, soft	Scaliness of scalp with crusting, seborrheic dermatitis (cradle cap) (Fig. 3-26) Ringworm or eczema of scalp

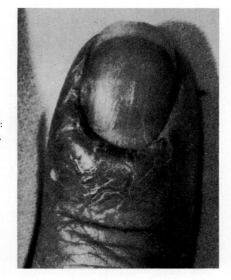

Fig. 3-25 Paronychia. (From Stewart WD, Danto JL, Maddin S: *Dermatology: diagnosis and treatment of cutaneous disorders,* ed 4, St Louis, 1978, Mosby—Year Book.)

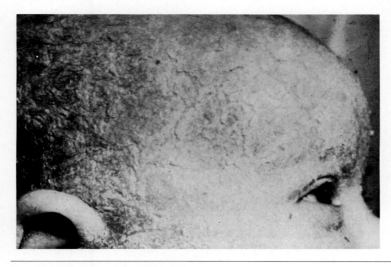

Fig. 3-26 Seborrheic dermatitis (cradle cap). (From Shirkey H: *Pediatric therapy,* ed 6, St Louis, 1979, Mosby—Year Book.)

CHARACTERISTIC OR AREA EXAMINED	NORMAL FINDINGS	DEVIATIONS FROM NORMAL
b. Scalp hair	Shiny, soft, fine texture; as child grows, hair takes on adult characteristics Irregularity in pigmentation	Brittle hair may be seen in children with hypothyroidism, ringworm of scalp, or other conditions Presence of nits
c. Distribution and configuration of body hair	Lanugo over body, mostly over shoulders and back; disappears during first 3 months of life Pubic hair develops between 8 and 12 years; smooth hair at first, changing to coarse, curly hair; followed approximately 6 months later by axillary hair; followed approximately 6 months later by facial hair in boys	Hairy trunk may be seen in children with Cushing syndrome Tufts of hair seen anywhere over spine, especially over sacrum (may mark spot of spina bifida) Absence of secondary hair characteristics

The Childbearing Woman

HISTORY AND CLINICAL STRATEGIES

- Incorporate observation of the integumentary system throughout the physical examination. Comfort of the pregnant woman should be encouraged. Aching and a heavy feeling may occur in pregnant women when they remain in the same position too long, which can lead to varicosities. Follow these guidelines for observing the skin:
  1. Have adequate lighting with sunlight or an overhead, diffuse light.
  2. Use drapes as appropriate and as preferred by individual clients; allow adequate exposure to examine the skin.
  3. Place the client in a semiupright position, especially during the last trimester.
- Drug addictions occur in all socioeconomic groups. Look for marks near possible injection sites that could indicate drug use. Nasal areas may be irritated if the client ingests drugs through the nose.

CLINICAL VARIATIONS: THE CHILDBEARING WOMAN

CHARACTERISTIC OR AREA EXAMINED	NORMAL FINDINGS	DEVIATIONS FROM NORMAL
1. Skin	Temperature may increase slightly early in pregnancy Striae gravidarum: pinkish- to silvery-white stretch lines (from distended connective tissue, especially on breasts and abdomen) Linea nigra: pigmented dark line from umbilicus to mons pubis External genitalia darken Chloasma, melasma: mask-type spots on face Complexion becomes sallow and later turns florid Pruritus (from bile salt buildup resulting from increased estrogen level)	Pallor: general skin color (may be caused by anemia)

Continued.

CLINICAL VARIATIONS: THE CHILDBEARING WOMAN—cont'd

CHARACTERISTIC OR AREA EXAMINED	NORMAL FINDINGS	DEVIATIONS FROM NORMAL
2. Vascularity	Vascular spiders: small red spots, especially on thighs	
	Varicosities may develop over legs, thighs	Deep venous thrombosis—edema above knee, skin feels hot, redness
	No change in old scars; new scars have dark pigment	Unusual color, warmth, excoriation (may be fibrosis, cellulitis, ulcerations)
	Molluscum fibrosum gravidarum: pinhead skin tags, usually disappear after delivery	
3. Nails and hair	Increased function of sweat and sebaceous glands and hair follicles	
	Nails thin during pregnancy	Spoon-shaped nails (may be from iron deficiency)
	Increased hair growth about third month; more fine, lanugo-type hair on chest and face	
	Hair texture coarser	
4. After delivery	Temperature increase and chilling may occur (caused by exertion, dehydration, hormonal and intraabdominal shifts); striae fade, turn silvery	Fever over 100.4° F (38° C) (suggests infection)
	Linea nigra fades, but light line may remain	
	Chloasma often disappears	
	Vascular spiders fade, but may remain visible	
	Hair loss may occur 2 to 4 months after delivery (from decreased thyroid function); hair will regrow	

 The Older Adult

HISTORY AND CLINICAL STRATEGIES

- Differentiating normal from abnormal skin changes may be difficult when assessing elderly clients. A novice examiner should consult regularly with an experienced clinician.
- "Normal" lesions must be considered a problem if they are causing distress (e.g., cosmetic concern, clothing rubbing, or irritating lesion).
- Elderly clients sometimes exhibit a more intense response to skin irritations. The client may feel more pain or more severe itching. Lesions or dermatitis may respond more slowly to treatment.
- Elderly clients may manifest a *reduced* pain response to lesions (especially in extremities); they may be unable to feel pain, or they may accept chronic discomfort as part of aging and fail to report it.
- If a client complains of itching and scratching (a fairly common complaint among elderly clients), assess the fingernails. Dirty, jagged fingernails often contribute to the problem.

- The integumentary system reflects an individual's relationship to the outer as well as the inner environment. Some of the variables affecting the skin, hair, and nails follow:
  1. External environment
     a. Cold weather conditions: increased sensitivity to cold.
     b. Humidity and moisture: low humidity (especially in winter) will irritate dry skin; individuals who habitually soak in warm water (to relieve arthritic pain) may develop dry skin.
     c. Sun: chronic exposure (especially with light-skinned individuals) results in a higher incidence of precancerous and cancerous growths. Sun sensitivity may develop; certain drugs and chemicals contribute to phototoxic reactions: sulfonamides, thiazide diuretics, antibacterial soaps.
     d. Skin irritants: soaps, detergents, lotions with high alcohol content, disinfectants, and woolen clothing may aggravate dry skin.

e. Allergic reactions (occur fairly often): jewelry, dark blue or black dyes in clothing or shoes, chemicals in crease-resistant clothing, and linens or clothing containing residual soap or detergent are some of the more common causative factors.

f. Decreased activity (pressure friction): will stress the system.

g. Hazards: clients who exhibit multiple bruises or excoriations should be assessed for safety hazards and related falls (Chapter 1, pp. 31 and 32).

h. Abuse or neglect: bruises (in various stages of healing), burns, cuts, scratches, rope burns, gag marks, choke marks, and welts are common indicators of possible abuse or neglect.

2. Internal environment
   a. Medications (often numerous with the elderly) may create problems (rash, itching).
   b. Systemic/chronic disease (itching).
   c. Nutritional deficiencies (e.g., vitamin A deficiency may result in rough, dry skin).
   d. Decreased circulation lowers skin resistance to infection.

CLINICAL VARIATIONS: THE OLDER ADULT

CHARACTERISTIC OR AREA EXAMINED	NORMAL FINDINGS	DEVIATIONS FROM NORMAL
1. Skin color a. General tone b. Uniformity	Caucasian skin appears white More freckles, uneven tanning, or pigment deposits in sun-exposed areas (more evident on fair skin) (Fig. 3-27) Hypopigmented patches	Pallor associated with anemia Hypersensitivity to sun (marked reddening, eczematous changes)

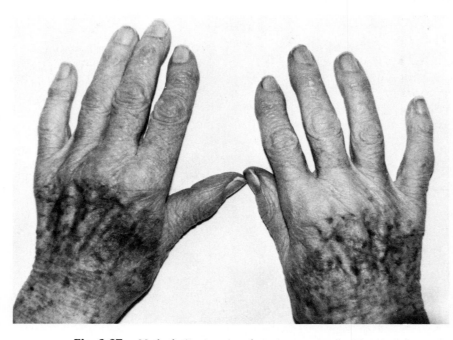

Fig. 3-27 Marked pigmentation deposits associated with aging.

Continued.

CLINICAL VARIATIONS: THE OLDER ADULT—cont'd

CHARACTERISTIC OR AREA EXAMINED	NORMAL FINDINGS	DEVIATIONS FROM NORMAL
2. Moisture	Increased dryness (especially extremities) Decreased perspiration	Marked flaking
3. Texture	Flaking, scaling (associated with dry skin, especially over lower extremities	Scaling associated with dryness, itching, and scratching (erythema, excoriation may be present)
4. Thickness	Thinner skin (especially over dorsal surface of hands and feet, forearms, lower legs, bony prominences, such as scapula, trochanter, knees) Other skin areas may be thicker (abdomen, torso)	 Torso obesity distribution associated with disease
5. Mobility and turgor	General loss of elasticity; appears lax Increased wrinkle pattern (more marked in sun-exposed areas, in fair skin, in expressive areas of face) (Fig. 3-28)	 Marked wrinkling or sagging associated with weight loss (Fig. 3-29) Perlèche: deep wrinkling, fissures, or maceration at corners of mouth; monilial infection often develops in this moist area (associated with overclosure of mouth because of ill-fitting dentures or edentulous state) (Fig. 3-30)
	Pendulous parts sag or droop (skin under chin, earlobes, breasts, scrotum)	Pendulous scrotal tissue may become excoriated or damaged because of client sliding or sitting on it

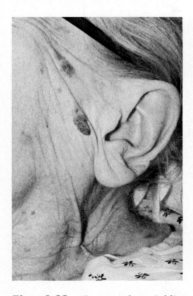

Fig. 3-28 Increased wrinkling and skinfolds associated with aging.

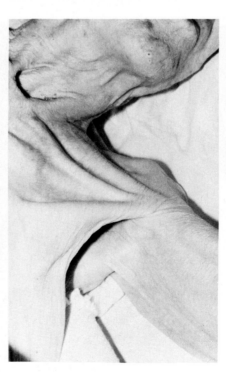

Fig. 3-29 Marked weight loss. Note bony prominences and sagging skinfolds.

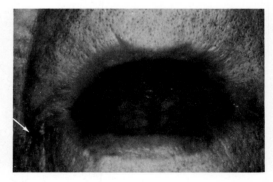

Fig. 3-30 Perlèche. (Courtesy Dr. George Blozis, The Ohio State University College of Dentistry.)

CHARACTERISTIC OR AREA EXAMINED	NORMAL FINDINGS	DEVIATIONS FROM NORMAL
6. Hygiene		Hard-to-reach areas may be less clean (e.g., feet, axillary area, buttocks, or inguinal skinfolds)
7. Skin surface a. Alterations or lesions	Nevi (common moles) often become lighter in color or disappear	Evaluated in the same manner as with adult client
(1) Seborrheic keratosis*		*Seborrheic dermatitis†*
(a) Location	Temples, neck, back, under pendulous breasts	Face, scalp, upper chest (oil-rich areas of body)
(b) Size	2 to 3 cm in diameter	Wide variation
(c) Color	Light tan to black	Red or yellow scaling
(d) Surface characteristics	Appears "stuck on"; lobulated or warty, scaly, thickened	Demarcated scaling, redness, and itching; may erupt into reddish-brown papules with yellow scaling
(e) Distribution	Often multiple (Fig. 3-31)	Singular or multiple (often associated with illness, confinement, and inability to maintain good hygiene) (Fig. 3-32)

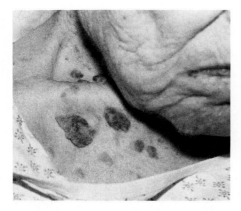

Fig. 3-31 Seborrheic keratosis.

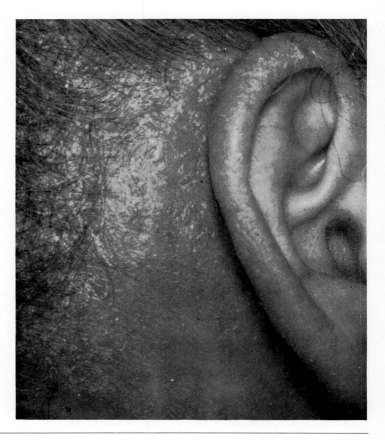

Fig. 3-32 Seborrheic dermatitis of postauricular area. (From Stewart WD, Danto JL, Maddin S: *Dermatology: diagnosis and treatment of cutaneous disorders,* ed 4, St Louis, 1978, Mosby—Year Book.)

*These lesions commonly occur in elderly adults. They are described by some authors as "normal," in that the chief concern for the client is cosmetic. Beginners in assessment should consider all lesions as problems until experience enables them to recognize common deviations within normal limits.

†These lesions are fairly common in elderly adults. They are all considered "abnormal" and should be treated.

Continued.

CLINICAL VARIATIONS: THE OLDER ADULT—cont'd

CHARACTERISTIC OR AREA EXAMINED	NORMAL FINDINGS	DEVIATIONS FROM NORMAL
(2) Skin tags (acrochordons)*		*Herpes zoster†*
(a) Location	Side of neck, face, axillary folds	Can be anywhere on body: thorax, abdomen (most common), forehead and temple, neck and shoulders
(b) Size	1 mm to 1 cm	Under 1 cm (multiple vesicles)
(c) Color	Pinkish-tan to light brown	Red
(d) Surface characteristics	Soft, pedunculated	Multiple, confluent vesicles preceded by pain and burning and followed by weeping, crusting, and healing; postzoster neuralgia (severe pain) may persist for week or months
(e) Distribution	Often multiple, may be singular (Fig. 3-33)	Over a segmented sensory nerve area (Fig. 3-34)
(3) Senile angiomas*		*Dry skin dermatitis†*
(a) Location	Trunk, proximal extremities, scrotum	Lower legs (most common), arms, hands, trunk
(b) Size	1 to 5 mm diameter	Wide variation
(c) Color	Purple or red	White flakes, redness with inflammation
(d) Surface characteristics	Smooth, soft, dome-shaped May bleed if traumatized	Flaking, redness, fissures, itching
(e) Distribution	Singular or multiple	Multiple

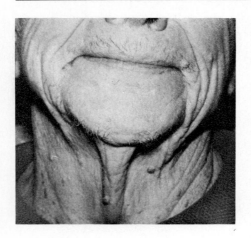

Fig. 3-33   Skin tags in the neck and bristly facial hair.

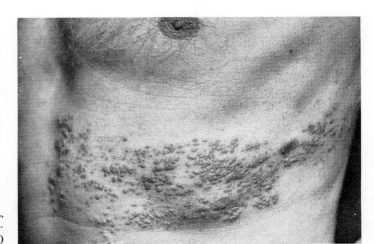

Fig. 3-34   Herpes zoster. (From Stewart WD, Danto JL, Maddin S: *Dermatology: diagnosis and treatment of cutaneous disorders,* ed 4, St Louis, 1978, Mosby–Year Book.)

---

*These lesions commonly occur in elderly adults. They are described by some authors as "normal," in that the chief concern for the client is cosmetic. Beginners in assessment should consider all lesions as problems until experience enables them to recognize common deviations within normal limits.

†These lesions are fairly common in elderly adults. They are all considered "abnormal" and should be treated.

CHARACTERISTIC OR AREA EXAMINED	NORMAL FINDINGS	DEVIATIONS FROM NORMAL
(4) Sebaceous hyperplasia* (more common in males)		*Actinic keratosis†*
(a) Location	Forehead, nose, cheeks	Dorsum of hands, forehead, ears, face, neck
(b) Size	2 to 3 mm diameter	Varies
(c) Color	Yellow	White scales, mild erythema
(d) Surface characteristics	Papular, flat, may be umbilicated or lobular	Small, macular with scales and varying degree of mild erythema (premalignant, slow growing)
(e) Distribution	Singular or multiple (Fig. 3-35)	May be singular or may erupt in multiple spots over sun-exposed areas *Basal cell carcinoma†* Location: lower lip, face (especially on eyelid, nose, earlobe); can occur anywhere Size: small; varies, but usually 0.5 to 1 cm Color: varies Surface: varies; usually begins as small, pearly-translucent papule that breaks down into an ulcer with bleeding and crusting; border of crater is elevated and pearly in appearance; painless

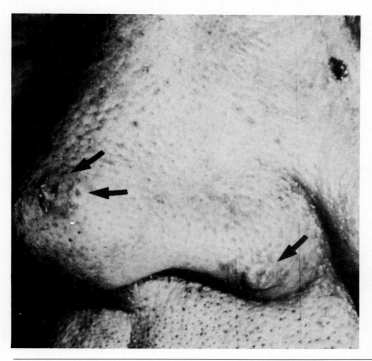

Fig. 3-35 Sebaceous hyperplasia. (From Steinberg FU, editor: *Care of the geriatric patient,* ed 6, St Louis, 1983, Mosby–Year Book.)

*These lesions commonly occur in elderly adults. They are described by some authors as "normal," in that the chief concern for the client is cosmetic. Beginners in assessment should consider all lesions as problems until experience enables them to recognize common deviations within normal limits.

†These lesions are fairly common in elderly adults. They are all considered "abnormal" and should be treated.   *Continued.*

CLINICAL VARIATIONS: THE OLDER ADULT—cont'd

CHARACTERISTIC OR AREA EXAMINED	NORMAL FINDINGS	DEVIATIONS FROM NORMAL
		Distribution: Usually singular (see Fig. 5-34)
		*Squamous cell carcinoma**
		Location: most often on lip, cheek, ear, temple, neck; can occur anywhere
		Size: varies, usually 1 cm
		Color: varies
		Surface: variety of forms; usually begins as reddish-brown nodule that breaks down into a necrotic ulcer (develops more rapidly than basal cell); may begin as a persistent scale that eventually ulcerates
		Distribution: usually singular, may be multiple
		Use extra caution in assessing lesions or changes in (1) sun-exposed areas, (2) moist folds (monilial infections frequently erupt in genital or inframammary areas), or (3) lower extremities (look for reddening, flaking, dusky appearance, blanching, mottling)
b. Skin alterations: trauma induced	Bruises, lacerations, excoriations may heal more slowly	Large number of bruises Tearing of thin skin Reddened areas from pressure (bony prominences) Fissures or hyperkeratosis associated with friction (heels, toes, side of foot rubbing against shoe) Evaluated in same manner as with adult client
8. Nails a. Configuration	Toenails may be thickened, distorted (toenails treated for fungal infection may not return to normal configuration) (Fig. 3-36)	Toenail thickening associated with fungal infection (yellow discoloration, granular surface)

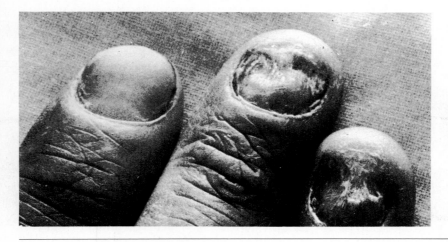

Fig. 3-36 Fungal infection of nails. (From Stewart WD, Danto JL, Maddin S: *Dermatology: diagnosis and treatment of cutaneous disorders,* ed 4, St Louis, 1978, Mosby—Year Book.)

*These lesions are fairly common in elderly adults. They are all considered "abnormal" and should be treated.

CHARACTERISTIC OR AREA EXAMINED	NORMAL FINDINGS	DEVIATIONS FROM NORMAL
b. Consistency	Fingernails may be more brittle, may peel	Uncut toenails curled over foot
c. Color	Toenails may lose translucency	
9. Hair and scalp		
a. Surface characteristics	Sebaceous hyperplasia may extend into scalp	Evaluated in same manner as with adult client
b. Distribution	Increased facial hair (especially women), bristly quality (Fig. 3-33)	
	Men may have coarse hair in ears, nose, eyebrows	
	Decreased scalp hair (scalp may be visible)	Sudden hair loss
	Symmetrical balding in men (most often frontal or occipital)	Patchy, asymmetrical hair loss
	Decreased pubic and axillary hair	
c. Texture	Facial hair coarse, body hair fine	Sudden change in texture
d. Color	Graying, whitening (hairs that do not lose pigment often become darker)	
e. Quantity	General decrease of body and scalp hair	

Study Questions

General

For questions 1 through 8, all the statements but one are true. Pick the false one.

1. The stratum corneum:
   - ☐ a. Contains keratin
   - ☐ b. Is part of the epidermis
   - ☐ c. Is composed of dead cells
   - ☐ d. Absorbs water readily
   - ☐ e. Lies under the subcutaneous layer

2. The epidermal layer:
   - ☐ a. Is avascular
   - ☐ b. Is uniformly paper thin
   - ☐ c. Is a barrier to external substances
   - ☐ d. Prevents excessive water loss

3. Keratin:
   - ☐ a. Cells are in calluses
   - ☐ b. Is the principal constituent of nails and hair
   - ☐ c. Cells are in corns
   - ☐ d. Produces pigment for skin color

4. Melanin:
   - ☐ a. Produces pigment for skin color
   - ☐ b. Serves as a shield against ultraviolet rays
   - ☐ c. Deposits are often lighter in the palms and nail beds
   - ☐ d. Production ceases with aging

5. The dermis:
   - ☐ a. Is well supplied with blood and lymph vessels
   - ☐ b. Contains the peripheral nervous system
   - ☐ c. Is nourished by the epidermis
   - ☐ d. Contains sebaceous glands

6. The subcutaneous layer:
   - ☐ a. Stores fat
   - ☐ b. Contributes to body heat conversion
   - ☐ c. Varies greatly in amounts among individuals
   - ☐ d. Supplies melanocytes for pigmentation
   - ☐ e. Acts as a cushion

7. Systematic integument evaluation is especially important when the client:
   - ☐ a. Is receiving treatments (e.g., topical medications, soaks) that involve the skin
   - ☐ b. Has impaired circulation
   - ☐ c. Depends on others for physical care or protection (e.g., infants, debilitated or immobilized individuals)
   - ☐ d. Has been living under unhygienic circumstances
   - ☐ e. Is known to have particularly sensitive or delicate skin
   - ☐ f. a, b, and c
   - ☐ g. All of the above
   - ☐ h. All except d
   - ☐ i. All except e

8. Which of the following statements are true:
   - ☐ a. Prolonged anoxemia will result in clubbing of the nails
   - ☐ b. Spider angiomas can be associated with pregnancy
   - ☐ c. Hypothyroidism can cause scalp hair to be dry and coarse
   - ☐ d. Acne is likely to be more prominent on the face, scalp, chest, and back
   - ☐ e. Scabies is likely to be more prominent on the wrists, hands, axillae, and inguinal area
   - ☐ f. All except b
   - ☐ g. a, d, and e
   - ☐ h. All of the above
   - ☐ i. All except c

Match the definitions in column B with the terms in column A.

Column A

9. ____ Macule
10. ____ Papule
11. ____ Nodule
12. ____ Vesicle
13. ____ Bulla
14. ____ Pustule
15. ____ Wheal
16. ____ Scale
17. ____ Crust
18. ____ Erosion
19. ____ Scar
20. ____ Fissure

Column B

a. Large, superficial, fluid-containing elevation greater than 0.5 cm
b. Loss of superficial epidermis, moist but not bleeding
c. Circumscribed, flat, change in skin color
d. Thin flakes of exfoliated epidermis
e. Deep linear crack in the skin
f. Solid elevated mass, usually less than 1 cm
g. Solid mass extending into subcutaneous or dermal tissue
h. Replacement of skin by fibrous tissue
i. Elevation containing purulent exudate
j. Small superficial elevation, less than 1 cm, containing serous fluid
k. Dried residue of serum, pus, or blood
l. Flat-topped, superficial, and well-circumscribed elevation

The Newborn

Match each term in column A with the one best description in column B.

Column A

Normal findings

21. ____ Acrocyanosis
22. ____ Erythema toxicum
23. ____ Harlequin sign
24. ____ Lanugo
25. ____ Milia
26. ____ Mottling
27. ____ Vernix caseosa

Column B

a. White sebaceous cysts
b. Cut-glass color
c. Waxy, greasy covering
d. Downy hair
e. Transitory skin marks
f. Transitory blue extremities
g. Side-to-side color difference

Deviations from normal

28. ____ Absent nails
29. ____ Desquamation
30. ____ Pallor
31. ____ Plethora
32. ____ Perpsiration
33. ____ Petechiae

a. Sign of polycythemia
b. Sign of anemia
c. Sign of birth trauma
d. Sign of drug withdrawal
e. Sign of postmaturity
f. Sign of fetal alcohol syndrome

The Child

Match each term in column A with the one best description in column B.

Column A

34. ____ Café au lait spots
35. ____ Mongolian spots
36. ____ Strawberry marks
37. ____ Storkbite
38. ____ Port-wine stains

Column B

a. Seen in dark-skinned children
b. Small, pink mark; usually disappears by age 5
c. 2 to 3 cm mark appears in first few months; gone by age 5
d. Purple area; does not disappear spontaneously
e. Cream-colored spots

The Childbearing Woman

Match each term in column A with the one best description in column B.

Column A

39. ____ Chloasma/melasma
40. ____ Linea nigra
41. ____ Striae gravidarum
42. ____ Varicosities
43. ____ Vascular spiders

Column B

a. Mask-type face spots
b. Red skin patterns
c. Silvery stretch lines
d. Dark lines from umbilicus to mons pubis
e. Dilated blood vessels

Select the *one* best answer to the following questions:

44. Increased hair growth occurs about the:
    □ a. First month of pregnancy
    □ b. Third month of pregnancy
    □ c. Second month postpartum
    □ d. Fourth month postpartum

45. Soon after childbirth, exertion and intraabdominal shifts may cause a woman to have:
    □ a. Fever
    □ b. Overhydration
    □ c. Chills
    □ d. Hallucinations

The Older Adult

For questions 46 through 48, all the statements are true except one. Pick the false statement.

46. A number of epidermal and dermal changes occur with aging.
    □ a. Outer skin moisture and suppleness often directly reflect the amount of moisture available in the environment
    □ b. Toenails may be thicker and somewhat disfigured
    □ c. The loss of melanocytes may contribute to a pale appearance in whites
    □ d. Precancerous lesions are a noted hazard for brown- and yellow-skinned people
    □ e. Pigment deposits (lentigines) may be more numerous in sun-exposed skin areas

47. Subcutaneous fat decreases with aging.
    □ a. Bony prominences emerge
    □ b. Sensitivity to cold weather increases
    □ c. Sensitivity to warm weather increases
    □ d. A folded, wrinkled, and lax appearance of the skin increases
    □ e. The abdomen may remain obese despite fat loss over arms and legs

48. A healthy elderly person might manifest the following integumentary changes.
    □ a. Hyperkeratosis
    □ b. Vitiligo
    □ c. Increased coarsening of facial hair
    □ d. Decrease and thinning of body hair
    □ e. Patchy balding (men)

SUGGESTED READINGS

General

Bates B: *A guide to physical examination,* ed 4, Philadelphia, 1987, JB Lippincott.

Cuzzel J: Clues: pain, burning and itching, *Am J Nurs* 90(7):15, 16, 1990.

Forbes EJ, Fitzsimons VM: *The older adult: a process for wellness,* St Louis, 1981, Mosby–Year Book.

Fowler E: Nursing diagnosis: potential for skin impairment in skin integrity, *J Gerontol Nurs* 12(3):34, 1986.

Malasanos L, Barkauskas V, Stoltenberg AK: *Health assessment,* ed 4, St Louis, 1990, Mosby–Year Book.

McCance L, Huether E: *Pathophysiology: the biological basis for disease in adults and children,* St Louis, 1990, Mosby–Year Book.

Potter P: *Pocket nurse guide to physical assessment,* ed 2, St Louis, 1990, Mosby–Year Book.

Seidel HM, Ball JW, Dains JE, Benedict GW: *Mosby's guide to physical examination,* ed 2, St Louis, 1991, Mosby–Year Book.

Shmunes E: The importance of pre-employment examinations in the prevention and control of occupational skin disease, *J Occup Med* 22(6):407, 1980.

Stewart WD, Danto JL, Maddin S: *Dermatology: diagnosis and treatment of cutaneous disorders,* ed 4, St Louis, 1978, Mosby–Year Book.

Thompson JM, McFarland GK, Hirsch JE, and others: *Mosby's manual of clinical nursing,* ed 2, St Louis, 1989, Mosby–Year Book.

The newborn

Auvenshine MA, Enriquez MG: *Maternity nursing: dimensions of change,* Belmont, Calif, 1985, Wadsworth.

Bobak IM, Jensen MD: *Essentials of maternity nursing,* ed 3, St Louis, 1991, Mosby–Year Book.

Judd JM: Assessing the newborn from head to toe, *Nursing '85* 15(12):34, 1985.

Kiernan BS, Scoloveno MA: Assessment of the neonate, *Top Clin Nurs* 8(1):1, 1986.

The Organization of Obstetrical, Gynecological and Neonatal Nurses (NAACOG): Physical assessment of the neonate, *OGN Nursing Practice Resource,* Oct. 1986, The Association.

Pillitteri A: *Maternal-newborn nursing: care of the growing family,* ed 3, Boston, 1985, Little, Brown.

Pritchard JA, MacDonald PC: *Williams' obstetrics,* ed 17, New York, 1985, Appleton-Century-Crofts.

Scanlon JW and others: *A system of newborn physical examination,* Baltimore, 1979, University Park Press.

Seidel HM, Ball JW, Dains JE, Benedict GW: *Mosby's guide to physical examination,* ed 2, St Louis, 1991, Mosby–Year Book.

Whaley LF, Wong DL: *Essentials of pediatric nursing,* ed 3, St Louis, 1989, Mosby–Year Book.

The child

Alexander M, Brown MS: *Pediatric history taking and physical diagnosis for nurses,* ed 2, New York, 1979, McGraw-Hill.

Barness L: *Manual of pediatric physical diagnosis,* ed 6, Chicago, 1990, Mosby–Year Book.

Cohen S: Skin rashes in infants and children: programmed instruction, *Am J Nurs* 78(6): 1041, 1978.

DeAngelis C: *Pediatric primary care,* ed 3, Boston, 1984, Little, Brown.

Verboc J, Morley N: *Color atlas of pediatric dermatology,* Philadelphia, 1983, JB Lippincott.

Whaley LF, Wong DL: *Essentials of pediatric nursing,* ed 3, St Louis, 1989, Mosby–Year Book

The childbearing woman

Auvenshine MA, Enriquez MG: *Maternity nursing: dimensions of change,* Belmont, Calif, 1985, Wadsworth.

Beischer NA, MacKay EV: *Obstetrics and the newborn: an illustrated textbook,* ed 2, Philadelphia, 1986, WB Saunders.

Bobak IM, Jensen MD: *Essentials of maternity nursing,* ed 3, St Louis, 1991, Mosby–Year Book.

Pillitteri A: *Maternal-newborn nursing: care of the growing family,* ed 3, Boston, 1985, Little, Brown.

Pritchard JA, MacDonald PC: *Williams' obstetrics,* ed 17, New York, 1985, Appleton-Century-Crofts.

Seidel HM, Ball JW, Dains JE, Benedict GW: *Mosby's guide to physical examination,* ed 2, St Louis, 1991, Mosby–Year Book.

Whitley N: *A manual of clinical obstetrics,* Philadelphia, 1985, JB Lippincott.

The older adult

Berliner H: Aging skin, *Am J Nurs* 86(10):1138, 1986.

Brozena J, Waterman G, Fenske NA: Pigmented skin lesions in the elderly: considerations in the differential diagnosis, *Geriatrics* 45(5):38, 1990.

Burnside IM, editor: *Nursing and the aged,* ed 3, New York, 1988, McGraw-Hill.

DeVillez RL: Externally and internally caused skin problems of aging, *Geriatrics* 38(1):71, 1983.

Ebersole P, Hess P: *Toward healthy aging,* ed 3, St Louis, 1990, Mosby–Year Book.

Fenske NA, Lober CW: Skin changes of aging: pathological implications, *Geriatrics* 45(3):27, 1990.

Malasanos L, Barkauskas V, Stoltenberg-Allen K: *Health assessment,* ed 4, St Louis, 1990, Mosby–Year Book.

Quinn MJ, Tomita SK: *Elder abuse and neglect,* New York, 1986, Springer Publishing.

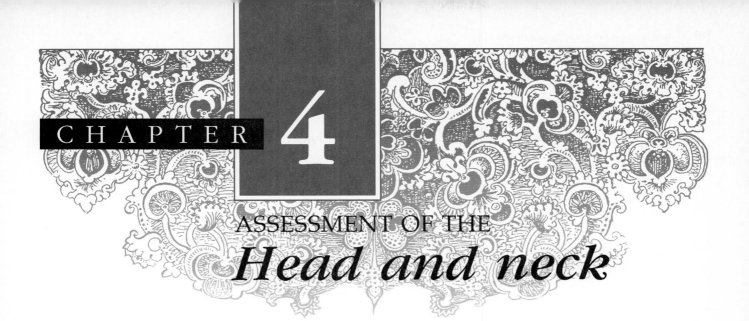

CHAPTER 4

ASSESSMENT OF THE
Head and neck

VOCABULARY

alopecia Absence or loss of hair.

anterior triangle (of neck) Landmark area for palpating the submaxillary, submental, and anterior cervical lymph nodes; sectioned by the anterior surface of the sternocleidomastoid muscle, the mandible, and an imagined line running from the chin to the sternal notch.

cricoid cartilage Lowermost cartilage of the larynx.

fontanel Unossified space or soft spot lying between the cranial bones of an infant.

frontal bone Forehead bone.

goiter Hypertrophy of the thyroid gland, usually evident as a pronounced swelling in the neck.

hirsutism Excessive body hair, usually in a masculine distribution, owing to heredity, hormonal dysfunction, porphyria, or medication.

hyoid Single bone suspended from the styloid process of the temporal bone.

isthmus (glandulae thyroideae) Narrow portion of the thyroid gland connecting the left and right lobes.

lymphadenitis Inflammation of the lymph nodes.

lymphoma General term for growth of new tissue in the lymphatic area; ordinarily a malignant growth.

manubrium Uppermost of the three bones of the sternum.

mastoid process Conical projection of the temporal bone extending downward and forward behind the external auditory meatus.

occipital bone Bone in the lower back part of the skull between the parietal and temporal bones.

parietal bone One of the pair of bones that form the sides of the cranium.

posterior triangle (of neck) Landmark area for palpating the posterior cervical chain, the supraclavicular chain, and the occipital lymph chain; sectioned along the anterior border by the sternocleidomastoid muscle, the posterior border by the trapezius muscle, and the bottom by the clavicle.

shotty node Lymph node that feels hard and nodular; generally movable and nontender; may show evidence of having been infected many times in the past.

sternocleidomastoid muscle Major muscle that rotates and flexes the head; originates by two heads from the sternum and clavicle and inserts on the mastoid process and the occipital bone.

trapezius muscle Major muscle that rotates and extends the head; originates along the superior curved line of the occiput and the spinous processes of the seventh cervical and all thoracic vertebrae and inserts at the clavicle, acromion, and base of the scapula.

ANATOMY AND PHYSIOLOGY REVIEW

The seven bones of the head are the frontal (2), parietal (2), temporal (2), and occipital (1), as shown in Fig. 4-1. The bones are covered with the scalp and hair. The face consists of 8 bones—the nasal, frontal, lacrimal, sphenoid, zygomatic, ethmoid, and maxillary bones and the movable mandible.

The eyes, ears, nose, and mouth are basically symmetrical. However, characteristics of the face are unique to each individual. Sensory and facial muscles are innervated by the fifth and seventh cranial nerves. For cranial nerve V, the sensory branches are the ophthalmic, maxillary, and mandibular. Cranial nerve VII innervates the muscles of facial expression.

The neck can be divided into two triangles—the anterior triangle and the posterior triangle (Fig. 4-2). The anterior triangle is bordered above by the mandible, laterally by the sternocleidomastoid, and medially by the trachea. The posterior triangle is bordered by the sternocleidomastoid and the trapezius muscles and below by the clavicle.

Major structures of the neck are seen in Fig. 4-3. These

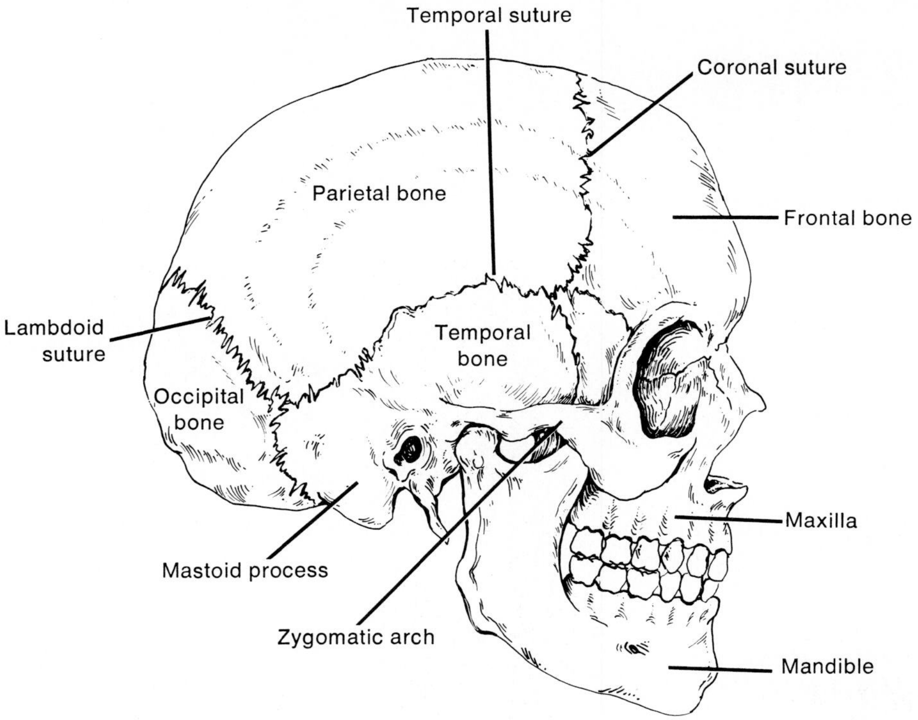

Fig. 4-1 Lateral view of adult skull.

Temporal suture

Coronal suture

Parietal bone

Frontal bone

Lambdoid suture

Temporal bone

Occipital bone

Maxilla

Mastoid process

Zygomatic arch

Mandible

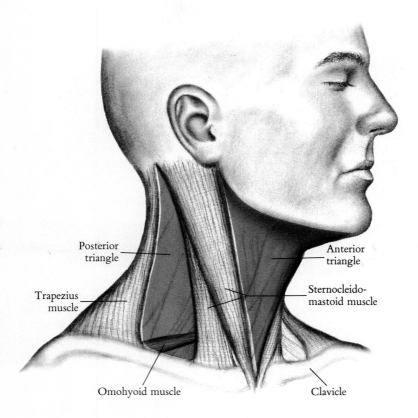

Posterior triangle

Anterior triangle

Trapezius muscle

Sternocleido-mastoid muscle

Omohyoid muscle

Clavicle

Fig. 4-2 Anterior and posterior triangles of neck. (From Seidel HM, Ball JW, Dains JE, Benedict GW: *Mosby's guide to physical examination,* ed 2, St Louis, 1991, Mosby—Year Book.)

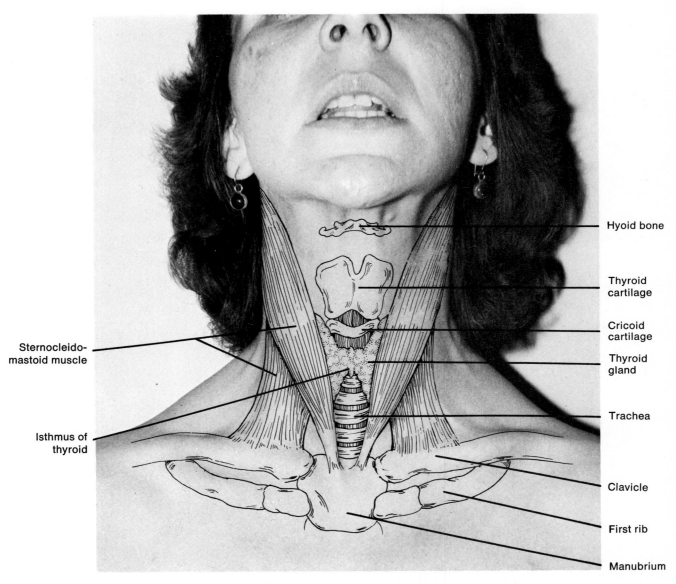

Hyoid bone

Thyroid cartilage

Cricoid cartilage

Thyroid gland

Trachea

Clavicle

First rib

Manubrium

Sternocleido-mastoid muscle

Isthmus of thyroid

Fig. 4-3 Anatomical structure of neck.

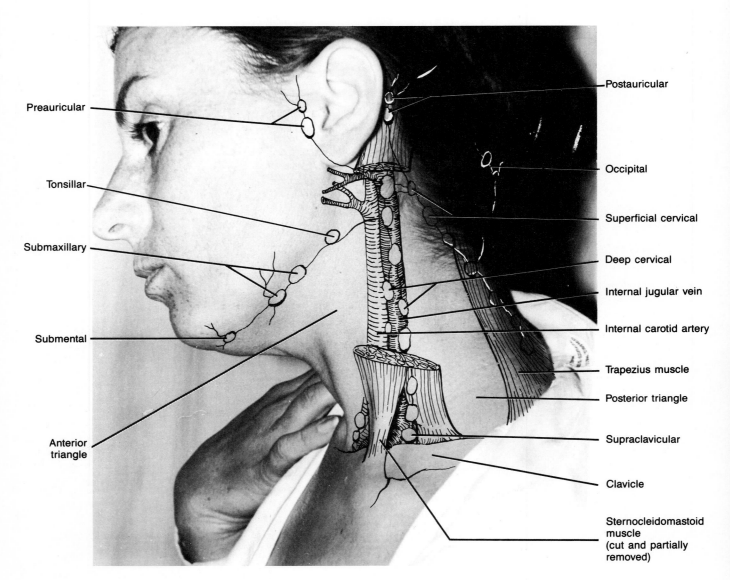

Preauricular

Tonsillar

Submaxillary

Submental

Anterior
triangle

Postauricular

Occipital

Superficial cervical

Deep cervical

Internal jugular vein

Internal carotid artery

Trapezius muscle

Posterior triangle

Supraclavicular

Clavicle

Sternocleidomastoid
muscle
(cut and partially
removed)

Fig. 4-4 Lateral view of anatomical lymph structures of neck with nodes.

are the sternocleidomastoid muscle, the hyoid bone, the thyroid cartilage, the cricoid cartilage, the thyroid gland, and the trachea. The thyroid gland lies across the trachea and tucks back behind the sternocleidomastoid muscle. The middle section of the thyroid is called the *isthmus* of the thyroid.

Lymph nodes of the head and neck occur in chains and clusters. Superficial nodes are located in subcutaneous connective tissue, and deeper nodes lie beneath the muscles (Fig. 4-4). The deep cervical chain lies beneath the sternocleidomastoid muscle. Other cervical chains can be palpated. Lymph nodes are round and smooth and normally not palpable.

• • •

Assessment of the head and neck requires a firm understanding of the underlying anatomy. The practitioner must be able to visualize the structures of the neck and the lymph nodes and should use the fingerpads to gently palpate the designated areas. The thyroid may or may not be palpable; the lymph nodes generally are not palpable.

COGNITIVE OBJECTIVES

At the end of this chapter the learner will demonstrate knowledge of assessment of the head and neck by the ability to do the following:

- Apply the terms that are listed in the vocabulary section.
- Systematically list structures of the head and neck evaluated during the physical examination.
- Describe the characteristics of a lymph node that must be evaluated.
- Describe the lymphatic drainage of the head and neck.
- Explain the significance of and methods for examining the thyroid gland and trachea.
- Identify selected elements of the head and neck examination for the newborn, the child, the childbearing woman, and the older adult.
- Identify selected elements of the head and neck examination of the older adult.

CLINICAL OUTLINE

At the end of this chapter the learner will perform a systematic assessment of the head and neck, demonstrating the ability to do the following:

- Obtain a pertinent health history from the client.
- Demonstrate and describe the results of inspection and palpation of the following aspects of the head:
  1. Skull for contour and size
  2. Scalp for texture and color
  3. Hair for distribution, quality, and quantity
  4. Facies for symmetry, quality, color, expression, and movements
  5. Head movements
- Demonstrate and describe the results of inspection and palpation of neck and thyroid gland for the following:
  1. Symmetry
  2. Muscular development and movement
  3. Landmarks and location of the trachea
  4. Location, size, shape, delineation, mobility, consistency, and surface characteristics of the faciocervical lymph nodes
  5. Placement, symmetry, and characteristics of the thyroid gland
- Summarize results of the assessment with a written description of findings.

HISTORY

- Head injury profile
  1. Events associated with the injury
     a. Predisposing factors leading to injury, such as epilepsy or a seizure disorder, blackout, poor vision, dizziness, light-headedness
     b. Precipitating factors leading to injury, such as unsafe conditions, wet floors, getting up too fast
  2. If possible, description of the exact details of the injury
     a. Specifically, what happened
     b. How client appeared immediately after injury (unconscious, dazed, crying, convulsive)
     c. How client was 5 minutes later (vomited, complained of headache, appeared fine, same as immediately after, or different)
     d. Client's general condition (gotten progressively worse or better or been unchanged) since injury
  3. Associated symptoms
     a. State of consciousness: unconscious (momentary vs. prolonged—describe), dazed, sleepy
     b. Neck or head pain (see headache profile that follows)
     c. Visual problems: droopy eyes, blurred or double vision
     d. Vomiting: number of times, associated distress, projectile in nature
     e. Motor or sensory changes: staggered gait, tremors, numbness of limbs
     f. Ear or nasal discharge: serous or bloody discharge from nose or ears
     g. Loss of urine or bowel control since injury
     h. Loss of memory: recent or long term
  4. Medications
     a. Those routinely being taken

b. Any discontinued within 1 week before injury
- Headache profile

Because of the vast complexity of headaches, profile questioning will incorporate the symptom analysis format presented in Chapter 1.

1. When client was last entirely well
   a. When *this type* of headache started occurring
   b. How long client has been bothered with headaches in general
2. Date of current problem onset: If headache has been going on for some time, try to determine beginning date.
3. Character
   a. Constant bandlike pressure
   b. Throbbing, pounding
   c. Single-area pressure
   d. Single-area pain (dull vs. sharp)
   e. Shooting pains (dull vs. sharp)
   f. Severity of headache
4. Nature of problem onset
   a. Slowly over several weeks, days, hours
   b. Abrupt onset over several minutes
5. Client's hunch of precipitating factors
   a. Stress
   b. Sudden movement or exercise
   c. Alcohol
   d. Medication
6. Course of problem
   a. Lasts for minutes, hours, days, weeks before disappearing; relieved by medication
   b. Lasts for minutes, hours, days, weeks before disappearing; medication not necessary for relief
   c. Appears in clusters (several over given time period), then disappears for extensive period before returning
7. Location of problem
   a. Occipital region
   b. Frontal region
   c. Temporal region
   d. Neck region
   e. Maxillary sinus region
   f. Behind eyes
   g. Unilateral or bilateral
   h. Generalized or specific
8. Relation to other entities
   a. Visual changes (decreased acuity or blurring, tearing)
   b. Nausea and vomiting (which came first—headache or nausea and vomiting)
   c. Nasal stuffiness and discharge
   d. Muscle aches and pains
   e. Cough, sore throat
   f. Neck pain and/or stiffness
   g. Fever
   h. Change in level of consciousness as headache increases
   i. Headache symptoms aggravated by movement
9. Patterns
   a. Timing
      (1) Worse in morning or evening
      (2) Occurs only during sleep
      (3) Worse or better as day progresses
   b. Duration
      (1) Episodes getting closer together and worse
      (2) Getting worse but no closer together
      (3) Lasting longer
10. Efforts to treat
    a. Physician help sought for headache
    b. Current medications taken—prescription and over-the-counter
    c. Body positions that help headache
    d. Other remedies that help headache
11. How headaches interfere with client's activities of daily living
- Complaints of neck pain
1. Head or neck injury or strain
2. Swelling of neck
3. Limitations of neck movement (continuous vs. sporadic)
4. Neck movement aggravates or alleviates neck pain
5. Radiation patterns to arms, shoulders, hands, down back
- Complaints of dizziness
1. Important to determine exactly what is meant; the term *dizziness* means the inability to maintain equilibrium. In the objective type the room seems to spin; in the subjective type the client feels as though he is moving.
- Thyroid dysfunction
1. Changes in sleep pattern or energy level: fatigue, drowsiness
2. Changes in emotional patterns: mood changes, irritability, nervousness
3. Altered sensitivity to heat or cold
4. Hair loss, change in texture of hair or skin, or brittleness of nails
5. Changes in appetite, weight loss, bowel habits, thirst, or frequency of urination
6. Changes in menstrual pattern
7. Hoarseness, difficulty swallowing, swelling, or pain or tenderness in the neck

Text continues on p. 104.

CLINICAL GUIDELINES

ASSESSMENT PROCEDURE	EVALUATION	
	NORMAL FINDINGS	DEVIATIONS FROM NORMAL

1. Ask client to sit and remove wig or hairpiece
2. Inspect and palpate:
  a. Skull (Fig. 4-5)
    (1) Contour
	Rounded and symmetrical with frontal, parietal, and bilateral occipital prominences	Lumps, marked protrusions, depressions

(2) Size	Wide variety of sizes	Greatly enlarged Abnormally small Protruding mandible
b. Scalp (Fig. 4-6) (1) Texture	Skin intact	Lesions, scabs Tenderness Scaliness Superficial nodules
	Smooth and even skin	Thickening of skin, which becomes coarse, leathery, and oily and develops thick folds

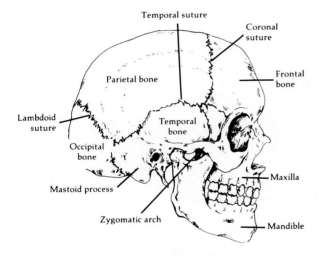

Fig. 4-5 Anatomical landmarks of skull.

Temporal suture
Coronal suture
Frontal bone
Parietal bone
Lambdoid suture
Temporal bone
Occipital bone
Maxilla
Mastoid process
Zygomatic arch
Mandible

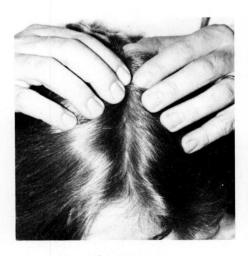

Fig. 4-6 Scalp palpation.

Continued.

CLINICAL GUIDELINES—cont'd

| | EVALUATION | |
ASSESSMENT PROCEDURE	NORMAL FINDINGS	DEVIATIONS FROM NORMAL
		Skin and bone changes also seen in jaw and facial bones, hands, feet (acromegaly) (Fig. 4-7)

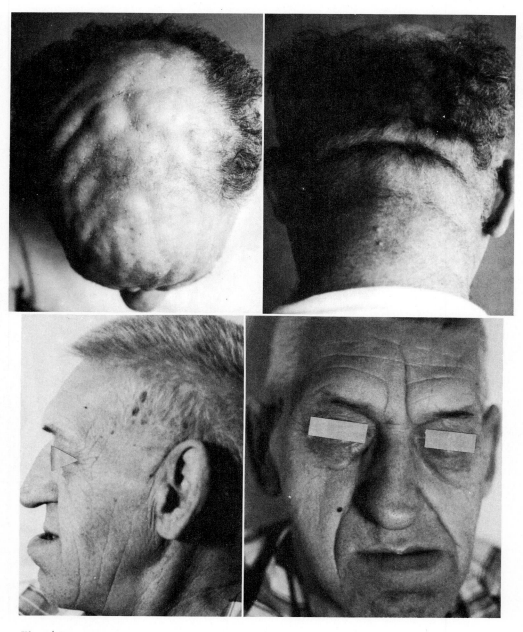

Fig. 4-7 Scalp and facial changes noted with acromegaly. (From Prior JA, Silberstein JS, Stang JM: *Physical diagnosis: the history and examination of the patient,* ed 6, St Louis, 1981, Mosby—Year Book.)

ASSESSMENT PROCEDURE	EVALUATION	
	NORMAL FINDINGS	DEVIATIONS FROM NORMAL
(2) Color	Pigmentation will vary according to race	Reddened areas Areas of increased or decreased pigmentation
c. Hair (1) Foreign bodies		Flaking Nits
(2) Distribution	Even Bilateral, symmetrical balding (Fig. 4-8, *A*)	Patchy, asymmetrical alopecia (Fig. 4-8, *B*)
(3) Quantity	Thick, thin, sparse	Excessive loss
(4) Quality	Shiny, smooth	Dull, brittle Excessive coarseness or dryness
(5) Hygiene	Clean	Odor; matted, dirty
d. Face (1) Symmetry	Symmetrical placement and shape of eyes, ears, mouth, eyebrows, nasolabial folds	Marked asymmetry
(2) Quality	Facial qualities vary according to race and body build	Edema (especially of eyelids) (Fig. 4-9)

A **B**

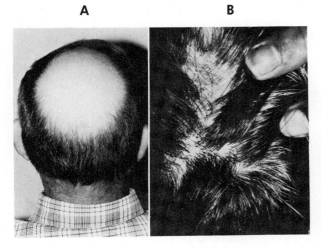

Fig. 4-8 **A,** Normal balding pattern. **B,** Abnormal balding pattern. (From Stewart WD, Danto JL, Maddin S: *Dermatology: diagnosis and treatment of cutaneous disorders,* ed 4, St Louis, 1978, Mosby–Year Book.)

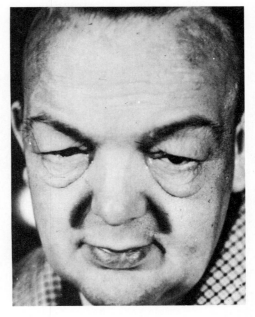

Fig. 4-9 Periorbital edema and facial puffiness as seen in myxedema. (From Prior JA, Silberstein JS, Stang JM: *Physical diagnosis: the history and examination of the patient,* ed 6, St Louis, 1981, Mosby–Year Book.)

Continued.

CLINICAL GUIDELINES—cont'd

| | EVALUATION | |
ASSESSMENT PROCEDURE	NORMAL FINDINGS	DEVIATIONS FROM NORMAL
	(Note slight facial asymmetry in Fig. 4-10, *A*)	Exceptionally coarse features Puffiness Excessive perspiration Waxy pallor Lesions Lip lesions, fissures, swelling Acne, scarring
(3) Color	Pigmentation varies with race	Jaundice Cyanosis (especially around lips) Pigmentation variations
(4) Expression	Alert; response appropriate to conversation	No responsiveness Tense, drawn muscles Inappropriate expression
(5) Movements 3. Evaluate head and neck a. Instruct client to:	Controlled, smooth	Involuntary

(1) Move chin to chest
   (2) Move head back so that chin is pointing toward ceiling
   (3) Move head so that ear is moved toward shoulder (do not allow client to move shoulder up to ear)
	Controlled and smooth throughout series of movements
	Movement of neck from neutral upright position
	  Chin toward chest, 45-degree flexion
	  Chin upward toward ceiling, 55-degree extension
		Ratchety movement
		Bounding (up and down), synchronizes with pulse
		Rhythmic movement or tremor

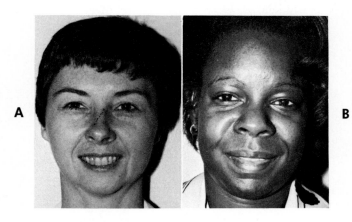

Fig. 4-10   Variations of facial structures.

ASSESSMENT PROCEDURE	EVALUATION	
	NORMAL FINDINGS	DEVIATIONS FROM NORMAL
(4) Move head and neck in lateral rotation so that while head is upward and pointed forward, the client's chin is placed on first one shoulder and then the other	Lateral bending, 40 degrees each way Rotation 70 degrees for both right and left directions No discomfort or limitation of movement (Fig. 4-11)	Pain throughout movement Pain at particular points during movement Spasms or tics Limited range of motion Unable to touch points (as indicated)
b. Neck range of motion may be evaluated by a single rotary movement incorporating the four touch points		

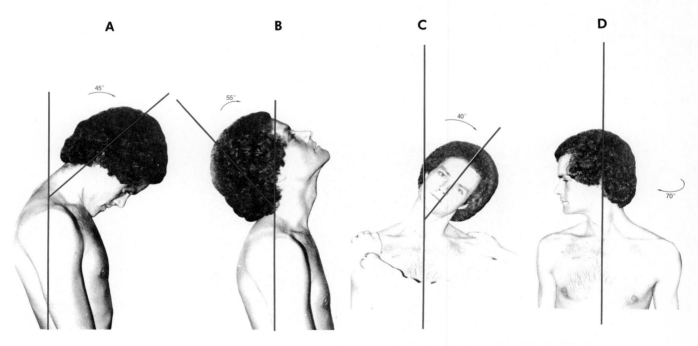

Fig. 4-11   Normal range of motion of neck. **A,** Flexion. **B,** Extension. **C,** Lateral bending. **D,** Rotation.

Continued.

CLINICAL GUIDELINES—cont'd

ASSESSMENT PROCEDURE	EVALUATION	
	NORMAL FINDINGS	DEVIATIONS FROM NORMAL
c. Neck symmetry (Fig. 4-12)	Head position centered Bilateral symmetry of trapezius and sternocleidomastoid muscles	Head tilted Muscle shortening, wasting Tenderness on palpation Masses, scars
4. Palpate trachea (easiest just above suprasternal notch) a. Location	Central placement	Lateral displacement Tenderness on palpation
b. Landmarks	Tracheal rings Cricoid cartilage Thyroid cartilage	
5. Inspect thyroid a. Instruct client to: (1) Put chin up as if drinking from glass (2) Swallow		
b. Note symmetry and placement	Gland usually not visible Normal lobe may be seen as slight thickening when client swallows	Unilateral or bilateral lobe enlargement* (Fig. 4-13)
c. Palpate thyroid (1) Stand behind client (a) Instruct client to flex head slightly (b) Tilt chin slightly toward side you are examining		

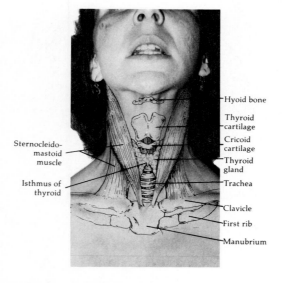

Fig. 4-12   Anatomical landmarks of anterior neck.

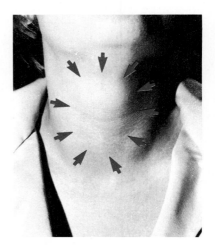

Fig. 4-13   Minimum thyroid enlargement encroaching on sternocleidomastoid muscle. Note full appearance of neck.

Auscultate the thyroid gland if enlargement is found (use bell of stethoscope). Evidence of abnormality is systolic bruit or continuous venous hum in supraclavicular areas.

| | EVALUATION | |
ASSESSMENT PROCEDURE	NORMAL FINDINGS	DEVIATIONS FROM NORMAL
(c) Place your fingers anteriorly with finger pads over client's trachea		
(d) Instruct client to swallow periodically (it may be necessary to give client a small glass of water to facilitate swallowing) so that you can locate identifying landmarks, including:		
—Thyroid cartilage	Smooth; centrally located	
—Cricoid cartilage	Smooth, ringlike structure	
—Isthmus	Smooth tissue found approximately 1 cm below cricoid cartilage May not be felt With swallowing may feel smooth tissue slide under skin	
—Thyroid lobes on lateral border of gland		
–Right lobe felt with chin slightly flexed to right	Lobes may not be felt If felt, lobes are small, smooth, nontender, and rise freely with swallowing	Enlarged lobes Palpated easily without swallowing Nodular or irregular lobe consistency Tender to palpation Gland not freely moving with swallowing
–Place right fingertips directly behind sternocleidomastoid muscle		
–Fingertips of left hand slightly displace trachea to right		
–Instruct patient to swallow (Fig. 4-14)	Right lobe larger than left	

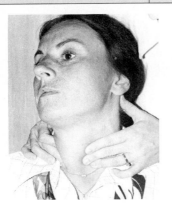

Fig. 4-14　Palpating thyroid behind the client. Displace trachea with left hand. Palpate thyroid lobe with right hand behind sternocleidomastoid muscle.

CLINICAL GUIDELINES—cont'd

ASSESSMENT PROCEDURE	EVALUATION	
	NORMAL FINDINGS	DEVIATIONS FROM NORMAL

—Main body of gland
  –Right lobe felt with chin slightly to right
  –Place right fingertips directly in front of sternocleidomastoid muscle
  –Fingertips of left hand slightly displace trachea to right
  –Instruct patient to swallow
 —Reverse procedure for left lobe evaluations
(2) Stand in front of the client
  (a) Instruct client to flex neck forward and to right		

	Lobes may not be felt If felt, lobes are small, smooth, nontender, and rise freely with swallowing	Enlarged lobes Palpated easily without swallowing Nodular or irregular lobe consistency Tender to palpation Gland not freely moving with swallowing

(b) Use second and third fingers to feel over cricoid cartilage and thyroid isthmus
  (c) Move fingers laterally and deep into medial borders of sternocleidomastoid muscle; identify landmarks, including:
   —Thyroid cartilage
 	
   —Cricoid cartilage
   —Isthmus		

	Smooth Centrally located Smooth ringlike structure Smooth tissue found approximately 1 cm below cricoid cartilage May not be felt With swallowing may feel smooth tissue slide under skin	
(d) Hook tips of second and third fingers of left hand behind sternocleidomastoid muscle; palpate lobes of thyroid with pad of thumbs (e) Reverse procedure for left lobes		

ASSESSMENT PROCEDURE	EVALUATION	
	NORMAL FINDINGS	DEVIATIONS FROM NORMAL

6. Lymph nodes
  a. Inspect side of neck (Fig. 4-15)
  b. Palpate the following nodes:
    (1) Preauricular (Fig. 4-16)
    (2) Postauricular and occipital (Fig. 4-17)
    (3) Tonsillar, submaxillary, and submental (Fig. 4-18)
    (4) Superficial and deep cervical (Fig. 4-19)		

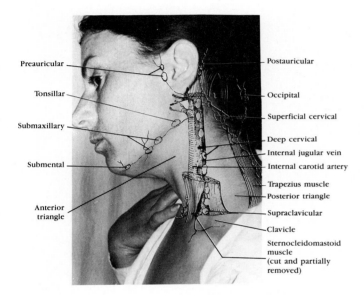

Fig. 4-15   Anatomical landmarks of lateral head and neck.

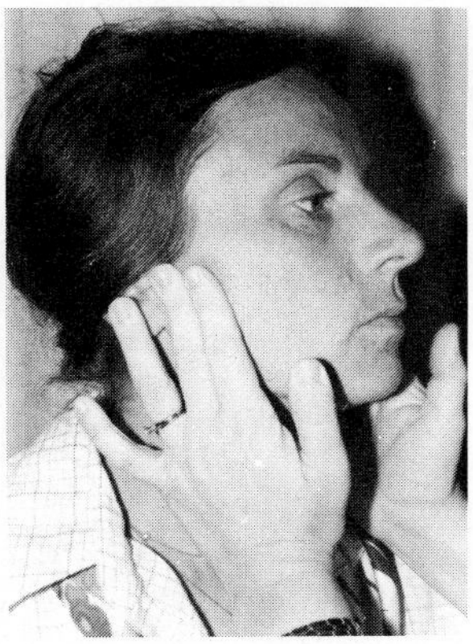

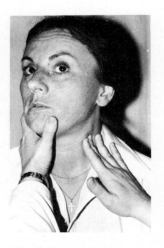

Fig. 4-16   Palpating preauricular lymph nodes.

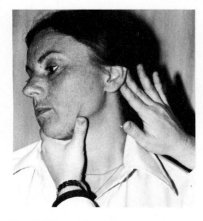

Fig. 4-17   Palpating posterior auricular chain of lymph nodes.

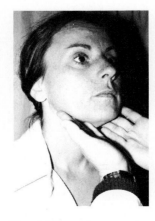

Fig. 4-18   Palpating submaxillary lymph nodes.

Fig. 4-19   Palpating deep cervical chain of lymph nodes.

Note: Inspection and palpation of the jugular vein and carotid arteries and auscultation of the carotid arteries are described in Chapter 9.
Continued.

CLINICAL GUIDELINES—cont'd

	EVALUATION	
ASSESSMENT PROCEDURE	NORMAL FINDINGS	DEVIATIONS FROM NORMAL
(5) Posterior cervical (Fig. 4-20) (6) Supraclavicular (Fig. 4-21) c. Size (cm) and shape	Nodes usually not palpable If palpable, they are small, mobile, discrete, nontender	Palpable nodes Large, round, cylindrical, irregular
d. Delimitation e. Mobility		Multiple discrete or matted nodes Fixed to underlying tissue Fixed to overlying tissue Induration
f. Consistency g. Surface characteristics h. Tenderness i. Heat j. Erythema		Hard, firm; soft, spongy Smooth, nodular Tender on palpation Present Present

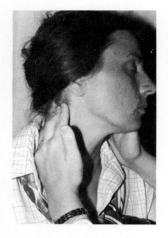

Fig. 4-20 Palpating posterior cervical chain of lymph nodes.

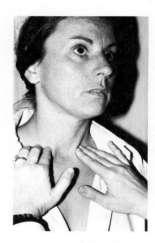

Fig. 4-21 Palpating supraclavicular chain of lymph nodes.

CLINICAL TIPS AND STRATEGIES

- **Abnormal quantity of hair and abnormal hair or scalp texture should be explored:** Most clients are aware of recent or marked changes in texture. Thinning hair, loss of elasticity, or changing pigmentation may be part of the normal aging process. Change in hair care habits can contribute to hair texture changes.
- **Nits can be confused with dandruff:** Nits are creamy, yellow, ovoid, and smooth. They cling to a strand of hair. Dandruff flakes will shake away from scalp or hair and are irregularly shaped.

- **When palpating the skull/scalp, use the palmar surface of finger pads:** Some beginning examiners tend to use the distal tips of the fingers instead of the finger pads. The finger pads are much more sensitive to subtle changes.
- **Have the client flex the neck slightly forward for thyroid and trachea palpation:** This permits muscle relaxation in this area so that the examiner's fingers can probe more effectively.
- **When palpating the neck and thyroid, have the**

client comfortably seated so that the neck is relaxed: Some examiners actually encourage the client to rest the back of the head against the examiner's chest.

- **Some textbooks present both anterior and posterior thyroid palpation:** Posterior position thyroid palpation is presented here because it is the easiest technique for the beginner to master.
- **There are many teaching techniques for cervical lymph node palpation:** Each text the beginning student reads may give slightly different locations for the nodes and use slightly different names. The important points for the student to remember follow:
  1. Find the text you believe best describes node locations, and stick to that text for memorization and practice.
  2. Although general anatomical node positions are described in texts, individual locations vary.
  3. When palpating for lymph nodes, the examiner must screen the *entire area* of the anticipated nodes before summarizing clinical findings.
  4. *Light* palpation is necessary to pick up smaller, more superficial nodes.
  5. At times it is helpful for the examiner to place one hand on the client's head and to palpate with the

other. In this way the client's head can be moved into any desired position.
- **If you find identifiable lymph nodes,** note the following:
  1. Node size, shape, perimeters, mobility, consistency, and tenderness.
  2. Systemic symptoms that may be related to node enlargement. Table 4-1 describes node locations and the areas of the body drained by them.

SAMPLE RECORDING: NORMAL FINDINGS

Skull: Normocephalic. No tenderness, lesions, or masses.
Hair: Dark-brown natural color with beginning graying. No nits or flaking noted.
Face: Symmetrical. Skin smooth and moist. No involuntary movements noted.
Neck: Symmetrical and supple. Trachea midline; thyroid not palpable. No palpable nodes or masses. Full and strong range of motion without discomfort.

TABLE 4-1   Lymphatic drainage pattern for cervical lymph nodes

NODE	LOCATION	RECEIVES DRAINAGE FROM
Preauricular	In front of tragus of external ear	Scalp, external auditory canal, forehead or upper facial structures, lateral portion of eyelids
Postauricular	Behind ear on mastoid process	Parietal region of scalp, external auditory canal
Occipital	Midway between external occipital protuberance and mastoid process	Parietal region of scalp
Tonsillar	At angle of mandible	Tonsils, posterior palate, thyroid, floor of mouth
Submaxillary	Halfway between angle and tip of mandible	Tongue, submaxillary glands, mucosa of lips and mouth
Submental	In midline behind tip of mandible	Tongue, mucosa of lips and mouth, floor of mouth
Superficial cervical chain	Superficial to sternocleidomastoid muscle	Skin of neck, ear
Posterior cervical chain	Along anterior edge to trapezius muscle	Posterior scalp, thyroid, posterior skin of neck
Deep cervical chain	Under sternocleidomastoid muscle; includes four separate chains extending over larynx, thyroid gland, and trachea	Larynx, thyroid, trachea, ear, and upper part of esophagus
Supraclavicular	Deep in angle formed by sternocleidomastoid muscle and clavicle	Upper abdomen, lungs, breast, arm

The Newborn

HISTORY AND CLINICAL STRATEGIES

- The examiner must remember that even though babies are born with six fontanels, generally only the frontal and occipital fontanels are palpated.
  1. The examiner must have a firm understanding of normal findings so that there can be early identification of deviations.
  2. The examiner should palpate fontanels when the infant is quiet; fontanels may bulge slightly when the infant cries.

- It is easiest to perform a head and neck examination when the newborn is in an upright position.
  1. Compare palpation findings with the birth history. Molding is more noticeable over the occiput area in vertex presentations unless there was a brow or chin presentation.
  2. Full range of motion in the neck should be observed. Resistance should not be felt. Do not force movement.

CLINICAL VARIATIONS: THE NEWBORN

CHARACTERISTIC OR AREA EXAMINED	NORMAL FINDINGS	DEVIATIONS FROM NORMAL

1. Shape and size	Symmetrical
	Molding; long, narrow head with overriding sutures from vaginal birth; should disappear a few days after birth
	Caput succedaneum (edema from birth)
	Head circumference (33 to 37 cm), about 2 cm more than chest
	Usually silky, fine hair over scalp
		Asymmetrical (may be from intrauterine position)
		Displacement of cranial bones (may be intracranial hemorrhage)
		Cephalhematoma (hemorrhage from traumatic birth)
		Circumference by gestational age:
		  Macrocephaly: over 90th percentile
		  Microcephaly: under 10th percentile
		  Large head, thin cerebral mantle (may be hydrocephalus)
		  Small head (may be anencephaly)
		Skull depression, irregularity (may be fracture)
		Cranial bruit (suggests arteriovenous malformation)
		Soft bones indenting with light pressure (may be craniotabes)
		Saclike structures (may be meningocele or encephalocele)

2. Sutures and fontanels	Palpable sutures
	Fontanels: flat, soft
	  Diamond-shaped anterior; one fingertip (2 to 3 cm) wide, 3 to 4 cm long; between parietal and frontal bones
	  Triangular posterior; may be nearly closed at birth; 1 to 2 cm if measurable
		Suture closure (suggests craniosynostosis)
		Full, bulging (may be intracranial pressure, hematoma, meningitis, hydrocephalus)
		Indented, sunken (may be dehydration)
		Large posterior fontanel (suggests Down syndrome)

3. Face and neck	Small, round, symmetrical Cheeks have fat pads Chin recedes Neck symmetrical, chubby, short with even skinfolds Head moves backward and forward without difficulty Newborn can move head slightly when prone Possible pronounced trachea, enlarged thymus gland	Asymmetry (may be facial paralysis) Back neck fat pad (suggests Down syndrome) Webbing, masses, skin breaks, bruises, swelling, abrasions Rigid neck (may be torticollis or meningitis) Torticollis (may be from breech position)

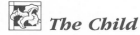

The Child

HISTORY AND CLINICAL STRATEGIES

- Head and neck examination of a child is usually easy to do because it is not considered an intrusive procedure; however, it may be difficult if the examiner's hands are too large to accurately assess the tiny structures of a child's head and neck.
    1. The fontanels usually present no difficulty in palpation.
    2. Head circumference should be evaluated for every child during each visit until the age of 2 years. Because cloth tape measures can stretch, the examiner should use either a metal or paper tape measure. The tape measure should be placed in front at midforehead level and in the back at the level of the occipital protuberance.
    3. For successful evaluation of the child's cervical lymph nodes, the neck muscles must be relaxed. We have found it most helpful to palpate both sides of the child's neck at the same time. This permits comparison of unilateral or bilateral findings.
    4. The techniques for evaluating the thyroid are the same as those for the adult. The examiner should use only two fingers of each hand as the tracheal stabilizer and lobe palpator, as opposed to all four fingers as with an adult client.
    5. Because of the lack of neck muscle stability in the infant, the examiner may elect to evaluate the thyroid from an anterior position with the infant supine.
- Lymph node presence in children seems to be the norm rather than the exception. The important point is to draw a relationship between the presence of lymph nodes and the general wellness or illness of the child. Barness states: "Shotty, discrete, movable, cool, nontender nodes up to 1 cm in the cervical region are normal when found in the child under 12 years of age."*
- When examining the child's head and neck, evaluate also the range of motion of the neck. Although an older child is instructed to perform this maneuver, younger children and infants should be passively moved through the ranges of neck motion.
- Before remarking on any unusual facial characteristics of a child, be sure to take a careful look at the parents.

RISK FACTORS FOR THE PEDIATRIC CLIENT

- Child whose fontanels close earlier than scheduled or remain open longer than scheduled
- Fontanels with diameters larger than 4 or 5 cm
- Child with overriding suture lines or suture lines that remain separated for a prolonged period
- Child whose head and chest circumferences are disproportionate before age 2
- Any bulge areas noted on the scalp or skull
- Child with multiple lymph nodes palpated (unexplained presence)
- Child with any supraclavicular nodes palpated
- Child whose neck does not seem to be growing in proportion to the body
- Any neck stiffness or crying with range-of-motion exercise
- Child who maintains a tonic neck reflex beyond 3 to 5 months
- Infant unable to hold head up by 2 months
- Infant, when in sitting position, unable to hold head steady by 4 months

---

*From Barness L: *Manual of pediatric physical diagnosis,* ed 5, Chicago, 1981, Mosby–Year Book, p 55.

CLINICAL VARIATIONS: THE CHILD

CHARACTERISTIC OR AREA EXAMINED	NORMAL FINDINGS	DEVIATIONS FROM NORMAL
a. Contour	Symmetry noted with frontal, parietal, and bilateral occipital prominences Long head in Nordic child Broad head in Oriental child	Asymmetry, marked depressions or protrusions Flattening of part of head Odd-shaped head that does not follow racial heritage Frontal bulging
b. Size (Measure during every visit until age 2 years.)	By age 2 years both chest and head circumferences are same size; during childhood chest becomes 5 to 7 cm larger than head (Table 4-2, p. 108)	Any sudden increase in head size Failure of head to grow

Continued.

CLINICAL VARIATIONS: THE CHILD—cont'd

CHARACTERISTIC OR AREA EXAMINED	NORMAL FINDINGS	DEVIATIONS FROM NORMAL
2. Sutures and fontanels (Fig. 4-22)	Suture ridges may be palpated until approximately 6 months Anterior fontanel: small or absent at birth; then enlarges to average 2.5 × 2.5 cm; normally closes between 9 months and 2 years	Sutures that are overriding or remain open beyond 6 months Late closure of fontanel (beyond 2 years)

TABLE 4-2   Head circumference norms for young children*

	BOYS (by percentile)			GIRLS (by percentile)		
AGE	10	50	90	10	50	90
Birth	33.5†	35.3	37.0	33.4	34.7	36.0
3 mo	39.2	40.9	42.1	38.5	40.0	41.7
6 mo	42.7	43.9	45.4	41.3	42.8	44.5
9 mo	44.5	46.0	47.1	43.1	44.6	46.3
12 mo	45.5	47.3	48.4	44.3	45.8	47.7
15 mo	46.3	48.0	49.2	44.9	46.3	48.4
18 mo	47.0	48.7	49.9	45.4	47.1	49.0
2 yr	48.0	49.7	51.0	46.4	48.1	50.1
2½ yr	48.5	50.2	51.6	47.0	48.8	50.8
3 yr	48.9	50.4	51.9	47.5	49.3	51.1

Data from Waring WW, Jeansone IO III: Practical manual of pediatrics: a pocket reference for those who treat children, *ed 2, St Louis, 1982, Mosby—Year Book.*

Head circumference growth rates:
    Full-term newborn-3 mo   2 cm/mo
    3-6 mo   1 cm/mo
    6 mo-1 yr   0.5 cm/mo
†*Measurements are given in centimeters.*

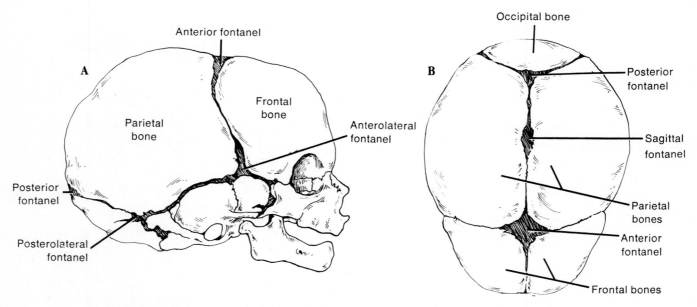

Fig. 4-22   Anatomical structures of infant's skull. **A,** Lateral view. **B,** Superior view.

CHARACTERISTIC OR AREA EXAMINED	NORMAL FINDINGS	DEVIATIONS FROM NORMAL
	Posterior fontanel: may or may not be able to palpate at birth; usually closes between 1 and 2 months	
a. Palpate fontanel for quality (Infant should be sitting and *not* crying; lying or crying may give fontanel a full or bulging appearance.)	No bulging Slight depression normal Slight palpitations	Bulging or significant depression Bounding palpitations
3. Scalp texture	Skin intact	Crusting Lesions, scabs Tenderness Ringworm patches Superficial nodules
4. Hair		White streaks from forehead toward crown (Waardenburg syndrome symptom) Lack of hair pigment Flaking
a. Foreign bodies	None present	Nits
b. Distribution	Even	Patchy, asymmetrical alopecia
c. Quantity	Thick, thin, sparse	Excessive loss
d. Quality	Shiny, smooth	Dull, brittle Excessive coarseness or dryness
e. Hygiene	Clean	Odor; matted, dirty
5. Face		
a. Symmetry	Eyes same level Symmetrical placement and shape of eyes, ears, mouth, eyebrows, nasolabial folds	Wide-set or close-set eyes Marked asymmetry Wide bulge at base of nose
b. Quality		Edema (especially of eyelids) Markedly coarse features Puffiness Excessive perspiration Waxy pallor Lesions Lip lesions, fissures, swelling Acne, scarring
c. Color	Pigmentation will vary with race	Jaundice Cyanosis (especially around lips) Pigmentation variations
d. Expression	Alert; response appropriate to conversation	No responsiveness Tense, drawn muscles Inappropriate expression
e. Movements	Controlled, smooth	Involuntary
6. Head and neck movements		
a. Passive range of motion with infants	Able to hold head up from prone position by 2 months Infants younger than 3 months have head lag when pulled into sitting position	Unable to hold head up by 2 months Head lag present beyond 3 months

CLINICAL VARIATIONS: THE CHILD—cont'd

CHARACTERISTIC OR AREA EXAMINED	NORMAL FINDINGS	DEVIATIONS FROM NORMAL
b. Active range of motion with older children (1) Ask child to look in each direction	Tonic neck reflex up to 5 months Infant in sitting position able to hold head steady by 4 months Controlled and smooth throughout series of movement No discomfort or limitations of movement	Tonic neck beyond 5 months Unable to hold head steady by 4 months Ratchety movement Bounding (up and down), synchronizes with pulse Pain throughout movement Pain of particular points during movement Spasms or tics Limited range of motion Unable to touch points
7. Neck a. Symmetry	Head position centered Bilateral symmetry of trapezius and sternocleidomastoid muscles Neck short with skinfolds between chin and shoulders during infancy; lengthens during next 3 to 4 years	Head tilted Muscle shortening, wasting Masses, scars Webbing (seen as extra folds of skin)
b. Palpate (Slightly extend chin upward to expose as much anterior neck as possible.) (1) Location	Central placement	Lateral displacement Tenderness on palpation
(2) Landmarks	Tracheal rings Cricoid cartilage Thyroid cartilage	
8. Thyroid (Palpation should be done using two or three fingers; evaluation will depend on cooperation of child.) a. Thyroid cartilage	Smooth Centrally located	
b. Cricoid cartilage	Smooth ringlike structure	
c. Isthmus	Smooth tissue found below cricoid cartilage May not be felt With swallowing may feel smooth tissue slide under skin	
d. Thyroid lobes	Lobes may not be felt If lobes are felt, they are small, smooth, nontender, and rise freely with swallowing	Enlarged lobes Palpated easily without swallowing Nodular or irregular lobe consistency Tender on palpation Gland not freely moving with swallowing
9. Lymphatic nodes a. Palpate the following nodes: (1) Preauricular (2) Postauricular (3) Occipital (4) Tonsillar (5) Submaxillary (6) Submental		

CHARACTERISTIC OR AREA EXAMINED	NORMAL FINDINGS	DEVIATIONS FROM NORMAL
(8) Posterior cervical (9) Deep cervical (10) Supraclavicular		
b. Size and shape	Usually not palpable or may be small, mobile, discrete, nontender Single nodes up to 1 cm; may appear as shotty, discrete, movable, cool, nontender	Palpable Large, round, cylindrical, irregular Multiple discrete or matted nodes Similar findings in children over 12 years of age
c. Mobility		Fixed to underlying or overlying tissue Induration
d. Consistency		Hard, firm, soft, spongy
e. Surface characteristics		Smooth, nodular
f. Tenderness		Tender on palpation
g. Heat		Present
h. Erythema		Present

 ## The Childbearing Woman

HISTORY AND CLINICAL STRATEGIES

- Note any history of goiter, neck surgery, or head and neck problems.
  1. Emergency general anesthesia is always a possibility, so prenatal examinations should include any structural defects or dental work that may interfere with intubation.
  2. Oral hygiene and diet should be noted so that problems during pregnancy can be avoided.
- Some women have headaches, especially during the first trimester of pregnancy. Any discomfort should be investigated, especially later in pregnancy when toxemia or another systemic problem may cause head pain.

CLINICAL VARIATIONS: THE CHILDBEARING WOMAN

CHARACTERISTIC OR AREA EXAMINED	NORMAL FINDINGS	DEVIATIONS FROM NORMAL
1. Characteristics	May develop blotchy, pigmented spots on face that disappear or fade after delivery (see Chapter 3)	
	Some enlargement of thyroid from hyperplasia and vascularity	Preexisting thyroid conditions require management
	Facial edema during last trimester	Edema may be sign of toxemia Higher incidence of Bell palsy during pregnancy
	Headaches (from hormonal influence on intracranial vascular system, usually subside after first trimester)	Severe, persistent headaches need investigation
2. After delivery	Characteristics such as edema, thyroid enlargement, and facial spots usually disappear soon after delivery	

The Older Adult

HISTORY AND CLINICAL STRATEGIES

- Mild tremors (rhythmic) of the head are reported by some authors as normal for some elderly people. However, beginning examiners should report any finding of this nature on the problem list.
- Head and neck range of motion should be assessed slowly and carefully. The single rotary movement, recommended on p. 99, for this assessment should not be performed with elderly individuals. Each movement should be evaluated separately for the following symptoms:
  1. Pain on movement
  2. Limited movement
  3. Jerky or "cogwheel" motion
  4. Dizziness accompanying or resulting from movement
  5. Crepitation
  6. Tension of muscles in neck during movement
- If neck pain and/or limitation of movement is a complaint, get full information about the following:
  1. Duration of problem
  2. Association of problem with trauma (e.g., from lifting, falling)
  3. Any additional discomfort or sensation (e.g., pain radiating to shoulders, arms, or chest or numbness in fingers or hands)

  4. Aggravating factors (e.g., necessity for stooping, lifting at home or work)
  5. Interference with activities of daily living (e.g., housework, driving automobile, discomfort during sleep, inability to look down while climbing or descending stairs)
- Dizziness associated with head and neck movements can pose a serious safety problem for the client. Inquire about client's ability to drive an automobile and to move about in the home and community safely.
- The submandibular salivary glands are rather large, palpable, soft, and symmetrical and lie approximately midway between the chin and the mandible angles on either side.
- A complaint of sudden (i.e., within 10 to 30 minutes) swelling under the mandible (usually just anterior to the ear) may be associated with parotid gland response to obstruction of a duct, duct spasm, or a stone in the duct. Clarify the timing of onset of swelling, duration (swelling may subside within 30 to 60 minutes), and whether swelling is associated with eating (during or immediately after). The gland may remain enlarged or may swell periodically. This should be considered a problem for referral, but the preceding information assists with the final differential diagnosis.
- Refer to pp. 104-105 for additional history and clinical strategy considerations.

CLINICAL VARIATIONS: THE OLDER ADULT

CHARACTERISTIC OR AREA EXAMINED	NORMAL FINDINGS	DEVIATIONS FROM NORMAL
1. Skull		
a. Contour	Rounded and symmetrical with frontal, parietal, and bilateral occipital prominences	Lumps, marked protrusions, depressions Lateral expansion of skull
b. Size	"Normal" encompasses a wide variety of sizes	Noticeably enlarged Abnormally small Protruding mandible
2. Scalp		
a. Surface characteristics	Skin intact and smooth	Lesions, scabs Tenderness Scaliness Superficial nodules
b. Color	Pigmentation varies with race	Reddened areas Areas of increased or decreased pigmentation
3. Hair		
a. Foreign bodies	None present	Flaking Nits, pediculi
b. Distribution	Even Bilateral, symmetrical balding	Patchy, asymmetrical alopecia

CHARACTERISTIC OR AREA EXAMINED	NORMAL FINDINGS	DEVIATIONS FROM NORMAL
	Women may exhibit increased facial hair over upper lip or on chin	
c. Quantity	Often less hair; appears thin or sparse	Sudden or excessive loss
d. Quality	Smooth; may have less luster than younger adult	Brittle Excessive coarseness or dryness
e. Hygiene	Clean	Odor; matted, dirty
4. Face		
a. Symmetry	Usually symmetrical; however, dentures or loss of some teeth may alter facial arrangement	Marked asymmetry (especially eyelids, nasolabial folds, smile pattern)
b. Quality	Expression is alert, responsive Wrinkling of skin, especially at forehead, mouth, eyes	Flat or expressionless (limited eye blinking) Edema (especially of eyelids) Markedly coarse features Puffiness Excessive perspiration Waxy pallor Lesions Lip lesions, fissures Swelling Cachectic Acne, scarring
c. Color	Pigmentation varies with race Color evenly distributed	Jaundice Cyanosis (especially around lips) Pigmentation variations
d. Expression	Alert; eye contact in response to conversation	Tense, drawn muscles Inappropriate expression
e. Movements	Controlled, smooth	Tremors, twitches, tics, involuntary movements (e.g., grinding motion of jaws, tremors either localized to lips or eyes or over entire head)
5. Head and neck position		
a. Observe head and neck while client is relaxed and looking straight ahead	Head, neck, and lower jaw may be thrust slightly forward (particularly if client manifests a kyphotic stance) Females may show a "dowager's hump," an accumulation of posterior fat over the cervical vertebrae	Head and neck held rigidly (diminished or absent cervical concavity); inability to thrust head forward normally
b. Involuntary movements	None present	Tremors (coarse or fine) Bounding (up and down) Synchronizes with pulse
c. Instruct client to: (1) Move chin to chest (Examiner places one hand over back of neck.)	Many elderly clients with cervical arthritis cannot touch chin to chest No discomfort or marked limitation	Pain with movement (*Note:* Pain may be referred to the ear.) Crepitation (felt by examiner) Gross limitation of movement or jerky motion

Continued.

CHARACTERISTIC OR AREA EXAMINED	NORMAL FINDINGS	DEVIATIONS FROM NORMAL
(2) Move chin toward right shoulder	Movement smooth and easily controlled	Client experiences pain, dizziness with side movements
(3) Move chin to left shoulder (Do not permit client to shrug or elevate shoulders.)	Smooth, easy motion No gross limitation (movement approximately 70 degrees from straight-ahead gaze in both directions)	Crepitation or limitation
(4) Move head toward right shoulder (so that client's ear is directed toward shoulder)	Client should be able to move head 40 degrees from midline in either direction	Pain, grossly limited movement Crepitation
(5) Move head toward left shoulder		
(6) Move head back so chin points toward ceiling	30 degrees back from straight-up position	Pain, grossly limited movement Crepitation
6. Neck a. Symmetry	Head position centered Bilateral symmetry of trapezius and sternocleidomastoid muscles	Head tilted Muscle asymmetry or shortening
b. Surface	Neck veins prominent; loss of subcutaneous fat Overlying skin is thin Smooth, symmetrical, and nontender on palpation	Marked muscle wasting or tension Tenderness, masses
7. Trachea a. Location	Central placement	Lateral displacement Tenderness on palpation
b. Landmarks	Tracheal rings Cricoid cartilage Thyroid cartilage	
8. Thyroid a. Symmetry	Gland usually not visible	Unilateral or bilateral lobe enlargement
b. Palpate along trachea for:	Smooth	
(1) Thyroid cartilage	Centrally located	
(2) Cricoid cartilage	Smooth ringlike structure	
(3) Isthmus	Smooth tissue found approximately 1 cm below cricoid cartilage May not be felt With swallowing may feel smooth tissue slide under skin	
(4) Thyroid lobes	Lobes may not be felt If lobes are felt, they are small, smooth, rise freely with swallowing Nontender	Enlarged lobes Palpated easily without swallowing Nodular or irregular lobe consistency Tender to palpation Gland not freely moving with swallowing
9. Lymphatic nodes a. Inspect and palpate the following nodes: (1) Preauricular (2) Postauricular (3) Occipital (4) Tonsillar (5) Submaxillary		

CHARACTERISTIC OR AREA EXAMINED	NORMAL FINDINGS	DEVIATIONS FROM NORMAL
(6) Submental		
(7) Superficial cervical		
(8) Posterior cervical		
(9) Deep cervical		
(10) Supraclavicular		
b. Size and shape	Usually not palpable	Palpable
c. Delimitation		Large, round, cylindrical, irregular
		Multiple discrete, or matted nodes
d. Mobility		Fixed to underlying or overlying tissue
		Induration
e. Consistency		Hard, firm, soft, spongy
f. Surface characteristics		Smooth, nodular
g. Tenderness		Tender on palpation
h. Heat		Present
i. Erythema		Present

 Study Questions

General

1. Which *one* of the following statements about cervical lymph nodes is *not* true:
   - ☐ a. The deep cervical chain is largely obscured by the sternocleidomastoid muscle
   - ☐ b. Normally, fasciocervical lymph nodes are not palpable in an adult
   - ☐ c. Lymphatics from the thorax drain up to the supraclavicular nodes
   - ☐ d. Deep, firm palpation is necessary to effectively reach the tonsillar nodes
   - ☐ e. Nodes enlarged as a consequence of prior inflammation are frequently palpable

2. An ear infection might involve all the following lymph nodes except one. Identify the *one not involved.*
   - ☐ a. Preauricular
   - ☐ b. Superficial cervical
   - ☐ c. Posterior cervical chain
   - ☐ d. Deep cervical chain
   - ☐ e. Postauricular

3. An infected tooth might involve all of the following lymph nodes except one. Identify the *one not involved.*
   - ☐ a. Posterior cervical
   - ☐ b. Submental
   - ☐ c. Submaxillary
   - ☐ d. Tonsillar
   - ☐ e. Deep cervical

4. The anterior triangle of the neck includes all but one of the following structures. Identify the *one not included.*
   - ☐ a. Thyroid gland
   - ☐ b. Anterior cervical nodes
   - ☐ c. Trachea
   - ☐ d. Carotid artery
   - ☐ e. Omohyoid muscle

5. The largest endocrine gland in the body is the:
   - ☐ a. Adrenal gland
   - ☐ b. Parotid gland
   - ☐ c. Thyroid gland
   - ☐ d. Ovary
   - ☐ e. Submaxillary gland

6. Swallowing causes the lateral parts of the thyroid tissue to _____ against the examiner's fingers.
   - ☐ a. Fall
   - ☐ b. Rise
   - ☐ c. Bulge
   - ☐ d. Remain stationary

7. The thyroid isthmus is not easily palpated:
   - ☐ a. Just above the cricoid cartilage
   - ☐ b. Just below the cricoid cartilage
   - ☐ c. Just below the thyroid cartilage
   - ☐ d. Just above the thyroid cartilage
   - ☐ e. Just below the hyoid bone

The Newborn

Select the *one* best answer to the following questions.

8. What is a usual finding of a newborn's head:
   - ☐ a. Asymmetrical shape
   - ☐ b. Cephalhematoma
   - ☐ c. Cranial bruit
   - ☐ d. Caput succedaneum

9. A bulging fontanel suggests:
   - ☐ a. Dehydration
   - ☐ b. Intracranial pressure
   - ☐ c. Craniotabes
   - ☐ d. Brain tumor

10. Which of the following characteristics would you expect to find when examining a newborn's head and neck:
    - ☐ a. Pronounced trachea, receding chin
    - ☐ b. Rigid neck, asymmetrical cheeks
    - ☐ c. Small thymus, torticollis
    - ☐ d. Neck webbing, thin cheeks

The Child

11. When palpating the skull of a 4-month-old child, the examiner would *expect* the following *normal findings:*
    - ☐ a. Skull size of 36 cm
    - ☑ b. Sagittal suture palpated
    - ☐ c. Coronal suture palpated
    - ☐ d. Anterior fontanel approximately 2 × 2 cm; soft, not full
    - ☐ e. Posterior fontanel approximately 1 × 1 cm; soft, not full
    - ☐ f. All except b
    - ☐ g. All except c
    - ☐ h. All except a
    - ☐ i. All except e
    - ☐ j. All of the above

The Childbearing Woman

Select the *one* best answer to the following questions.

12. Hyperplasia and vascularity during pregnancy may result in an enlarged:
    - ☐ a. Nasal septum
    - ☐ b. Parotid cyst
    - ☐ c. Thyroid gland
    - ☐ d. Intracranial space

The Older Adult

13. When assessing an elderly client for head and neck range of motion:
    - ☐ a. A single rotary motion is a good screening mechanism
    - ☐ b. Assess for dizziness associated with movement
    - ☐ c. Crepitation may be felt by the examiner
    - ☐ d. Assess for jerky motions
    - ☐ e. Ask client to shrug shoulders to complete full range of motion testing
    - ☐ f. All of the above
    - ☐ g. b, c, and d
    - ☐ h. a, c, and e
    - ☐ i. All except b

14. Painful limited head and neck motion:
    - ☐ a. Can be accompanied by pain radiating to shoulders and arms
    - ☐ b. Can impose safety risks on client
    - ☐ c. Can always be resolved with proper exercises and rest
    - ☐ d. All of the above
    - ☐ e. a and b

SUGGESTED READINGS
General

Bates B: *A guide to physical examination,* ed 5, Philadelphia, 1991, JB Lippincott.

Examination of the head and neck, *Am J Nurs* 75(5):1, 1975.

Malasanos L, Barkauskas V, Stoltenberg AK: *Health assessment,* ed 4, St Louis, 1990, Mosby—Year Book

Long BC, Woods NF, Cassmeyer VL: *Medical-surgical nursing: concepts and clinical practice,* ed 4, St Louis, 1991, Mosby—Year Book.

Prior JA, Silberstein JS, Stang JM: *Physical diagnosis: the history and examination of the patient,* ed 6, St Louis, 1981, Mosby—Year Book.

Werner SC, Ingbar SH: *The thyroid: a fundamental and clinical text,* ed 4, New York, 1978, Harper & Row.

The newborn

Auvenshine MA, Enriquez MG: *Maternity nursing: dimensions of change,* Belmont, Calif, 1985, Wadsworth.

Beischer NA, MacKay EV: *Obstetrics and the newborn: an illustrated textbook,* ed 2, Philadelphia, 1986, WB Saunders.

Bobak IM, Jensen MD: *Essentials of maternity nursing,* ed 3, St Louis, 1991, Mosby—Year Book.

Judd JM: Assessing the newborn from head to toe, *Nurs '85* 15(12):34, 1985.

Kiernan BS, Scoloveno MA: Assessment of the neonate, *Top Clin Nurs* 8(1):1, 1986.

The Organization for Obstetrical, Gynecological and Neonatal Nurses (NAACOG): *Physical assessment of the neonate,* OGN Nursing Practice Resource, Oct. 1986, The Association.

Pillitteri, A: *Maternal-newborn nursing: care of the growing family,* ed 3, Boston, 1985, Little, Brown.

Pritchard JA, MacDonald PC: *Williams' obstetrics,* ed 17, New York, 1985, Appleton-Century-Crofts.

Scanlon JW and others: *A system of newborn physical examination,* Baltimore, 1979, University Park Press.

Seidel HM, Ball JW, Dains JE, Benedict GW: *Mosby's guide to physical examination,* ed 2, St Louis, 1991, Mosby—Year Book.

Whaley LF, Wong DL: *Nursing care of infants and children,* ed 4, St Louis, 1991, Mosby—Year Book.

The child

Barness L: *Manual of pediatric physical diagnosis,* ed 6, Chicago, 1990, Mosby—Year Book.

Brown MS, Alexander M: Physical examination. IV. The lymph system, *Nurs '73* 3(10):49, 1973.

Brown MS, Alexander M: Physical examination. VI. The head, face, and neck *Nurs '74* 4(1):47, 1974.

DeAngelis C: *Pediatric primary care,* ed 3, Boston, 1984, Little, Brown.

Whaley LF, Wong DL: *Essentials of pediatric nursing,* ed 3, St Louis, 1989, Mosby—Year Book.

The childbearing woman

Auvenshine MA, Enriquez MG: *Maternity nursing: dimensions of change,* Belmont, Calif, 1985, Wadsworth.

Beischer NA, MacKay EV: *Obstetrics and the newborn: an illustrated textbook,* ed 2, Philadelphia, 1986, WB Saunders.

Bobak IM, Jensen MD: *Essentials of maternity nursing,* ed 3, St Louis, 1991, Mosby—Year Book.

Pilletteri A: *Maternal-newborn nursing: care of the growing family,* ed 3, Boston, 1985, Little, Brown.

Pritchard JA, MacDonald PC: *Williams' obstetrics,* ed 17, New York, 1985, Appleton-Century-Crofts.

Seidel HM, Ball JW, Dains JE, Benedict GW: *Mosby's guide to physical examination,* ed 2, St Louis, 1991, Mosby—Year Book.

Whitley N: *A manual of clinical obstetrics,* Philadelphia, 1985, JB Lippincott.

The older adult

Caird FI, Judge TG: *Assessment of the elderly patient,* London, 1977, Pitman Medical Publishing.

Carotenuto R, Bullock J: *Physical assessment of the gerontologic client,* Philadelphia, 1980, FA Davis.

Seidel HM, Ball JW, Dains JE, Benedict GW: *Mosby's guide to physical examination,* ed 2, St Louis, 1991, Mosby—Year Book.

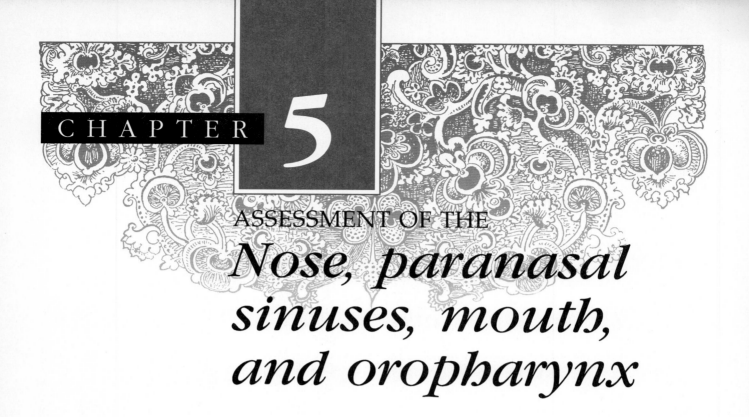

CHAPTER 5

ASSESSMENT OF THE
Nose, paranasal sinuses, mouth, and oropharynx

VOCABULARY

alveolar ridge Bony prominences of the maxilla and mandible that support the teeth; in edentulous clients these structures support dentures.

aphthous ulcer (canker sore) A painful ulcer on the mucous membrane of the mouth.

attrition of teeth Wearing away of the occlusal surfaces of the teeth from many years of chewing or excessive grinding.

bruxism Grinding of the teeth; usually an unconscious act occurring during sleep.

buccal Pertaining to the inside of the cheek.

epistaxis Bleeding from the nose.

epulis Any growth on the gum.

Fordyce spots Small, yellow spots on the buccal membrane that are visible sebaceous glands; a normal phenomenon seen in many adults, but sometimes mistaken for abnormal lesions; also called *Fordyce granules*.

frenulum (lingual) Band of tissue that attaches the ventral surface of the tongue to the floor of the mouth.

gingiva Pertaining to the gum.

glossitis An inflammation of the tongue.

leukoplakia Thickened, white, well-circumscribed patch that can appear on any mucous membrane; sometimes precancerous; often a response to chronic irritation, such as pipe smoking.

nares (singular: naris) Nostrils; the anterior openings of the nose.

papilla General term for a small projection; dorsal surface of the tongue is composed of a variety of forms of papillae that contain openings to the taste buds.

periodontitis (pyorrhea) Inflammation and deterioration of the gums and supporting alveolar bone; occurs in varying degrees of severity; if neglected, this condition will result in loss of teeth.

perlèche (cheilosis, cheilitis) Fissures at the corners of the mouth that become inflamed; causes are overclosure of the mouth in an edentulous client, marked loss of alveolar ridge, or riboflavin deficiency; saliva irritates the area, and moniliasis is a common complication.

plaque Film that accumulates on the surface of teeth; made up of mucin and colloidal material from saliva, plaque is subject to bacterial invasion.

ptyalism Excessive salivation.

rhino- Combining form pertaining to the nose.

> EXAMPLE: *Rhinitis* is an inflammation of the mucous membrane of the nose.

stoma General term that means opening or mouth.

> EXAMPLE: *Stomatitis* refers to a general inflammation of the oral cavity.

torus palatinus Exostosis, or benign outgrowth of bone, located on the midline of the hard palate; a fairly common finding that appears in a variety of shapes and sizes.

turbinates Extensions of the ethmoid bone located along the lateral wall of the nose; these fingerlike projections are covered with erectile mucosal membranes that become swollen or inflamed in response to allergy or viral invasion.

vermilion border Demarcation point between the mucosal membrane of the lips and the skin of the face; common site for recurrent infections, such as herpes infections, and carcinoma; blurring of this border may be an early sign of lesion development.

xerostomia Dryness of the mouth.

ANATOMY AND PHYSIOLOGY REVIEW
The Nose and Paranasal Sinuses

The upper third of the nose is encased in bone, which attaches to the forehead (frontal bone). The bone extends to the lower two thirds of the nose, which is composed of cartilage (Fig. 5-1). The septal cartilage maintains the shape of the nose and separates the nares (nostrils), which maintain an open passage for air. The nasal cavity is lined with a highly vascular mucous membrane that contains cilia (nasal hairs), which trap airborne particles and prevent them from reaching the lungs. The lateral walls of the nasal cavity are lined with the inferior, middle, and superior turbinates (bony protrusions covered with mucous membrane), which contain openings, or meatuses (Fig. 5-2). The inferior meatus drains tears from the nasolacrimal duct, and the middle meatus serves as an outlet for paranasal sinus drainage.

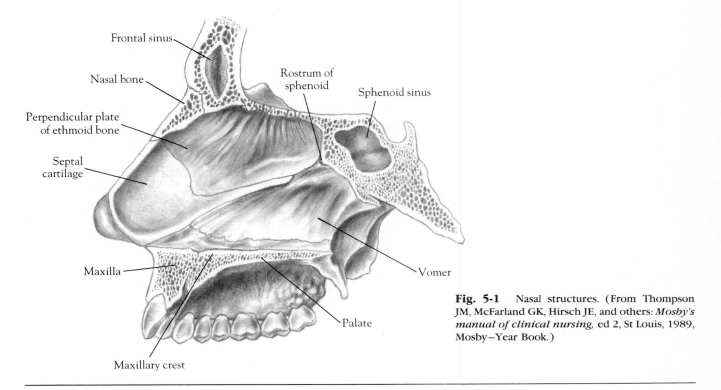

Fig. 5-1 Nasal structures. (From Thompson JM, McFarland GK, Hirsch JE, and others: *Mosby's manual of clinical nursing,* ed 2, St Louis, 1989, Mosby—Year Book.)

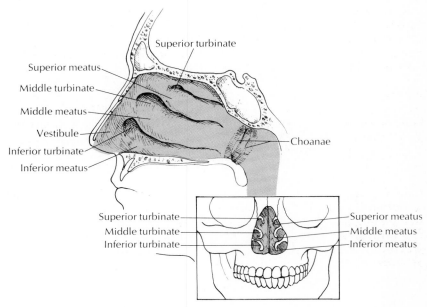

Fig. 5-2 Nasal turbinates. (From Malasanos L, Barkauskas V, Stoltenberg-Allen K: *Health assessment,* ed 4, St Louis, 1990, Mosby—Year Book.)

The paranasal sinuses extend out of the nasal cavities through narrow openings into the skull bones to form bilateral (paired), air-filled, mucous membrane–lined pockets. The sphenoidal, frontal, ethmoidal, and maxillary sinuses constitute the paranasal sinuses (Fig. 5-3).

The Mouth

The mouth contains the tongue, which has hundreds of taste buds (papillae) on its dorsal surface. The taste buds distinguish sweet, sour, bitter, and salty tastes. The ventral surface is smooth and very vascular. Three pairs of salivary glands—the submandibular, the sublingual, and the parotid—release saliva through small openings (ducts) in response to the presence of food particles, to begin the process of digestion (Fig. 5-4). The submandibular glands are tucked under the mandible and lie approximately midway between the chin and the posterior mandibular angle. They are soft, symmetrical, and

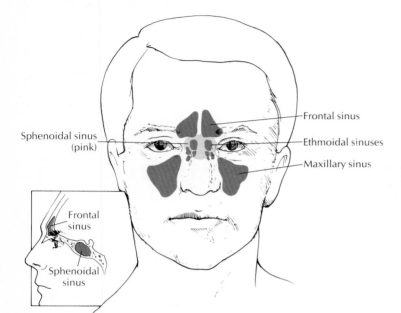

Sphenoidal sinus (pink)

Frontal sinus

Ethmoidal sinuses

Maxillary sinus

Frontal sinus

Sphenoidal sinus

Fig. 5-3   Paranasal sinuses. (From Malasanos L, Barkauskas V, Stoltenberg-Allen K: *Health assessment,* ed 4, St Louis, 1990, Mosby–Year Book.)

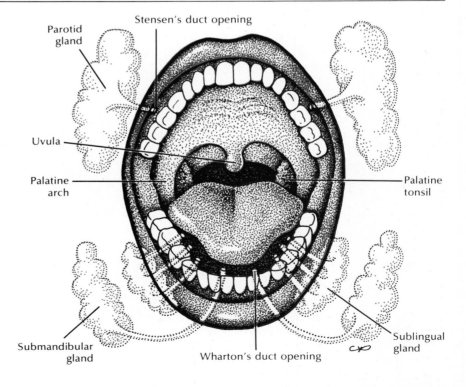

Parotid gland

Stensen's duct opening

Uvula

Palatine arch

Palatine tonsil

Submandibular gland

Wharton's duct opening

Sublingual gland

Fig. 5-4   Structures of the mouth. (From Malasanos L, Barkauskas V, Stoltenberg-Allen K: *Health assessment,* ed 4, St Louis, 1990, Mosby–Year Book.)

palpable and are sometimes mistaken for lymph nodes by the beginning examiner. The parotid glands are anterior to the ears immediately above the mandibular angle. They are not palpable unless they are enlarged. The sublingual glands lie on the floor of the mouth and are not palpable or visible. Wharton's duct, the opening for the submandibular gland, is visible on both sides of the floor of the mouth under the tongue. Stensen's ducts (parotid gland openings) are visible on both sides of the cheek adjacent to the second molars.

The normal adult has 32 teeth, which are tightly en-cased in mucous membrane–covered, fibrous gum tissue and rooted in the alveolar ridges of the maxilla and mandible (Fig. 5-5). The third molars are congenitally absent in some adults.

The Oropharynx

The oropharynx includes the structures behind the mouth that are visible on examination: the uvula, the anterior and posterior pillars, the tonsils, and the posterior pharyngeal wall (Fig. 5-6). The uvula is suspended, midline, from the soft palate, which extends out to either

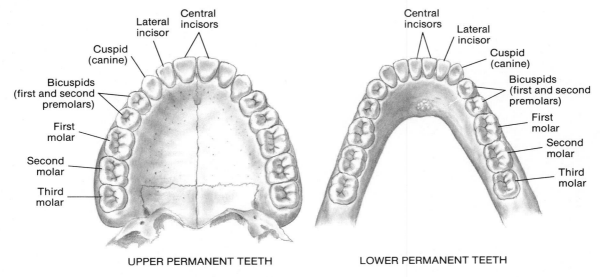

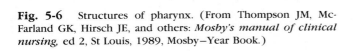

Fig. 5-5   Upper and lower permanent teeth. (From Seidel HM, Ball JW, Dains JE, Benedict GW: *Mosby's guide to physical examination,* St Louis, 1987, Mosby–Year Book.)

Fig. 5-6   Structures of pharynx. (From Thompson JM, Mc-Farland GK, Hirsch JE, and others: *Mosby's manual of clinical nursing,* ed 2, St Louis, 1989, Mosby–Year Book.)

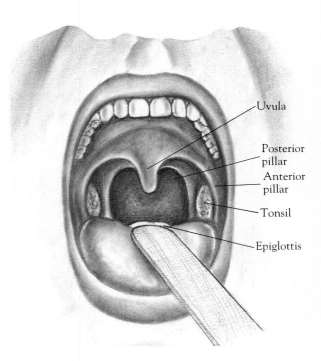

side to form the anterior pillar. The tonsils are tucked in between the anterior and posterior pillars and may be normally atrophied in adults to the point of being barely visible. The posterior pharyngeal wall is visible when the tongue is extended and depressed. The wall is highly vascular and may show color variations of red and pink because of the presence of small vessels and lymphoid tissue. The epiglottis, a cartilagenous structure that protects the laryngeal opening, sometimes projects into the pharyngeal area and is visible as the tongue is depressed.

COGNITIVE OBJECTIVES

At the end of this chapter the learner will demonstrate knowledge of assessment of the nose, paranasal sinuses, mouth, and oropharynx by the ability to do the following:

- Apply the terms that are listed in the vocabulary section.
- List inspection criteria and processes for evaluating the external and internal nose, including nasal structure, turbinates, meatuses, and septum.
- List inspection and palpation criteria for evaluating the maxillary and frontal sinuses.
- Discuss a systematic method to test intactness of the olfactory nerve (cranial nerve [CN] I).
- Identify the anterior and posterior boundaries of the mouth.
- Describe characteristics of the lips, gums, tongue, teeth, and buccal mucosa that are relevant to assessment.
- Point out characteristics of the oropharynx that are relevant to assessment.
- Identify selected common physical variations with the newborn, the child, the childbearing woman, and the older adult.

CLINICAL OUTLINE

At the end of this chapter the learner will perform a systematic assessment of the nose, paranasal sinuses, mouth, and oropharynx by demonstrating the ability to do the following:

- Obtain a pertinent health history from a client.
- Demonstrate and describe results of inspection and palpation of the following:
  1. External and internal nose for structure, septum position, patency, turbinates, and meatuses
  2. Frontal and maxillary sinuses
  3. Temporomandibular joint for mobility, tenderness, crepitus, referred pain, and occlusion
  4. Lips for color, symmetry, moisture, and surface characteristics
  5. Gingivobuccal fornices and buccal mucosa for color, landmarks, and surface characteristics
  6. Gums for color and surface characteristics

  7. Teeth for number, color, form, surface characteristics, and insertion
  8. Tongue for symmetry, movement, color, surface characteristics, and texture
  9. Floor of mouth for color and surface characteristics
  10. Hard and soft palates for color and surface characteristics
- Describe results of inspection and observation of the mouth and the oropharynx for landmarks, color, surface, and odor.
- Summarize results of the assessment with a written description of the findings.

HISTORY

- If client complains of nasal passage obstruction, ask the following questions:
  1. Is there a history of nasal surgery?
  2. Is there a history of blow or injury to nose?
  3. Are both nares usually obstructed, or just one?
  4. Is it often necessary to breathe through the mouth (especially at night)?
  5. Is there a history of discharge followed by crusting and localized pain? Is nose picking or scratching contributing to the problem?
  6. Are nose drops or nasal spray used? Clarify type, amount, frequency, and how long client has used medication.
- If client has a history of nosebleeds, ask the following questions:
  1. Does bleeding usually occur from both nostrils, or just right or left naris?
  2. Is bleeding aggravated by crusting? Is pain followed by picking or scratching?
  3. Do full symptom analysis with this complaint.
- Is there a history of repeated sinusitis? General treatment?
- Is there a history of chronic postnasal drip? Is it associated with seasons or weather changes?
- If mouth or dental problems are observed, the following inquiries are appropriate:
  1. Do you experience pain? If so, how severe and how often? Do you treat the pain? What medications? How often? Do you apply anything locally to teeth or gums? What and how often?
  2. Do your mouth problems interfere with or alter food intake? Describe foods that you can no longer eat.
  3. Are other members of the family having dental or mouth problems?
- If lesions are observed on mouth or lips, inquire about:
  1. Efforts to treat (medications or local applications).
  2. Whether lesions disappear and reappear. Identify pattern, if possible, associated with foods, stress, seasons, fatigue.

3. Whether others close to client have lesions.
4. Whether client smokes a pipe.
- If client wears dentures, inquire about their effectiveness:
    1. Are they worn all the time? Just for meals?
    2. Do they permit the eating and chewing of all foods?
    3. Are they loose or wobbly?
    4. Do they click or whistle or interfere with talking?
    5. Are adhesives used to retain dentures in place?
    6. Ask about denture cleaning habits.
    7. Are gums or palate ever irritated or tender?
    8. Does client feel that the dentures are cosmetically satisfactory?
- If client complains of or offers a history of sore throat, ask the following questions:
    1. Are others in your home ill at present time or do others close to you often have colds or sore throats?
    2. Do you have to inhale dust or fumes at work?
    3. Does it feel as though you have a lump in your throat?

4. Does it hurt to swallow?
5. Is the sore throat associated with fever, cough, headache, decreased appetite?
6. Is your nose obstructed ("stopped up"); do you have to breathe through your mouth?
7. Is your throat more tender in the morning? Evening?
8. Is your home dry (humidity level)?
9. Is sore throat associated with hoarseness?
10. Treatment (medications, gargling)?
- If client complains of a hoarse voice (either acute, intermittent, or chronic), ask:
    1. Do you use your voice a lot?
    2. Is hoarseness associated with fever, sore throat, or cold symptoms?
    3. Does the weather affect your voice?
    4. In addition to hoarseness, has your voice changed (e.g., weak, husky, higher, or lower pitch)?
    5. Do you have a constant urge to clear your throat?

Text continues on p. 134.

CLINICAL GUIDELINES

ASSESSMENT PROCEDURE	EVALUATION	
	NORMAL FINDINGS	DEVIATIONS FROM NORMAL

1. Assemble necessary equipment
  a. Gloves
  b. Penlight
  c. Otoscope with broad-tipped nasal speculum or nasal speculum		

2. Inspect general appearance of nose		
a. Surface/skin	Smooth, intact Skin color same as face	Lesions, warty appearance Redness, discoloration Vascularization
b. Contour	External alignment symmetrical (or nearly symmetrical)	Marked asymmetry Swelling or hypertrophy (bulbous appearance)
c. Nares	Symmetrical Dry, no crusting No flaring or narrowing associated with breathing	Discharge present, crusting Narrowing on inspiration (associated with chronic obstruction and mouth breathing)
3. Press finger on side of client's nose to occlude one naris, and ask client to close mouth and breathe through opposite side to test for patency; repeat with other naris	Noiseless, free exchange of air through each naris	Breathing noisy or obstructed
4. Palpate external nose for: a. Stability	Firm	Unstable

Continued.

ASSESSMENT PROCEDURE	EVALUATION	
	NORMAL FINDINGS	DEVIATIONS FROM NORMAL
b. Tenderness	Nontender	Tender on palpation; masses
5. Evaluate olfactory nerve (CN I): ask client to close eyes and mouth; occlude one naris at a time, and hold aromatic substance (lemon extract, coffee) under each nostril for odor identification	Client able to identify odor	Incorrect identification of odor
6. Inspect internal nasal cavity using nasal speculum: hold speculum in left hand and stabilize with index finger against side of nose; insert speculum approximately 1 cm, and dilate outer naris as much as possible (Fig. 5-7); use right hand to adjust client's head and to hold penlight, or use otoscope with nasal speculum attached; observe naris:		
a. With client's head erect (Fig. 5-8)	Floor of nose (vestibule) Inferior turbinate	Furuncle (most often present in vestibule)

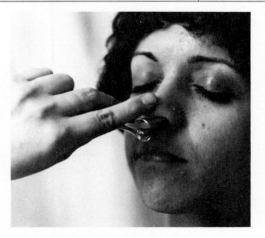

Fig. 5-7 Nasal speculum insertion.

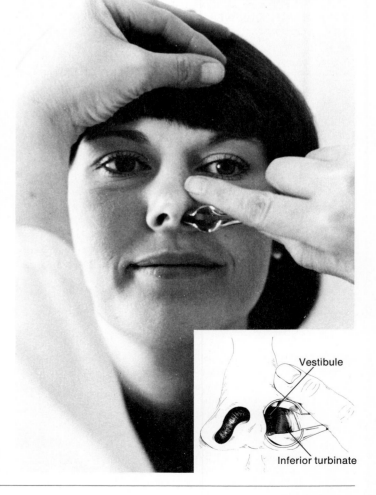

Fig. 5-8 Nasal speculum inserted; view of naris with head in upright position.

	EVALUATION	
ASSESSMENT PROCEDURE	**NORMAL FINDINGS**	**DEVIATIONS FROM NORMAL**
	Nasal hairs present Mucosa slightly darker (redder) than oral mucosa	Tenderness Marked redness Crusting, discharge Lesions or masses
b. With client's head back (Fig. 5-9)	Middle meatus Middle turbinate Turbinates same color as surrounding nasal mucosa	Sinus drainage Polyps, masses Turbinates appear pale, swollen (allergic responses) Mucosa markedly red with copious discharge
c. With client's head to side (Fig. 5-10); repeat with opposite naris	Film of clear discharge (small amount) Lower third is vascular area (Kiesselbach area)	Yellow, thick, green discharge Bleeding, crusting Tenderness Lesions

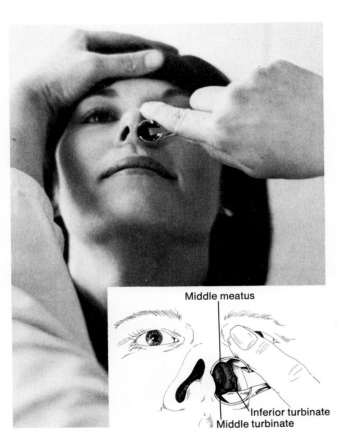

Fig. 5-10 Nasal speculum inserted; view of naris with head turned to side.

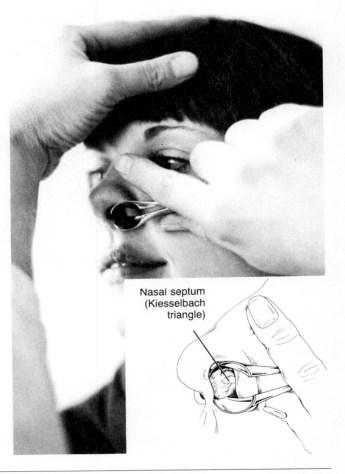

Fig. 5-9 Nasal speculum inserted; view of naris with head tilted back.

Continued.

CLINICAL GUIDELINES—cont'd

ASSESSMENT PROCEDURE	EVALUATION	
	NORMAL FINDINGS	DEVIATIONS FROM NORMAL
	Septum midline and straight (*Note:* Many normal individuals show a slight deviation of the septum without symptoms of occlusion.)	Marked deviation of septum

d. Inspect and palpate paranasal sinuses for tenderness and swelling
       1. Frontal (Fig. 5-11)
       2. Maxillary (Fig. 5-12)
	Nontender
	No swelling
		Tender on palpation
		Swelling of soft tissue over sinus area

7. Assemble equipment for examination of mouth and pharynx:
    a. Penlight
    b. Two tongue blades
    c. Two 4 × 4–inch gauze sponges
    d. Gloves or finger cots		

8. Inspect, palpate, and maneuver temporomandibular joint: place fingers in front of each ear and ask client to open and close mouth slowly (Fig. 5-13) a. Mobility	Smooth jaw excursion, 3.5 to 4.5 cm (1⅓ to 1¾ inches)	Limited excursion
b. Tenderness	Absent on palpation	Present on palpation
c. Crepitus	Absent	Present
d. Referred pain	Absent	Present (especially on closure of jaw)

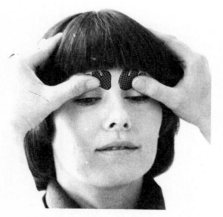

Fig. 5-11 Palpating frontal sinuses.

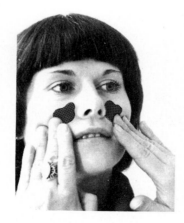

Fig. 5-12 Palpating maxillary sinuses.

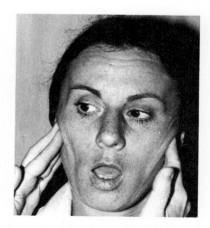

Fig. 5-13 Palpating the temporomandibular joint.

ASSESSMENT PROCEDURE	EVALUATION	
	NORMAL FINDINGS	DEVIATIONS FROM NORMAL
9. Inspect closed mouth: ask client to clench teeth and smile a. Occlusion	Top back teeth rest directly on lower teeth; upper incisors slightly override lowers (Fig. 5-14)	Protrusion of upper incisors Protrusion of lower incisors Upper incisors do not overlap lowers on closure (Fig. 5-15) Lateral displacement of teeth; back teeth do not occlude Separation or malalignment of individual teeth
10. Inspect and palpate lips for: a. Color	Pink	Pale, cyanotic, reddened
b. Symmetry	Vertical and lateral symmetry at rest or on movement	Swelling (general or localized), induration
c. Moisture	Smooth and moist	Dry, flaking, cracked

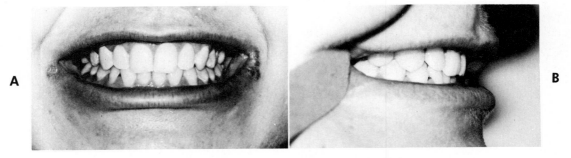

Fig. 5-14 Normal occlusion. **A,** Front view. Note vesicular and ulceration patterns at the corners of the mouth. **B,** Lateral view.

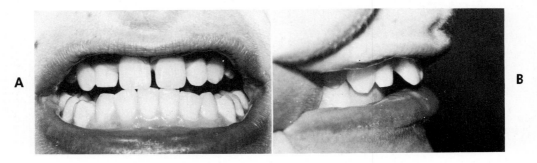

Fig. 5-15 Example of malocclusion. **A,** Front view. **B,** Profile.

Continued.

CLINICAL GUIDELINES—cont'd

	EVALUATION	
ASSESSMENT PROCEDURE	NORMAL FINDINGS	DEVIATIONS FROM NORMAL
d. Surface characteristics	Slight vertical linear markings	Lesions: plaques, vesicles (Fig. 5-16), nodules, ulcerations Inflamed fissures at corners
11. Ask client to remove any dental appliances and to open mouth partially; inspect and palpate inner lips and upper and lower gingivobuccal fornices; ask client to open mouth wide, and inspect buccal mucosa; use tongue blade and penlight		
a. Color	Pale coral, pink Increased pigmentation (general or localized) with dark-skinned individuals	Pale, cyanotic, reddened Local deposits of brown pigmentation
b. Landmarks	Parotid duct (pinpoint red marking); may be slightly elevated (Fig. 5-17)	
c. Surface characteristics	Smooth Where teeth meet, occlusion line may appear on adjacent mucosa (Fig. 5-17) Clear saliva over surface	Ulcers White patches White plaques Swelling (local/general) Bleeding Excessively dry mouth Excessive salivation
12. Inspect and palpate gums for: a. Color	Pink, coral	Reddened, pale

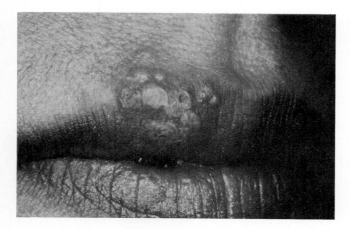

Fig. 5-16 Herpes simplex I. (Courtesy Dr. George Blozis, The Ohio State University College of Dentistry, Columbus, Ohio.)

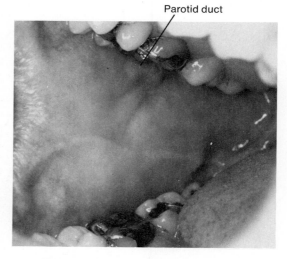

Parotid duct

Fig. 5-17 Occlusion line on buccal membrane. Note parotid (Stensen) duct. (Courtesy Dr. George Blozis, The Ohio State University College of Dentistry, Columbus, Ohio.)

ASSESSMENT PROCEDURE	EVALUATION	
	NORMAL FINDINGS	DEVIATIONS FROM NORMAL
b. Surface characteristics	Slightly stippled (Fig. 5-18) Clearly defined, tight margin at tooth Patchy brown pigmentation (usually with dark-skinned individuals)	Swelling (stippling disappears) Bleeding with slight pressure Enlarged crevice between teeth and gums Pockets containing debris at tooth margin (Fig. 5-19) Gingivitis and edema can develop into advanced pyorrhea, with erosion of gum tissue, destruction of underlying bone, and loosening of teeth (Fig. 5-20)

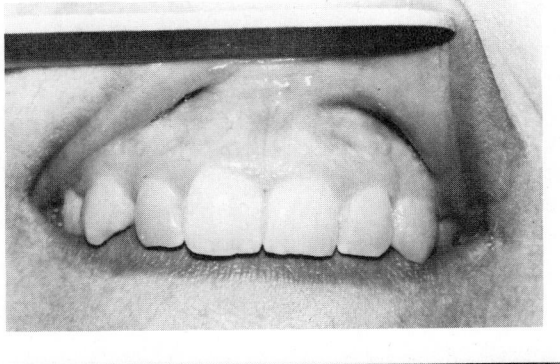

Fig. 5-18   Slightly stippled gum surface is a normal characteristic.

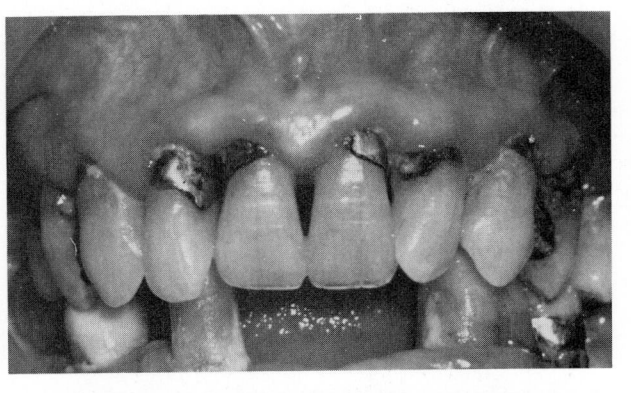

Fig. 5-19   Pockets containing debris at tooth margin.

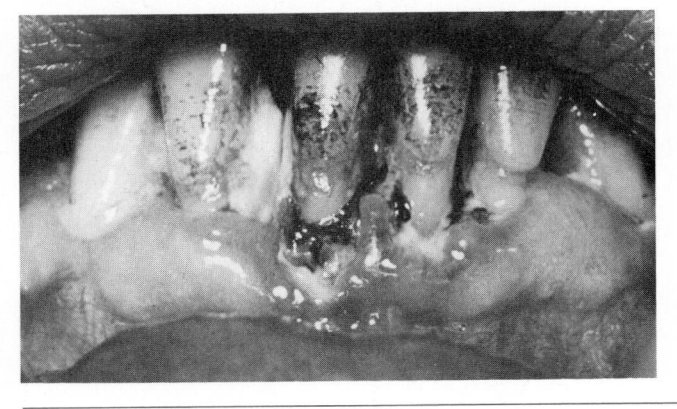

Fig. 5-20   Advanced pyorrhea. (From DeWeese DD, Saunders WH, Schuller DE, Schleuning AJ II: *Otolaryngology—head and neck surgery,* ed 7, St Louis, 1988, Mosby–Year Book.)

Continued.

CLINICAL GUIDELINES—cont'd

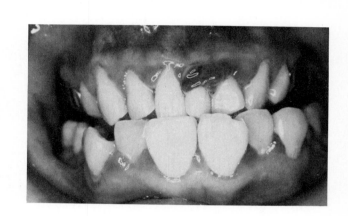

Fig. 5-21 Pregnancy gingivitis with hypertrophy. (Courtesy Dr. George Blozis, The Ohio State University College of Dentistry, Columbus, Ohio.)

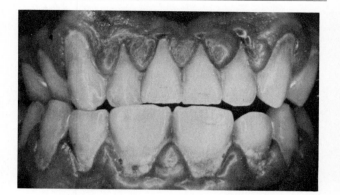

Fig. 5-22 Marked enlargement of gums. (Courtesy Dr. Leonard K. Ebel, The Ohio State University College of Dentistry, Columbus, Ohio.)

EVALUATION		
ASSESSMENT PROCEDURE	NORMAL FINDINGS	DEVIATIONS FROM NORMAL
	Hypertrophy may appear at puberty or during pregnancy (Fig. 5-21) If inflammation (gingivitis) appears, client should be referred for evaluation by dentist	Ulcer, epulis Blue-black line at gum margin Marked enlargement (Fig. 5-22) Tenderness on palpation White patches (especially with edentulous clients)
13. Inspect teeth for: a. Number	Thirty-two teeth (full adult) (see Fig. 5-5) Upper and/or lower third molars sometimes congenitally absent	Missing teeth
b. Color	White, yellow, or gray hues	Darkened, stained (individual teeth or all)
c. Form	Smooth edges	Central incisor notching Irregular notching Broken Peglike Debris present (especially at gum line)
d. Surface characteristics	Smooth Dental restorations present	

ASSESSMENT PROCEDURE	EVALUATION	
	NORMAL FINDINGS	DEVIATIONS FROM NORMAL
		Caries (Fig. 5-23)
		Much tooth neck exposed, with receding gums
14. Maneuver teeth for tightness	No movement or slight movement	Marked movement (generalized or localized)
15. Inspect and palpate tongue: ask client to protrude tongue		
a. Symmetry and movement	Forward thrust smooth and symmetrical	Unilateral atrophy
		Lateral movement
	Appearance of tongue symmetrical	Fasciculation
b. Color	Pink	Red
c. Surface characteristics	Dorsal and lateral:	
	Moist, glistening coating	
	Papillae present	Papillae absent
	Elongated vallate papillae	Lesions

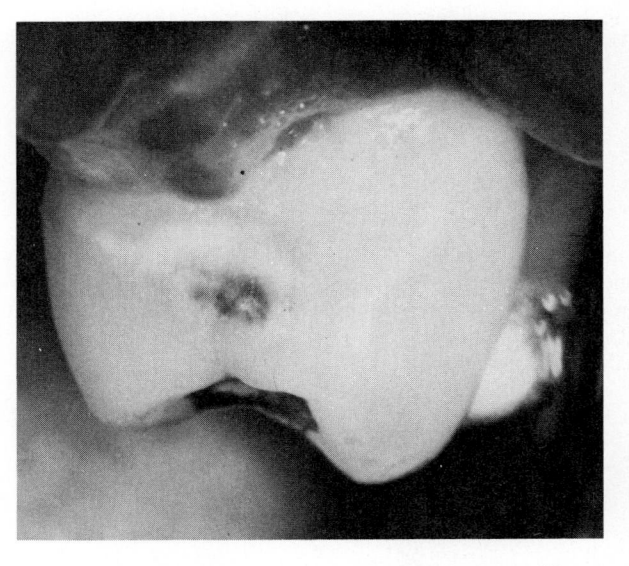

Fig. 5-23   Early tooth decay with surface intact. (Courtesy Dr. George Blozis, The Ohio State University College of Dentistry, Columbus, Ohio.)

Continued.

	EVALUATION	
ASSESSMENT PROCEDURE	NORMAL FINDINGS	EVIATIONS FROM NORMAL
16. Grasp tongue with 4 × 4 -inch gauze pad, and palpate all sides for texture	Fissures present (Fig. 5-24) Smooth, even tissue	Lumps, nodules Induration
17. Ask client to put tongue to roof of mouth; inspect and palpate	Pink and smooth, with large veins (Fig. 5-25)	Lesions, patches

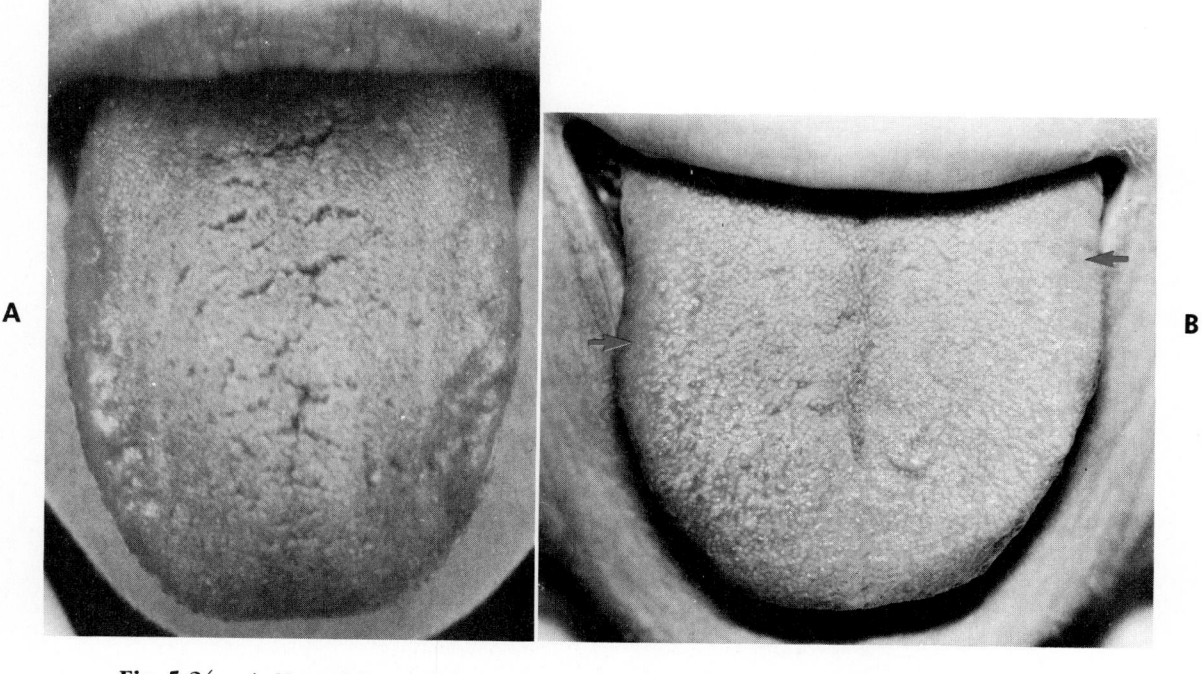

Fig. 5-24 **A,** Normal dorsal surface of tongue. Note papillae, small fissures, and scalloped effect along left lateral border, a normal deviation caused by adjacent teeth. **B,** Dorsal surface on elderly individual's tongue. Arrows indicate smoothness (papillary atrophy) on lateral borders.

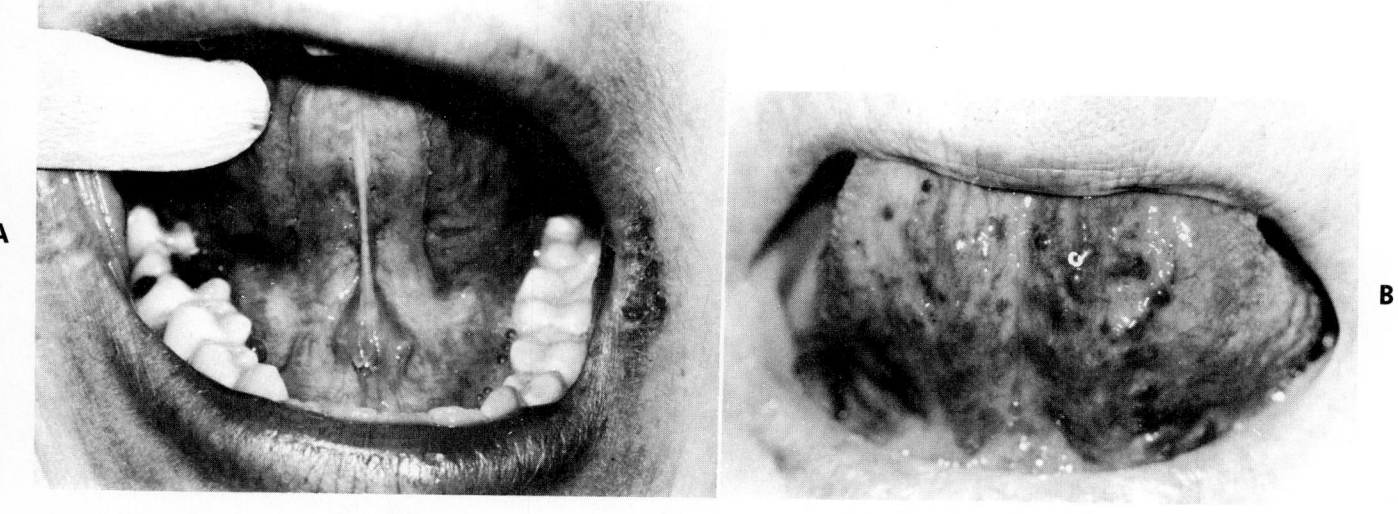

Fig. 5-25 **A,** Normal ventral surface of tongue showing vessels, septum, and floor of mouth. **B,** Ventral surface of elderly individual's tongue. Note engorged and nodular vessels.

ASSESSMENT PROCEDURE	NORMAL FINDINGS	DEVIATIONS FROM NORMAL
ventral surface and floor of mouth for:		
a. Color	Pale, coral, pink	Pallor, redness
b. Surface characteristics	Frenulum (centered)	Lesions, lumps
	Submaxillary duct opening	
18. Inspect and palpate hard and soft palates for:		
a. Color	Hard palate: pale	Reddened
	Soft palate: pink	Pallor, redness
	(*Note:* Heavy smokers may show small red dots on surface of hard palate as shown in Fig. 5-26)	
b. Surface characteristics	Hard palate immovable, with irregular transverse rugae	Patches, lesions
		Petechiae
	Midline exostosis (torus palatinus) may be present (Fig. 5-27)	
	Soft palate movable	Lesions
	Symmetrical elevation	
	Smooth	
19. Observe for mouth odor	Absent or sweet	Fetid, musty, or acetonic
20. Inspect oropharynx for:		
a. Landmarks	Anterior and posterior pillars symmetrical	
	Uvula midline	Pulled laterally

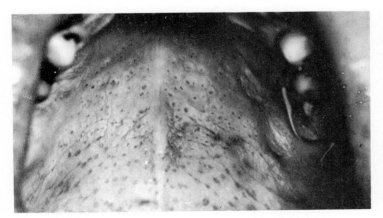

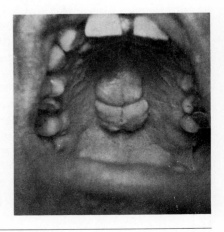

Fig. 5-26 Nicotine stomatitis. (From DeWeese DD, Saunders WH, Schuller DE, Schleuning AJ II: *Otolaryngology—head and neck surgery,* ed 7, St Louis, 1988, Mosby–Year Book.)

Fig. 5-27 Torus palatinus. (From DeWeese DD, Saunders WH: *Textbook of otolaryngology,* ed 6, St Louis, 1982, Mosby–Year Book.)

Note: Gag reflex is tested at this time (CN IX, CN X). This is covered in the neurological assessment (Chapter 15).

Continued.

CLINICAL GUIDELINES—cont'd

ASSESSMENT PROCEDURE	EVALUATION	
	NORMAL FINDINGS	DEVIATIONS FROM NORMAL
	Tonsils (may be partially or totally absent); may also be called *tonsil tag* (Fig. 5-28)	Hypertrophied (adult)
b. Color	Posterior wall pink	Reddened
c. Surface characteristics	Smooth	Lesions, plaques
	Tonsils may be cryptic (see Fig. 5-28)	Increased vascularity
	Posterior wall: slight vascularity may be present	Crypts inflamed or filled with debris or exudate
		Vertical reddened lines or general redness
		Swelling, exudate
		Gray membrane

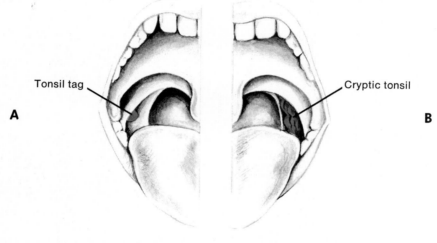

Tonsil tag

Cryptic tonsil

A

B

Fig. 5-28 **A,** Tonsil tag. **B,** Cryptic tonsil.

CLINICAL TIPS AND STRATEGIES

- **A prolonged examination of the nose or mouth should be carried out with client comfort in mind:** The head should be supported. Having the client lie down may be easiest for both him and the examiner. (Remember that the head must be tilted at various angles for viewing the nose.)
- **Correct technique is necessary to properly visualize the lower and the middle turbinates:** The examiner must insert the nasal speculum at least 1.3 cm (½ inch) into the nares.
- **Stabilize the nasal speculum:** Place the index finger against the side of the patient's nose to avoid jiggling the speculum unnecessarily while it is in the naris.
- **The nasal speculum (if otoscope not in use) is to be inserted with the blades up and down:** This prevents pressure of the speculum blades against the septum, which can cause much discomfort. Open the blades as wide as possible for optimum viewing.
- **Be aware of the presence of nasal hair:** Be careful not to pinch hair as you remove the speculum.
- **Angled mouth mirrors are used by some practitioners:** They are helpful for viewing posterior angles.
- **Early dental caries cannot be recognized without the use of radiography:** An examination of teeth with the use of a penlight, mirror, and tongue blade does not constitute adequate screening for dental caries.
- **The tongue blade on the posterior dorsal surface of the tongue will usually cause a gag reflex:** For most of the examination the tongue blade, when used, should rest lightly on the anterior part of the tongue.
- **Many clients can elevate their soft palate and de-**

SAMPLE RECORDING: NORMAL FINDINGS

Nose: Appears straight and symmetrical with nostrils patent. Odors properly identified. Nasal mucosa pink, moist, with no discharge or lesions. Sinuses nontender on palpation.

Mouth and pharynx:

Temporomandibular joint fully mobile, without tenderness or crepitus.

Lips pink, moist, without lesions.

Buccal mucosa, gingivae, and hard and soft palates pink with no lesions, inflammation, patches, or swelling.

Teeth: 28 (all third molars absent). Firmly seated, with five gold restorations. No debris, staining, obvious caries. No inflammation at gingivae.

Tongue: midline, symmetrical. No lesions or fasciculations.

Floor of mouth without lesions.

Uvula midline, *tonsils* absent. *Pharyngeal wall* pink with no lesions, exudate, or swelling. *Mouth odor* faintly sweet.

---

press their own tongue for viewing of the pharyngeal wall: The examiner does not have to use a tongue depressor.

- **Explain *all* procedures to the client:** This should be done *before* beginning (especially when grasping the tongue).
- **Gloves should be worn for all mouth examinations.**

 The Newborn

HISTORY AND CLINICAL STRATEGIES

- Do not place objects in the mouths of newborns. Gently open the jaws by placing fingers onto the cheeks and pressing inward. Use a flashlight to examine the mouth and throat.
  1. A short tongue is a common finding.
  2. Note any abnormalities (e.g., protruding tongue, lip notches, palate deformities).
- Test nares patency by holding one nostril closed and then the other one. Evaluate and report any breathing difficulty or nasal discharge. Drainage may be symptomatic of drug withdrawal or syphilis.

CLINICAL VARIATIONS: THE NEWBORN

CHARACTERISTIC OR AREA EXAMINED	NORMAL FINDINGS	DEVIATIONS FROM NORMAL
1. Nose	In midline, symmetrical, flat, no movement with breathing Nasal breathing; mouth breathing when crying Ethmoidal, sphenoidal sinuses and maxillary antrums present Milia may be present	Nasal flaring is sign of respiratory difficulty Hypertelorism—wide nose base (greater than 2.5 cm in term infant) with widely spaced eyes Choanal atresia—nasal passage obstruction with membrane or bone Nasal discharge
2. Mouth	Mouth symmetrical when crying and sucking Lips pink; tongue does not protrude Frenulum close to tongue tip Bohn nodules (Epstein pearls)—small, white, epithelial cells on palate or gums Ranulas—small whitish-blue benign mucous gland cysts Mucocele, mucous retention cyst—clear, elevated cysts on tongue or inside lips	Microstomia—small opening (suggests trisomy disorder) Cleft lip and palate Frenulum linguae Excessive salivation Whitish-gray thrush—*Candida* infection Macroglossia, aglossia, (tongue variations associated with Down syndrome, Beckwith syndrome, cretinism, hyperpituitarism) Mouth and chin disorders—micrognathia, mandibular hypoplasia, Pierre-Robin syndrome Pterygoid ulcers, Bednar aphthae—gray lesions on soft or hard palate (caused by trauma, malnourishment)

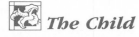 *The Child*

HISTORY AND CLINICAL STRATEGIES

- It is important to assess individually the nose, mouth, teeth, and oropharynx of all children. The frontal and maxillary sinuses are routinely palpated in children over 8 years of age.
- Because of the intrusive nature of these examinations, the examiner should delay assessment until the end of the entire examination.
- Although it is desirable to assess the nose, mouth, and throat while the child is sitting, a young or uncooperative child will need to be firmly restrained. Following are examination strategies:
  1. Infants to 1 year are usually restrained in a supine position with the child's arms extended over the head and secured in position by a parent or helper.
  2. Toddlers may be restrained in either a supine po-

sition as just described or when sitting on the parent's lap. If the second method is used, the child's legs are trapped between the parent's knees, and the arms and chest are restrained with one of the parent's arms while the other hand is used to restrain the child's head firmly against the parent's chest (Fig. 5-29).

  3. For preschoolers, spend time getting to know the child; allow him to play with the tongue blade during the examination, and play smiling and "aah" games as a buildup to the actual mouth and throat examination. Although these techniques may work for some children, others will need to be restrained with one of the techniques just described. Regardless of the technique used for the throat examination, we have discovered that it may be helpful to divide the examination of the mouth and throat

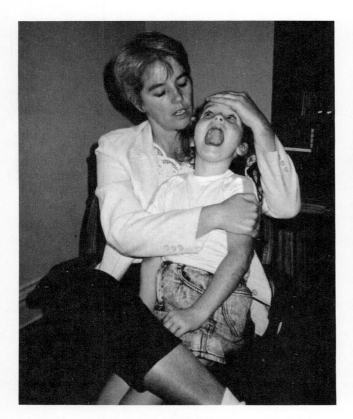

Fig. 5-29 Technique to restrain child for mouth examination.

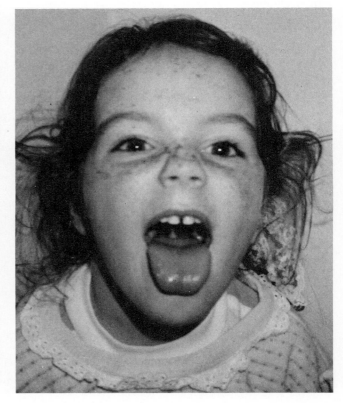

Fig. 5-30 Cooperative preschooler participating in mouth examination.

into two phases and evaluate each at different times during the total assessment. The mouth evaluation is easily done early in the examination process. If the examiner simply approaches the sitting child with a flashlight and asks the child to show lips, teeth and tongue, an initial assessment can be made. A more thorough evaluation of unexposed spots and the throat should be postponed until the end of the examination (Fig. 5-30).

4. School-age children are usually cooperative and willing to show off their new teeth or the absence of their teeth. The mouth and throat are easiest to evaluate if the child is sitting upright on the examination table.

- It is a universal problem to attempt to open the mouth of an uncooperative child whose teeth are clenched tight. Although not every technique will work on every child, the following might be helpful:
  1. Slowly advance the tongue blade along the lips to the posterior teeth.
  2. Carefully ease the blade between the teeth toward the pharynx.
  3. If possible, maintain a downward motion on the tongue blade so that the tongue is pushed forward and the base of the tongue is pressed downward. The child will suddenly gag, and the mouth will open wide.
  4. During what appears to be a split second of visibility, the examiner must view all the structures therein.

Repeated practice is necessary to develop the inclusive scanning view required during mouth and throat evaluation.

- Several techniques can be used to facilitate the posterior pharynx viewing while avoiding the gag reflex:
  1. A common one is to instruct the child to pant like a puppy while sticking the tongue far forward. This technique lowers the posterior tongue and raises the uvula.
  2. The second technique requires placing the tongue blade along the lateral aspect of the tongue instead of down the middle.

- Whenever the nose is inspected or whenever there is a history of unilateral nasal drainage or a "strange" odor about the child's head or mouth, a foreign body in the nose must be considered.

- Bruising or lacerations about the lips, gums, frenulum, or buccal mucosa of an infant or young child must be further evaluated as a possible sign of child abuse. Forced feedings by either a bottle or spoon may cause such bruising.

- It is important to inquire about tooth brushing from the time the first tooth appears. Brushing habits, as well as who brushes the child's teeth, are important.

- In young children with extensive caries of the central upper teeth, the examiner should inquire about the child's continuing use of a bottle, especially as a nighttime routine.

- When inspecting the child's occlusion, instruct the child to bite down as if chewing food. If the examiner instructs the child to show his teeth, a purposeful malocclusion might be noted.

- The clinical evaluation of the pediatric client's sinuses differs from that of the adult. Because of the difficulty and reliability of clinical assessment, the frontal and maxillary sinuses are not normally evaluated until about age 8. From that age on the technique of evaluation is the same as for the adult client, testing for such disorders as puffiness or tenderness to palpation.

- Because of the smallness of the subject and the difficulty in adult technique instrumentation, the nasal evaluation may best be done using the otoscope with the nasal speculum.

- In trying to evaluate the patency or possibility of a naris obstruction, the examiner may either listen for patency by using a stethoscope at the naris opening or by using a small mirror to detect spot fogging during exhalation.

- Risk factors of the pediatric client include the following:
  1. History of recurrent nosebleeds
  2. Obvious nasal septal deviation after trauma
  3. Obvious malocclusion
  4. History of thumb sucking, especially as secondary teeth erupt
  5. "Bottle babies," those who routinely have access to a bottle especially after teeth erupt; continue to evaluate for caries.
  6. Children with poor hygiene habits or those who do not routinely have preventive dental care.
  7. Recurrent mouth infections, thrush, gingivostomatitis, or canker sores
  8. Recurrent tonsil infections
  9. Noted bruising to the gums, lips, or hard palate
  10. No teeth by age 12 months

Text continues on p. 143.

CLINICAL VARIATIONS: THE CHILD

CHARACTERISTIC OR AREA EXAMINED	NORMAL FINDINGS	DEVIATIONS FROM NORMAL
1. Nose		
a. Outer surface	Smooth, intact	Lesions
	Skin color same as face	Eczema
	May have some redness around nares openings if child has a cold	Acne
b. Contour	External alignment symmetrical or nearly symmetrical	
c. Form	Some children with allergies may show transverse ridge from chronic upward wiping of nares (called the *allergic salute*)	Flaring with inhalation
d. Patency of nares	Noiseless, free exchange of air through each naris	Breathing noisy or obstructed
		Unilateral patency (evaluate for foreign body or polyps)
e. Evaluation of olfactory nerve (CN I) not normally conducted in children		
2. Internal nasal cavity—observe nares:		
a. With client's head erect	Floor of nose (vestibule)	Septal deviation
	Inferior turbinate	Septal perforation (noted by viewing spot of light in other naris)
	Nasal hairs present	Furuncle (most often present in vestibule)
	Mucosa slightly darker (redder) than oral mucosa	Tenderness
		Marked redness
		Crusting, discharge
		Lesions or masses
b. With client's head back	Middle meatus	Sinus drainage
	Middle turbinate	Polyps, masses
	Turbinates same color as surrounding nasal mucosa	Turbinates appear pale, swollen (allergic responses)
		Mucosa markedly red with copious discharge present
	Film of clear discharge (small amount)	Yellow, thick, green discharge
c. With client's head to side	Septum	Bleeding, crusting
	Lower third is vascular area (Kiesselbach area)	Tenderness
		Lesions
	Septum midline and straight	Marked deviation of septum
3. Frontal and maxillary sinuses (See Clinical Tips and Strategies," p. 134)	Nontender	Tender on palpation
	No swelling	Swelling of soft tissue over sinus area
4. Temporomandibular joint (to be evaluated if the child is cooperative)		
a. Mobility	Smooth jaw excursion	Limited excursion
b. Tenderness	Absent on palpation	Present on palpation
c. Crepitus	Absent	Present (especially on closure of jaw)
d. Referred pain	Absent	Present (especially on closure of jaw)
5. Occlusion	Top back teeth rest directly on top of lower teeth; upper incisors slightly override lowers	Protrusion of upper incisors
		Protrusion of lower incisors
		Upper incisors do not overlap lowers on closure

CHARACTERISTIC OR AREA EXAMINED	NORMAL FINDINGS	DEVIATIONS FROM NORMAL
		Lateral displacement of teeth
6. Jaw size	Appears appropriate for face size	Very *small* or *large* mandible, seen in numerous congenital diseases
7. Lips		
a. Color	Pink	Pale, cyanotic Cherry pink Marked circumoral pallor
b. Symmetry	Vertical and lateral symmetry at rest or on movement	Swelling (general or localized), induration, twisting, drooping clefts
c. Moisture	Smooth and moist	Dry, flaking, cracking corners are especially common (evaluate for impetigo)
d. Surface characteristics	Slight vertical linear markings Breast- or bottle-fed babies may develop a sucking tubercle in middle of upper lip	Fissures Lesions: plaques, vesicles, nodules, ulcerations
8. Inner lips and buccal mucosa		
a. Color	Pale coral, pink Increased pigmentation (general or localized) with dark-skinned individuals	Pale, cyanotic, reddened Local deposits of brown pigmentation Black, blue areas
b. Landmarks	Parotid duct (pinpoint red marking) may be slightly elevated	Puffy, reddened area
c. Surface characteristics	Smooth Fine gray ridge Where teeth meet, occlusion line may appear Salivation in children between 3 months and 2 years may be normal If child also appears ill, salivation should be considered abnormal until proved otherwise	Ulcers White patches (*Candida albicans,* or thrush) where scraped-off patches are reddened and tend to bleed White plaques Swelling Bleeding Excessively dry mouth (observe for other signs of dehydration, fever, or possible atropine ingestion) Excessive salivation may be seen in gingivostomatitis (child appears ill and usually drools) or in child with multiple caries)
9. Gums		
a. Color	Pink, coral	Reddened, pale
b. Surface characteristics	Slightly stippled Sharp margin at tooth Patchy brown pigmentation (usually with dark-skinned individuals) Hypertrophy may appear at puberty May see downward extension of alveolar frenulum as child's central incisors separate; should self-correct Small pearly white cysts (Epstein pearls) may be seen along gums of infants; usually disappear by age 2 or 3 months; called *Bohn nodules* when on midpalate	Swelling (stippling disappears) Bleeding (with slight pressure) Enlarged crevice between teeth and gums Pockets containing debris at tooth margin Ulcers, epulis Blue-black line at gum margin Marked hypertrophy Tenderness on palpation Hypertrophy of gum tissue may be indicative of mouth breathers, vitamin deficiency, or phenytoin (Dilantin) ingestion

Continued.

CLINICAL VARIATIONS: THE CHILD—cont'd

CHARACTERISTIC OR AREA EXAMINED	NORMAL FINDINGS	DEVIATIONS FROM NORMAL
10. Teeth		
a. Number: note eruption timing, sequence of eruption, and positioning of teeth	See Fig. 5-31 for normal number of teeth at given age	No teeth by age 1 year Missing teeth inappropriate for age
b. Color	White, yellow, or gray hues	Darkened teeth Brown teeth (may indicate decay) Mottled or pitted permanent teeth (may indicate decreased fluoride or tetracycline ingestion) Green or black teeth (if caused by iron ingestion, discoloration will dissipate after iron supplement is discontinued)
c. Surface characteristics	Smooth, regularly formed teeth	Excessive smoothness (may indicate grinding of teeth) Debris present, especially at gum line Caries
11. Tongue		
a. Symmetry and movement	Smooth and even tissue Able to touch tongue to upper lips	Fissures Tongue appearing too large for mouth (protusion of tongue) Glossoptosis: tongue attached farther forward than usual Tongue-tied: child unable to advance tongue forward to lips
b. Color	Pink	Red, strawberry tongue (may be seen with scarlet fever)
c. Surface characteristics	Dorsal and lateral: moist, glistening coating Papillae present Elongated vallate papillae Fissures present Texture smooth, even Ventral: pink and smooth, with large veins	Papillae absent Lesions Furrows in tongue Lumps, nodules, induration Lesions, patches
12. Floor of mouth		
a. Color	Pale, coral, pink	Pallor, reddened
b. Surface characteristics	Frenulum (centered) Submaxillary duct opening	Lesions, lumps
13. Hard palate		
a. Color	Pale pink	Reddened
b. Surface characteristics	Immovable with irregular transverse rugae Bohn nodules (gone by 2 or 3 months) Very high or narrow arch requires further evaluation; may be linked to multiple other syndromes	Patches Lesions Petechiae Clefts Bruising
14. Soft palate		
a. Color	Pink	Reddened Pallor
b. Surface characteristics	Movable Symmetrical elevation Smooth	Discharge Edema Patches Lesions

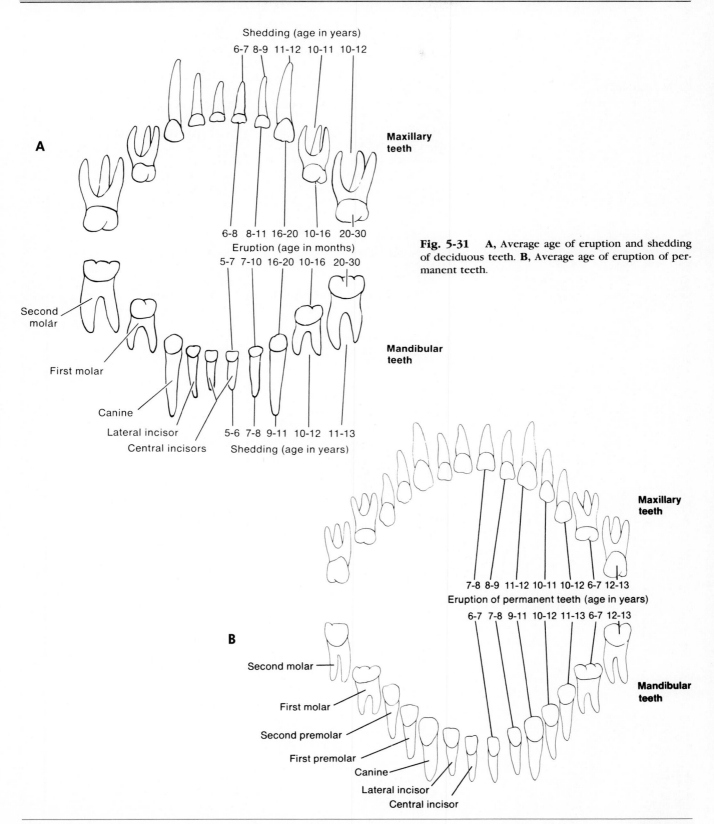

Fig. 5-31 **A,** Average age of eruption and shedding of deciduous teeth. **B,** Average age of eruption of permanent teeth.

CLINICAL VARIATIONS: THE CHILD—cont'd

CHARACTERISTIC OR AREA EXAMINED	NORMAL FINDINGS	DEVIATIONS FROM NORMAL
15. Mouth odor	Absent	Fetid, musty (further investigate poor hygiene, local or systemic infections, sinusitis, mouth breathers)
		Foreign body in nose
		Acetonic or very sweet smell
16. Oropharynx		
a. Landmarks	Anterior and posterior pillars symmetrical	Lateral deviation
	Uvula midline	Bifid uvula
	Tonsils pink	Uvula with lateral deviation
	Size may vary from barely visible to very large (Fig. 5-32)	Reddened; pus, coating, exudate present
	Cryptic	Tonsils occluding swallowing or breathing
		White or yellow follicles filling cryps
		Ulcerative
b. Color	Posterior wall pink	Reddened
c. Surface characteristics	Posterior wall may show slight vascularity	Vertical reddened lines or general redness
		Swelling, exudate, gray membrane

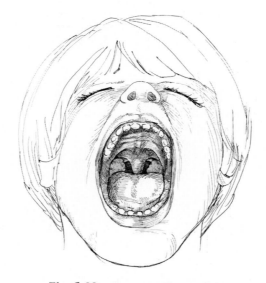

Fig. 5-32   Large tonsils in a child.

The Childbearing Woman

HISTORY AND CLINICAL STRATEGIES

- Nosebleeds are a common occurrence during pregnancy. Use of a humidifier may help prevent drying of mucosa.

- Gums may bleed more easily during pregnancy. Use of a soft toothbrush, daily flossing, and regular dental appointments should be encouraged.
- The history should include diet and oral hygiene habits.

CLINICAL VARIATIONS: THE CHILDBEARING WOMAN

CHARACTERISTIC OR AREA EXAMINED	NORMAL FINDINGS	DEVIATIONS FROM NORMAL
1. Nose	Congestion, stuffiness of nasopharynx from increased estrogen level Epistaxis—nosebleeds common during pregnancy (from engorged veins) Swollen turbinates, mucosa (may be rhinitis)	Increased nasal discomfort (may be sinusitis, infection) Severe bleeding, nasal symptoms (needs investigation)
2. Mouth	Epulis—vascular Gingivitis—swelling, bleeding Gums soften, may be hyperemic, hyperplastic Varicose veins of tongue may occur With proper care and diet, teeth condition should remain unchanged Ptyalism—increased salivary perception in first trimester (may be from increased swallowing from nausea)	Teeth and gum deterioration (not from pregnancy but from trauma, dietary insufficiency, infection)
3. After delivery	Gums regress after delivery; nasal symptoms soon subside	

The Older Adult

HISTORY AND CLINICAL STRATEGIES

- A number of variables contribute to mouth problems in elderly adults.
  1. Bone resorption is considered a normal aging process, but it can be escalated by systemic disease or local factors within the mouth.
  2. The diminished flow of saliva decreases the self-cleaning process within the mouth.
  3. Slower healing processes decrease the oral tissue's potential for repairing minor trauma from food, cold, or other assaults from the external environment.
  4. The presence of systemic disease (more common with geriatric clients) often manifests local changes or problems in the mouth.
  5. Physical disability (especially loss of manual dexterity or visual problems) decreases the individual's potential for a high level of self-care.
  6. Time itself has an effect: (1) old dental restorations deteriorate; (2) tooth enamel calcifies, erodes, and deteriorates from years of overly vigorous brushing; (3) gum tissue resorbs and exposes the neck of the tooth, which is vulnerable to decay; (4) attrition of the teeth (wearing down of the occlusal surface) occurs; and (5) gingival tissue becomes less elastic and more vulnerable to trauma.
  7. Other problems sometimes associated with aging interfere with mouth care: nutritional deficiency, emotional or mental changes, financial concerns.
- The practitioner must take a careful history of self-care habits, frequency of visits to the dentist, and client's concerns about problems that interfere with self-care. (See "History," p. 122, for specific questions related to nose, sinus, mouth, and throat assessment.)

RISK FACTORS FOR MOUTH AND DENTAL DISEASE

- Confusion (even transient confusion or a shortened attention span can drastically alter client's self-care habits)
- Physical disability (client unable to provide adequate self-care)
- Poor eating habits: no intake of "cleaning" foods, high sugar content, limited intake of foods that require chewing
- Chronic mouth breathing (increases vulnerability of oral tissue to trauma, inflammatory response)
- History of chronic smoking (associated with higher incidence of oral cancer)
- History of chronic use of alcohol (higher associated incidence of cancer)
- Systemic diseases (only a sample of relevant diseases included)
  1. Osteoporosis (associated with bone resorption)
  2. Cirrhosis of liver (higher associated incidence of cancer of mouth)
  3. Any disease disrupting protein metabolism
  4. Anemia; blood dyscrasias
  5. Diabetes mellitus
- Illness that creates general disability (e.g., fatigue, weakness) and thus interferes with self-care
- Local irritants chronically assaulting oral tissues (e.g., pipe smoking, chewing tobacco)
- History of poor dental care habits

CLINICAL VARIATIONS: THE OLDER ADULT

CHARACTERISTIC OR AREA EXAMINED	NORMAL FINDINGS	DEVIATIONS FROM NORMAL
1. General appearance of nose		
a. Surface/skin	Smooth, intact Skin color same as face	Lesions, warty appearance Redness, discoloration Vascularization
b. Contour	External alignment symmetrical (or nearly symmetrical)	Marked asymmetry Swelling or hypertrophy (bulbous appearance)
c. Nares	Symmetrical Dry, no crusting No flaring or narrowing associated with breathing Increase in bristly hairs (especially men)	Marked asymmetry Discharge present, crusting Narrowing on inspiration (associated with chronic obstruction and mouth breathing)
d. Patency	Noiseless, free exchange of air through each naris	Patency may be occluded because of nose drying out and crusting; associated with inflammatory response Breathing noisy or obstructed
e. Stability	Firm	Unstable
f. Tenderness	Nontender	Tender on palpation; masses
2. Sense of smell and odor identification	Sense of smell somewhat decreased with aging, but client should be able to identify strong odor	Unable to identify strong odor

CHARACTERISTIC OR AREA EXAMINED	NORMAL FINDINGS	DEVIATIONS FROM NORMAL
3. Internal nasal cavity—observe nares		
a. With client's head erect	Floor of nose (vestibule)	Furuncle (most often present in vestibule)
	Inferior turbinate	
	Nasal hairs present	Tenderness
	Mucosa slightly darker (redder) than oral mucosa	Marked redness
		Crusting, discharge
		Lesions or masses
b. With client's head back	Middle meatus	Sinus drainage
	Middle turbinate	Polyps, masses
	Turbinates same color as surrounding nasal mucosa	Turbinates appear pale, swollen (allergic responses)
	Mucosa tends to be dryer	Increased friability of tissues
		Increased vulnerability to inflammatory response
		Mucosa markedly red with copious discharge present
c. With client's head to side	Film of clear discharge (small amount)	Yellow, thick, green discharge
	Lower third is vascular (Kiesselbach area)	Bleeding, crusting
		Tenderness
	Septum midline and straight	Lesions
		Marked deviation of septum
4. Sinuses (frontal and maxillary)	Nontender	Tender on palpation
	No swelling	Swelling of soft tissue over sinus area
5. Temporomandibular joint		
a. Mobility	Smooth jaw excursion, 3.5 to 4.5 cm (1⅓ to 1¾ inches)	Joint may dislocate when mouth opened wide (associated with loss of elasticity of joint ligaments)
		Limited excursion
b. Tenderness	Absent on palpation	Present on palpation
c. Crepitus	Absent	Present
d. Referred pain	Absent	Present (especially on closure of jaw)
6. Occlusion	May be changed because of missing teeth	Protrusion of upper incisors
		Protrusion of lower incisors
	Marked overclosure of jaws may be associated with edentulous client	Upper incisors do not overlap lowers on closure
	Individuals who stoop and thrust head forward tend to habitually protrude lower jaw	Later displacement of teeth; back teeth do not occlude
7. Lips		
a. Color	Pink	Pale, cyanotic, reddened
b. Symmetry	Vertical and lateral symmetry at rest or on movement	Swelling (general or local), induration
c. Moisture	Decreased supply of saliva may contribute to dryer lips	Dry, flaking, cracked
d. Surface	Increased vertical markings	Marked, deep wrinkling and fissures at corner of mouth (perlèche) associated with inflammatory response to severe overclosure or vitamin deficiency)
	"Purse-string" appearance associated with edentulism or overclosure of jaws	

Continued.

CLINICAL VARIATIONS: THE OLDER ADULT—cont'd

CHARACTERISTIC OR AREA EXAMINED	NORMAL FINDINGS	DEVIATIONS FROM NORMAL
8. Inner lips and buccal mucosa; ask client to remove any dental appliance		Lesions at vermilion border (Figs. 5-33 and 5-34) or development of indistinct border Fissures radiating across lip border Lesions: plaques, vesicles, nodules, ulcerations Inflamed fissures at corners
a. Color	Pale coral, pink Increased pigmentation (general or local) with dark-skinned individuals	Pale, cyanotic, reddened Local deposits of brown pigmentation
b. Landmarks	Parotid duct (pinpoint red marking); may be slightly elevated	
c. Surface characteristics	Mucosa becomes thinner and less vascular; may appear shinier than in younger adult	White or gray patches (leukoplakia) Monilial patches fairly common problem

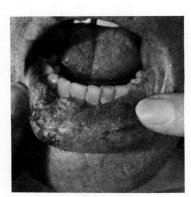

Fig. 5-33   Squamous cell carcinoma. (From Stewart WD, Danto JL, Maddin S: *Dermatology: diagnosis and treatment of cutaneous disorders,* ed 4, St Louis, 1978, Mosby–Year Book.)

Fig. 5-34   Basal cell carcinoma. (From Steinberg FU, editor: *Care of the geriatric patient,* ed 6, St Louis, 1983, Mosby–Year Book.)

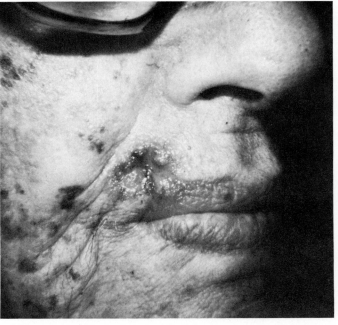

CHARACTERISTIC OR AREA EXAMINED	NORMAL FINDINGS	DEVIATIONS FROM NORMAL
	Fordyce granules common (Fig. 5-35)	Hyperkeratotic response (white areas, may be raised, rough); might be normal response to trauma, but should be referred for validation
		Petechiae
		Swelling (local/general)
		Bleeding
		Ulcers
		Excessively dry mouth
		Excessive salivation
9. Gums		
a. Color	May appear slightly paler	Reddened, excessively pale
b. Surface characterisitics	Stippling may be somewhat decreased	Increased friability of gums; bleeding with slight pressure
		Lesions, redness, uneven ridges, spurs, white patches, or tenderness of edentulous gums
		Marked pallor (fibrotic changes) of gums
	Clearly defined, tight margin at tooth	Enlarged crevices between teeth and gums
	Patchy brown pigmentation (usually with dark-skinned individuals)	Pockets containing debris at tooth margin
10. Teeth		
a. Number	Thirty-two (full adult)	Missing teeth
	Third molars, upper and/or lower, sometimes congenitally absent	
b. Color	May appear more yellow or slightly darker (uniformly)	Darkened, stained (individual teeth or all)

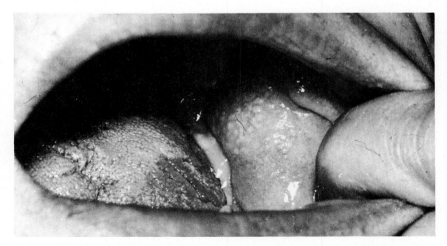

Fig. 5-35 Fordyce granules on buccal mucosa. (From DeWeese DD, Saunders WH, Schuller DE, Schleuning AJ II: *Otolaryngology—head and neck surgery,* ed 7, St Louis, 1988, Mosby–Year Book.)

Continued.

CLINICAL VARIATIONS: THE OLDER ADULT—cont'd

CHARACTERISTIC OR AREA EXAMINED	NORMAL FINDINGS	DEVIATIONS FROM NORMAL
c. Form and surface characteristics	Teeth may appear elongated (increased root surface or neck of tooth exposure associated with resorption of supporting bone) (see Fig. 5-19)	Enamel of old teeth may display cracks with stains (see Fig. 5-19) Old dental restorations may be deteriorated (especially at margins) Dentin surface may appear abraded Occlusal surfaces markedly worn down (leaving hollow surface appearance) Cusps of teeth may break off
d. Maneuverability	No movement or slight movement	Loosening of teeth a special hazard, associated with periodontal disease, bone resorption
11. Tongue a. Symmetry and movement	Forward thrust smooth and symmetrical Appearance of tongue is symmetrical	Unilateral atrophy Lateral movement Fasciculation Tongue lies limp on floor of mouth
b. Color	Pink	Red
c. Surface characteristics	Dorsal and lateral: Moist, glistening coating Papillae may appear slightly smoother, shinier (Fig. 5-19, *B*) Fissures present	Papillae absent Lesions Very smooth tongue (associated with vitamin deficiency)
d. Texture	Smooth, even tissue Ventral Epithelium thin and loosely attached Veins often varicosed (see Fig. 5-26, *B*)*	Lumps, nodules Induration Lesions, patches
12. Floor of mouth a. Color and surface	Pale coral, pink Frenulum (centered) Submaxillary duct opening	Pallor, redness Lesions, lumps Watch for retention cysts at salivary duct opening
13. Hard and soft palates a. Color	Hard palate pale Soft palate pink	Reddened Pallor, redness
b. Surface characteristics	Hard palate immovable, with irregular transverse rugae Midline exostosis (torus palatinus) may be present Soft palate movable Symmetrical elevation Smooth	Patches, lesions Petechiae Watch for injuries, lesions related to denture trauma Mucosal glands may become inflamed in heavy smokers
14. Mouth odor	Absent or sweet	Fetid, musty, or acetonic
15. Oropharynx a. Landmarks	Anterior and posterior pillars symmetrical Uvula midline	Pulled laterally

*The beginning examiner should consider varicosities a condition for referral for consulation.

Note: Gag reflex is tested at this time (CN IX, CN X). This is covered in the neurological assessment (Chapter 15).

CHARACTERISTIC OR AREA EXAMINED	NORMAL FINDINGS	DEVIATIONS FROM NORMAL
	Tonsils may be partially or totally absent; may also be called *tonsil tag*	Hypertrophied (adult)
b. Color	Posterior wall pink	Reddened
c. Surface characteristics	Smooth	Crypts inflamed or filled with debris or exudate
	Tonsils may be cryptic (see Fig. 5-28, *B*)	
	Slight vascularity may be present on posterior wall	Increased vascularity
		Vertical reddened lines or general redness
		Swelling, exudate
		Gray membrane

 Study Questions

General

1. With a nasal speculum and penlight, an examiner is able to view the:
   - ☐ a. Vestibule
   - ☐ b. Anterior septum
   - ☐ c. Inferior turbinate
   - ☐ d. Middle turbinate
   - ☐ e. a and c
   - ☐ f. All of the above
2. A nasal speculum is inserted:
   - ☐ a. 0.5 cm (⅕ inch)
   - ☐ b. 1 cm (⅓ inch)
   - ☐ c. 2 cm (¾ inch)
3. It is then opened:
   - ☐ a. Transversely
   - ☐ b. Vertically
   - ☐ c. Transversely, initially; then vertically
4. The _____ of the nose is bone.
   - ☐ a. Upper third
   - ☐ b. Upper two thirds
   - ☐ c. Lower half
   - ☐ d. Entire middle portion
5. The paranasal sinuses directly evaluated are:
   - ☐ a. Sphenoidal
   - ☐ b. Frontal
   - ☐ c. Splanchnic
   - ☐ d. Ethmoidal
   - ☐ e. Maxillary
   - ☐ f. a, c, and d
   - ☐ g. c and e
   - ☐ h. b and c
   - ☐ i. b and e
   - ☐ j. b, c, and d

6. The paranasal sinuses drain into the:
   - ☐ a. Superior turbinate
   - ☐ b. Middle turbinate
   - ☐ c. Middle meatus
   - ☐ d. Vestibule
7. Which statement(s) is/are true about the lips:
   - ☐ a. Overclosure of the mouth can cause fissuring at the mouth angles
   - ☐ b. A chancre on the lip might resemble a carcinoma or a cold sore
   - ☐ c. There is a rich blood and lymphatic supply to the lips
   - ☐ d. Aging tends to diminish the pattern on the vermilion surface
   - ☐ e. Herpetic vesicles of the lip are common
   - ☐ f. All of the above
   - ☐ g. All except d
   - ☐ h. b, c, and e
   - ☐ i. All except b
8. Which statement is false about the gums:
   - ☐ a. The gums are composed of fibrous tissue covered with mucous membrane
   - ☐ b. The most common irritant to gums is calculus deposits around the necks of teeth
   - ☐ c. Stippling of gums is an early indicator of periodontal disease
   - ☐ d. Gingival enlargement (hypertrophy) can occur in healthy as well as disease states

9. Which statement is false about the buccal mucosa:
   - ☐ a. Leukoplakia may be a precancerous lesion
   - ☐ b. The Wharton duct opens into the buccal membrane opposite the second molar
   - ☐ c. Cheek biting can result in a hyperkeratotic reaction
   - ☐ d. A generalized increased pigmentation is a precancerous condition

10. Which statement is false about the teeth:
    - ☐ a. Congenital absence of third molars is usually indicative of other congenital disorders
    - ☐ b. The biting surface of incisors may become abraded by opening bobby pins
    - ☐ c. Radiography is necessary for early detection of caries
    - ☐ d. Teeth can darken because of some systemic medications, local exposure (e.g., smoking), or trauma

11. Which statement is false about the oropharynx:
    - ☐ a. Smoking may result in a generalized redness of the oropharynx
    - ☐ b. Tonsils may be enlarged without being infected
    - ☐ c. Streptococcal pharyngeal infection produces classic signs and is easily diagnosed
    - ☐ d. Red and pink color variations of the pharyngeal surface are normal

The Newborn

Select the *one* best answer to the following questions.

12. Newborns normally breathe:
    - ☐ a. Through their nose
    - ☐ b. By flaring their nostrils
    - ☐ c. Through their mouths
    - ☐ d. By retracting their xiphoid

13. A normal finding related to a newborn's mouth would be the presence of:
    - ☐ a. Aglossia
    - ☐ b. Thrush
    - ☐ c. Epstein pearls
    - ☐ d. Micrognathia

The Child

14. Transverse creasing across the bridge of a child's nose is most often indicative of:
    - ☐ a. A chromosomal abnormality
    - ☐ b. An allergic child
    - ☐ c. A child with Down syndrome
    - ☐ d. Trauma to the nose
    - ☐ e. A birth defect

15. Normally salivation in the child is noted about age:
    - ☐ a. Birth
    - ☐ b. 1 month
    - ☐ c. 3 months
    - ☐ d. 5 months
    - ☐ e. None of the above

16. Which of the following findings indicates an abnormality requiring additional assessment and referral:
    - ☐ a. Pink tonsils extending almost to midline of throat; no difficulty swallowing or breathing
    - ☐ b. Cryptic tonsils
    - ☐ c. Transverse tongue fissures
    - ☐ d. Epstein pearls
    - ☐ e. None of the above

The Childbearing Woman

Select the *one* best answer to the following questions.

17. Engorged veins may cause a pregnant woman to experience:
    - ☐ a. Vertigo
    - ☐ b. Lethargy
    - ☐ c. Epistaxis
    - ☐ d. Anorexia

18. The perception of increased salivation during the first trimester is called:
    - ☐ a. Gingivitis
    - ☐ b. Hyperplasia
    - ☐ c. Hyperemesis
    - ☐ d. Ptyalism

The Older Adult

19. Some studies show that the most common reason for loss of teeth with elderly clients is:
    - ☐ a. Dental caries
    - ☐ b. Root canal problems
    - ☐ c. Soft enamel
    - ☐ d. Periodontal disease

20. Lesions commonly found in the mouth of geriatric clients are:
    - ☐ a. Fordyce granules
    - ☐ b. Hyperkeratosis
    - ☐ c. Petechiae
    - ☐ d. Purpura
    - ☐ e. All except d
    - ☐ f. a and b
    - ☐ g. a and c
    - ☐ h. All except c

21. Xerostomia:
    - ☐ a. Is caused by bone resorption
    - ☐ b. Is rare and occurs in people over age 80
    - ☐ c. Interferes with self-cleaning of the mouth
    - ☐ d. Only occurs after poor oral self-care habits

22. Some of the risk factors that could alert a practitioner to potential mouth or dental problems are:
    - ☐ a. Cirrhosis of the liver
    - ☐ b. Use of chewing tobacco
    - ☐ c. Severe arthritis of the hands
    - ☐ d. Osteoporosis
    - ☐ e. Chronic heavy smoking
    - ☐ f. All of the above
    - ☐ g. All except d
    - ☐ h. a, b, and e
    - ☐ i. b and e

SUGGESTED READINGS
General

Bates B: *A guide to physical examination,* ed 4, Philadelphia, 1987, JB Lippincott.

Judge R, Zuidema G, Fitzgerald F: *Clinical diagnosis,* ed 4, Boston, 1982, Little, Brown.

Malasanos L, Barkauskas V, Stoltenberg-Allen K: *Health assessment,* ed 4, St Louis, 1990, Mosby—Year Book.

McCance KL, Huether SE: *Pathophysiology: the biological basis for disease in adults and children,* St Louis, 1990, Mosby—Year Book.

Phipps WJ, Long BC, Woods NF, Cassmeyer VL: *Medical surgical nursing: concepts and clinical practice,* ed 4, St Louis, 1991, Mosby—Year Book.

Prior JA, Silberstein JS, Stang JM: *Physical diagnosis: the history and examination of the patient,* ed 6, St Louis, 1981, Mosby—Year Book.

Seidel HM, Ball JW, Dains JE, Benedict GW: *Mosby's guide to physical examination,* ed 2, St Louis, 1991, Mosby—Year Book.

Thompson JM, McFarland GK, Hirsch JE, and others: *Clinical nursing,* ed 2, St Louis, 1989, Mosby—Year Book.

The newborn

Auvenshine MA, Enriquez MG: *Maternity nursing: dimensions of change,* Belmont, Calif, 1985, Wadsworth.

Judd JM: Assessing the newborn from head to toe, *Nurs '85* 15(12):34, 1985.

Kiernan BS, Scoloveno MA: Assessment of the neonate, *Top Clin Nurs* 8(1):1, 1986.

The Organization for Obstetrical, Gynecological and Neonatal Nurses (NAACOG): *Physical assessment of the neonate,* OGN Nursing Practice Resource, Oct. 1986, The Association.

Pillitteri A: *Maternal-newborn nursing: care of the growing family,* ed 3, Boston, 1985, Little, Brown.

Scanlon JW and others: *A system of newborn physical examination,* Baltimore, 1979, University Park Press.

Seidel HM, Ball JW, Dains JE, Benedict GW: *Mosby's guide to physical examination,* ed 2, St Louis, 1991, Mosby—Year Book.

Whaley LF, Wong DL: *Nursing care of infants and children,* ed 4, St Louis, 1991, Mosby—Year Book.

The child

Barness L: *Manual of pediatric physical diagnosis,* ed 6, Chicago, 1990, Mosby—Year Book.

DeAngelis C: *Pediatric primary care,* ed 3, Boston, 1984, Little, Brown.

McDonald RE, Avery DR: *Dentistry for the child and adolescent,* ed 5, St Louis, 1987, Mosby—Year Book.

Waring WW, Jeansonne LO: *Practical manual of pediatrics,* ed 2, St Louis, 1982, Mosby—Year Book.

Whaley LF, Wong LD: *Essentials of pediatric nursing,* ed 3, St Louis, 1989, Mosby—Year Book.

The childbearing woman

Auvenshine MA, Enriquez MG: *Maternity nursing: dimensions of change,* Belmont, Calif, 1985, Wadsworth.

Bobak IM, Jensen, MD: *Essentials of maternity nursing,* ed 3, St Louis, 1991, Mosby—Year Book.

Pillitteri A: *Maternal-newborn nursing: care of the growing family,* ed 3, Boston, 1985, Little, Brown.

Pritchard JA, MacDonald PC: *Williams' obstetrics,* ed 17, New York, 1985, Appleton-Century-Crofts.

Seidel HM, Ball JW, Dains JE, Benedict GW: *Mosby's guide to physical examination,* ed 2, St Louis, 1991, Mosby—Year Book.

Whitley N: *A manual of clinical obstetrics,* Philadelphia, 1985, JB Lippincott.

The older adult

Carotenuto R, Bullock J: *Physical assessment of the gerontologic client,* Philadelphia, 1980, FA Davis.

Ebersole P, Hess P: *Toward healthy aging,* ed 3, St Louis, 1990, Mosby—Year Book.

Hauk L: Enabling clients to manage dentures, *Geriatr Nurs,* Sept/Oct, 1986, p 254.

Ofstehage JC, Magilvy K: Oral health and aging, *Geriatr Nurs,* Sept/Oct, 1986, p 238.

Steinberg FU, editor: *Care of the geriatric patient,* ed 6, St Louis, 1983, Mosby—Year Book.

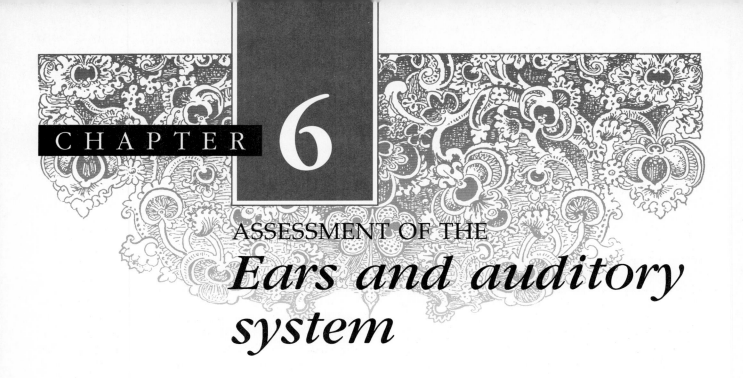

CHAPTER 6

ASSESSMENT OF THE
Ears and auditory system

VOCABULARY

anulus Dense fibrous ring surrounding the tympanic membrane.

auricle Flap of the external ear; also called the *pinna.*

cerumen Waxy secretion of the glands of the external acoustic meatus; earwax.

cochlea Conical bony structure of the inner ear; perforated by numerous appertures for passage of the cochlear division of the acoustic nerve.

Darwinian tubercle Blunt point projecting up from the upper part of the helix of the ear.

dizziness Disturbed sense of relationship to space.

eustachian tube Tube, lined with mucous membrane, that joins the nasopharynx and the tympanic cavity, allowing equalization of air pressure with atmospheric pressure.

helix Margin of the external ear.

incus One of three ossicles in the middle ear; resembling an anvil, it communicates sound vibrations from the malleus to the stapes.

injection Redness or congestion of the tympanic membrane caused by dilation of blood vessels secondary to an inflammatory or infectious process.

labyrinth Complex structure of the inner ear that communicates directly with the acoustic nerve, transmitting sound vibrations from the middle ear through the fluid-filled network of three semicircular canals that join at a vestibule connected to the cochlea.

light reflex Triangular landmark area on the tympanic membrane that most brightly reflects the examiner's light source.

malleus Innermost ossicle of the middle ear; resembling a hammer, it is connected to the tympanic membrane and transmits sound vibrations to the incus, which communicates with the stapes.

mastoid process Conical projection of the caudal posterior portion of the temporal bone.

nystagmus Involuntary rhythmical movement of the eyes; oscillations may be horizontal, vertical, rotary, or mixed.

otalgia Pain in the ear.

otitis Inflammation or infection of the ear.

otitis externa Inflammation on infection of the external canal or auricle of the external ear.

otitis media Inflammation or infection of the middle ear.

pars flaccida Small portion of the tympanic membrane between the mallear folds.

pars tensa Larger portion of the tympanic membrane.

pinna Auricle or projected part of the external ear.

presbycusis Impairment of hearing in old age.

stapes One of the ossicles in the middle ear; it resembles a tiny stirrup and transmits sound vibrations from the incus to the internal ear.

tinnitus Tinkling or ringing sound heard in one or both ears.

tophus Calculus, containing sodium urate deposits, that develops in periauricular fibrous tissue.

tragus Cartilaginous projection in front of the exterior meatus of the ear.

umbo Central depressed portion of the concavity on lateral surface of the tympanic membrane; marks the spot where the malleus is attached to the inner surface.

vertigo Sensation of a whirling motion, involving either oneself or external objects.

vestibule Middle part of the inner ear, located behind the cochlea and in front of the semicircular canals.

ANATOMY AND PHYSIOLOGY REVIEW

The ear is a sensory organ that functions both in equilibrium and hearing. It is divided into three sections: the outer ear, the middle ear, and the inner ear (Fig. 6-1).

The outer ear is made up of the auricle and the auditory ear canal. The auricle, or pinna, is composed of cartilage covered with skin. The auditory ear canal is a curved canal that extends for approximately 2.4 cm (Fig. 6-2). The ear canal is covered with cerumen-producing glands.

The middle ear is separated from the external ear canal by the tympanic membrane. The tympanic membrane is shiny, translucent, and pearl gray. The middle ear is an air-filled cavity across which sound is transmitted by way of three tiny bones—the ossicles (malleus, incus, and stapes). The inner ear is connected by the eustachian tube to the nasopharynx. The eardrum is visualized as an oblique membrane pulled inward at its center by the handle and short process of the malleus. The cone of light may be seen downward and anteriorly. Above the short process is the pars flaccida. The remainder of the drum constitutes the pars tensa (Fig. 6-3).

The inner ear is a curved cavity inside a bony labyrinth consisting of the vestibule, the semicircular canals, and the cochlea. The vestibule and the semicircular canals make up the organs that coordinate equilibrium.

The cochlea is a coiled structure containing the organ of Corti, which transmits sound impulses to the eighth cranial nerve.

Hearing occurs when sound waves enter the external auditory ear canal and strike the tympanic membrane. The ossicles are then put into vibration, after which the hair cells of the organ of Corti are set into motion and the eighth cranial nerve is stimulated. The impulses are transmitted to the temporal lobe of the brain for interpretation.

Hearing Loss
Conductive Hearing Loss

This type of hearing loss occurs when a change in the outer and/or middle ear impairs conduction of sound from the outer to the inner ear. Air conduction is impeded. Common causes of conductive hearing loss include impaction by cerumen, foreign bodies lodged in the ear canal, tumors of the middle ear, and otitis media. Symptoms of conductive hearing loss include diminished hearing and low-volume speaking voice.

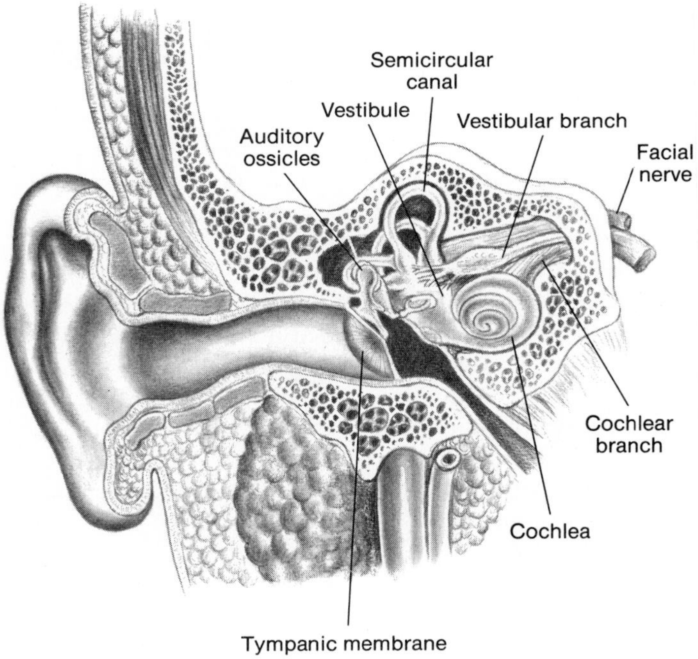

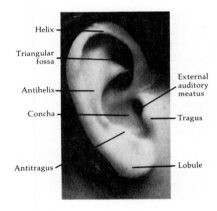

Fig. 6-2 Ear landmarks.

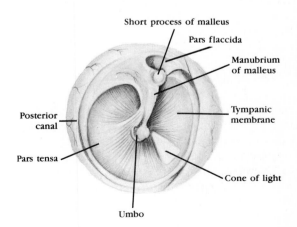

Fig. 6-3 Tympanic membrane landmarks.

Fig. 6-1 Anatomy of external, middle, and inner ear. (Modified from Thompson JM, McFarland GK, Hirsch JE, and others: *Mosby's manual of clinical nursing*, ed 2, St Louis, 1989, Mosby–Year Book.)

Sensorineural Hearing Loss

This type of hearing loss is caused by impairment of the organ of Corti. Conditions that commonly cause this are Meniere disease, ototoxicity, and systemic diseases, such as syphilis and diabetes mellitus. Presbycusis is the most common form of sensorineural hearing loss and is especially common in the elderly.

COGNITIVE OBJECTIVES

At the end of this chapter the learner will demonstrate knowledge of assessment of the ear and auditory system by the ability to do the following:

- Apply the terms that are listed in the vocabulary section.
- Systematically list examination criteria for evaluating the external ear, including the following:
  1. Anatomical positioning
  2. Surface characteristics of the external ear and ear canal
  3. Tympanic membrane (TM) (see Fig. 6-1)
- Describe the technique of manipulating the external ear and canal for otoscopic examination of the adult and the child.
- List six methods to screen for hearing problems, three for the adult and three for the child.
- Identify selected common variations for the child and the older adult.
- Differentiate testing methods for evaluating conductive and perceptive hearing loss; describe the Rinne and Weber tests, and discuss normal and abnormal findings for each.
- List descriptors for evaluating the TM. Describe normal findings and the suggested significance of deviations from normal.

CLINICAL OUTLINE

At the end of this chapter the learner will perform a systematic assessment of the ear and auditory system, demonstrating the ability to do the following:

- Obtain a pertinent health history from a client.
- Demonstrate inspection of the external ear and relate findings concerning:
  1. Ear position, size, and symmetry
  2. Skin color, intactness, deformities, and lesions
  3. Patency of external canal
- Palpate the external ear and mastoid process and relate findings relevant to skin texture, tenderness, nodules, and swelling.
- Demonstrate inspection of the external canal and tympanic membrane (TM) and relate findings concerning:
  1. Color of canal tissue, evidence of tissue intactness, discharge, deformities, masses or lesions, cerumen presence, and characteristics

2. Landmark identification, including umbo, malleus, light reflex, pars tensa, pars flaccida, and anulus
3. Color of the TM
4. Tension of the TM
5. Intactness, scars, or deformities of the TM
- Evaluate the client's auditory system by using screening techniques, including the Rinne and Weber tests, and interpret findings.
- Summarize results of the assessment with a written description of the findings.

HISTORY

- Is there a family history of hearing problems or hearing loss?
- Is there history of frequent ear problems or infections during childhood? Describe typical treatment techniques and course of the problem.
- Is there history of any ear injury or hearing problems related to trauma?
- If the client complains of painful ears, the examiner should collect descriptive data using the analysis of a symptom format. In addition, the possibility of trauma to the ears— either by foreign body, harsh cleaning, or environmental noise—must be investigated, and related complaints, including recent problems with mouth, teeth, paranasal sinuses, or throat, must be inquired about.
- If itching of the ears is a complaint, ask the client where the sensation is felt, what the duration of the sensation is, and what he has done to correct the problem. In addition, inquire about swimming, showering, and ear-cleansing techniques.
- Medication history is especially important if the client has any complaints of tinnitus or extra noise in the ears. Special emphasis should be placed on collecting information about ototoxic drugs, including acetyl-salicylic acid, quinine, streptomycin, neomycin, gentamicin, or nitrofurantoin.
- If the client complains of dizziness or vertigo, the examiner must collect detailed information to describe the exact nature of the problem.
  1. Vertigo is the sensation of whirling motion: with eyes open, the client states that the surroundings are moving; with eyes closed, the client feels himself in motion. Dizziness is the disturbed sense of relationship to space.
  2. How does the sensation change with the client's change in position (e.g., lying down, bending, standing)?
  3. Is the client taking medications, or does he have a systemic disease?
  4. Does the symptom (e.g., falling, losing balance) interfere with the client's activities of daily living?

- If the client complains of a hearing loss, the examiner should inquire about the following:
  1. Sudden or slow onset of hearing problem
  2. Environmental factors, such as factory noise
  3. Specific types of sounds or tones that the client has difficulty hearing, such as conversation or a telephone ringing
  4. To what degree the hearing problem interferes with the client's activities of daily living; whether it causes a problem on the job, in television viewing, phone conversations, etc.
  5. What types of corrective devices the client has tried; where and from whom the devices were obtained
- If environmental or employment noise is a problem, what precautions, if any, are taken? Head sets or ear plugs? What is the extent of the environmental exposure?

Text continues on p. 161.

CLINICAL GUIDELINES

ASSESSMENT PROCEDURE	EVALUATION	
	NORMAL FINDINGS	DEVIATIONS FROM NORMAL

1. Collect equipment
  a. Otoscope with bright light, several sizes of ear specula, pneumatic bulb
  b. Tuning fork (500 to 1000 cycles per second [cps])
2. Perform physical assessment of the ear
  a. Inspect both ears for alignment and configuration
	Ears of equal height and size
	Located so that pinna is on line with corner of eye (Fig. 6-4, *A*)
	Ear within 10° angle of vertical position
		Abnormal configuration
		Low-set or unequal positioning (Fig. 6-4, *B*)

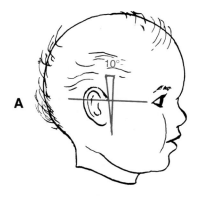 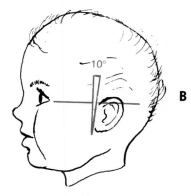

Fig. 6-4　Ear alignment. **A,** Normal alignment. **B,** Low-set alignment.

Continued.

CLINICAL GUIDELINES—cont'd

ASSESSMENT PROCEDURE	EVALUATION	
	NORMAL FINDINGS	DEVIATIONS FROM NORMAL
b. Inspect external ear (anterior and posterior bilateral and mastoid areas) (Fig. 6-5)	Skin color pink, uniform Skin intact	Redness Swelling Deformities, lesions, nodules such as Darwinian tubercle Tophi (Fig. 6-6) Cauliflower ear (Fig. 6-7) Furuncles
c. Palpate external ear (auricles and mastoid areas)	Intact Smooth, nontender	Tenderness Pain Swelling Nodules

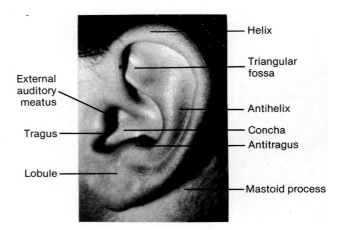

External auditory meatus — Tragus — Lobule —

— Helix

— Triangular fossa

— Antihelix

— Concha
— Antitragus

— Mastoid process

Fig. 6-5   Landmarks of ear.

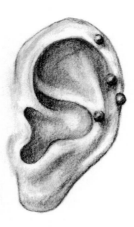

Fig. 6-6   Tophi.

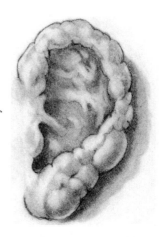

Fig. 6-7   Cauliflower ear.

	EVALUATION	
ASSESSMENT PROCEDURE	**NORMAL FINDINGS**	**DEVIATIONS FROM NORMAL**
d. Use otoscope to examine: (1) External auditory canal (see clinical strategies for technique and Fig. 6-8 for structures)	Cerumen present; note color (may vary: black, brown, dark red, creamy, brown-gray); texture (may vary from moist waxy to dry flaky or hard texture); no odor Caucasians and blacks: generally have wet cerumen that is tan or brown Asians and American Indians: generally have dry cerumen that is light to brown-gray Hair present (Fig. 6-9) Canal skin intact Uniform pink color Tenderness with deep speculum insertion	Cerumen impacting ear canal; unable to visualize canal or TM (Fig. 6-10) Lesions, bleeding, discharge (note appearance and odor), foreign bodies (Fig. 6-11), inflammation, growths (Fig. 6-12), pain, tenderness, swelling, infection Partial occlusion of auditory canal caused by improper retraction of auricle; can usually be remedied by correct traction (Fig. 6-13)

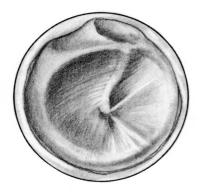

Fig. 6-8   Structures of ear.

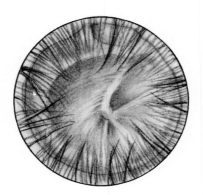

Fig. 6-9   Hairy ear canal.

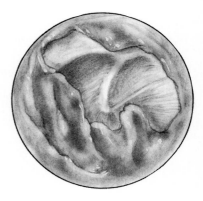

Fig. 6-10   Cerumen in ear canal.

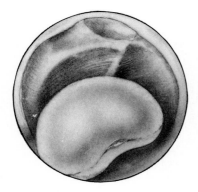

Fig. 6-11   Foreign object in ear canal.

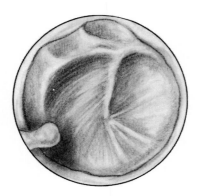

Fig. 6-12   Polyp in external ear canal.

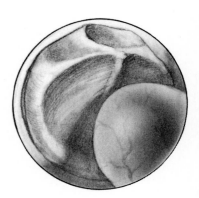

Fig. 6-13   Wall of ear canal obstructing view.

Continued.

CLINICAL GUIDELINES—cont'd

ASSESSMENT PROCEDURE	EVALUATION	
	NORMAL FINDINGS	DEVIATIONS FROM NORMAL
(2) Tympanic membrane (Fig. 6-14)		
(a) Characteristics	Drum intact	Membrane not intact (Fig. 6-15) or showing scarring (Fig. 6-16)
	Slight fluctuation present when swallowing	Membrane fixed and nonfluctuating or jerky fluctuation present
(b) Color	Shiny, pearly gray, translucent appearance	Other TM colors indicating abnormality: Serum—yellow-amber Blood—blue or deep red Pus—chalky white Infection—red or pink Fibrosis—dull surface Diffuse or spotty light Obliteration of some or all landmarks Increased vascularization (injection)

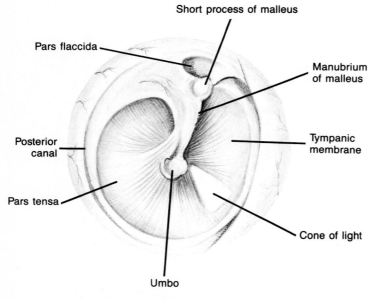

Fig. 6-14   Tympanic membrane landmarks.

Short process of malleus

Pars flaccida

Manubrium of malleus

Posterior canal

Tympanic membrane

Pars tensa

Cone of light

Umbo

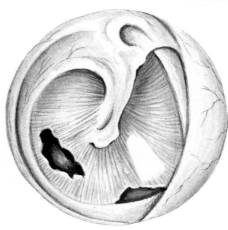

Fig. 6-15   Perforated membrane.

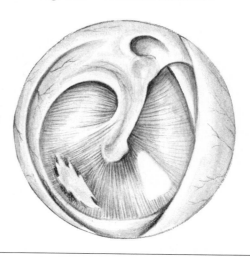

Fig. 6-16   Scarring of membrane.

| | EVALUATION | |
ASSESSMENT PROCEDURE	NORMAL FINDINGS	DEVIATIONS FROM NORMAL
(c) Landmarks: follow anulus around periphery of pars tensa	Cone of light (pars tensa) Umbo Handle of malleus Short process of malleus Malleolar folds Pars flaccida	Accentuated landmarks (indicating negative pressure behind TM) Bulging membrane (indicating buildup of pressure behind TM)
3. Perform screening evaluation of auditory function		
a. Whispered voice: stand 30 to 60 cm (1 to 2 feet) from client, mask client's opposite ear, exhale, then whisper in very low voice; increase intensity until client responds correctly at least 50% of time; use both monosyllabic and bisyllabic words; repeat other side	Able to hear softly whispered words at distance of 30 to 60 cm (1 to 2 feet) Bilaterally equal response	Unilateral response or bilaterally unequal response Unable to repeat words until whispered voice is louder
b. Watch tick: place ticking watch 2 to 5 cm (1 to 2 inches) from ear; mask opposite ear; repeat other side	Able to hear ticking watch at distance of 2 to 5 cm (1 to 2 inches)	Clients with high-frequency hearing loss unable to hear ticking
c. Tuning fork		
(1) **Rinne test** (compares air conduction to bone conduction): softly strike tuning fork and place on client's mastoid process; when client is no longer able to hear tone, remove tuning fork and place it in front of same ear; tone should be heard approximately twice as long in this position (Fig. 6-17)	Air-conducted sound heard twice as long as bone-conducted sound (AC > BC); called *positive result*	Bone-conducted sound heard as long as or longer than air-conducted sound (BC ≥ AC); called *negative result;* a sign of conductive loss

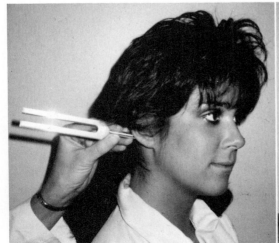 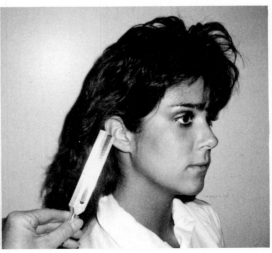

Fig. 6-17   Rinne test. **A,** Behind ear, on mastoid process. **B,** In front of ear.

Continued.

CLINICAL GUIDELINES—cont'd

ASSESSMENT PROCEDURE	EVALUATION	
	NORMAL FINDINGS	DEVIATIONS FROM NORMAL
(2) **Weber test** (assesses bone conduction by testing lateralization of sounds): softly strike tuning fork and place on midline of forehead (Fig. 6-18)	Bilaterally equal sound	If client has conductive loss, sound lateralizes to poorer ear If client has sensorineural loss, sound lateralizes to good ear
4. Evaluate vestibular portion of auditory nerve (CN VIII) a. Test for nystagmus using cold caloric test (procedure is *not normally* done during screening examination and should not be performed if client is thought to have acute middle ear infection or perforated eardrum): client sits with head tilted 60° in extension (backward) position; irrigate against eardrum with 10 ml of ice water (32°-50° F) over 20-second period; test one ear at a time and note response	Nausea, dizziness, and nystagmus appearing in about 30 seconds and lasting approximately 1½ minutes (Fig. 6-19)	Bilaterally unequal response Unduly prolonged unilateral nystagmus
b. Test for vestibular functioning (Romberg sign): client stands with feet together, eyes closed, arms to side; watch for steadiness of stance (stand near in case client loses balance) (Fig. 6-20)	Swaying but able to maintain body and feet positioning for 5 seconds	Unable to maintain positioning Need to widen base support Unable to keep from falling

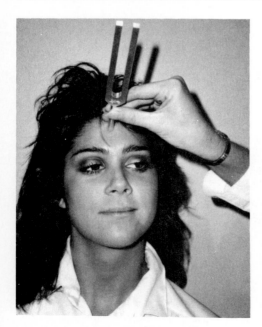

Fig. 6-18 Weber test. Tuning fork is placed on forehead.

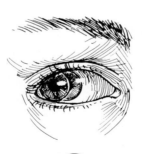

Fig. 6-19 Nystagmus associated with CN VIII vestibular malfunction.

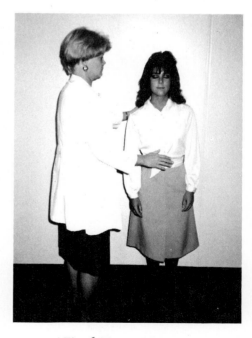

Fig. 6-20 Romberg test.

CLINICAL TIPS AND STRATEGIES

- **Hearing evaluation should begin from the moment you meet the client:** Note how the individual responds to your speaking; note *posturing of head* or types of words that need repeating.
- **When using the otoscope consider the following guidelines:**
  1. Use the largest speculum that will fit comfortably into the ear canal (Fig. 6-21)

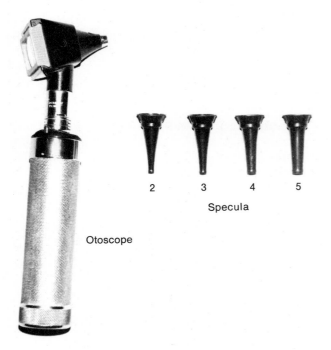

2
3
4
5

Specula

Otoscope

2. The otoscope must have good batteries or adequate illumination of the landmarks of the ear will be impossible. (Bulb should give off white, *not* yellow, light)
3. The adult client should be sitting with the head tilted toward the opposite shoulder.
4. Hold the otoscope between the palm and the first two fingers of one hand. The handle may be positioned either downward (Fig. 6-22) or upward (see Fig. 6-27). The examiner must determine which position provides better immobility between the otoscope and the client's head.
5. With the other hand, grasp the pinna with the thumb and fingers and pull out, up, and back to straighten the canal (see Fig. 6-22).
6. Remember, the inner two thirds of the external ear

Fig. 6-21   Otoscope with all sizes of available specula.

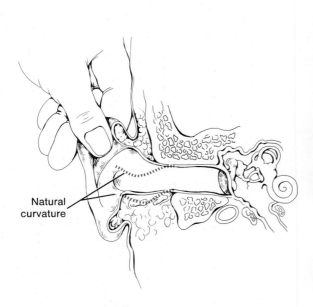

Natural
curvature

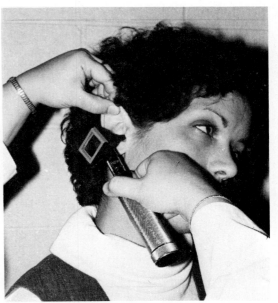

Fig. 6-22   Straighten external canal of adult ear by pulling helix up and out.

canal are bony. It will *hurt* if the speculum is pressed against either side (Fig. 6-23). If the examiner is having difficulty seeing the TM, a combination of repositioning the head, pulling the auricle in a slightly different position, and reangling the otoscope should be attempted.

7. When placing the speculum in the client's ear, make sure to steady your hand against the client's head by extending one or two fingers from the hand holding the otoscope.

- **A cerumen spoon or irrigation may be used to remove cerumen from the external ear canal:** If the cerumen is wet and waxy, a cerumen spoon works best; if it is dry, irrigation is preferable. The examiner must see the TM in any client with a history suggestive of hearing or ear problems.

- **Sometimes only about half of the TM is visualized because of bone structure or excessive hair in the ear canal:** If that half appears healthy and without disease, one can assume that the other half is healthy also.

- **When striking a tuning fork, be careful not to make the tone too loud:** If this happens, it will take so long to quiet the tone enough for auditory testing that the client may become tired. It is usually sufficient to tap the fork gently on the knuckle or stroke the fork between the thumb and the index finger (Fig. 6-24).

- **The examiner's position is important during the whisper test:** Make sure to position yourself so that the client cannot read your lips.

- **The technique of masking is very important:** The examiner should simply instruct the client to insert a finger into the ear that is not being tested and then wiggle it back and forth slightly to occlude hearing in that ear by masking it with noise. The technique is reversed during examination of the opposite ear.

- **Carefully interpret findings:** Although ear and hearing examination may appear to be a simple task, it is important that you slow down and thoughtfully evaluate your findings.

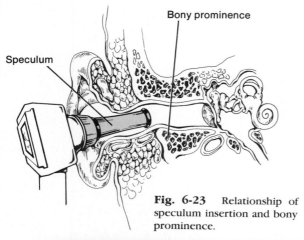

Fig. 6-23 Relationship of speculum insertion and bony prominence.

SAMPLE RECORDING: NORMAL FINDINGS

Ear: Positioning bilaterally symmetrical; smooth auricles without lesions or discharge.
External canal: small amount of dark cerumen noted.
Tympanic membrane intact; all landmarks clearly identified.
Auditory: Can hear low whisper at 60 cm (2 feet).
Rinne: AC > BC.
Weber: equal lateralization.
Vestibular: CN VIII intact.

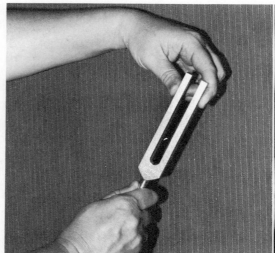
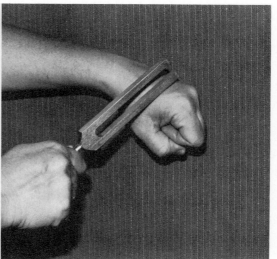

Fig. 6-24 Activating the tuning fork. Hearing is tested at *near-threshold* levels; therefore the fork should be made to ring softly. **A,** Stroking the fork. **B,** Tapping the fork gently on the knuckle.

The Newborn

HISTORY AND CLINICAL STRATEGIES

- Infants should not have any objects (e.g., cotton tips) inserted blindly into their ears. Use care if visualizing the inner ear with an otoscope. Pull ear gently downward to straighten canal.

- Low-set ears are associated with various anomalies, and further investigation is needed. To determine ear position, draw an imaginary line from the middle of the eye to the first crease or top of the ear. If the ear is below the level of the eyes, the ears are in a low position.

CLINICAL VARIATIONS: THE NEWBORN

CHARACTERISTIC OR AREA EXAMINED	NORMAL FINDINGS	DEVIATIONS FROM NORMAL
1. Ear	Regular shape, symmetric	Asymmetry, auricular pits, skin tags (may relate to congenital anomaly)
	Dermal sinus and ear tags (possibly nonconsequential)	
	Patent ear canal	
	Tympanic membrane is superior, horizontal	
	Eardrum is duller, more gray than in older infant or child	Red color (may be otitis media)
	Reddish-blue color may be seen when crying	Blue-black color (suggests hemorrhage)
	Bulging membrane occurs rarely	
	Clear amber color is serous fluid	
	Pinna easily bends with instant recoil	Pinna is more folded, flat in premature infant
		Pinna is stiff with thicker cartilage in postterm infants
	Top of ear even with inner and outer eye canthus	Low-set ears (suggests chromosomal or renal congenital disorders)
2. Hearing	Infant startles with loud noises	Deafness is difficult to confirm
	Head turns toward voice, ringing bell	

 The Child

HISTORY AND CLINICAL STRATEGIES

- Evaluation of a child's ear is exactly like that of an adult's ear. For screening purposes the vestibular component is not evaluated.
- The examiner must evaluate the same anatomical structures in both an adult's and a child's ears. It is important for the examiner to scale down expectations to maintain a gentle approach (Fig. 6-25). Consequently, insert the speculum into the canal between 0.6 and 1.2 cm (¼ and ½ inch).

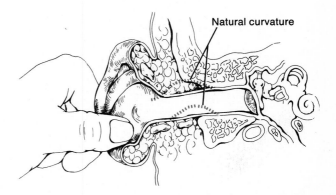

Fig. 6-25 Anatomical comparison of adult's and child's ear.

- One difference in examining a child's ear is the curvature of the external canal (Fig. 6-26). Because of the upward curvature of the canal in the infant and small child, the examiner must grasp the lower portion of the auricle and retract the ear downward and backward to straighten the canal. By age 3, the child's canal has changed to assume more of an adult position. Therefore with the child who is 3 years and older, the pinna should be pulled up and back to straighten the canal.

- Young children can be "squirmy;" we have found it best to examine the child's ear canal and TM in the following manner:

  1. Place the child in either a prone position with head to the side and arms downward (Fig. 6-27), or

  2. Place the child in a supine position on the cart with arms extended overhead and secured by the parent (Fig. 6-28).

  3. Hold the otoscope like a pencil, with the handle extending upward toward the top of the child's head. Brace the otoscope and your hand against the child's head by extending one or two fingers as securing forces (Fig. 6-27). This position will allow your hand and the instrument to go along with any sudden movements.

  4. The child *must* be securely immobilized during the ear examination.

- Because of the sensitive nature of the ear examination, it is best left until the last part of the physical exam-

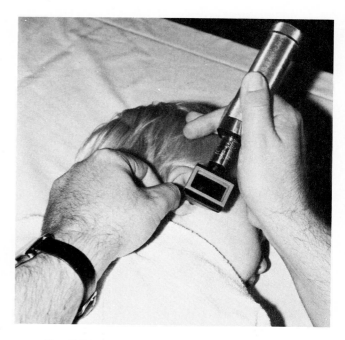

Fig. 6-27 Examination of child in prone position with arms to side.

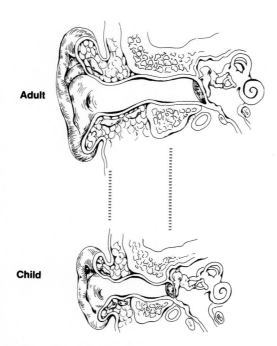

Fig. 6-26 Pull ear down and out to straighten ear canal.

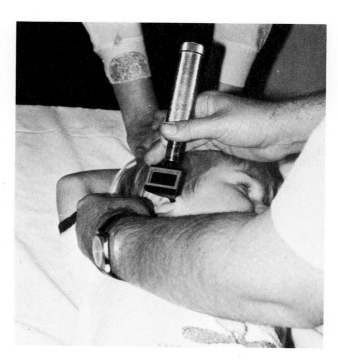

Fig. 6-28 Examination of child in supine position with arms overhead.

ination. Should the child become upset, this will permit immediate return to the parent for cuddling.

- During the TM evaluation the examiner may decide to evaluate the fluctuating capacity of the TM by injecting small puffs of air against the membrane. This is especially important if the child is thought to have fluid or pressure buildup behind the TM. Slight fluctuation of the membrane is a normal response; no movement or jerky movement is abnormal. There are several instruments and procedures to perform this assessment (Fig. 6-29). The examiner must choose the largest speculum that will fit into the child's ear canal; the secure, tight fit will allow air pressure to move the TM.

- Every child should have an ear evaluation. If the ear canal is occluded with wax, the examiner must use one of the common techniques to remove it. If the child is ill or running a fever, examination of the TM is an *absolute must*.

- History questions specifically related to the pediatric client include the following:

1. Recurrent infections of the throat or ears? Number during past 6 months? Usual treatment?
2. Ear problems becoming more frequent and/or severe?
3. History of ear surgery? If so, what and when?
4. Child play with his ears frequently or have tendency toward putting objects in his ears?
5. History of foreign body in ears?
6. How does the parent clean the child's ears?
7. Child ever had his ears tested? If so, by whom and where?
8. If the child has low-set ears, question extensively about kidney or other congenital problems.
9. If a child has symptoms of ear or auditory dysfunction, it is important to inquire specifically about any past disease or drug usage that is considered potentially ototoxic. Children who are at high risk are those who have had measles, mumps, otitis media, any disease with high fever, or drugs, including streptomycin, kanamycin, and neomycin.

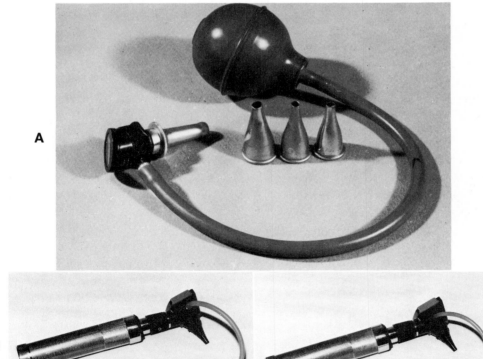

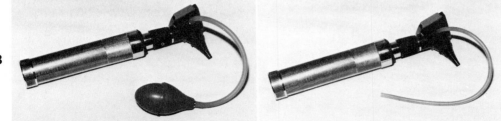

Fig. 6-29 **A,** Pneumatic otoscope. **B,** Regular otoscope with pneumatic bulb. **C,** Regular otoscope with pneumatic tube. End of the tubing is placed in the examiner's mouth, where small puffs of air are expelled against the child's tympanic membrane. (**A** from Prior JA, Silberstein JS, Stang JM: *Physical diagnosis: the history and examination of the patient,* ed 6, St Louis, 1981, Mosby–Year Book.)

CLINICAL VARIATIONS: THE CHILD

CHARACTERISTIC OR AREA EXAMINED	NORMAL FINDINGS	DEVIATIONS FROM NORMAL
1. External ear a. Alignment	Ears of equal height and size Located so that pinna is on line with corner of eye Ear within 10° angle of vertical position	Low-set or unequal positioning

b. Configuration		Abnormal configuration
		   Deformities, lesions, nodules such as Darwinian tubercle
		   Tophi
		   Cauliflower ear
		   Furuncles

2. External canal a. Color and surface	Skin color pink, uniform Skin intact Hair present Canal skin intact Tenderness with deep speculum insertion	Redness Swelling Lesions, bleeding, discharge (note appearance and odor), foreign bodies, inflammation, growths, pain, tenderness, swelling, infection Partial occlusion of auditory canal caused by improper retraction of auricle; can usually be corrected with traction
	Smooth, nontender	Tenderness Pain Swelling Nodules
b. Cerumen	Cerumen present; note color (may vary: black to brown to creamy pink), texture (may vary from moist waxy to dry flaky or hard texture); no odor	Cerumen impacting ear canal; unable to visualize canal or TM
3. Tympanic membrane a. Characteristics	Drum intact Presence of myringotomy tube (Fig. 6-30) in selected clients	Membrane not intact or showing scarring

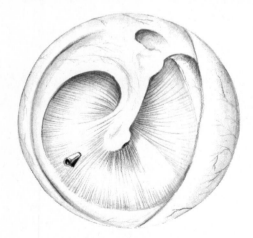

Fig. 6-30   Drainage tube inserted after myringotomy.

CHARACTERISTIC OR AREA EXAMINED	NORMAL FINDINGS	DEVIATIONS FROM NORMAL
b. Tension: use pneumatic or squeeze bulb to evaluate TM fluctuation	Slight fluctuation of drum with air puffs	Fixed, nonfluctuating or jerky fluctuation
c. Color	Shiny, pearly gray, translucent appearance	Other TM colors indicating abnormality: Serum—yellow-amber Blood—blue or deep red Pus—chalky white Infection—red or pink Fibrosis—dull surface
d. Landmarks	Cone of light (pars tensa) Umbo Handle of malleus Short process of malleus Malleolar folds Pars flaccida	Diffuse or spotty light Obliteration of some or all landmarks Increased vascularization (injection) Accentuated landmarks (indicating negative pressure behind TM) Bulging membrane (indicating buildup of pressure behind TM)
4. Auditory function a. Up to 2 months: at distance of approximately 30.5 cm (12 inches), and so that infant does not see, snap fingers loudly or ring bell (may need to repeat several times)	Startle reflex or eye blink	No response
b. 2 to 3 months: at distance of approximately 30.5 cm (12 inches), and so that infant does not see, snap fingers loudly or ring bell	Eye blink, or stopping movement to listen for sound	No response
c. 3 months and older: at distance of approximately 30.5 cm (12 inches), and so that infant does not see, snap fingers loudly or ring bell	Turns head toward noise	No response
d. Older infants and toddlers: have child sit on parent's lap; stand behind parent; first on one side and then the other, either ring bell, whisper "s" or "sh" words, or call child's name	Turns head toward noise	No response
e. Preschool and school age: should receive audiometric testing; for preschool and school-age client, if audiometry unavailable, use same screening as for adult client	Able to hear 1000, 2000, 4000, and 6000 cps at 25 decibels (db)	Unable to hear recommended levels
(1) Whispered voice	Able to hear whispered voice at 30 to 60 cm (1 to 2 feet)	Unilateral or unequal response Unable to repeat words until whispered voice is louder
(2) Watch ticking	Able to hear ticking watch at distance of 2 to 5 cm (1 to 2 inches)	Unable to hear ticking
(3) Tuning fork: Rinne test Weber test	AC > BC Bilaterally equal sound	AC = BC Lateralization of sound

The Childbearing Woman

HISTORY AND CLINICAL STRATEGIES

- Assess usual ear hygiene practices.
- If a woman inserts cotton tips into her ear, she should be instructed how to avoid causing trauma and pushing cerumen further into the ear. This may be a good time to discourage the use of cotton tips in her infant's ears.

CLINICAL VARIATIONS: THE CHILDBEARING WOMAN

CHARACTERISTIC OR AREA EXAMINED	NORMAL FINDINGS	DEVIATIONS FROM NORMAL
1. Characteristics	Hearing perception may decrease Engorged eustachian tubes (from capillary fullness) Tympanic membranes may have increased fluid	Otosclerosis and hearing loss may be aggravated by pregnancy
2. Postdelivery	Eustachian tubes and tympanic membranes return to state before pregnancy	

 The Older Adult

HISTORY AND CLINICAL STRATEGIES

- Formal hearing screening should be delayed until near the end of the assessment. Client anxiety or insecurity about ability to perform may exist at the beginning of the examination and may interfere with accurate assessment.
- Informal hearing screening should occur at the beginning and throughout the assessment. Noting whether the client is able to respond appropriately to questions or conversation, with and/or without direct eye contact, is an important clue for assessment of hearing acuity.
- Other clues or "red flags" indicating possible hearing difficulty follow:
  1. Client watches examiner's face and mouth movements closely.
  2. Client's speech volume control is erratic or constantly pronounced.
  3. Client's tone of voice is monotonous, unvaried.
  4. Client's speech is distorted (especially with use or omission of vowel sounds).
  5. Client's family describes changed behaviors, in the form of preoccupation, withdrawal, irritability, or alienation.
- A large percentage of older adults have never had their hearing checked for the following reasons:
  1. Hearing loss is often gradual and insidious.
  2. People are frequently sensitive about a suspected loss. "Sensitivity" can be exhibited in the form of denial, defensiveness, and paranoid beliefs about relationships with others.
  3. Resignation to a hearing loss may exist on the part of the client and his family. It is assumed that it is a nontreatable aspect of aging.
- If hearing loss is offered as a complaint, the following questions should be asked:
  1. Is the loss in both ears or one ear?
  2. Was the onset sudden or gradual? (*Note:* A sudden onset is a "red flag" for immediate referral to a physician.) "Sudden" should be clarified in terms of instant loss (may be indicative of vascular disruption) versus a loss that occurred over a few hours or days (may indicate a viral disorder).
  3. Is all hearing diminished or just certain types of

sounds (e.g., does conversation sound garbled, can you hear the telephone)?

4. Do outside or environmental noises interfere with or distort hearing (e.g., is it more difficult to understand conversation if a lot of people are talking at once)?
5. Do you have a history of exposure to loud or continuous noises (e.g., the whine of machinery on the job)?
6. Have you ever had any auditory training?
7. Does your hearing loss interfere with your daily life (e.g., responses of family or friends to loss, general social or family relationships, ability to function at work or at home)?
8. Have you ever used or do you now use a hearing aid?

- Obtain a drug history. Salicylates, aminoglycosides (e.g., gentamicin, streptomycin), furosemide, quinine, and ethacrynic acid are commonly used drugs that diminish hearing.
- Hearing aids are expensive and can be misused, nontherapeutic, or even damaging. Ebersole* notes the following recent federal regulations that require medical evaluation before an individual can purchase a hearing aid:
  1. Visible congenital or traumatic deformity of the ear.
  2. Active drainage from the ear in the last 90 days.
  3. Sudden or progressive hearing loss within the last 90 days.
  4. Acute or chronic dizziness.
  5. Unilateral sudden hearing loss within the last 90 days.
  6. Visible evidence of significant cerumen accumulation or a foreign body in the ear canal.
  7. Pain or discomfort in the ear.
  8. Audiometric air-bone gap equal to or greater than 15 db.
- If a hearing aid is used, the following questions should be asked:
  1. Do you feel it is effective? (*Note:* Adjustment to a new hearing aid may take 2 to 6 months.)
  2. How often do you wear it (all the time, on social occasions, rarely, never)?
  3. Do you have any difficulty operating it or using it (e.g., pushing small switches or buttons, inserting batteries, fastening aid to clothing, inserting earmold, untangling wires)?

4. Do you have difficulty keeping it in good repair, or are you concerned about expenses related to repair?
5. Do you have difficulty cleaning it? (*Note:* Cerumen or other debris can plug the tiny hole that carries sound through the earmolds.)
6. When was it purchased? Who prescribed it?

- Tinnitus may be interpreted by the client as a ringing, cracking, whistling, or buzzing sound. In addition to a full-symptom analysis, be certain to clarify the quality of the sound.
  1. Tinnitus may be a pulsatile sensation (possibly associated with carotid bruits), a steady noise, or a transient complaint.
  2. Chronic tinnitis (6 months or more) should be differentiated from a similar complaint of short duration and/or sudden onset.
- Vertigo must be differentiated from unsteadiness, which is fairly common with elderly people. If vertigo is established as a complaint, ask if it is associated with head or neck movement (in addition to doing a full-symptom analysis).
- Ear pain or a feeling of "fullness" may reflect a problem related to temporomandibular joint movement, cervical arthritis, or dental disease.
- See p. 154 in this chapter for further questions.

RISK FACTORS FOR POSSIBLE HEARING DEFICIENCY

- History of long exposure to loud or continuous noise
- History of chronic nasal allergy
- Systemic disease (some of the more commonly associated diseases: cardiovascular disease, diabetes mellitus, nephritis)
- Sensitivity to some medications (see list on p. 154)
- Chronic cigarette smoking
- General physical or emotional disability (some authors state there is a correlation between impaired physical and/or emotional well-being and diminished hearing acuity)
- Family history of deafness

---

*From Ebersole P, Hess P: *Toward healthy aging,* ed 3, St Louis, 1990, Mosby–Year Book.

CLINICAL VARIATIONS: THE OLDER ADULT

CHARACTERISTIC OR AREA EXAMINED	NORMAL FINDINGS	DEVIATIONS FROM NORMAL
1. External ear		
a. Alignment	Ears of equal height and size Located so that pinna is on line with corner of eye Ear within 10° angle of vertical position	Low-set or unequal positioning
b. Configuration	Earlobes may appear pendulous	Abnormal configuration
c. Surface characteristics	Skin color pink, uniform Skin intact	Redness Swelling Deformities, lesions, nodules such as Darwinian tubercle Tophi Cauliflower ear Furuncles
	Smooth, nontender	Tenderness Pain Swelling Nodules
2. External canal		
a. Color, surface characteristics, discharge	Canal skin intact Uniform pink color Tenderness with deep speculum insertion Cerumen present; note color (may vary from black to brown to creamy pink) and texture (may vary from moist waxy to dry flaky or hard texture) Impacted cerumen usually contains more keratin and may be more difficult to remove Hair present	Cerumen impacting ear canal (*Note:* In older adults cerumen can become very dry and totally obstruct canal; canal can also be obstructed with impacted skin and hair [keratoses].) Lesions, bleeding, discharge (note appearance and odor), foreign bodies (Fig. 6-11), inflammation, growths (Fig. 6-12), pain, tenderness, swelling, infection Be alert for sebaceous cysts, furuncles, dermatosis, or increase in granulation tissue (*Note:* Earmolds—part of hearing aids—may cause irritation of canal, especially if they do not fit well.)
3. Tympanic membrane		
a. Characteristics	Drum intact	Membrane not intact (Fig. 6-15) or showing scarring (Fig. 6-16)
	Slight fluctuation present with swallowing	Fixed, nonfluctuating or jerky fluctuation
b. Color	Shiny, pearly gray, translucent appearance	Other TM colors indicating abnormality: Serum—yellow-amber Blood—blue or deep red Pus—chalky white Infection—red or pink Fibrosis—dull surface

CHARACTERISTIC OR AREA EXAMINED	NORMAL FINDINGS	DEVIATIONS FROM NORMAL
c. Landmarks: follow anulus around periphery of pars tensa	Cone of light (pars tensa) Umbo Handle of malleus Short process of malleus Malleolar folds Pars flaccida Landmarks may appear slightly more pronounced with atrophic or sclerotic tympanic changes	Diffuse or spotty light Obliteration of some or all landmarks Increased vascularization (injection) Accentuated landmarks (indicating negative pressure behind TM) Bulging membrane (indicating buildup of pressure behind TM)
4. Screening evaluation of auditory function*		
a. Whispered voice	Able to hear softly whispered words at distance of 30 to 60 cm (1 to 2 feet) Bilaterally equal response	Unilateral response or bilaterally unequal response Unable to repeat words until whispered voice is louder
b. Watch tick	Able to hear ticking watch at distance of 2 to 5 cm (1 to 2 inches)	Clients with high-frequency hearing loss unable to hear ticking
c. Tuning fork		
(1) Rinne test	Air-conduction sound heard twice as long as bone conduction (AC > BC); called a *positive result*	Bone-conduction sound heard as long as or longer than air-conduction sound (*Note:* Air-conduction hearing time will exceed bone-conduction time with sensorineural loss but will be accompanied by unequal lateralization in Weber test.)
(2) Weber test	Bilaterally equal sound	If client has conductive loss, sound will lateralize to poorer ear If client has sensorineural loss, sound will lateralize to better ear
5. Vestibular portion of auditory (CN VIII) (evaluates labyrinth system)		
a. Test for nystagmus	Slow movement of eyes in one lateral direction until they reach their limit; steady gaze in that position	Rapid compensatory rhythmic movement in eyes in opposite direction (Fig. 6-19)
b. Test for falling (Romberg sign): client stands with feet together, eyes closed, arms to side; watch for steadiness of stance; stand nearby in case client loses balance	Swaying but able to maintain body and feet positioning	Unable to maintain positioning Need to widen base support Unable to keep from falling

A client with a suspected hearing loss should be referred for audiometric testing.

Study Questions

General

1. The eardrum divides the:
   - ☐ a. External ear from the inner ear
   - ☐ b. Middle ear from the inner ear
   - ☐ c. External ear from the middle ear
2. When choosing a tuning fork for testing auditory function, pick one with frequencies between:
   - ☐ a. 200 and 500 cps
   - ☐ b. 400 and 800 cps
   - ☐ c. 500 and 1000 cps
   - ☐ d. 1000 and 2000 cps
3. Functions of the middle ear are to:
   - ☐ a. Transmit sounds across the ossicle chain to the inner ear
   - ☐ b. Transmit stimuli to the cochlear branch of the auditory nerve
   - ☐ c. Maintain balance
   - ☐ d. Protect the auditory apparatus from intense vibrations
   - ☐ e. Equalize air pressure
   - ☐ f. a, c, and e
   - ☐ g. b, d, and e
   - ☐ h. a, c, d, and e
   - ☐ i. a, d, and e
   - ☐ j. All of the above
4. The cochlear branch of the auditory nerve responsible for hearing is:
   - ☐ a. CN II
   - ☐ b. CN IV
   - ☐ c. CN VIII
   - ☐ d. CN IX
   - ☐ e. None of the above
5. Which statements are true concerning the Rinne test:
   - ☐ a. It is a test of bone conduction only
   - ☐ b. It is a test of bone conduction and air conduction
   - ☐ c. The sound is referred to the better ear because the cochlea or the auditory nerve is functioning more effectively
   - ☐ d. A normal response would be that if the tuning fork were placed on the mastoid process until it were no longer heard and then placed in front of the auditory meatus, the sound would continue to be heard
   - ☐ e. A normal response would be that if the fork were placed in the middle of the forehead, the sound would radiate bilaterally and equally
   - ☐ f. a and d
   - ☐ g. b, c, and d
   - ☐ h. a, c, and e
   - ☐ i. b and d
   - ☐ j. None of the above

The Newborn

6. What ear structure is duller and more gray in a newborn than in a child:
   - ☐ a. Canal
   - ☐ b. Hammer
   - ☐ c. Stapes
   - ☐ d. Eardrum
7. An ear sign suggesting chromosomal disorders is:
   - ☐ a. Reddish-blue drum
   - ☐ b. Low-set ears
   - ☐ c. Instant pinna recoil
   - ☐ d. Symmetric shape

The Child

8. The external ear of the child is:
   - ☐ a. Normally at a position lower than the corner of the eye, but by the child's first birthday it is at its normal adult position
   - ☐ b. Slanted backward at about a 10° angle
   - ☐ c. Normally above the position of the corner of the eye, but by the child's first birthday it is at its normal adult position
   - ☐ d. Directly vertical to the position of the head
   - ☐ e. Normally at the same level as the corner of the eye
   - ☐ f. a and b
   - ☐ g. b and c
   - ☐ h. b and e
   - ☐ i. c and d
   - ☐ j. d and e

The Childbearing Woman

9. Altered hearing perception during pregnancy is the result of:
   - ☐ a. Decreased tympanic fluid
   - ☐ b. Thinner eardrums
   - ☐ c. Swollen oval windows
   - ☐ d. Engorged eustachian tubes

The Older Adult

10. Pick the false statement. Presbycusis:
   - ☐ a. Is a progressive, bilaterally symmetrical hearing loss
   - ☐ b. Can often be relieved with surgical repair
   - ☐ c. Often involves auditory loss of high tones initially
   - ☐ d. When advanced may cause speech to sound garbled or distorted
   - ☐ e. Can exist to a fairly advanced degree before a client will report it as a symptom

11. Pick the false statement. Tinnitus:
    - ☐ a. Might be caused by cerumen impaction
    - ☐ b. Can be associated with temporomandibular joint malfunction
    - ☐ c. Can be associated with chronic emotional upset
    - ☐ d. Is an early symptom of presbycusis
    - ☐ e. Might occur with an arthritic client who is taking regular doses of an analgesic

Mark each statement as either "T" for true or "F" for false.

12. _____ Speech can eventually become distorted with a client who has a prolonged severe hearing loss.

13. _____ A sudden hearing loss in an elderly client usually indicates mechanical obstruction and subsides quickly (within 3 days).

14. _____ Loss of general physical well-being may affect the client's auditory effectiveness.

15. _____ Earmolds (part of hearing aids) should fit very loosely when inserted into the canal to avoid friction or pressure irritation.

SUGGESTED READINGS

General

Bates B: *A guide to physical examination,* ed 4, Philadelphia, 1987, JB Lippincott.

Bierman C, Pierson E: Diseases of the ear, *J Allergy Clin Immunol* 5:1009, 1981.

DeWeese DD, Saunders WH: *Textbook of otolaryngology,* ed 6, St Louis, 1982, Mosby–Year Book.

Malasanos L, Barkauskas V, Stoltenberg-Allen K: *Health assessment,* ed 4, St Louis, 1990, Mosby–Year Book.

Patient assessment: examination of the ear, Programmed instruction, *Am J Nurs* 75(3), 1975.

Prior JA, Silberstein JS, Stang JM: *Physical diagnosis: the history and examination of the patient,* ed 6, St Louis, 1981, Mosby–Year Book.

Seidel HM, Ball JW, Dains JE, Benedict GW: *Mosby's guide to physical examination,* ed 2, St Louis, 1991, Mosby–Year Book.

Thompson JM, McFarland GK, Hirsch JE, and others: *Clinical nursing,* ed 2, St Louis, 1989, Mosby–Year Book.

Weir MR and others: Assessing middle ear disease: beyond visual otoscopy, *Am Fam Physician* 30(5):201, 1984.

The newborn

Auvenshine MA, Enriquez MG: *Maternity nursing: dimensions of change,* Belmont, Calif, 1985, Wadsworth.

Bobak IM, Jensen MD: *Essentials of maternity nursing,* ed 3, St Louis, 1991, Mosby–Year Book.

Judd JM: Assessing the newborn from head to toe, *Nurs '85* 15(12):34, 1985.

Kiernan BS, Scoloveno MA: Assessment of the neonate, *Top Clin Nurs* 8(1):1, 1986.

The Organization for Obstetrical, Gynecological and Neonatal Nurses (NAACOG): *Physical assessment of the neonate,* OGN Nursing Practice Resource, Oct, 1986, The Association.

Pillitteri A: *Maternal-newborn nursing: care of the growing family,* ed 3, Boston, 1985, Little, Brown.

Scanlon JW, and others: *A system of newborn physical examination,* Baltimore, 1979, University Park Press.

Seidel HM, Ball JW, Dains JE, Benedict GW: *Mosby's guide to physical examination,* ed 2, St Louis, 1991, Mosby–Year Book.

Whaley LF, Wong DI: *Nursing care of infants and children,* ed 4, St Louis, 1991, Mosby–Year Book.

The child

Barness L: *Manual of pediatric physical diagnosis,* ed 6, Chicago, 1990, Mosby–Year Book.

Bates H: *A guide to physical examination,* ed 5, Philadelphia, 1991, JB Lippincott.

Brown MS, Alexander M: Physical examination. VIII. Hearing acuity, *Nurs '74* 4(4):61, 1974.

DeAngelis C: *Pediatric primary care,* ed 3, Boston, 1984, Little, Brown.

Dichiara E: A sound method for testing child's hearing, *Am J Nurs* 84(9):1104, 1984.

Gershel J, and others: Accuracy of the Welch Allyn Audioscope and traditional hearing screening for children with known hearing loss, *J Pediatr* 106(1):15, 1985.

Grimes CT: Audiologic evaluation in infancy and childhood, *Pediatr Ann* 14(3):211, 1985.

Whaley LF, Wong DL: *Essentials of Pediatric Nursing,* ed 3, St Louis, 1989, Mosby–Year Book.

The childbearing woman

Pillitteri A: *Maternal-newborn nursing: care of the growing family,* ed 3, Boston, 1985, Little, Brown.

Seidel HM, Ball JW, Dains JE, Benedict GW: *Mosby's guide to physical examination,* ed 2, St Louis, 1991, Mosby–Year Book.

Whitley N: *A manual of clinical obstetrics,* Philadelphia, 1985, JB Lippincott.

The older adult

Ebersole P, Hess P: *Toward healthy aging,* ed 3, St Louis, 1990, Mosby–Year Book.

Holder L: Hearing aids: handle with care, *Nurs '82,* 12:64, 1982.

Palmore E, editor: *Normal aging II: reports from the Duke Longitudinal Studies,* Durham, NC, 1974, Duke University Press.

Pearson LJ, Kotthoff ME: *Geriatric clinical protocols,* Philadelphia, 1979, JB Lippincott.

Thompson JM, McFarland GK, Hirsch JE, and others: *Mosby's manual of clinical nursing,* ed 2, St Louis, 1989, Mosby–Year Book.

Turner JS: Treatment of hearing loss, ear pain, and tinnitus in older patients, *Geriatrics* 37(8):107, 1982.

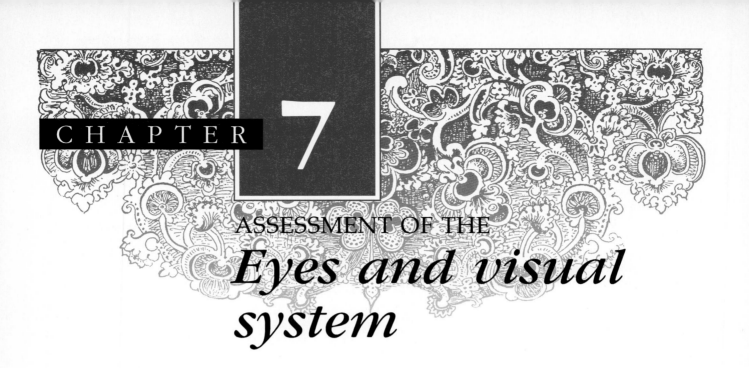

CHAPTER 7

ASSESSMENT OF THE
Eyes and visual system

VOCABULARY

accommodation Process of visual focusing from far to near; accomplished by contraction of the ciliary muscle, which thickens and increases the convexity of the crystalline lens.

amblyopia Reduced vision that occurs after deprivation of visual stimulation during visual maturation (birth to 2 years); eye appears normal during examination; also called *suppression amblyopia*.

ametropia General term denoting a condition involving a refractive error.
EXAMPLES: myopia, hyperopia.

aphakia Absence of the crystalline lens of the eye.

arcus senilis Gray ring composed of lipids deposited in the peripheral cornea; commonly seen in older adults; also called *arcus cornealis*.

asthenopia General eye discomfort or fatigue resulting from use of the eyes.

astigmatism Visual distortion resulting from an irregular corneal curvature that prevents light rays from being focused clearly on the retina.

blepharitis Inflammation of the eyelid.

bulbar conjunctiva Thin, transparent mucous membrane that covers the sclera and adjoins the palpebral conjunctiva, which lines the inner eyelid.

canthus Outer or inner angle between the upper and lower eyelids.

cataract Opacity of the crystalline lens of the eyes.

chalazion Small, localized swelling of the eyelid caused by obstruction and dilation of a meibomian gland.

cycloplegia Paralysis of the ciliary muscle resulting in a loss of accommodation and a dilated pupil; usually induced with medication to allow for examination or surgery of the eye.

diplopia Double vision; usually caused by an extraocular muscle malfunction or a muscle innervation disorder.

dyslexia Impairment of the ability to read (with no impairment of mental or intellectual function); letters or words may appear reversed, or the reader may have difficulty distinguishing right from left.

ectropion Abnormal outward turning of the margin of the eyelid.

enophthalmos Abnormal backward placement of the eyeball.

entropion Abnormal inward turning of the margin of the eyelid.

exophthalmos Abnormal forward placement of the eyeball.

glaucoma Eye disease characterized by abnormally increased intraocular pressure caused by obstruction of the outflow of aqueous humor.

hordeolum (stye) Infection of a sebaceous gland at the margin of the eyelid.

hyperopia (farsightedness) Refractive error in which light rays focus behind the retina.

miosis Condition in which the pupil is constricted; usually drug induced (agent is called a *miotic*).

mydriasis Dilation of the pupil; usually drug induced (agent is called a *mydriatic*).

myopia (nearsightedness) Refractive error in which light rays focus in front of the retina.

nicking Abnormal condition showing compression of a vein at an arteriovenous crossing; visible through an ophthalmoscope during a retinal examination.

O.D. (oculus dexter) Right eye.

O.S. (oculus sinister) Left eye.

O.U. (oculus uterque) Both eyes.

palpebral conjunctiva Thin, transparent mucous membrane that lines the inner eyelid and adjoins the bulbar conjunctiva, which covers the sclera.

palpebral fissure Opening between the upper and lower eyelids.

PERRLA Stands for "pupils equal, round, react to light, and accommodation."

photophobia Ocular discomfort caused by exposure of the eyes to bright light.

presbyopia Loss of accommodation (ability to focus on near objects) associated with aging.

ptosis Drooping of the upper eyelid; can be unilateral or bilateral; usually results from innervation or lid muscle disorder.

refraction Deviation of light rays as they pass from one transparent medium into another of different density.

scotoma Defined area of blindness within the visual field; can involve one or both eyes.

strabismus Condition in which the eyes are not directed at the same object or point.

ANATOMY AND PHYSIOLOGY REVIEW

The human eye lies in a bony orbit lined with fatty tissue. It is cradled in six oculomotor muscles, which surround and insert into the eyeball (Fig. 7-1). Three cranial nerves pass through a fissure in the posterior wall of the orbit and supply the oculomotor muscles as they stretch and contract to permit continuous eye movement. The oculomotor nerve (cranial nerve [CN] III) supplies the medial, inferior, and superior rectus muscles and the inferior oblique muscle, which control upward outer, lower outer, upward inner, and medial eye movements (Fig. 7-2). The trochlear nerve (CN IV) supplies the superior oblique muscle, which controls lower medial movement. The abducent nerve (CN VI) innervates the lateral rectus muscle, which controls lateral eye movement (see Fig. 7-2).

The eyelid protects the exposed part of the eye through closure and blinking, which keep out foreign objects and spread tears over the surface of the eyeball. The superior division of the oculomotor nerve (CN III) controls lid elevation, and the facial nerve (CN VII) controls lid closure. Sympathetic innervation controls involuntary blinking. The lid is lined with a thin, transparent mucous membrane (palpebral conjunctiva), which continues as an outer cover for the scleral surface of the eyeball (bulbar conjunctiva). The conjunctiva contains blood vessels, nerves, hair follicles, and sebaceous glands, which secrete material to lubricate the lids, prevent excessive evaporation of tears, and provide an airtight seal when the lid is closed.

The opening between the eyelids is called the *palpebral fissure*. Open lids reveal an inner (or medial)

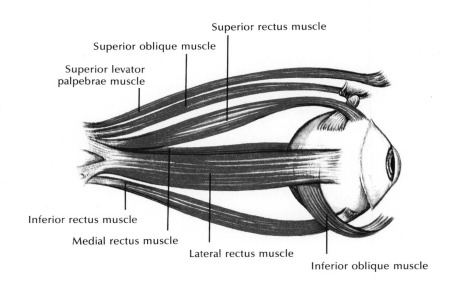

Fig. 7-1 Muscles of the right orbit as viewed from the side. (From Anthony CP, Thibodeau GA: *Textbook of anatomy and physiology,* ed 12, St Louis, 1987, Mosby–Year Book.

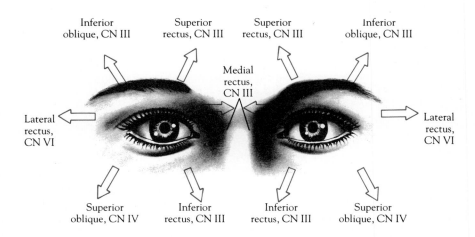

Fig. 7-2 Innervation and movement of extraocular muscles. (From Thompson JM, McFarland GK, Hirsch JE, and others: *Mosby's manual of clinical nursing,* ed 2, St Louis, 1989, Mosby–Year Book.)

canthus, where upper and lower lacrimal puncta (small openings) drain tears from the eyeball surface into the nasolacrimal duct (Fig. 7-3). The lacrimal gland, located in the anterior lateral fossa of the orbit, produces tears, which combine with sebaceous secretions to maintain a constant film over the cornea. The cornea covers the iris and the pupil and is transparent, avascular, and richly innervated with sensory nerves (trigeminal [CN V]). The cornea depends on a constant wash of tears for its oxygen supply and is subject to edema and a resultant blurring of vision with possible cell damage if the surface becomes dry. The cornea and sclera merge at a junction

called the *limbus* (see Fig. 7-3). The corneoscleral limbus has a rich vascular supply that encircles and nourishes the outer edges of the cornea. The sclera is the white, tough, fibrous outer coat that surrounds and covers the posterior five sixths of the eye.

The sclera, the outer layer of the eyeball, is adjacent to the middle layer (the uveal tract), which is composed of the choroid layer, the ciliary body, and the iris (Fig. 7-4). The choroid layer is highly vascular and supplies the retina with blood. The ciliary body contains muscles that control the shape of the lens for near and far vision, and secretes aqueous humor, which fills the anterior

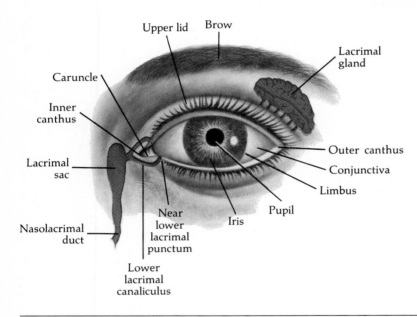

Fig. 7-3 Visible surface of eye. (From Thompson JM, McFarland GK, Hirsch JE, and others: *Mosby's manual of clinical nursing,* ed 2, St Louis, 1989, Mosby–Year Book.)

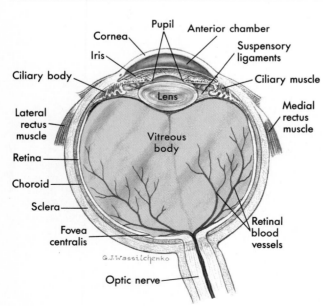

Fig. 7-4 Cross section of eye. (From Thompson JM, McFarland GK, Hirsch JE, and others: *Mosby's manual of clinical nursing,* ed 2, St Louis, 1989, Mosby–Year Book.)

chamber. The iris is a circular, muscular membrane that surrounds the pupil and regulates pupil dilation and constriction. The inner layer, the retina, is transparent and is an extension of the central nervous system. It contains rods and cones—photoreceptor cells—that are scattered throughout the retinal surface. Rods respond to low levels of light, and cones perceive images and colors in higher levels of light. On the posterior wall of the retina is the fovea centralis—a small depression that contains no rods but is densely packed with cones (see Fig. 7-4). Visual acuity is sharpest in this area in higher levels of light. The fovea is surrounded by the macula lutea—a pigmented area about 4.5 mm in diameter, which is visible to the examiner through an ophthalmoscope. Rods are densely packed in the periphery of this region. The optic disc (the head of the optic nerve) perforates the retina about 3 mm toward the nose from

the fovea. The disc is approximately 1.5 mm in diameter and contains no rods or cones. This results in a small blind spot for each eye, located about 15 degrees laterally from the center of vision. When viewed through the ophthalmoscope, the optic nerve appears as a pink or cream-colored circle with a white depression in the center. This depression is where the central retinal artery and central vein bifurcate, emerge, and feed into smaller branches throughout the retinal surface (see Fig. 7-4).

The eye contains three chambers: the anterior, the posterior, and the vitreous body. The anterior chamber rests between the cornea and the iris (Fig. 7-5). It is filled with approximately 0.2 ml of aqueous humor, which flows up from the posterior chamber and empties at the canal of Schlemm (Fig. 7-6). The posterior chamber is a narrow passage behind the iris and adjacent to

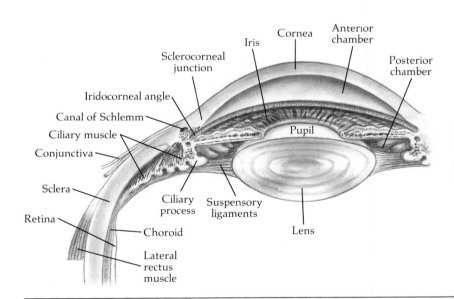

Fig. 7-5 Close-up view of ciliary body, lens, and anterior and posterior chambers. (From Thompson JM, McFarland GK, Hirsch JE, and others: *Mosby's manual of clinical nursing,* ed 2, St Louis, 1989, Mosby–Year Book.)

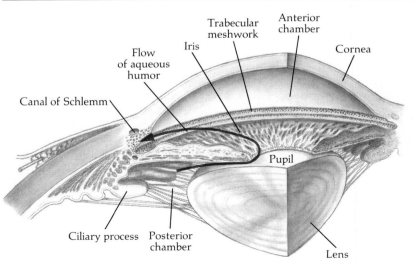

Fig. 7-6 Close-up view of flow of aqueous humor. (From Thompson JM, McFarland GK, Hirsch JE, and others: *Mosby's manual of clinical nursing,* ed 2, St Louis, 1989, Mosby–Year Book.)

the ciliary body (see Fig. 7-6). The vitreous body lies behind the lens and is filled with a gelatinous substance that adheres firmly to the surrounding retina (see Fig. 7-4).

The lens separates the posterior chamber from the vitreous body. It is biconvex and transparent and is held in suspension by suspensory ligaments attached to the ciliary body (see Fig. 7-4). The lens alters its shape for visual clarity when the eye is viewing an object at close range. It becomes thicker and more convex to accommodate near objects and is constantly adjusting to stimuli at different distances. Normally the lens is somewhat flattened and held tight by ligaments that attach to the circular ciliary muscle. Brain signals stimulate ciliary contraction and resultant lens shape alteration via the oculomotor nerve for this automatic response, called *accommodation.*

The optic nerve from each eye passes through the optic foramen, and they meet at the optic chiasm, which lies above and in front of the pituitary gland. Optic tracts emerge from the chiasm and encircle the hypothalamus

(Fig. 7-7). They terminate in the lateral geniculate bodies in the temporal lobes. Cells in the lateral geniculate bodies send fibers (optic radiation) to the occipital lobe of each cerebral hemisphere. The visual cortex in the posterior aspect of the occipital lobe receives most of the visual fibers for perception and interpretation.

Objects in the visual field stimulate the opposite side of the retina. When nerve fibers pass into the optic nerve, the nasal and temporal fibers are separate within the sheath. The nerves merge at the chiasm, and the nasal fibers cross over to the opposite optic tract. Temporal fibers do not cross, but continue to run laterally through the tract (see Fig. 7-7). Visual field defects can often be traced to disorders in specific anatomical locations because of the arrangement of nerve fibers. A left or right optic nerve lesion could cause a defect in the corresponding left or right eye. A common chiasm defect is bitemporal hemianopia, which results from a pituitary tumor. A left optic tract lesion would result in a bilateral right visual field defect. These defects are depicted in Fig. 7-8.

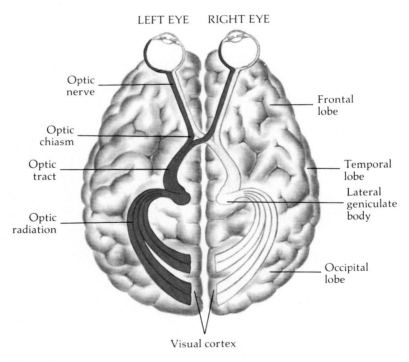

Fig. 7-7   Visual pathway. (From Thompson JM, McFarland GK, Hirsch JE, and others: *Mosby's manual of clinical nursing,* ed 2, St Louis, 1989, Mosby–Year Book.)

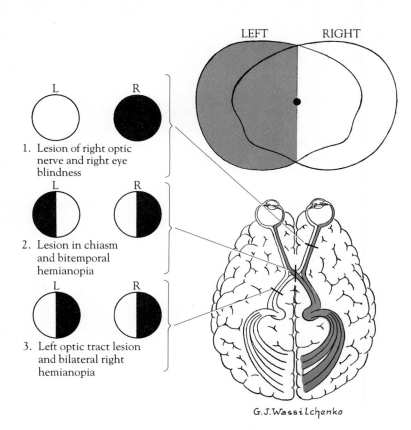

LEFT RIGHT

L R

1. Lesion of right optic nerve and right eye blindness

L R

2. Lesion in chiasm and bitemporal hemianopia

L R

3. Left optic tract lesion and bilateral right hemianopia

G.J.Wassilchenko

Fig. 7-8 Visual pathway defects. (From Thompson JM, McFarland GK, Hirsch JE, and others: *Mosby's manual of clinical nursing,* ed 2, St Louis, 1989, Mosby–Year Book.)

COGNITIVE OBJECTIVES

At the end of this chapter the learner will demonstrate knowledge of assessment of the eyes and visual system by the ability to do the following:

- Apply the terms that are listed in the vocabulary section.
- Identify the purposes for measuring distant and near visual acuity.
- Appropriately interpret the readings reporting distant visual acuity measurement.
- State the purposes for testing the corneal light reflex.
- Explain the purpose of the cover-uncover test.
- Identify the cranial nerves responsible for eyeball movement in the six fields of gaze.
- Identify the characteristics of normal anatomical structures of the external eye, including the following:
  1. Eyelids and lashes
  2. Spherical body in position within the socket
  3. Lacrimal apparatus
  4. Conjunctiva
  5. Cornea
  6. Iris and pupil
  7. Anterior chamber

- Describe the proper and effective techniques for handling the ophthalmoscope.
- Identify the characteristics of normal anatomical structures of the internal eye, including the following:
  1. Layers covering the eyeball
  2. Red reflex
  3. Retinal structures
     a. Disc and physiological cup
     b. Vessels
     c. Retina surface
     d. Macula and fovea centralis
- Identify selected common variations of the newborn, the child, the childbearing woman, and the older adult.

CLINICAL OUTLINE

At the end of this chapter the learner will perform a systematic assessment of the eyes and visual system, demonstrating the ability to do the following:

- Obtain a pertinent health history from the client.
- Demonstrate the correct procedures for testing a client for the following:
  1. Distant-vision acuity
  2. Near-vision acuity

3. Visual fields (confrontation method)
4. Extraocular movement control and parallel eye positioning by means of the following:
   a. Corneal light reflex
   b. Six fields of gaze
   c. Cover-uncover test
5. Corneal reflex
6. Direct and consensual pupillary response

- Demonstrate and describe the results of inspection and palpation of the following:
  1. Eyebrows for hair quality and distribution, skin surface, and bilateral movement
  2. Eyelids and lashes for height and bilateral dimension of palpebral fissures, lash formation and distribution, lid closure, blinking, tenderness, and surface characteristics
  3. Eyeball position in bony socket
  4. Lacrimal apparatus for puncta appearance and response to pressure at inner canthus
  5. Conjunctiva for color, tenderness, discharge, and surface characteristics
  6. Cornea for transparency, surface characteristics
  7. Anterior chamber and iris for transparency, iris color, surface and shape, and clearance between iris and cornea
  8. Pupil for shape and bilateral size

- Show proper use of the ophthalmoscope.
- Demonstrate a systematic inspection of the internal eye, including the following:
  1. Red reflex for color and shape
  2. Clear media of eye for transparency
  3. Optic disc for margin, shape, size, color, and physiological cup
  4. Retinal vessels for artery size, color, caliber, and distribution; vein size, color, caliber, and distribution
  5. Retinal surface for color and surface characteristics or alterations
  6. Macula and fovea centralis for color and surface characteristics

- Summarize results of the assessment with a written description of the findings.

HISTORY

- Is there a history of eye surgery, injury or trauma? Describe what and when.
- Is client currently taking or using any medications for eye problems? If so, describe. (*Note:* Eyedrops or ointments may not be reported as part of list of medications taken in original data base.)
- Is client subject to work or environmental conditions that could irritate or injure the eyes (e.g., irritating fumes, dust, smoke, flying sparks, or particles in air)? If so, does client wear goggles? If client rides a motorcycle, are goggles worn?
- Does client engage in any contact sport that creates problems with wearing corrective lenses or increases risk for eye injury?
- If client wears contact lenses, ask the following questions:
  1. When prescribed? By whom?
  2. Any difficulty with pain (mild, acute), burning, excessive tearing, photophobia (mild or severe), feeling of dryness, foreign body sensation, eye infections, swelling of eyelids or eyes (conjunctiva), excessive lens movement?
  3. Are lenses soft, hard, or extended-wear?
  4. How often are lenses checked by a physician?
  5. What are client's habits concerning the wearing of lenses?
     a. Duration (in a given day)?
     b. Ever sleep with lenses in place?

RISK FACTORS FOR CONTACT LENS COMPLICATIONS

- Poor blinking or poor lid function
- Diminished corneal sensation
- High astigmatism
- Disorganized life-style (difficulty storing, cleaning, wearing for appropriate periods)
- Swimming, contact sports
- Poor hygiene habits
- Susceptibility to infections (especially eye infections)
- Severe allergy (sneezing, eye watering)
- Limited or reduced manual dexterity
- Limited motivation to endure adjustment to new lenses or to tolerate foreign body in eye
- History of seizures
- Environment or work situation where fumes, smoke, or eye irritants exist
- Traveling (lens care and transport habits need to be considered, especially for soft lenses)

c. Worn every day or just for special occasions?

d. Lenses alternated with glasses?

e. Removed for special activities (e.g., contact sports, swimming)?

6. Ask client to describe the following:

a. Insertion/removal procedure

b. Cleaning/storage procedure

7. Does client have any special problems with lenses (e.g., keeping surface clean, free of scratches, or lenses popping out)?

8. *Note:* Soft and extended-wear lenses often present a different set of problems from hard lenses. The corneal surface is often more subject to edema resulting from deprivation of tears and oxygen. Symptoms of blurred vision, halos around lights, or slight redness may occur in the absence of pain. Corneal abrasion or breakdown will occur with prolonged or severe edema, and pain will accompany this sign. Palpebral conjunctivitis (of upper eyelid) is also a problem. The wearer may have great difficulty opening his eyes in the morning. Eventually redness, swelling, and discharge will appear. Soft lenses may also absorb fumes or dust and cause corneal irritation.

- *Note:* If client complains of *sudden onset* of any eye or visual symptoms (e.g., pain, loss of peripheral vision, blind spot, or any visual change), consider this an emergency for referral.

- If client complains of blurring, ask the following:

1. Does it involve one or both eyes?

2. Is it constant or transient?

3. Can it be cleared by blinking several times?

4. Does client have sensation that something is obstructing vision (e.g., cloudy or foggy interference) or are images out of focus?

5. Do images appear bent or warped?

6. Does squinting or frowning help to reduce blur?

7. Is blurring related to fatigue or eye strain?

- If client complains of eye strain, ask for a definition in terms of pain (localized in one or both eyes), headache (do symptom analysis), visual changes, association with time of day, use of corrective lenses, and reading or other vision use demands.

- If client complains of floaters or moving spots, ask the following:

1. Is the onset sudden (recent), or is this a chronic problem?

2. Are there large numbers, just a few, or do they occur singly?

3. Are they seen in one or both eyes?

- If client complains of redness, watering, or discharge around eyes, ask the following:

1. Is there a history of allergies? Is the problem seasonal, associated with sports activities, swimming?

2. Does anyone else in family or others in close contact with client have similar problems?

3. Any environmental factors that could serve as irritants?

- If client complains of diplopia (double vision), ask the following:

1. Is the onset sudden or gradual?

2. Is it present all the time?

3. Does it occur with both eyes open? Right eye closed? Left eye closed?

- If client complains of blind spot or peripheral vision loss, ask the following:

1. Is the onset sudden or gradual?

2. Does blind spot move with eye movement (i.e., does it remain in a constant position in relation to direction of gaze)?

- Does client have any unusual or different eye symptoms or sensations (e.g., flashes of light, distortion of color such as brownish-green or yellow hues, confusion about differentiating colors, halos around lights)?

- If client has a vision problem, how does it interfere with activities of daily living (e.g., getting around the house or community, caring for self, family, belongings, ability to read, driving a car, visualizing steps and curbs, maintaining job)?

- Diabetic clients of all ages should have regular eye examinations by an ophthalmologist. For people under 75 years of age, diabetes is the leading cause of blindness in the United States.* Diabetic retinopathy often progresses without symptoms; however, complaints of decreased or altered visual acuity, glare, or a shower of floaters warrants immediate referral to an ophthalmologist.

Text continues on p. 196.

---

*From Morbidity and Mortality Weekly Report: Perspectives in disease prevention and health promotion: guidelines for diabetic eye disease control, *N Engl J Med* 36(7):1987.

CLINICAL GUIDELINES

ASSESSMENT PROCEDURE	EVALUATION	
	NORMAL FINDINGS	DEVIATIONS FROM NORMAL

1. Gather equipment necessary to perform eye and vision assessment
  a. Snellen chart
  b. Near-vision chart or newsprint for testing near vision (Fig. 7-9)
  c. Cover card (opaque)
  d. Penlight
  e. Cotton wisp
  f. Cotton-tipped applicator
  g. Ophthalmoscope
 	
Acuity and function
 	
1. Perform measurement of distant vision (CN II)		

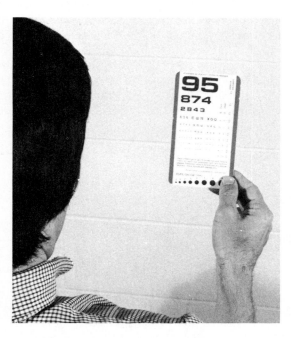

Fig. 7-9 Sample of a near-vision chart.

ASSESSMENT PROCEDURE	EVALUATION	
	NORMAL FINDINGS	DEVIATIONS FROM NORMAL
a. Stabilize Snellen chart on wall in well-lighted room (Fig. 7-10) b. Seat client comfortably 6 m (20 feet) from chart c. Ask client to cover one eye with cover card d. Ask client to repeat each letter as you point to it; begin pointing at letters in line where client is most comfortable reading—usually 20/30 or 20/20 line e. Urge client to read as many of smallest letters as possible, even if unable to complete a particular line f. Repeat procedure with other eye		

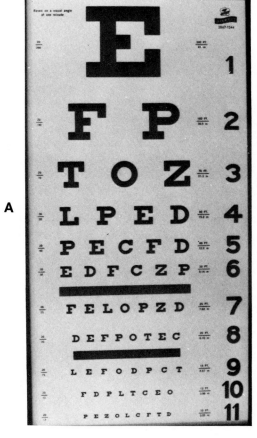
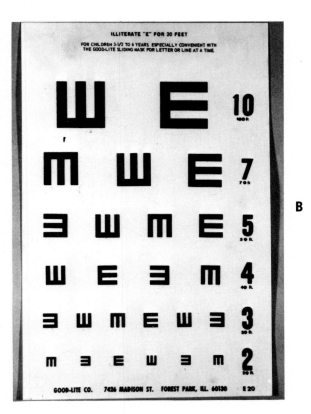

Fig. 7-10   Sample of charts used for distant-vision testing. (*Note:* The "E" chart can be used for illiterate clients.) (**A,** Courtesy Graham-Field Surgical Co, Inc, New Hyde Park, NY.)

CLINICAL GUIDELINES—cont'd

	EVALUATION	
ASSESSMENT PROCEDURE	NORMAL FINDINGS	DEVIATIONS FROM NORMAL
Acuity and function—cont'd		
g. Clients who wear corrective lenses for vision should be tested first while wearing glasses and then without*	20/20 O.D. and 20/20 O.S.	O.D. or O.S.: any letters missed in 20/20 line or above
h. Observe reading pattern and facial expression during acuity test	Reading pattern smooth, without hesitation Eyes remain open without frowning or squinting	Behaviors indicating reading difficulty: frowning, squinting, "cheating," leaning forward, tilting head, hesitancy or difficulty naming letters
2. Perform measurement of near vision		
a. Seat client comfortably		
b. Ask client to hold near-vision chart or newsprint 35 cm (14 inches) from face	Near-vision chart: 14/14 O.D. 14/14 O.S. Newsprint is read without hesitancy or attempt to position reading material closer or farther away	Unable to read letters at 35 cm (14 inch) distance Pushes reading material farther away (*Note:* Myopic [nearsighted] individuals may be able to read at a normal distance [14 inches] if they remove their glasses. They will report this as a change in vision. Formerly, they would have been able to read while wearing glasses.)
c. Ask client to read aloud letters or words in sentence	Eyes remain open without excessive blinking or facial distortions	Behaviors indicating difficulty: frowning, squinting, hesitancy, pulling reading material closer
d. If client wears corrective lenses for reading, perform test with glasses on		
3. Test for peripheral visual fields		
a. Examiner and client sit directly facing each other at distance of 60 to 90 cm (2 to 3 feet)		
b. Client covers one eye with cover card		
c. Examiner covers own eye directly opposite client's covered eye		
d. Client and examiner stare directly at each other's open eye		

Note: Reading glasses should not be used for testing far vision.

	EVALUATION	
ASSESSMENT PROCEDURE	**NORMAL FINDINGS**	**DEVIATIONS FROM NORMAL**
e. Examiner holds pencil or pen-light in hand and extends it to farthest periphery (Fig. 7-11) temporally and gradually brings object closer to midline point (equal distance between client and examiner) f. Ask client to report when object is first seen g. Procedure is repeated upward, toward nose, and downward h. Ask client to repeat entire procedure with other eye covered; examiner also covers other eye	Client and examiner report seeing object at approximately same time as it approaches from periphery; test assumes examiner has normal peripheral vision, described as: Temporal peripheral—90° Upward—50° Toward nose—60° Downward—70°	Client fails to report sighting object at same time as examiner in any one or in all directions (peripheral visual loss may involve both eyes or one eye) (*Note:* Confrontation method is a crude measurement for peripheral vision loss. A "blind spot" can occur within the central visual field [within 30° of central vision] and not be detected with this method.)
4. Test for extraocular muscle function a. Assess corneal light reflex (1) Ask client to stare straight ahead with both eyes open (2) Shine penlight, held at midline and directed toward corneas b. Test movement of eyes in six cardinal fields of gaze (CN III, IV, VI) (1) Client stabilizes head, looking directly ahead at examiner	Light reflections appear symmetrically in both pupils	Light reflections appear at different spots (asymmetrically) in each eye

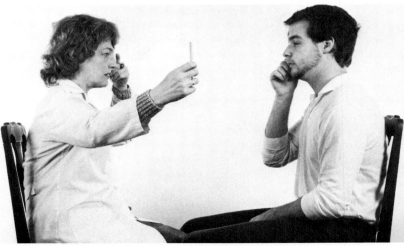

Fig. 7-11 Visual field testing: examiner holding object at midline.

Continued.

CLINICAL GUIDELINES—cont'd

ASSESSMENT PROCEDURE	EVALUATION	
	NORMAL FINDINGS	DEVIATIONS FROM NORMAL
Acuity and function—cont'd (2) Client is asked to move *eyes only* to follow object in examiner's hand (3) Examiner moves object from center position to upper and outer extreme (hold in position momentarily), back to center, and then to lower and inner extreme (Fig. 7-12) (4) Examiner moves object to temporal-nasal extremes, holding object in extreme positions momentarily (Fig. 7-13)		

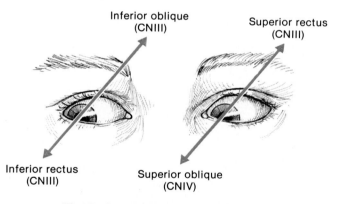

Fig. 7-12   Field testing position no. 1.

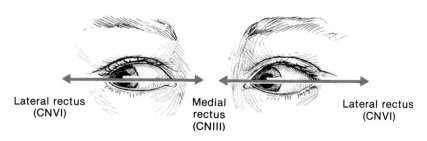

Fig. 7-13   Field testing position no. 2.

| | EVALUATION | |
ASSESSMENT PROCEDURE	NORMAL FINDINGS	DEVIATIONS FROM NORMAL
(5) Examiner moves object to opposite upper and outer extreme and back to opposite lower and inner extreme (Fig. 7-14)	Both eyes demonstrate coordinated, parallel movements in all directions End-point nystagmus may occur if eye is held in extreme gaze (mild rhythmic twitching with quick movement in direction of gaze with slow drift in other direction)	Eye movements are not coordinated or parallel; one or both eyes fail to follow examiner's hand in any given direction Sporadic or nonpurposeful eye movements Pathological nystagmus (quick movement always in same direction regardless of direction of gaze)

c. Perform cover-uncover test
  (1) Client is asked to stare straight ahead at fixed point
  (2) Examiner covers one eye with cover card and observes uncovered eye for movement to focus on designated point
	Uncovered eye does not move as examiner places card over other eye	Uncovered eye moves to focus on designated point (Fig. 7-15)

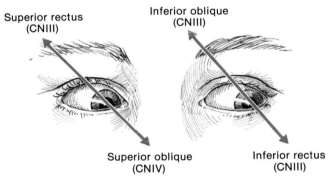

Superior rectus
(CNIII)

Inferior oblique
(CNIII)

Superior oblique
(CNIV)

Inferior rectus
(CNIII)

Fig. 7-14 Field testing position no. 3.

Fig. 7-15 Cover test for right eye demonstrating abnormal shift from lateral to central gaze.

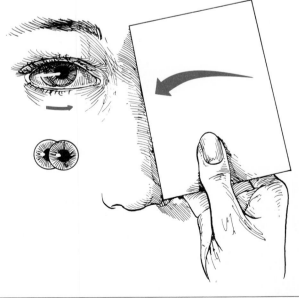

CLINICAL GUIDELINES—cont'd

ASSESSMENT PROCEDURE	EVALUATION	
	NORMAL FINDINGS	DEVIATIONS FROM NORMAL
Acuity and function—cont'd		
(3) Examiner removes card from same eye and observes newly uncovered eye for movement to focus	Newly uncovered eye does not move	Newly uncovered eye moves to focus on designated point (Fig. 7-16)
(4) Repeat steps 2 and 3 with other eye		
5. Test corneal reflex (CN V)		
a. Ask client to keep both eyes open and look up		
b. Examiner approaches from side with wisp of cotton		
c. Examiner lightly touches cornea (not conjunctiva) with cotton		
d. Repeat procedure with other eye	Lids of both eyes close when either cornea is touched*	Lids of one or both eyes fail to respond
6. Evaluate pupillary response (CN II, III)		
a. Evaluate direct and consensual reactions to light		
(1) Room should be partially darkened		
(2) Client holds both eyes open and fixes gaze straight ahead		

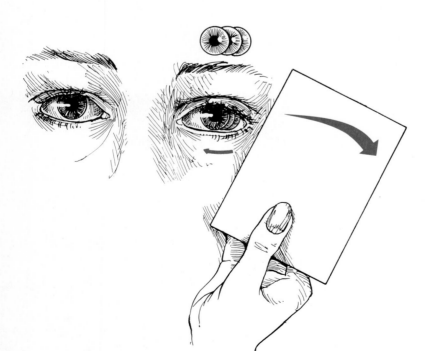

Fig. 7-16 Uncover test for left eye demonstrating abnormal shift from lateral to central gaze.

| | EVALUATION | |
ASSESSMENT PROCEDURE	NORMAL FINDINGS	DEVIATIONS FROM NORMAL
(3) Examiner approaches with penlight beam from side and shines light on pupil	Illuminated pupil constricts (direct response) Other eye (pupil) constricts simultaneously (consensual response)	Unequal (in size or speed) reflex responses or absent response
(4) Repeat procedure with other eye b. Test for accommodation (1) Client fixes gaze at object directly ahead at distant point (2) Examiner holds up object about 10 to 12 cm (4 or 5 inches) from client's nose	Speed of constrictive response (bilateral) may vary among clients	
(3) Ask client to adjust focus of gaze from distant object to object in front of nose	Pupils converge and constrict as eyes focus on near object Symmetrical response (Fig. 7-17) Client reports object in focus	Pupils fail to constrict or converge Asymmetrical response
External ocular structures		
1. Have client seated at eye level		
2. Inspect eyebrows, noting hair quality and distribution, skin quality, movement	Skin intact, without hair loss Equal alignment and movement	Flakiness, loss of hair, scaling Unequal alignment or movement
3. Inspect eyelids and lashes, noting the following:		
a. Height of palpebral fissures	Bilaterally equal in position	Asymmetrical positioning
b. Lid positioning	With eyes opened, lid margins overlie cornea at both superior and inferior borders	Sclera visible between upper lid(s); covers part of pupil
c. Lid closure	Complete, with smooth, easy motion	Incomplete, or closure with difficulty or pain

d. Blinking	Frequent involuntary, bilateral movements (average 15 to 20 blinks/min)	Rapid blinking
		  Monocular blinking
		  Absent or infrequent blinking

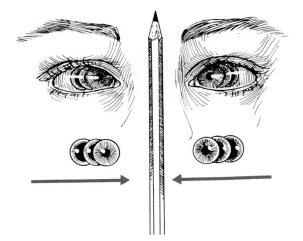

Fig. 7-17 Test for accommodation with convergence of eyes and pupil constriction.

Continued.

CLINICAL GUIDELINES—cont'd

ASSESSMENT PROCEDURE	EVALUATION	
	NORMAL FINDINGS	DEVIATIONS FROM NORMAL
External ocular structures—cont'd		

e. Surface characteristics	Skin intact, without discharge
	Lid margins flush against eyeball surface
	Lashes equally distributed and curled slightly outward
		Lesions, nodules, redness, flaking, crusting, excessive tearing, discharge
		Creamy or yellow plaques (xanthelasma) (Fig. 7-18)
		Lid edema
		Lid deformity
		    Lower lid pulled away, or drooping, from eyeball (Fig. 7-19)
		    Lower lid turned inward (Fig. 7-20)
		Lashes absent
		Lashes turned inward

4. Observe position of globe in bony socket	White persons: eyeball does not protrude beyond supraorbital ridge of frontal bone Black persons: eyeball may protrude slightly beyond supraorbital ridge	Asymmetrical placement Forward placement (exophthalmos) Backward placement (enophthalmos)
5. Inspect and palpate lacrimal apparatus (puncta) and eyelids		

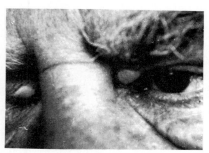

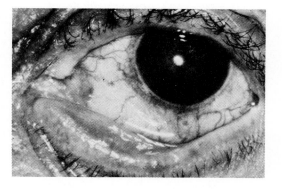

Fig. 7-18 Xanthelasma. (From Stewart W, Danto J, Maddin S: *Dermatology: diagnosis and treatment of cutaneous disorders,* ed 4, St Louis, 1978, Mosby–Year Book.)

Fig. 7-19 Ectropion: atonic lower lid with excessive tearing and exposed conjunctiva. (From Newell FW: *Ophthalmology: principles and concepts,* ed 5, St Louis, 1982, Mosby–Year Book.)

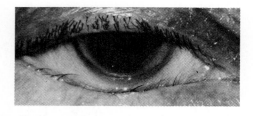

Fig. 7-20 Entropion: lower lid is turned inward (spastic), resulting in irritation of eye. (From Newell FW: *Ophthalmology: principles and concepts,* ed 5, St Louis, 1982, Mosby–Year Book.)

ASSESSMENT PROCEDURE	EVALUATION	
	NORMAL FINDINGS	DEVIATIONS FROM NORMAL
a. Examiner presses index finger against lower orbital rim near inner canthus (Fig. 7-21); pressure slightly everts lower lid	Puncta seen on tiny elevations on nasal side of upper and lower lid margins Mucosa pink and intact with no response to pressure	Puncta red, swollen, with response of tenderness to pressure Fluid or purulent material discharged from puncta in response to pressure
b. Gently palpate upper and lower lids for tenderness and nodules Exert minimal pressure over eyeball with examining finger*	No tenderness or nodules	Tenderness, nodules, or irregularities
6. Inspect bulbar conjunctiva and sclera and palpebral conjunctiva		
a. Separate lids widely with thumb and index finger, exerting pressure over bony orbit surrounding eye; ask client to look up, down, and to both sides	Bulbar conjunctiva clear; tiny red vessels may be visible Sclera appears white Tiny black dots (pigmentation) may appear near limbus (in dark-skinned individuals) Slight yellow cast (in dark-skinned individuals)	Blood vessels dilated Conjunctiva reddened Lesions or nodules Sclera yellow (jaundice) or significantly blue Foreign body Tenderness (especially in eye movement)
b. Pull down and evert lower lid; ask client to look up	Palpebral conjunctiva pink, intact, without discharge No tenderness or itching	Redness, lesions, nodules, discharge, tenderness, crusting
c. Eversion of upper lid is not ordinarily performed in screening examination; if indicated, the following steps should be performed†: (1) Explain entire procedure to the client before beginning		

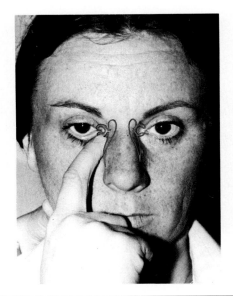

Fig. 7-21   Palpating the lacrimal puncta.

---

*If client complains of scratching or localized tenderness of eye, do not palpate over lid.

†Points (2) through (7) from Malasanos L, Barkaukas V, Stoltenberg-Allen K: Health assessment, ed 4, St Louis, 1990, Mosby–Year Book.

Continued.

CLINICAL GUIDELINES—cont'd

	EVALUATION	
ASSESSMENT PROCEDURE	**NORMAL FINDINGS**	**DEVIATIONS FROM NORMAL**
External ocular structures—cont'd (2) Ask the client to look down but to keep his eyes slightly open. This relaxes the levator muscle, whereas closing the eyes contracts the orbicularis muscle, preventing lid eversion. (3) Gently grasp the upper eyelashes and pull gently downward. Do not pull the lashes outward or upward; this, too, causes muscle contraction (Fig. 7-22, *A*). (4) Place a cotton-tipped applicator about 1 cm above the lid margin on the upper tarsal border and push gently downward with the applicator while still holding the lashes. This everts the lid (Fig. 7-22, *B*). (5) Hold the lashes of the everted lid against the upper ridge of the bony orbit, just beneath the eyebrow, never pushing against the eyeball (Fig. 7-22, *C*). (6) Examine the lid for swelling, infection, a foreign object, and so on.		

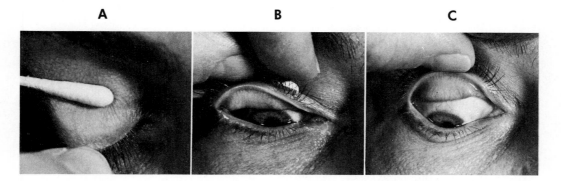

Fig. 7-22   Eversion of the upper eyelid, **A,** Lashes pulled gently downward and applicator positioned. **B,** Lid everts over applicator. **C,** Everted lid lashes stabilized against bony ridge. (From Newell FW: *Ophthalmology: principles and concepts,* ed 6, St Louis, 1986, Mosby—Year Book.)

| | EVALUATION | |
ASSESSMENT PROCEDURE	NORMAL FINDINGS	DEVIATIONS FROM NORMAL
(7) To return the lid to its normal position, move the lashes slightly forward and ask the client to look up and then to blink. The lid returns easily to a normal position.		
7. Inspect cornea, using oblique lighting; slowly move light reflection over corneal surface and check for:		
a. Transparency	Transparent	Opacities
b. Surface characteristics	Smooth Clear, shiny	Irregularities appearing in light reflections on surface Lesions, abrasions Foreign body Arcus senilis: white, opaque ring that encircles the limbus: may be abnormal in younger (under age 40) clients; often an insignificant sign with older clients Tissue growth from periphery toward corneal center (pterygium)
8. Inspect anterior chamber using oblique lighting for:		
a. Transparency	Transparent	Cloudy or any visible material, blood
b. Iris surface	Iris flat (Fig. 7-23, *A*)	Iris bulging toward cornea (crescent-shaped shadow may appear on far side of iris) (Fig. 7-23, *B*)
c. Chamber depth	Adequate (approximately 3.3 mm) clearance between cornea and iris	Chamber appears shallow

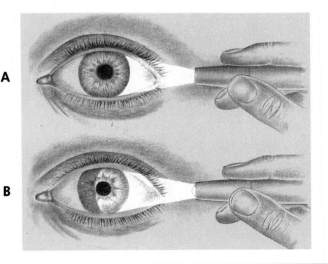

Fig. 7-23   A, Normal anterior chamber; iris is flat. **B,** Shallow anterior chamber; iris is bulging and crescent shadow appears on far side. (Modified from Seidel HM, Ball JW, Dains JE, Benedict GW: *Mosby's guide to physical examination,* ed 2, St Louis, 1991, Mosby–Year Book.)

Continued.

CLINICAL GUIDELINES—cont'd

ASSESSMENT PROCEDURE	EVALUATION	
	NORMAL FINDINGS	DEVIATIONS FROM NORMAL
External ocular structures—cont'd		
9. Inspect iris for:		
a. Shape	Round	Irregular shape
b. Color and consistency	Consistent coloration	Inconsistent coloration in one eye or between two eyes
10. Inspect pupil for:		
a. Shape	Round	Other than round
b. Bilateral size	Equal in size	Unequal in size
Internal eye		
1. Use ophthalmoscope (see "Clinical Tips and Strategies," p. 196, for technique) to observe:		
a. Red reflex from about 30 cm (1 foot) away, at 0 setting	Bright, round, red-orange glow seen through pupil	Decreased redness or roundness of reflex
b. Retinal structures (lens wheel usually remains at 0; it may need to be adjusted to allow for refractive errors: focus on a vessel and adjust lens until borders of image appear sharp and clear) (Fig. 7-24)		Dark spots or any opacities
(1) Optic disc margin	Regular, distinct Sharp outline Scattered or dense pigment deposits may be visualized at border Gray crescent may appear at temporal border	Margin blurred
— Shape	Round or slightly vertically oval	Irregular
— Size	Approximately 1.5 mm diameter (appears magnified 15 times to examiner) Marked myopic refractive errors may make disc appear larger	Shape and size of discs not equal in both eyes

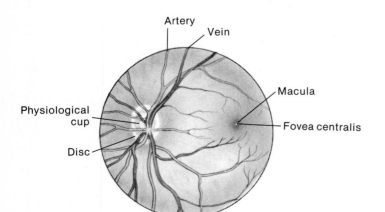

Fig. 7-24 Visible retinal structures of left eye.

ASSESSMENT PROCEDURE	EVALUATION	
	NORMAL FINDINGS	**DEVIATIONS FROM NORMAL**
	Hyperopic errors may make it appear smaller	
— Color	Creamy pink Lighter than retina Tiny vessels may be visible on disc surface	Diffuse pallor or pallor of section of disc, which always extends from center of disc to border Hyperemic disc with engorged, tortuous vessels on surface
— Physiological cup	Small depression just temporal of center of disc, does *not* extend to disc border Usually appears paler than disc, sometimes gray Usually occupies four tenths to five tenths of diameter of disc Vessels entering disc may drop abruptly into cup or may appear to fade gradually (Discs are more pronounced in some clients than others)	Cup extends to border of disc Cup occupies more than five tenths of diameter of disc Cup size or placement not equal in both eyes
(2) Retinal vessels: follow from disc to periphery, dividing retina into four quadrants		
— Arteries	Usually about 25% narrower than veins (2:3 or 4:5 ratio; size varies with number of branches) Narrow band of light may appear at center Light red	Arteries become narrow (2:4 or 3:5 ratio or less) Width of light reflex increases to cover over one third of artery Opaque or pale
— Veins	Larger than arteries No light reflection Darker in color Venous pulsation may be visible	Veins become larger
— Distribution and pattern (*Note:* Vessel abnormalities are not evenly distributed; scan all quadrants in orderly fashion for observation.)	Vessel caliber should be regular and uniformly decreasing in size as it branches and moves toward periphery	Irregularities of caliber; dilation or constriction Neovascularization (appears as compact patches of tortuous, narrow vessels)
	Artery/vein crossings should not alter (or pinch) caliber of underlying vessel	Indentations or nicks of vessels at artery/vein crossing
(3) Retinal background: scan the four quadrants in orderly fashion		
— Color	Pink, usually uniform throughout The fundi of black persons are often heavily pigmented and uniformly dark	Pallor of fundus (general or localized) Hemorrhage (may be linear, flame-shaped, round, dark or red, large or small)

Continued.

CLINICAL GUIDELINES—cont'd

	EVALUATION	
ASSESSMENT PROCEDURE	**NORMAL FINDINGS**	**DEVIATIONS FROM NORMAL**
Internal eye—cont'd		
— Surface characteristics	Fine granular texture Choroidal vessels may be visible through retinal layer (appear as linear, light orange streaks) Movable light reflections may appear on retinal surface (more prominent in young persons)	Microaneurysms (appear as discrete, tiny red dots) Soft or hard exudates (fuzzy or well-defined white patches)
(4) Macula and fovea centralis (located 2 disc diameters [DD] temporal to disc) — Color	Appears slightly darker than remainder of retina	Any abnormalities or lesions described for remainder of retinal surface
— Surface	Fovea may appear as tiny bright light in center of macula Tiny vessels may appear on surface Fine pigmentation and granular appearance may be visible	
c. Observe vitreous body (slowly move lens wheel into the positive numbers, from 0 to 15)	Clear Transparent	Floating particles Cloudiness
d. Observe cornea, anterior chambers, and lens (+15 to +20 setting)	Clear	Cloudiness or any visible material, blood

CLINICAL TIPS AND STRATEGIES

- **When testing with the Snellen chart, remember the following:**
  1. Always use an opaque card for covering the client's eyes (in lieu of client's hand).
  2. Client "cheating" may not be deliberate; it may be an unconscious attempt to resolve the frustration of not being able to perform the test.
  3. Be certain that the client can read or identify the letters; an illiterate client may simply indicate an inability to see the letters.
  4. Proceed slowly enough to permit the client sufficient time to follow directions.
  5. Far-vision errors should be recorded in the following manner—if the client misses two letters in the 20/20 line with the left eye: O.S. 20/20 − 2; if the client reads only one letter correctly in the 20/20 line with the right eye: O.D. 20/25 + 1.
- **When testing by confrontation for visual fields, hold the object in the midline between you and the client:** Beginning students often extend the object too far toward the client (this enables the examiner to spot the object first); or they hold the object too far back (Fig. 7-25). This gives the client the advantage in spotting the object.

- **When using the ophthalmoscope, the following procedures are helpful:**
  1. Turn the diaphragm dial so that the small, round, white light can be used. Turn on light to maximum brightness (old or defective batteries will reduce lighting).
  2. Client should be comfortably seated. Either stand or be seated facing the client.
  3. Client and examiner remove glasses. Removal of client's contact lenses is optional. It might help to reduce light reflection.
  4. The room should be darkened.
  5. Ask the client to hold both eyes open and to direct gaze slightly upward and straight ahead. Gaze should be fixed on some distant object and maintained even if the examiner's head gets in the way.
  6. For examination of the client's right eye, hold the ophthalmoscope in your right hand, over your right eye. Stand slightly to the right, at about a 15-degree angle (temporally) from the client.
  7. The ophthalmoscope is held with the index finger on the lens wheel. Rotate the lens wheel to 0 diopter setting (a lens that neither converges nor diverges light rays) (Fig. 7-26).
  8. Place left hand over the client's right eye, with thumb on upper brow.

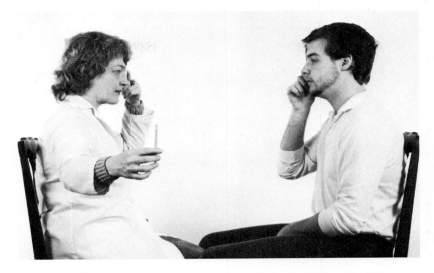

Fig. 7-25   Visual field testing; examiner fails to hold object at midline.

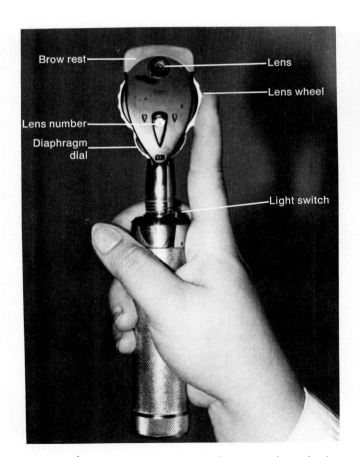

Brow rest

Lens

Lens wheel

Lens number

Diaphragm dial

Light switch

Fig. 7-26   Ophthalmoscope. Index finger is on lens wheel.

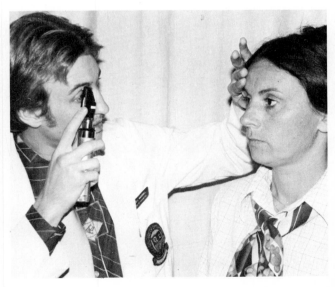

Fig. 7-27   Distance: 30.5 cm (12 inches); focus on pupil; red reflex visualized.

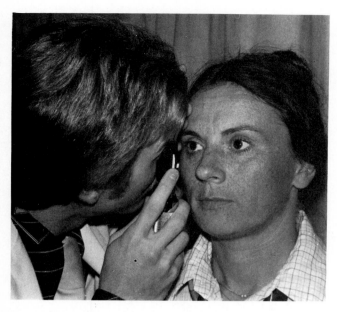

Fig. 7-28 Distance: 3 to 5 cm; lens wheel setting moves from + 20 to 0; focuses from cornea to retina.

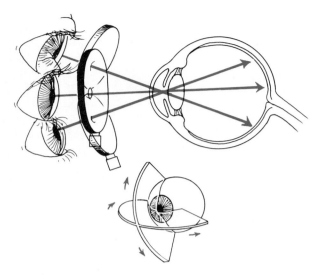

Fig. 7-29 Examiner directs opthalmoscope light through client's pupil onto the retina. Ophthalmoscope must be stabilized against examiner's own eye as he moves to view different retinal surfaces. (*Note:* Examiner moves in two dimensions—not just up and down.)

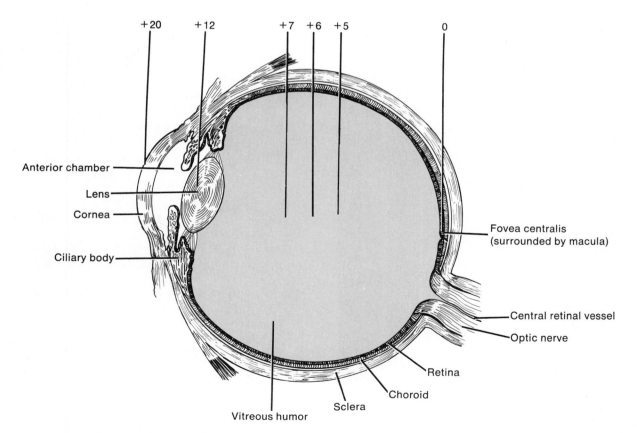

+20   +12   +7 +6 +5   0

Anterior chamber

Lens

Cornea

Ciliary body

Fovea centralis (surrounded by macula)

Central retinal vessel

Optic nerve

Retina

Choroid

Sclera

Vitreous humor

Fig. 7-30 Longitudinal cross section of eye showing focused ophthalmoscope lens setting.

9. Hold the ophthalmoscope firmly against your head, and approach to within 30 cm (12 inches) of the client (Fig. 7-27). Direct ophthalmoscope light into the pupil. Continue approach, and red reflex will appear. Try to keep both eyes open.

10. Continue the approach until 3 to 5 cm (1 to 2 inches) from client's eye (Fig. 7-28). Retinal structures should come into view. Clear focus can be established by looking closely at a vessel to see if the borders are sharp. Wheel adjustments need to be made for refractive errors. The myopic client's eyeball may be longer than normal, requiring rotation of the lens wheel into the red (minus) numbers for clarity. The hyperopic or aphakic client will require lens wheel movement into the black (plus) numbers for clarity.

11. The examiner may not initially focus on the disc. It is helpful to follow vessel bifurcations that lead toward the disc.

12. After inspection of the disc, follow the vessels peripherally in each of four directions. Light must always be shown *through* the pupil as the examiner inspects in different directions. Beginning examiners often lose their view as they begin to scan the fundus. The client's pupil serves as a stable fulcrum while the examiner and ophthalmoscope move *as a unit* in viewing the retinal periphery (Fig. 7-29).

13. Inspect the retinal background and the macula (2 disc diameters temporal to the disc).

14. After retinal inspection is completed, rotate the lens wheel slowly into the black numbers (0, +5, +10, +15, +20). As the numbers become larger, the anterior surfaces (vitreous, lens) come into view (Fig. 7-30).

15. Slowly rotate the lens wheel up to +20. This should bring the cornea and anterior chamber into focus.

16. Now change to the left eye. Start at client's left, holding the ophthalmoscope with the left hand and over the left eye.

17. *Note:* Clients who talk during the examination often tend to blink and move their eyes more often.

18. *Note:* Absence of the red reflex may indicate an abnormal eye, an improperly positioned ophthalmoscope, or that the client moved his eyes. If the red reflex is lost, back away and start over.

19. *Note:* It is extremely important that you consider your head and the ophthalmoscope as a unit. Be certain that the instrument is stabilized against your brow and cheek.

SAMPLE RECORDING: NORMAL FINDINGS

Distant vision: 20/20 O.U.: near vision: 14/14 O.U., no glasses.
Visual fields intact (by confrontation).
Parallel corneal light reflex, EOM intact, no nystagmus.
Eyes symmetrical without deviation of gaze with cover test.
Brows, lids, and lashes intact without deformity, ptosis, or lesions.
Conjunctiva/sclera clear; puncta patent; no discharge.
Cornea smooth and clear.
Iris flat, round, PERRLA.
Ophthalmoscopy
 Full bilateral red reflex; discs round, cream color, well-defined margins.
 Vessels—2:3 (A/V ratio); arteries light red with narrow light reflex and even caliber.
 Retina uniform red-orange without exudates or lesions.
 Maculae 2 DD from discs; no lesions.

 The Newborn

HISTORY AND CLINICAL STRATEGIES

- When examining a newborn who was vaginally delivered, the practitioner should carefully inquire about vaginal infections the mother may have had before delivery. This is of particular importance if the baby shows conjunctival irritation, pus, redness, or granular development.

- Although it is impossible to perform an accurate vision screening on a newborn, the examiner must perform some method of visual screening to rule out gross vision problems. For example, use a penlight at a distance of about 25 cm (10 inches), blink it on and off several times, and then move it around slightly. The infant should indicate recognition of the light and should follow it momentarily. No recognition or following requires further vision evaluation.

- Scleral color should be white. Hyperbilirubinemia may cause jaundiced, or yellow, eye appearance in newborns.

- Eye prophylaxis may cause red and irritated-looking eyelids in newborns. If there is purulent drainage, it should be cultured.

- It is difficult to examine a newborn's eyes. Holding or rocking infants into an upright position will usually elicit eye opening. Sterile gauze can be used to gently hold eyelids open, especially if eyelids are slippery.

CLINICAL VARIATIONS: THE NEWBORN

CHARACTERISTIC OR AREA EXAMINED	NORMAL FINDINGS	DEVIATIONS FROM NORMAL
1. External eye	Usually kept closed Symmetric appearance Blink reflex Spontaneous ocular movements (especially when held upright) No eyebrows Lashes (may be long) Conjunctivitis Puffy eyelids (from medication) Conjunctival hemorrhage Eyelid capillary hemangiomas (from birth) No tears for 2 weeks (immature lacrimal glands) Strabismus (random eye movements) Nystagmus (irregular movements) Gaze moves toward contoured object	Asymmetry Epicanthal folds (skin over inner canthus) Hypertelorism (wide-set eyes) Hypotelorism (eyes close together) Pronounced slant (suggests chromosomal defect) Purulent discharge (possible infection) Preterm clients susceptible to hyperoxia and retrolental fibroplasia (RLF) Eyes that search and oscillate Continual strabismus or nystagmus
2. Internal eye	Pupil size about 2-4 mm; round, equal diameter Whitish-blue sclera Subconjunctival hemorrhage (red spot on cornea [from delivery pressure]) Clear, transparent, lustrous cornea Ophthalmoscopic light: Bilateral red reflex—circular redorange spot; pale reflex in dark-skinned newborns	Dilated, constricted, or unequal pupils (may be brain damage) White pupil (may be retinoblastoma) Retinal hemorrhage (from traumatic birth) Enlarged, cloudy cornea (suggests glaucoma) White pupil, cloudy cornea of anterior chamber (suggests cataracts) Coloboma: irregular lid or pupil (missing iris may affect eyesight)

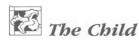 *The Child*

HISTORY AND CLINICAL STRATEGIES

- The practitioner should inquire about the developmental maturation of the child's visual system. Table 7-1 indicates developmental milestones. Numerous studies have shown that mothers are *most commonly* the ones who identify vision problems in their children.
- There is much controversy regarding novice practitioners using the ophthalmoscope with small children. We encourage the beginning examiner to attempt its use with all children. Although the findings may not equal the effort, repeated practice will increase the examiner's skill so that when there is a child who needs an ophthalmoscopic examination, the likelihood of seeing the internal structures will be increased. Following is a list of suggested techniques for use with infants and small children:

1. Babies up to about 18 months should be lying on their backs on the examining table. The overhead examination room lights should be off, but some type of side-room lighting should be on.
2. Hold a penlight or lighted object at arm's length (using left hand) above the baby's head to attract his focus while using the right hand on the ophthalmoscope to perform the internal eye examination. Assistance will be necessary to immobilize baby's head or to hold light.
3. Do not attempt to pry the child's eye open. If this technique is necessary, the child will not cooperate by focusing during the funduscopy examination.

TABLE 7-1   Sequence of visual development

AGE	CHARACTERISTICS OF DEVELOPMENT
Birth	Pupils react to light Moderate photophobia Eyes usually kept closed Blink reflex in response to light stimulus Corneal reflex in response to touch Retinoscopy indicates 1 to 3 diopters of hyperopia Nystagmus may be present Rudimentary fixation on objects with ability to follow to midline Visual acuity approximately 20/300
2 to 4 weeks	Fixation ability advances; stares at light source Follows to midline more readily Tear glands begin to function
4 to 12 weeks	Infant becoming alert to moving objects, but convergence and following are jerky and inexact Fascination for light objects and bright colors Tear glands begin to display response to emotion Binocular fixation established Follows moving object with head and eyes through 180°
12 to 20 weeks	Infant inspects hands One-inch colored cubes stimulate immediate fixation within 60 cm (2 feet) of eyes Accommodative convergence reflexes organizing Able to fixate on objects more than 90 cm (3 feet) distant Foveal pit becomes distinguishable as macular development proceeds Pigmentation of fundus not developed; appearance of fundus is pale Visual acuity 20/200
20 to 28 weeks	Color preference for bright reds and yellows develops Ciliary muscle function begins; accommodation convergence reflexes start to organize Coordination between hand and eye developing True blinking appears Binocular fixation clearly established Ultimate color of iris can now be determined Able to rescue dropped block
28 to 44 weeks	About 36 weeks, depth perception begins development Very interested in small objects and can accurately pick up 7-mm pellet Follows in both vertical and horizontal planes Tilts head backward to see upward Visual acuity exceeds 20/200
44 weeks to 12 months	Central acuity approaches 20/100 Readily discriminates simple geometrical forms and gazes intently at facial expressions Transverse diameter of cornea is 12 mm, the adult size Full binocular vision has developed Amblyopia may develop with lack of binocularity
12 to 18 months	Keen interest in pictures Can identify forms and associate simple visual experience Associates with visual experiences Able to scribble on paper Convergence becomes well established Depth perception remains crude
18 months to 2 years	Depth perception still immature Accommodation well developed Visual acuity 20/40

Modified from Chinn P, Leitch C: Child health maintenance: a guide to clinical assessment, *ed 2, St Louis, 1979, Mosby–Year Book.*

Continued.

TABLE 7-1   Sequence of visual development—cont'd

AGE	CHARACTERISTICS OF DEVELOPMENT
2 to 3 years	Convergence smooth Fixation on small objects or pictures should approach 50 seconds Able to recall visual images Visual acuity 20/40
3 to 5 years	Acuity appears well established, but amblyopia can occur from disuse Able to copy geometrical figures Reading readiness may be present
5 years	Only small potential for reduction of acuity from disuse (amblyopia development unlikely) Color recognition well established
6 years	Central acuity unconditionally established Physiological hyperopia decreases Visual acuity approaches 20/20 Gross attention span lengthened to 20 minutes, and detailed attention lasts about 2 minutes Color shading can be differentiated Depth perception fully developed

TABLE 7-2   Vision screening schedule

AGE	SCREENING	ANTICIPATED RESULTS	REFERRAL CRITERIA
Newborn	General vision ability	Should follow short distance	No recognition or blink
3 months	Strabismus screen	May be positive	
6 months to 1 year	Strabismus screen	Should be negative	Positive screen
3 years	"E" test	20/30 to 20/40	Grossly abnormal results
4 years	Color vision screening for boys (Ishihara test if possible)	Normal color identification	Abnormal color identification
	Visual field-confrontation screening	Sees objects at same time as examiner	Grossly abnormal results
5 to 8 years (test each year)	"E" test or Snellen test	20/30 to 20/40	20/40 results after two screening periods Unequal results (e.g., 20/20 O.D., 20/40 O.S.)
9 to 11 years (test each year)	Snellen test	20/20 to 20/30	>20/30 results after two screening periods Unequal results

4. Older children are likely to assist in the funduscopy examination if the examiner offers proper instructions and actually involves the child in the examination. These activities may include the following:
   a. Letting the child know in advance that the room lights will be turned out but that some small light will be left on
   b. Informing the child during the time the light is out that the examiner will be using a small flashlight to look into the child's eyes
   c. Reassuring him that the procedure will not hurt
   d. Instructing the child to look at a particular picture on the wall or providing the child with a penlight to shine onto a picture on the wall and then to look at the "lighted picture"
   e. Remembering that older children prefer to sit
5. The findings of the ophthalmoscopic examination for a child are very similar to those for an adult. The primary difference is the length of time the examiner has to survey the internal structures. The comparison is several seconds for the adult to split seconds for the child. During this time the examiner should at least attempt to do the following:
   a. Focus on the retina (most likely for children under 6 years old the lens wheel will be between 0 and −5).
   b. Observe disc and note flatness and sharpness of disc edges.
   c. Note color and gross characteristics of the retina.

- Vision screening begins informally with the newborn examination as the examiner notes the child's following and fixation capabilities. This should continue during each physical assessment period. Although there is some disagreement about the exact age children should receive formalized vision screening, Table 7-2 serves as a guide.
- By age 3 to 4 months the infant achieves the ability to fixate on one visual field with both eyes (binocularity). One of the most important tests for binocularity is alignment of the eyes to detect nonbinocular vision or strabismus.
- When using either the Snellen "E" chart or the Snellen alphabet chart with children, it is necessary to have two examiners: one to show the various lines of the chart and to point to the desired item, and the other to assist the child to stand or sit in the correct spot and correctly cover the eye not being tested.
- The alphabet chart is by far the more accurate, and whenever possible, it should be used. Directions for using the Snellen chart have been discussed previously.

- The mechanics of the "E" chart are generally the same as with the alphabet chart. The child is instructed to point with his finger and entire arm to the direction in which the "legs of the table" are pointing. This evaluates not only the ability to see the letter but also the ability to comprehend the idea of direction. Table 7-3 provides information about a variety of vision acuity tests.
- If the child wears glasses, vision screening should be done with glasses both on and off.
- Problems with strabismus or heterophoria should be carefully evaluated in every child over the age of 6 months. Infants younger than 6 months may have intermittent eye crossing, which can be normal. Such a finding in any child over the age of 6 months is considered abnormal, and the client should be referred. The two techniques for evaluating the situation in which the child's eyes do not focus to transmit good coordinated binocular vision are the cover test and the corneal light reflex test. Both have been described previously; they should be evaluated at near-point (35 cm [14 inches]) and far-point (6 m [20 feet]) distances. The age and cooperation of the child will determine the success of the evaluation.
- The importance of color vision screening is disputed among authorities. We believe it can be easily incorporated into a well-child examination and should therefore be done. Because color blindness is extremely rare among girls, only boys need to be tested. Before beginning the evaluation, the examiner must first evaluate the child's knowledge and correct recognition of colors. Color testing needs to be done only once.
- The eyesight of a child is so precious that the examiner should refer any questionable finding to a physician for further evaluation.

• • •

The overall success of this evaluation depends on the cooperation of the child. It is desirable to evaluate each component during every well-child visit. If the child is uncooperative, the examiner must decide whether to postpone the component being evaluated until later during the examination or to wait until the child's next visit.

There are five components of the pediatric vision screening examination that are most important: visual acuity, testing for farsightedness, strabismus screening, color vision screening, and visual field evaluation. These five components are incorporated into the clinical guidelines, which begin on p. 205.

Text continues on p. 213.

TABLE 7-3   Letter or symbol vision acuity tests

TEST	DESCRIPTION	COMMENTS*
Snellen Letter†	Uses letters of the English alphabet for testing at 20 feet	Suitable for most children above the second grade who are familiar with reading the alphabet
Snellen E†	Uses the capital letter E pointing in four directions; children "read" the chart by showing the direction of the letter E or using a large duplicate E to match the chart E at 20 feet	For illiterate or non–English speaking people and preschool children and grade 1 Preschool children often have difficulty with direction despite adequate vision
Home Eye Test for Preschoolers‡	Uses a large letter E for demonstration and an E chart for testing at 10 feet	Designed for use by parents for children 3 to 6 years
Blackbird Preschool Vision Screening Systems§	Uses a modified E to resemble a flying bird; children identify which way the bird is flying Uses flash cards, story-telling, and disposable cardboard eyeglass occluders	Designed for children as young as 3 years
Blackbird Storybook Home Eye Test§	Similar to above	Designed for use by parents for children as young as 2½ years
HOTV or Matching Symbol†	Uses the four letters H, O, T, and V on a chart for testing at 10 or 20 feet Child names the letters on the chart or matches them to a demonstration card	Suitable for children as young as 3 years Avoids the problem with image reversal and eye-hand coordination, which can occur with the letter E
Faye Symbol Chart†	Uses pictures of a house, apple, and umbrella on a chart for testing at 10 feet	Suitable for children as young as 27 to 30 months
Denver Developmental Screening Test (DDST)‖	Uses single cards for the letter E, one for demonstration and one for testing at 15 feet Also uses Allen Picture Cards (a tree, birthday cake, horse and rider, telephone, car, house, and teddy bear) for testing at 15 feet	Suitable for children 2½ years and older May be reliably used with cooperative children from the age of 24 months
Dot Test‡	Uses a series of different-sized dots; child points to one of the nine dots randomly positioned on a disk	Suitable for children as young as 24 months

From Whaley LF, Wong DL: Nursing care of infants and children, ed 3, St Louis, 1987, Mosby–Year Book.
*Ages for testing are based on published reports. In actual practice only a small percentage of young children may be successfully screened with many of these tests.
†Available from Good-Life Company, 1540 Hannah Ave, Forest Park, IL 60130.
‡Available from the National Society for the Prevention of Blindness, Inc, 79 Madison Ave, New York, NY 10016.
§Blackbird Vision Screening System, PO Box 7424, Sacramento, CA 95826.
‖Available from Denver Development Materials, Inc, PO Box 20037, Denver, CO 80220.

CLINICAL VARIATIONS: THE CHILD

CHARACTERISTIC OR AREA EXAMINED	NORMAL FINDINGS	DEVIATIONS FROM NORMAL
1. Distant vision (CN II) in children over age 3 years	3 years: 20/20 to 20/40 5 to 8 years: 20/30 to 20/40 9 to 11 years: >20/20 to 20/30	>20/40 results after two screening periods or unequal results in either eye (5 to 8 years) >20/30 results after two screening periods or unequal results in either eye (9 to 11 years)

2. Near vision: not routinely used until *older school-age evaluation;* when used, directions are same as for adult	Near-vision chart:
	  14/14 O.D.
	  14/14 O.S.
	Newsprint is read without hesitancy or attempt to pull it closer or push it farther away
	Eyes remain open without excessive blinking or facial distortions
		Client unable to read letters at 35 cm (14 inch) distance
		
		Note any other behaviors indicating difficulty (frowning, squinting, hesitancy, pulling reading material closer)

3. Peripheral visual fields: should be evaluated from age 3 years on or as soon as child is able to cooperate by *maintaining his position* throughout procedure	Client and examiner report seeing object at approximately same time as it approaches from periphery; this test assumes that the examiner has normal peripheral vision Another affirmative response is noting exact moment child changes head position to gaze toward object, indicating that child did see object coming into view (examiner must be alert to judge if this is same instance that examiner saw object) Temporal peripheral vision: 90° Upward: 50° Toward nose: 60° Downward: 70°	Client fails to report sighting object at same time as examiner, in any one direction or in all directions (peripheral visual loss may involve both eyes or one eye)
4. Extraocular muscle function (also a test for strabismus); eye muscle coordination is not fully mature until 1 year; at this time it shows mature adult function		
a. Corneal light reflex	Light reflections appear symmetrically in pupils	Light reflections appear at different spots (asymmetrically) in each eye
Because infants are unable to cooperate, examiner must use penlight to attract infant's attention; while infant focuses on light, examiner must evaluate light reflection position	If child is under 6 months of age, asymmetry of image may be normal	Refer for further evaluation if child is over 6 months

CLINICAL VARIATIONS: THE CHILD—cont'd

CHARACTERISTIC OR AREA EXAMINED	NORMAL FINDINGS	DEVIATIONS FROM NORMAL
b. Movement of eyes in six cardinal fields of gaze: test in children over 2 years of age; examiner may need to stabilize child's chin with hand to prevent entire head movement Newborns can have the cardinal fields of gaze assessed by passively moving the infant's head into the various positions	Both eyes demonstrate coordinated, parallel movements in all directions End-point nystagmus may occur if eye is held in extreme gaze (mild rhythmic twitching with quick movement in direction of gaze with slow drift in other direction)	Eye movements not coordinated or parallel (Fig. 7-31) One or both eyes fail to follow examiner's hand in any given direction Sporadic or nonpurposeful eye movements Pathological nystagmus (quick movement always in same direction regardless of direction of gaze)
c. Cover-uncover test: performed on all children 3 months and older until school age; test should be done with child looking at object about 35 cm (14 inches) away and then repeated as he viewed object approximately 6 m (20 feet) away	Uncovered eye does not move as examiner places card over other eye Newly uncovered eye does not move	Uncovered eye moves to focus on designated point Newly uncovered eye moves to focus on designated point Refer if child is over 6 months of age
5. Corneal reflex (CN V): not routinely tested in preschool children; when tested, technique is same as for adult	Lids of both eyes close when either cornea is touched	Lid(s) of one or both eyes fails to respond
6. Pupillary response: direct and consensual reaction to light	Pupil with light shining on it constricts (direct response) Other eye (pupil) constricts simultaneously (consensual response) Pupils converge and constrict as eyes focus on near object Response symmetrical	Unequal (in size or speed) reflex responses or absent response Pupils fail to constrict or converge Asymmetrical response
7. Color vision: use Ishihara test if possible; single line testing for preschool boys	Able to correctly differentiate colors	Unable to differentiate colors correctly

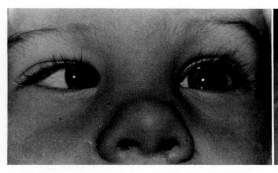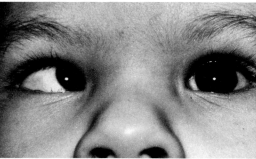

Fig. 7-31   Abnormal alignment of eyes. (From Helveston EM, Ellis FD: *Pediatric ophthalmology practice,* St Louis, 1980, Mosby–Year Book.)

CHARACTERISTIC OR AREA EXAMINED	NORMAL FINDINGS	DEVIATIONS FROM NORMAL
External ocular structures		
1. Have client seated at eye level. Note the following:		
a. Position and alignment of eyes on face	Outer canthus of eye aligns with pinna of ear	Outer canthus does not align with pinna of ear; may be higher or lower than pinna
b. Symmetry	See Fig. 7-32 for measurement criteria	Large spacing between eyes (hypertelorism) is frequent sign of mental retardation (*Note:* Even though large spacing may be normal, examiner should refer child to specialist for verification.)
2. Eyebrows		
a. Hair quality/distribution and skin quality	Skin intact, without hair loss	Flakiness, loss of hair, scaling
b. Movement	Equal alignment and movement	Unequal alignment or movement

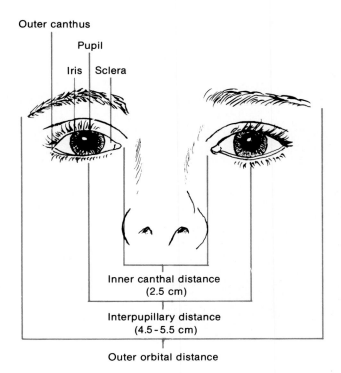

Outer canthus

Pupil

Iris Sclera

Inner canthal distance
(2.5 cm)

Interpupillary distance
(4.5 - 5.5 cm)

Outer orbital distance

Fig. 7-32 Anatomical landmarks for distance measurements.

Continued.

CLINICAL VARIATIONS: THE CHILD—cont'd

CHARACTERISTIC OR AREA EXAMINED	NORMAL FINDINGS	DEVIATIONS FROM NORMAL
3. Eyelids and eyelashes		
a. General slant of palpebral fissures: draw imaginary line through two points of medial canthus and across outer orbit of eyes with each eye on the line (Fig. 7-33)	Horizontal Oriental children may have slightly upward slant	Upward slant in non-Oriental children and children with Down syndrome (Fig. 7-34)
b. Lid positioning	With eyes opened, lid margins overlie cornea at both superior and inferior borders	Sclera visible between upper lid(s) and part of iris
c. Lid closure	Complete with smooth, easy motion	Incomplete or closure with difficulty or pain
d. Blinking	Frequent involuntary, bilateral movements (average 15 to 20 blinks/min)	Rapid blinking Monocular blinking Absent or infrequent blinking
e. Surface characteristics	Skin intact, without discharge Lid margins flush against eyeball surface Lashes equally distributed and curled slightly outward	Lesions, nodules, redness, flaking, crusting, excessive tearing, discharge Creamy or yellow plaques (xanthelasma)

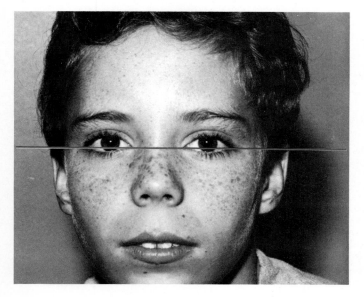

Fig. 7-33   Normal alignment of eyes.

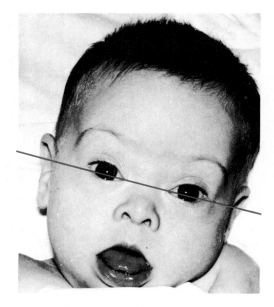

Fig. 7-34   Abnormal slanting seen in eyes of child with Down syndrome. (Modified from Reisman LF, Matheny AP: *Genetics and counseling in medical practice,* St Louis, 1969, Mosby–Year Book.)

CHARACTERISTIC OR AREA EXAMINED	NORMAL FINDINGS	DEVIATIONS FROM NORMAL
	Epicanthal folds (vertical folds of skin covering inner canthus of eye): may be considered normal in Oriental children (Fig. 7-35); should decrease greatly by age 10; position and degree of folds must be evaluated (Fig. 7-36)	Lid edema, lid deformity (pulled away from eyeball or turned inward) Lashes absent Lashes turned inward Large epicanthal folds in non-Oriental children, or folds that remain past age 10 Any sign of ptosis needs referral
4. Position of globe in socket	White persons: eyeball does not protrude beyond supraorbital ridge of frontal bone Black persons: eyeball may protrude slightly beyond supraorbital ridge	Forward displacement (exophthalmos) Backward displacement (enophthalmos) Sunken eyes may need further evaluation for dehydration or malnutrition
5. Lacrimal apparatus	No tearing during first month	Excessive tearing before third month No tearing by second month

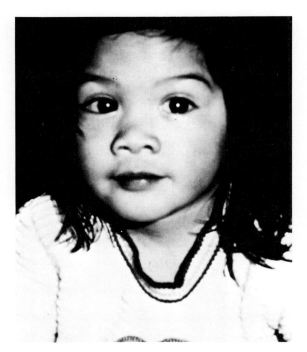

Fig. 7-35 Inner epicanthal folds may be normally seen in Oriental children. Note that this may give the appearance of pseudostrabismus. (From Whaley LF, Wong DL: *Nursing care of infants and children,* ed 3, St Louis, 1987, Mosby—Year Book.)

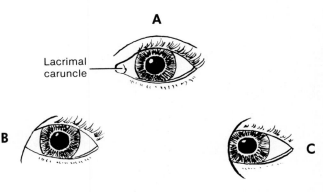

Fig. 7-36 Position and degree of epicanthal folds. **A,** Normal eye without epicanthal fold. **B,** Partial epicanthal fold of eye. **C,** Epicanthal fold completely covering lacrimal caruncle.

Continued.

CLINICAL VARIATIONS: THE CHILD—cont'd

CHARACTERISTIC OR AREA EXAMINED	NORMAL FINDINGS	DEVIATIONS FROM NORMAL
External ocular structures—cont'd		
a. Examiner presses index finger against lower orbital rim near inner canthus; pressure slightly everts lower lid	Puncta seen on tiny elevations on nasal side of upper and lower lid margins Mucosa pink and intact with no response to pressure	Puncta red, swollen, with tenderness on pressure Fluid or purulent material discharged from puncta in response to pressure
b. Gently palpate upper and lower lids for tenderness and nodules; exert minimal pressure over eyeball with examining finger	No tenderness or nodules	Tenderness, nodules, or irregularities
6. Bulbar conjunctiva and sclera	Infant sclera may have blue tinge caused by thinness Bulbar conjunctiva clear; tiny red vessels may be visible Sclera appears white Tiny black dots (pigmentation) may appear near limbus in dark-skinned persons Some pigmented deposits may appear Slight yellow cast in dark-skinned persons Palpebral conjunctiva pink, intact, without discharge No tenderness or itching	Darker blue sclera Blood vessels dilated Conjunctiva reddened Lesions or nodules Sclera yellow (jaundice) Foreign body Tenderness (especially on eye movements) Redness, lesions, nodules, discharge, tenderness, crusting
a. Lower lid eversion: not routinely performed in children unless examiner expects irritation, infection, or foreign body		
b. Upper lid eversion: not ordinarily performed in screening examination unless examiner expects irritation, infection, or foreign body; when performed, techniques are same as for adult		
7. Cornea (using oblique lighting)		
a. Transparency	Transparent	Opacities
b. Surface characteristics	Smooth Clear, shiny	Irregularities appearing in light reflections on surface Lesions, abrasions Foreign body Arcus senilis Tissue growth from periphery toward corneal center (pterygium) Corneal ulcerations

CHARACTERISTIC OR AREA EXAMINED	NORMAL FINDINGS	DEVIATIONS FROM NORMAL
8. Anterior chamber: child must be old enough to cooperate		
a. Transparency	Transparent	Cloudiness or any visible material, blood
b. Iris surface	Iris flat	Iris bulging toward cornea (crescent-shaped shadow may appear on far side of iris)
c. Chamber depth	Adequate clearance between cornea and iris	Chamber appears shallow
9. Iris		
a. Shape	Round	Irregular shape
b. Color and consistency	Coloration from newborn to 6 months may be blue Generally between 6 and 9 months permanent color is determined By 1 year all children should have permanent iris color	Inconsistency of coloration (in one eye or between two eyes) Black and white speckling (Brushfield spots) may be seen in children with Down syndrome
10. Pupil		
a. Shape	Round	Other than round
b. Bilateral size	Equal in size	Unequal in size
Internal eye (See both adult and child "Clinical Tips and Strategies," pp. 196-197, for techniques)		
1. Red reflex	Bright, round, red-orange glow seen through pupil (even in infants)	Decreased redness or roundness of reflex Dark spots or any opacities
2. Retinal structures (lens wheel at − 5 to 0)		
a. Optic disc margin	Regular, distinct Sharp outline scattered or dense pigment deposits may be visualized at border Gray crescent may appear at temporal border	Margin blurred
(1) Shape	Round or slightly vertically oval	Irregular
(2) Size	Approximately 1.5 mm diameter (appears magnified 15 times to examiner) Marked myopic refractive errors may make disc appear larger Hyperopic errors may make it appear smaller	Shape and size of discs not equal in both eyes
(3) Color	Creamy pink Lighter than retina Tiny vessels may be visible on disc surface	Diffuse pallor or pallor of section of disc, which always extends from center of disc to border Hyperemic disc (with engorged, tortuous vessels on disc surface)
(4) Physiological cup	Small depression just temporal of center of disc; does *not* extend to disc border Usually appears paler than disc; sometimes gray	Cup extends to border of disc

Continued.

CLINICAL VARIATIONS: THE CHILD—cont'd

CHARACTERISTIC OR AREA EXAMINED	NORMAL FINDINGS	DEVIATIONS FROM NORMAL
Internal eye—cont'd		
	Usually occupies four tenths to five tenths of diameter of disc	Cup occupies more than five tenths of diameter of disc
	Vessels entering disc may drop abruptly into cup or may appear to fade gradually	Cup size or placement not equal in both eyes
	Discs are more pronounced in some people than others	
b. Retinal vessels: follow from disc to periphery, dividing retina into four quadrants		
(1) Arteries	Usually about 25% narrower than veins (2:3 or 4:5 ratio; size varies with number of branches)	Arteries become narrow (2:4 or 3:5 ratio or less) (hypertension)
	Narrow band of light may appear at center	Width of light reflex increases to cover over one third of artery
	Light red	Opaque or pale in color
(2) Veins	Larger than arteries	Veins become larger
	No light reflection	
	Darker in color	
	Venous pulsations may be visible	
(3) Distribution and pattern (*Note:* Vessel abnormalities are not evenly distributed; scan all quadrants in orderly fashion for observation.)	Vessel caliber should be regular and uniformly decreasing in size as it branches and moves toward periphery	Irregularities of caliber; dilation constriction
	Artery/vein crossings should not alter (or pinch) caliber of underlying vessel	Neovascularization (appears as compact patches of tortuous, narrow vessels)
		Indentations or nicks of vessels at artery/vein crossing
c. Retinal background: scan four quadrants in orderly fashion		
(1) Color and surface characteristics	Pink, usually uniform throughout	Pallor of fundus (general or localized)
	Fundi of black clients often are heavily pigmented or uniformly dark	Hemorrhage (may be linear, flame shaped, rounded, dark or red, large or small)
	Choroidal vessels may be visible through retinal layer (appear as linear, light orange streaks)	Microaneurysms (appear as discrete, tiny red dots)
	Movable light reflections may appear on retinal surface (more prominent in young persons)	Soft or hard exudates (fuzzy or well-defined white patches)
d. Macula and fovea centralis: not fully mature until end of first year		
(1) Color and surface	Appears slightly darker than remainder of retina	Any abnormalities or lesions described for remainder of retinal surface
	Fovea may appear as tiny bright light in center of macula	
	Tiny vessels may appear on surface	
	Fine pigmentation and granular appearance may be visible	
(2) Vitreous body (lens wheel from 0 to +15)	Clear	Floating particles
	Transparent	Cloudy
(3) Cornea, anterior chamber, and lens (lens wheel from +15 to +20)	Clear	Cloudy
		Blood

The Childbearing Woman

HISTORY AND CLINICAL STRATEGIES

- When examining the eyes of a pregnant client, note pupil size and shape. Slightly unequal pupils may be a normal finding if the woman has always had this asymmetry. Unusual pupils may suggest drug addiction.
- Changes in eyesight occur during pregnancy and should be monitored by an ophthalmologist. Pregnancy-induced hypertension (toxemia) can cause several eyesight abnormalities:

1. Spots seen even with eyes closed
2. Chromatopsia (distorted color perception)
3. Blurred or double vision
4. Homonymous hemianopsia or temporary blindness
5. Retinal vessel constriction and edema seen during examination

These symptoms should not be ignored, since the underlying cause requires treatment.

- It may be difficult to see a red reflex if a woman's pupils are small.

CLINICAL VARIATIONS: THE CHILDBEARING WOMAN

CHARACTERISTIC OR AREA EXAMINED	NORMAL FINDINGS	DEVIATIONS FROM NORMAL
1. Characteristics	Eyelids darken from melanin pigment May have discomfort wearing contact lenses Eyesight and corrective prescription may change (caused by corneal fluid shifts during pregnancy; occasionally caused by enlarged pituitary gland compromising visual fields)	Pale conjunctivae (may mean anemia) Signs of toxemia: blurred, double vision Chromatopsia: unusual color perception, seeing spots, blindness in lateral eye halves, retinal arteriole constriction, sheen, disc edema, retinal detachment (emergency)
2. Postdelivery	Eyelids lighten Cornea curves change as fluid levels or pituitary gland return to prepregnant state	

 ## *The Older Adult*

HISTORY AND CLINICAL STRATEGIES

- Glaucoma symptoms and information follow:
  1. Open-angle, or chronic simple, glaucoma is the most common type of glaucoma in elderly clients.
  2. Early symptoms are absent or subtle:
     a. Vague loss of peripheral vision (which client may not notice or just attribute to aging)
     b. Aching or discomfort around eyes
     c. Difficulty adjusting to darkness (a common complaint *not* associated with glaucoma, caused by normal pupillary decrease in size)
  3. May be familial (tonometry screening should be performed with other family members)
  4. Usually bilateral
  5. Noncompliancy with treatment prescribed for glaucoma may be a problem because:
     a. The disease itself is often asymptomatic, and the miotic drops create difficulty in adjusting to darkness.
     b. Clients may have difficulty administering medication.
  6. Clients with acute closed-angle glaucoma have acute symptoms, and it is regarded as an emergency medical problem. The symptoms are:
     a. Severe eyeball pain and headache
     b. Colored halos around lights
     c. Sudden decrease in visual acuity
     d. Nausea, vomiting
  7. Clients with closed-angle (or narrow-angle) glaucoma can also have acute intermittent attacks alternating with remissions.
- Cataract symptoms and information follow:
  The extent of client visual loss or blurring may not correlate with the extent of opacity viewed by the examiner.

2. Opacities may be nuclear (central) (which tend to interfere with central vision), peripheral, or scattered.

3. Lens opacities increase glare (e.g., lights at night, bright sunlight, highly polished floors).

4. Cataracts are usually bilateral; however, they can progress at different rates in each eye.

5. Common symptoms accompanying cataracts are:
   a. General darkening of images
   b. Glare
   c. Sense of dimness
   d. Image distortion

6. If the cataracts have been removed and corrective lenses are worn, the client may have good central vision, but images appear closer and larger than they really are. Peripheral vision will be diminished. Safety concerns, such as using stairs, learning to turn head to side to view peripheral images, maneuvering in traffic, and adjusting to visual change, should be discussed.

7. Corneal contact lenses can be prescribed for individuals who have had cataracts removed. Peripheral vision is more accurate with these lenses. However, adjustment to wearing lenses is difficult (see pp. 180-181 for some details).

8. Intraocular lens implantation is being performed increasingly for clients who have had cataracts removed. The implantation offers more normal central and peripheral vision. Miotic eyedrops are prescribed to ensure that the lens remains in place.

• The examiner will probably be working with clients who are chronically visually handicapped. Some common problems follow:

1. Blurred or diminished vision acuity
2. Decreased ability to perceive depth
3. Difficulty adjusting to darkness; light, in general, appears dimmer
4. Increased glare
5. Diminished peripheral vision
6. Loss of color perception acuity (lens becomes more yellow with aging, and objects appear more yellow; difficulty differentiating blue/green hues)

• The problems just mentioned may be perceived by the client as mild inconveniences or as major problems. The practitioner must take an adequate history to cover safety concerns and successful and satisfactory performance of activities of daily living (see original data base screening, p. 26, for details). Particular safety and convenience concerns to inquire about follow:

1. Sufficient lighting available in home (dark hallways, stairways, night light)
2. Sufficient lighting for close work (reading, sewing, writing)
3. Safety concerns at night or in the dark (driving, walking on irregular surfaces)
4. Reduction of glare and excess lighting ("neon" lighting contributes to glare), windows without curtains, highly polished floors
5. If depth perception is altered, concerns about using stairs, stepping off curbs
6. If necessary, client access to special materials available for visually handicapped (e.g., large-print books, magazines, and calendars, special dials for telephone)
7. Resources available for help (e.g., relatives, neighbors, local community agencies)
8. Difficulty with administration of medication
9. Adequacy of *total* sensory input with visually handicapped clients (e.g., is client alone for long periods; able to use television or radio as a means of receiving information?)

• When interviewing visually handicapped clients, the following behaviors are helpful:

1. Remember that this individual is probably in a strange environment and is receiving a multitude of sensory stimuli. New sounds, odors, environmental temperatures, and a busy, crowded environment may overload a client whose vision is diminished to the extent that he cannot accommodate. Privacy, a quiet area, and the use of touch to communicate are helpful.
2. Questions should be worded distinctly and slowly, allowing client sufficient time to respond.
3. The examiner must explain every activity *before* it happens.

• Review "History" and "Clinical Tips and Strategies" (pp. 180, 196) for additional information related to eye and visual examination.

• *Note:* Testing for intraocular pressure with a tonometer has not been covered in this chapter. However, it is considered a necessary component of regular eye/vision screening for adults over 40 years of age.

CLINICAL VARIATIONS: THE OLDER ADULT

CHARACTERISTIC OR AREA EXAMINED	NORMAL FINDINGS	DEVIATIONS FROM NORMAL
Visual acuity and function		
1. Distant-vision measurement (CN II)	20/20 to 20/30 O.D., O.S. (with corrective lenses)	O.D. or O.S.: any letters missed in 20/20 to 20/30 line or above*
a. Reading patterns	Smooth, without hesitation Eyes remain open without frowning or squinting	Behaviors indicating difficulty reading (frowning, squinting, "cheating," leaning forward, tilting head, hesitancy or difficulty naming letters)

2. Near-vision measurement	One author states that average individual over age 60 cannot focus more closely than 3 feet without corrective lenses
	With corrective lenses:
	   14/14 O.D.
	   14/14 O.S.
		Inability to read newsprint or near-vision chart at 35 cm (14 inches) with corrective lenses
		Tendency to push reading material farther away
		(*Note:* Myopic (nearsighted) individuals may be able to read at normal (14-inch) distance if they *remove* their glasses. They will report this as a change in vision. Formerly they should have been able to read while wearing glasses. *Older adults* may report sudden improvement in near vision. This may result from cataract formation, which causes lens contraction and increases lens curvature. Such a change should be referred.)

a. Reading patterns	Newsprint or chart is read without hesitancy or attempt to pull it closer or push it farther away Eyes remain open without excessive blinking or facial distortions	Note any other behaviors indicating difficulty (frowning, squinting, hesitancy, pulling reading material closer)

3. Peripheral visual fields (confrontation method)	Client and examiner report seeing object at approximately same time as it approaches from periphery; this test assumes that examiner has normal peripheral vision
	Normal described as:
	   Temporal peripheral vision: 90°
	   Upward: 50°
	   Toward nose: 60°
	   Downward: 70°
		Client fails to report sighting object at same time as examiner in any one direction or in all directions (peripheral visual loss may involve both eyes or one eye)
		
		(*Note:* Confrontation method is a crude measurement for peripheral visual loss. Central visual loss [e.g., blind spots or scotomas] will not be detected with this method.)

4. Extraocular muscle function a. Corneal light reflex	Light reflection appears symmetrically in the two pupils	Light reflection appears at different spots (asymmetrically) in each eye
b. Movement of eyes in six cardinal fields of gaze (CN III, IV, VI)	Both eyes demonstrate coordinated, parallel movements in all directions	Eye movements not coordinated or parallel

*Several authors state that distant visual acuity begins to decrease in the sixth decade and that only about 15% of the individuals over 80 years measure at 20/20. However, for screening purposes any measurement less than 20/20 to 20/30 is considered a problem for referral regardless of client age.

Continued.

CLINICAL VARIATIONS: THE OLDER ADULT—cont'd

CHARACTERISTIC OR AREA EXAMINED	NORMAL FINDINGS	DEVIATIONS FROM NORMAL
Visual acuity and function—cont'd		
	End-point nystagmus may occur if eye is held in extreme gaze (mild rhythmic twitching with quick movement in direction of gaze with slow drift in other direction)	One or both eyes fail to follow examiner's hand in any given direction Sporadic or nonpurposeful eye movements Pathological nystagmus (quick movement always in same direction regardless of direction of gaze) (*Note:* Clients with Parkinson disease tend to manifest restriction of conjugate upward gaze.)
c. Cover-uncover test	Uncovered eye does not move as examiner places card over other eye	Uncovered eye moves to focus on designated point
	Newly uncovered eye does not move	Newly uncovered eye moves to focus on designated point
5. Corneal reflex (CN V)	Lids of both eyes close when either cornea is touched	Lid(s) of one or both eyes fails to respond
6. Pupillary response (CN II, III) a. Direct and consensual reaction to light	Constriction response (bilateral) somewhat delayed: pupil with light shining on it constricts (direct response); other pupil constricts simultaneously (consensual response)	Unequal (in size or speed) reflex response or absent response
b. Accommodation	Pupil constriction remains intact in response to accommodation Client will probably report that near object is out of focus (near-vision reading test measures client's ability to focus on near objects)	Pupils fail to constrict Asymmetrical response
External ocular structures		
1. Eyebrows a. Hair quality and distribution, skin quality	Skin intact, without marked or patchy hair loss Moderate thinning of brows (especially at temporal side) Brows in equal alignment	Flaking, scaling, lesions Marked or patchy hair loss Unequal alignment
b. Movement	Equal (bilateral)	Asymmetrical
2. Eyelids/lashes a. Height of palpebral fissures	Bilaterally equal in position	Asymmetrical positioning
b. Lid positioning	Upper lids may droop to greater extent than in young adult (lids overlie cornea at both superior and inferior borders)	Lids droop to extent of interfering with vision Sclera visible between upper and/or lower lid margins and iris
c. Lid closure	Complete with smooth, easy motion	Incomplete, or closure with difficulty or pain
d. Blinking	Frequent involuntary, bilateral movements (average 15 to 20 blinks/min)	Rapid blinking Monocular blinking Absent or infrequent blinking

CHARACTERISTIC OR AREA EXAMINED	NORMAL FINDINGS	DEVIATIONS FROM NORMAL
e. Surface characteristics	Numerous wrinkles, thin skinfolds Skin intact, without discharge Lower lid margins may droop slightly away from eyeball surface Lashes curled outward (lashes may be sparse) Creamy yellow plaques, sometimes raised, may appear (especially near inner canthus) (xanthelasma, see Fig. 7-18)	Flaking, crusting Lesions (basal cell carcinoma most commonly found in this area (Fig. 7-37) Ectropion, with tearing (see Fig. 7-19) (may become infected) Entropion (may become infected), lashes curled inward or absent (see Fig. 7-20)
3. Position of globe in socket	Globe sinks deeper into socket (loss of fat cushion)	Forward displacement (exophthalmos) Marked backward displacement (enophthalmos) Asymmetrical placement
4. Lacrimal apparatus a. Puncta and eyelids (on palpation)	Puncta seen on tiny elevations on nasal side of upper and lower lid margins Mucosa pink and intact with no response to pressure Occasionally lacrimal gland can be viewed if upper eyelid is raised or everted (loss of circumorbital fat)	Puncta red, swollen, with tenderness on pressure Fluid or purulent material discharged from puncta in response to pressure
b. Upper and lower lids	No tenderness or nodules	Tenderness, nodules, or irregularities
5. Bulbar conjunctiva, sclera, palpebral conjunctiva	Bulbar conjunctiva may appear somewhat dry, lacking luster of younger adult Bulbar conjunctiva clear; tiny red vessels may be visible Sclera appears white Tiny black dots (pigmentation) may appear near limbus in dark-complexioned persons Some pigmented deposits may appear Slight yellow cast in dark-complexioned persons Palpebral conjunctiva pink, intact, without discharge No tenderness or itching	Profuse tearing Blood vessels dilated Conjunctiva reddened Lesions or nodules Sclera yellow (jaundice) or significantly blue Foreign bodies Tenderness (especially on eye movement) Redness, lesions, nodules, discharge, tenderness, crusting

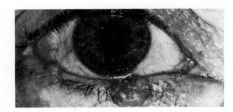

Fig. 7-37   Basal cell carcinoma of the lower lid. (From Newell FW: *Ophthalmology: principles and concepts,* ed 6, St Louis, 1986, Mosby–Year Book.)

Continued.

CLINICAL VARIATIONS: THE OLDER ADULT—cont'd

CHARACTERISTIC OR AREA EXAMINED	NORMAL FINDINGS	DEVIATIONS FROM NORMAL
External ocular structures—cont'd		
6. Cornea (use oblique lighting)		
a. Transparency	Transparent	Opacities
b. Surface characteristics	Smooth Clear, shiny Arcus senilis (deposit of white-yellow material around periphery of cornea; may be slightly elevated) (Fig. 7-38)	Irregularities appearing in light reflections on surface Lesions, abrasions, foreign body Tissue growth from periphery toward corneal center (pterygium)
7. Anterior chamber (use oblique lighting)		
a. Transparency	Transparent	Cloudy or any visible material, blood
b. Iris surface	Iris flat	Iris bulging toward cornea (crescent-shaped shadow may appear on far side of iris)
c. Chamber depth	Chamber becomes shallower with aging; however, clearance between cornea and iris is maintained	Marked shallowness
8. Iris		
a. Shape	Round (wedge or portion of iris may be absent in clients who have had cataract removal)	Irregular
b. Color and consistency	May be some irregularity of density of pigmentation (bilateral) Normal pigment replaced by pale brown coloration	Inconsistency of coloration between eyes

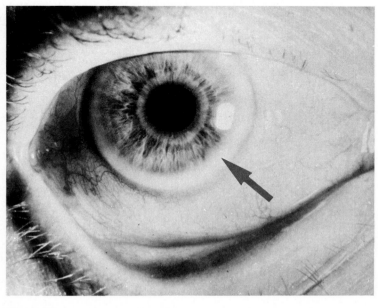

Fig. 7-38   Arcus senilis. (From Steinberg FU, editor: *Care of the geriatric patient,* ed 6, St Louis, 1983, Mosby—Year Book.)

CHARACTERISTIC OR AREA EXAMINED	NORMAL FINDINGS	DEVIATIONS FROM NORMAL
9. Pupil		
a. Shape and size	Round (shape may appear somewhat irregular or square with intraocular lens implant after cataract surgery) Aged pupils often smaller in size (sometimes markedly so) Elderly client receiving topical miotic agents (for glaucoma) will have constricted pupils	Irregular shape
b. Bilateral size	Equal	Unequal
Internal eye		
1. Red reflex	Bright, round, red-orange glow seen through pupil Increasing opacities of lens viewed as part of normal aging; examiner may commonly see various patterns of dark spots or clouds (either central, peripheral, or scattered) in aged client's reflex For screening purposes all opacities should be viewed as problem for referral	Opacities or decreased redness or roundness of reflex
2. Cornea, anterior chamber, lens	Clear	Cloudy or any visible materials; blood
3. Vitreous body	Clear Transparent	Cloudy Floating particles
4. Retinal structures		
a. Optic disc margin	Regular, distinct Sharp outline; scattered or dense pigment deposits may be visualized at border Gray crescent may appear at temporal border	Margin blurred
(1) Shape	Round or slightly vertically oval	Irregular
(2) Size	Approximately 1.5 mm diameter (appears magnified 15 times to examiner) Marked myopic refractive errors may make disc appear larger After cataract extraction, disc appears very small Hyperopic errors may make it appear smaller	Shape and size of discs not equal in both eyes
(3) Color	Creamy pink Lighter than retina Tiny vessels may be visible on disc surface	Diffuse pallor or pallor of section of disc, which always extends from center of disc to border Hyperemic disc (with engorged, tortuous vessels on disc surface)
(4) Physiological cup	Small depression just temporal of center of disc; does *not* extend to disc border	Cup extends to border of disc

Continued.

CLINICAL VARIATIONS: THE OLDER ADULT—cont'd

CHARACTERISTIC OR AREA EXAMINED	NORMAL FINDINGS	DEVIATIONS FROM NORMAL
Internal eye—cont'd	Usually appears paler than disc, sometimes gray	
	Usually occupies four tenths to five tenths of diameter of disc	Cup occupies more than five tenths of diameter of disc
	Vessels entering disc may drop abruptly into cup or may appear to fade gradually	Cup size or placement not equal in both eyes
	Discs are more pronounced in some clients than others	
b. Retinal vessels		
(1) Arteries	Arteriolar reflex is slightly widened	Arteries become narrow (2:4 or 3:5 ratio or less) (hypertension)
	Arteriolar column may appear slightly narrower, straighter with slight irregularities in caliber (Fig. 7-39)	Width of light reflex increases to cover over one third of artery
	Arteries may appear more opaque, gray	Opaque or pale in color
	Adult arteries usually about 25% narrower than veins (2:3 or 4:5 ratio; size varies with number of branches)	
	Narrow band of light may appear at center	
	Light red	
(2) Veins	Larger than arteries	Veins become engorged
	No light reflection	
	Darker in color	
(3) Distribution and pattern	Vessel caliber should be regular and uniformly decreasing in size as it branches and moves toward periphery	Irregularities of caliber; dilation or constriction
		Neovascularization (appears as compact patches of tortuous, narrow vessels)
	Artery/vein crossings should not alter (or pinch) caliber of underlying vessel	Indentations or nicks of vessels at artery/vein crossing

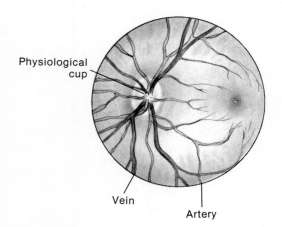

Fig. 7-39 Retinal changes in the aging eye. Arteriolar columns are narrower, straighter with slight irregularities in caliber. Retina may appear paler and more transparent (showing choroidal vessels).

CHARACTERISTIC OR AREA EXAMINED	NORMAL FINDINGS	DEVIATIONS FROM NORMAL
c. Retinal background (1) Color	Pink, usually uniform throughout	Pallor of fundus (general or localized)
	Fundi of black persons are often heavily pigmented and uniformly dark	White choroid and vessels clearly visible through thinned or absent retina
(2) Surface characteristics	Fine granular surface Choroidal vessels may be visible through retinal layer (appear as linear, light orange streaks) Movable light reflections may appear on retinal surface (more prominent in young clients)	Hemorrhage (may be linear, flame-shaped, rounded, dark or red, large or small) Microaneurysms (appear as discrete, tiny red dots) Drusen commonly seen (usually located symmetrically in both eyes) Any fuzzy or well-defined white or yellow patches
d. Macula and fovea centralis	Appears slightly darker than rest of retina (slight dispersion of granular pigment) Foveal (light) reflex may be less bright than in young adult Tiny vessels may appear on surface	Macular degeneration manifests small areas or clumps of black pigment in and around macula (degree of pigmentation does not always correlate with visual loss symptoms) May be hemorrhage visible in area

 Study Questions

General

1. Distant-vision acuity results are reported in fraction form. Mrs Jones's medical record states that she measured 20/40 O.D. and 20/40 O.S. This means that:
   - ☐ a. She was standing 40 feet from the eye chart and could read the line that someone with normal vision could read standing 20 feet from the chart
   - ☐ b. She was standing 20 feet from the chart and could read the line that someone with normal vision could read standing 40 feet from the chart
   - ☐ c. She was able to read 20 of the 40 letters on the chart
   - ☐ d. She has presbyopia
   - ☐ e. None of the above

2. The corneal light reflex:
   - ☐ a. Tests for alignment of the anteroposterior axes of the two eyes
   - ☐ b. Tests for corneal reflex
   - ☐ c. Demonstrates bilateral pupillary convergence
   - ☐ d. Might indicate a weak extraocular muscle if asymmetry is present
   - ☐ e. Will help to differentiate epicanthus and crossed eyes
   - ☐ f. c and e
   - ☐ g. a, d, and e
   - ☐ h. All except b
   - ☐ i. None of the above

3. Visual field defects may:
   - ☐ a. Occur laterally
   - ☐ b. Occur bilaterally
   - ☐ c. Occur in the form of a blind spot
   - ☐ d. Involve temporal field loss of both eyes
   - ☐ e. Involve temporal field loss of one eye and nasal field loss of the other eye
   - ☐ f. a and c
   - ☐ g. b, d, and e
   - ☐ h. All except a
   - ☐ i. All except d
   - ☐ j. All of the above

4. The cover-uncover test:
   - ☐ a. Is a test for nystagmus
   - ☐ b. When successfully performed, demonstrates that CN VIII is intact
   - ☐ c. Is a test for maintenance of parallel eyes
   - ☐ d. Is a test to demonstrate near-vision acuity
   - ☐ e. None of the above

5. Eye orbit movement is controlled by six muscles and three cranial nerves. The cranial nerves involved are the:
   - ☐ a. Optic (CN II), oculomotor (CN III), and abducens (CN VI)
   - ☐ b. Oculomotor (CN III), trochlear (CN IV), and abducens (CN VI)
   - ☐ c. Oculomotor (CN II), trigeminal (CN V), and facial (CN VII)
   - ☐ d. Optic (CN II), trigeminal (CN V), and abducens (CN VI)

6. The pupil of the eye:
   - ☐ a. Normally constricts in response to a bright light
   - ☐ b. Dilates in response to accommodation for near objects
   - ☐ c. May normally be slightly irregular in shape
   - ☐ d. Tends to be larger in myopic clients
   - ☐ e. Constricts in response to parasympathetic stimulation of the iris muscles
   - ☐ f. All of the above
   - ☐ g. a, d, and e
   - ☐ h. b and d
   - ☐ i. All except c

7. The eyelids:
   - ☐ a When open, normally cover a small portion of the iris
   - ☐ b. Are lined with palpebral conjunctiva
   - ☐ c. When open, form the palpebral fissure, the distance between the lid margins
   - ☐ d. Contain sebaceous glands
   - ☐ e. Are normally flush against the eyeball when open
   - ☐ f. All of the above
   - ☐ g. c and e
   - ☐ h. a, b, and d
   - ☐ i All except b
   - ☐ j. All except c

8. The eyeball is a sphere suspended within a bony orbit by means of:
   - ☐ a Muscles
   - ☐ b. Ligaments
   - ☐ c. Fat cushion
   - ☐ d. Scleral tissue
   - ☐ e. Nasolacrimal ducts
   - ☐ f. All of the above
   - ☐ g. a, b, and c
   - ☐ h. a, c, and d
   - ☐ i. b and e

9. When examining the lacrimal apparatus, only one portion is actually observed; it is the:
   - ☐ a. Lacrimal gland
   - ☐ b. Puncta
   - ☐ c. Lacrimal sac
   - ☐ d. Nasolacrimal duct

10. The conjunctiva:
   - ☐ a. Is the transparent lining of the eyelids
   - ☐ b. Is the transparent covering of the anterior portion of the eyeball
   - ☐ c. Is the white, porcelain-like covering of the eyeball
   - ☐ d. Normally contains a few visible vessels
   - ☐ e. Surfaces are kept moist and clean by a film of tears
   - ☐ f. a and e
   - ☐ g. c and d
   - ☐ h. a, b, and e
   - ☐ i. All except b
   - ☐ j. All except c

11. The cornea:
    □ a. Is normally transparent
    □ b. May normally show a somewhat irregular surface
    □ c. Covers the pupil and meets the scleral layer at the pupillary border
    □ d. Surface, when touched, transmits the sensation through CN V (trigeminal nerve)
    □ e. Abrasions can often be detected through oblique light reflections on its surface
    □ f. All of the above
    □ g. a, b, and e
    □ h. c and e
    □ i. a, d, and e
    □ j. All except b

12. You are holding the ophthalmoscope 4 cm from the client's eye. You want to examine the anterior chamber of the lens. You should set the lens wheel at _____ for the best focus.
    □ a. −3
    □ b. 0
    □ c. −10 to −15
    □ d. +5 to +2
    □ e. +15 to +20

13. When using the ophthalmoscope:
    □ a. Approach the client about 15° temporally
    □ b. Move the ophthalmoscope forward and backward in front of your eye until the red reflex comes into focus
    □ c. Stabilize the client's head with your free hand
    □ d. Ask the client to look at the ophthalmoscope light
    □ e. Keep the client talking to distract him from the examination
    □ f. All of the above
    □ g. b, c, and d
    □ h. a and c
    □ i. a, d, and e
    □ j. All except d

14. The normal color of the optic disc is:
    □ a. Creamy pink
    □ b. Pinkish-red
    □ c. Pale gray
    □ d. Bluish-gray

15. The physiological depression (cup) within the disc:
    □ a. Is just temporal of the center of the disc
    □ b. May normally extend to the disc border with hyperoptic clients
    □ c. Normally appears paler than the disc
    □ d. Usually occupies approximately half the diameter of the disc
    □ e. May normally be more pronounced in one eye
    □ f. All of the above
    □ g. a and d
    □ h. b and e
    □ i. All except e
    □ j. a, c, and d

16. Normal retinal arteries visible to the examiner are:
    □ a. About 25% narrower than the veins
    □ b. Darker in color than the veins
    □ c. Opaque in appearance
    □ d. About 50% narrower than the veins
    □ e. None of the above

17. Normal retinal veins visible to the examiner:
    □ a. Are about 25% narrower than the arteries
    □ b. Are lighter in color than the arteries
    □ c. Often manifest a band of light at the center of the vessel
    □ d. Are over twice as wide as the arteries
    □ e. None of the above

18. The normal retinal surface visible to the examiner:
    □ a. May show a fine granular texture
    □ b. May show marked dark-pigmented spots
    □ c. May show light orange streaks (choroidal vessels)
    □ d. a and b
    □ e. a and c

The Newborn

19. A newborn normally has:
    □ a. No tears
    □ b. Continual strabismus
    □ c. Epicanthal folds
    □ d. Pronounced eye slants

20. Usual internal eye characteristics of a newborn include:
    □ a. White pupil
    □ b. Coloboma
    □ c. Absent red reflex
    □ d. Transparent cornea

The Child

21. Which of the following findings alone indicate referral of the child for further physician evaluation:
    - ☐ a. Four-month-old-child whose eyes periodically cross
    - ☐ b. Four-year-old child whose visual acuity was 20/40 O.U.
    - ☐ c. Six-year-old child whose visual acuity was 20/30 O.D.; 20/40 O.S.
    - ☐ d. Ten-month-old child who demonstrates right eye drifting with cover test
    - ☐ e. Five-year-old boy who excessively blinks but shows no signs of corneal irritation or infection
    - ☐ f. All except b
    - ☐ g. b and c
    - ☐ h. a, d, and e
    - ☐ i. c and d
    - ☐ j. None of the above

22. All the following are true but one. Identify the *false* statement. When performing vision screening on kindergarten children using the Snellen "E" chart, the examiner should:
    - ☐ a. Test each eye separately
    - ☐ b. Test both eyes together
    - ☐ c. Evaluate only those children who have never been tested before
    - ☐ d. Place the child 20 feet from the chart
    - ☐ e. Retest any child who scores over 20/40

23. If you were to develop a vision screening program for 4-year-olds, which of the following techniques would you include:
    - ☐ a. Peripheral visual field testing
    - ☐ b. Cover test
    - ☐ c. Near-vision screening
    - ☐ d. Snellen visual acuity testing using either alphabet or "E" chart
    - ☐ e. Color vision screening using Ishihara test; test boys only
    - ☐ f. All of the above
    - ☐ g. a, c, and d
    - ☐ h. b, d, and e
    - ☐ i. All except c
    - ☐ j. All except e

The Childbearing Woman

24. Eye prescription changes during pregnancy are usually related to:
    - ☐ a. Pregnancy-induced hypertension
    - ☐ b. Retinal constriction
    - ☐ c. Corneal fluid shifts
    - ☐ d. Chromatopsia dilation

The Older Adult

25. Cataracts:
    - ☐ a. Are inherited
    - ☐ b. Are chiefly associated with diabetic clients
    - ☐ c. Do not create any visual problems until they become "ripe"
    - ☐ d All of the above
    - ☐ e. None of the above

26. Glaucoma:
    - ☐ a. Is readily recognized in elderly clients because of the associated acute symptoms
    - ☐ b. Can be diagnosed in its early stages by careful examination of the optic disc
    - ☐ c. Is usually bilateral
    - ☐ d. All of the above
    - ☐ e. None of the above

27. Presbyopia:
    - ☐ a. Is synonymous with hyperopia
    - ☐ b. Affects most individuals over 60 years of age
    - ☐ c. Does not occur if the individual is myopic
    - ☐ d. Is rare
    - ☐ e. None of the above

28. If an elderly client complains of difficulty adjusting to darkness, this difficulty might mean:
    - ☐ a. That his pupil is smaller and admits less light to the retina
    - ☐ b. Advanced macular degeneration
    - ☐ c. Optic atrophy
    - ☐ d. Retinal detachment

SUGGESTED READINGS
General

Bates B: *A guide to physical examination*, ed 4, Philadelphia, 1987, JB Lippincott.

Binder PS: The physiologic effects of extended wear soft contact lenses, *Ophthalmology* 87(8):745, 1980.

Houde WL, Rubin ML: Extended-wear lenses: an update, *Surv Ophthalmol* 26(2):103, 1981.

Malamed M: Complications of contact lenses, *Emerg Med* 12:218, 1982.

Malasanos L, Barkauskas V, Stoltenberg-Allen K: *Health assessment*, ed 4, St Louis, 1990, Mosby–Year Book.

Morbidity and mortality weekly report: Perspectives in disease prevention and health promotion: guidelines for diabetic eye disease control, *N Engl J Med* 36(7):1987.

Moses RA, Hart WM, editors: *Adler's physiology of the eye: clinical application*, ed 8, St Louis, 1987, Mosby–Year Book.

Newell FW: *Ophthalmology: principles and concepts*, ed 6, St Louis, 1986, Mosby–Year Book.

Seidel HM, Ball JW, Dains JE, Benedict GW: *Mosby's guide to physical examination*, ed 2, St Louis, 1991, Mosby–Year Book.

Thompson JM, McFarland GK, Hirsch JE, and others: *Mosby's manual of clinical nursing*, ed 2, St Louis, 1989, Mosby–Year Book.

The newborn

Auvenshine MA, Enriquez MG: *Maternity nursing: dimensions of change*, Belmont, Calif, 1985, Wadsworth.

Bobak IM, Jensen MD: *Essentials of maternity nursing*, ed 3, St Louis, 1991, Mosby–Year Book.

Judd JM: Assessing the newborn from head to toe, *Nurs '85* 15(12):34, 1985.

Kiernan BS, Scoloveno MA: Assessment of the neonate, *Top Clin Nurs* 8(1):1, 1986.

The Organization for Obstetrical, Gynecological and Neonatal Nurses (NAACOG): *Physical assessment of the neonate*, OGN nursing practice resource, Oct, 1986, The Association.

Pillitteri A: *Maternal-newborn nursing: care of the growing family*, ed 3, Boston, 1985, Little, Brown.

Scanlon JW and others: *A system of newborn physical examination*, Baltimore, 1979, University Park Press.

Seidel HM, Ball JW, Dains JE, Benedict GW: *Mosby's guide to physical examination*, ed 2, St Louis, 1991, Mosby–Year Book.

Whaley LF, Wong DL: *Nursing care of infants and children*, ed 4, St Louis, 1991, Mosby–Year Book.

The child

Alexander M, Brown MS: *Pediatric history taking and physical diagnosis for nurses*, ed 2, New York, 1979, McGraw-Hill.

Alexander M, Brown MS: Physical examination. V. Examining the eye, *Nurs '73* 3(12):41, 1973.

Chinn P, Leitch C: *Child health maintenance: a guide to clinical assessment*, ed 2, St Louis, 1979, Mosby–Year Book.

DeAngelis C: *Basic pediatrics for the primary health care provider*, ed 2, Boston, 1984, Little, Brown.

Helveston EM, Ellis FD: *Pediatric ophthalmology practice*, ed 2, St Louis, 1984, Mosby–Year Book.

Kirschen D, Rosenbaum A, Ballard E: The dot visual acuity test: a new acuity test for children, *J Am Optom Assoc* 54(12):1055, 1983.

Newell FW: *Ophthalmology: principles and concepts*, ed 7, St Louis, 1991, Mosby–Year Book.

Powell ML: *Assessment and management of developmental changes and problems in children*, ed 2, St Louis, 1981, Mosby–Year Book.

Sato-Viacrucis K: The evaluation of the Snellen E to the Blackbird, *School Nurse*, Spring, 1985, p 18.

Whaley LF, Wong DL: *Essentials of Pediatric Nursing*, ed 3, St Louis, 1989, Mosby–Year Book.

The childbearing woman

Auvenshine MA, Enriquez MG: *Maternity nursing: dimensions of change*, Belmont, Calif, 1985, Wadsworth.

Kinyoun J, Kalina R: Visual loss from choroidal ischemia, *Am J Ophthalmol* 101:650, 1986.

Pillitteri A: *Maternal-newborn nursing: care of the growing family*, ed 3, Boston, 1985, Little, Brown.

Whitley NA: *Manual of clinical obstetrics*, Philadelphia, 1985, JB Lippincott.

The older adult

Burnside IM, editor: *Nursing and the aged*, ed 3, New York, 1988, McGraw-Hill.

Carotenuto R, Bullock J: *Physical assessment of the gerontologic client*, Philadelphia, 1980, FA Davis.

Ebersole P, Hess P: *Toward healthy aging*, ed 3, St Louis, 1990, Mosby–Year Book.

Newell FW: *Ophthalmology: principles and concepts*, ed 7, St Louis, 1991, Mosby–Year Book.

Pesci BR: When the patient's problem is really poor vision, *RN* 49:22, 1986.

Pizzarello LD: The dimensions of the problem of eye disease among the elderly, *Ophthalmology* 94:1191, 1987.

Steinberg FU, editor: *Care of the geriatric patient*, ed 6, St Louis, 1983, Mosby–Year Book.

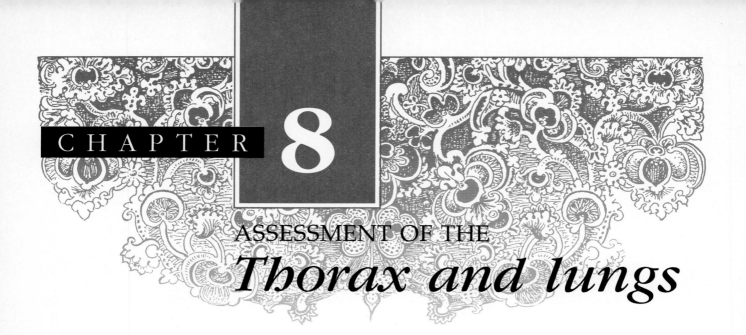

CHAPTER 8

ASSESSMENT OF THE
Thorax and lungs

VOCABULARY

adventitious sounds Sounds that are not normal within the lungs.

angle of Louis Point of tracheal bifurcation.

asthma Paroxysmal dyspnea that is accompanied by wheezing and caused by spasm of the bronchial tubes or by swelling of their mucous membranes.

Biot breathing Breathing characterized by several short breaths followed by long, irregular periods of apnea.

bradypnea Breathing that is abnormally slow.

bronchitis Inflammation of the bronchi.

bronchophony Increased vocal resonance detected over a bronchus that is surrounded by consolidated lung tissue.

bronchovesicular breathing Refers to breath sounds at a pitch intermediate between bronchial or tracheal sounds and alveolar sounds.

consolidation Increasing density of lung tissue caused by pathological engorgement.

costal angle Costal margin angle formed on the anterior chest wall at the base of the xiphoid process, where the ribs separate.

cyanosis Bluish-gray discoloration of the skin resulting from the presence of or abnormal amounts of reduced hemoglobin in the blood.

diaphragmatic excursion The extent of movement of the lungs.

dyspnea Breathing that is labored or difficult.

egophony Bleating nasal sound heard during auscultation of the chest when the client speaks in a normal tone.

emphysema A chronic pulmonary disease characterized by overdistended lung tissue.

friction rub Sound produced by the rubbing of the pleura of the lung.

hemoptysis The expectoration of blood from the lungs or bronchial tubes.

hyperpnea Respiration that is deeper and more rapid than that usually experienced during normal activity.

hyperresonance Sound elicited by percussion; its pitch lies between that of resonance and tympany.

Kussmaul respiration Deep, gasping type of respiration, often associated with diabetic acidosis.

kyphosis Exaggeration or angulation of the normal posterior curve of the spine.

manubrium of sternum Upper segment of the sternum that articulates with the clavicle and the first pair of costal cartilages

orthopnea Difficulty in breathing in any position other than an upright one.

pectus carinatum Abnormal prominence of the sternum.

pectus excavatum Abnormal depression of the sternum.

pleximeter Finger placed on the skin surface to receive the blow from the percussion hammer or plexor.

rale Abnormal wet or dry respiratory sound heard during auscultation of the chest.

rhonchus Coarse, dry rale heard in the bronchial tubes.

scoliosis Lateral curvature of the spine.

singultus Hiccup.

stridor Shrill, harsh sound heard during inspiration and caused by laryngeal obstruction.

tactile fremitus Vibratory sensations of the spoken voice felt through the chest wall on palpation.

tympany Low-pitched note heard on percussion of the distended thorax.

vesicular breathing The normal breath sounds heard over most of the lungs.

vocal fremitus The sensation of vibrations produced when the client speaks.

whispered pectoriloquy Transmission of whispered words through the chest wall, heard during auscultation; indicates solidification of the lungs.

ANATOMY AND PHYSIOLOGY REVIEW

The primary function of the respiratory system is to supply oxygen to the body cells and to remove carbon dioxide from the cells.

The anatomy of the respiratory system is discussed from a functional perspective within each of the four respiratory levels, which follow:

1. Ventilation: the movement of air from outside to inside the body and the distribution of the air within the tracheobronchial system to the gas exchange units of the lungs.

2. Diffusion and perfusion: the movement of oxygen and carbon dioxide across the alveolar-capillary membrane to the blood in the pulmonary capillaries.

3. Blood flow: the transportation of respiratory gases through the pulmonary and arterial circulation, the distribution and exchange of oxygen and carbon dioxide at the peripheral tissues, and the return of respiratory gases to the lungs.

4. Control of breathing: the regulation of ventilation to maintain adequate gas exchange, usually in accord

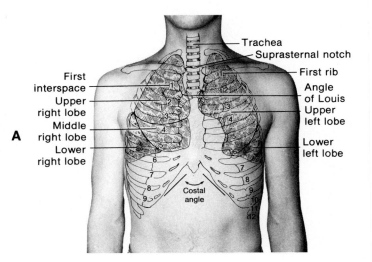
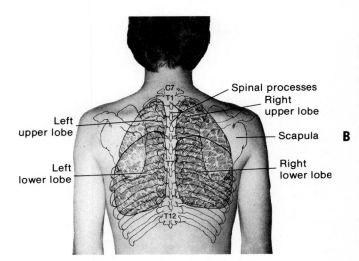

Fig. 8-1 **A,** Anterior view of anatomy of thorax. **B,** Posterior view of anatomy of thorax.

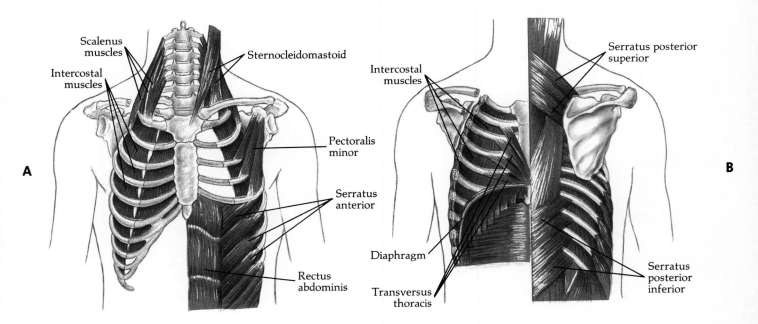

Fig. 8-2 Muscles of ventilation. **A,** Anterior view. **B,** Posterior view. (From Thompson JM, McFarland GK, Hirsch JE, and others: *Mosby's manual of clinical nursing,* ed 2, St Louis, 1989, Mosby—Year Book.)

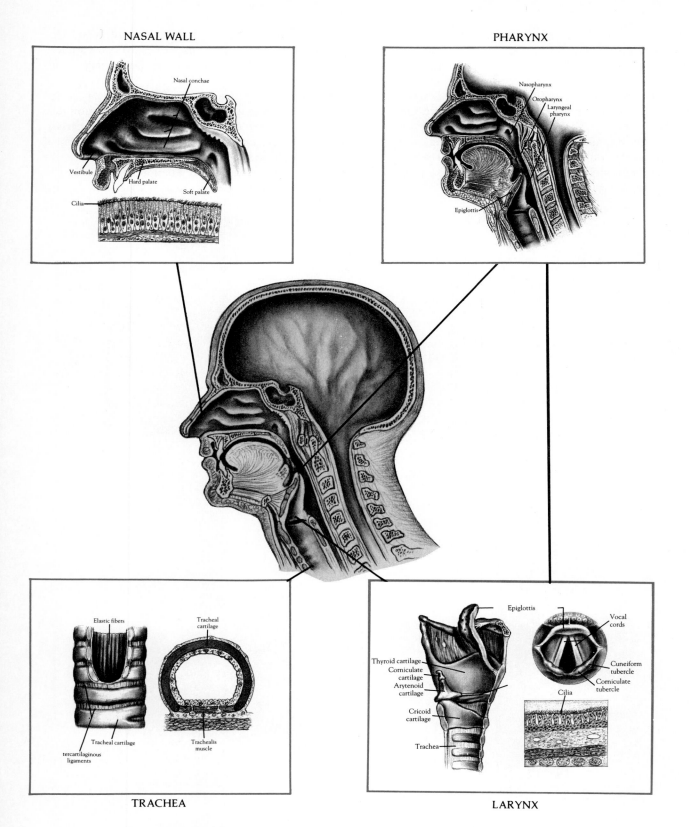

Fig. 8-3 Structures of upper airway. (From Thompson JM, McFarland GK, Hirsch JE, and others: *Mosby's manual of clinical nursing,* ed 2, St Louis, 1989, Mosby—Year Book.)

with changing metabolic demands or other special needs.

Only the first function of respiration (ventilation) is discussed in this anatomy and physiology section. The reader is directed to a physiology text for more details.

Ventilation is the process that moves air from the outside of the body to the gas exchange units of the lungs. The sternum, manubrium, and xiphoid process form the anterior border of the thorax. The posterior portion is formed by 12 thoracic vertebrae. The lateral boundaries are formed by 12 pairs of ribs, which have a posterior connection directly to the thoracic vertebrae. The first seven ribs are also connected to the sternum by the costal cartilages (Fig. 8-1). The major muscle groups used in the ventilatory process are the diaphragm and the intercostal muscles (Fig. 8-2).

The diaphragm is the principal muscle of inspiration. During a deep inspiration the diaphragm contracts and moves downward. This contraction, which occurs because of stimulation by the phrenic nerve, forces two major movements that facilitate ventilation: the first raises the lower ribs upward and laterally, increasing both the transverse and lateral intrathoracic space; the second action of the diaphragmatic contraction forces the abdominal contents downward. Both actions facilitate ventilation. The intercostal muscles are divided into the external and internal muscles. The external intercostal muscles contract to increase the anterioposterior

diameter of the thoracic cavity during inspiration. With deep and purposeful breathing, internal intercostal muscles contract to decrease the transverse diameter during expiration.

The upper airway, consisting of the nose, pharynx, larynx, and extrathoracic trachea (Fig. 8-3), has three major functions, which follow:
- To conduct air to the lower airway
- To protect the lower airway from foreign matter
- To warm, filter, and humidify inspired air

The lower airway, consisting of the trachea, mainstem bronchi, segmental bronchi, subsegmental bronchioles, terminal bronchioles, and gas exchange units, has three functions, as follows:
- Air conduction to the alveolar level of the lungs
- Mucociliary clearance
- Pulmonary surfactant production by the type II cells of the alveoli

The most distal section of the lower respiratory tract consists of the terminal respiratory units (acini), which include the respiratory bronchioles, the alveolar ducts, the alveolar sacs, and the terminal air sacs themselves, called *alveoli*. Fig. 8-4 shows the cluster arrangement of these terminal respiratory units.

It is important to identify topographical landmarks of the thorax. This provides a method by which to identify positive findings. Important landmarks include those shown in Fig. 8-5.

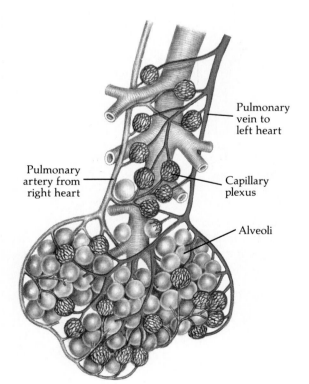

Pulmonary vein to left heart

Pulmonary artery from right heart

Capillary plexus

Alveoli

Fig. 8-4   The terminal respiratory units. (From Thompson JM, McFarland GK, Hirsch JE, and others: *Mosby's manual of clinical nursing,* ed 2, St Louis, 1989, Mosby–Year Book.)

Fig. 8-5 **A,** Topographical landmarks of anterior thorax. **B,** Topographical landmarks of posterior thorax. **C,** Topographical landmarks of thorax (lateral view).

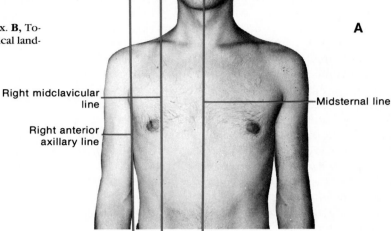

Right midclavicular line

Right anterior axillary line

Midsternal line

A

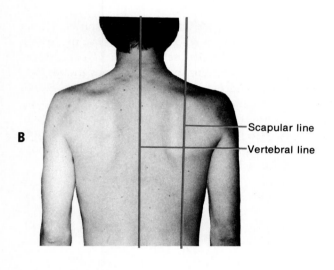

B

Scapular line

Vertebral line

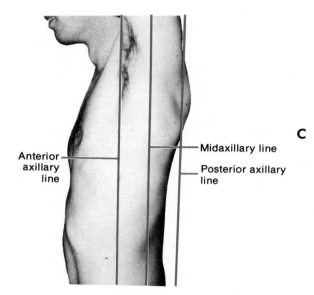

C

Anterior axillary line

Midaxillary line

Posterior axillary line

• • •

Examination of the thorax and lungs is a systematic process that can be learned fairly quickly. The most important findings, however, are subtle tissue perfusion findings. We are interested not only in the findings of auscultation and percussion, but also in oxygenation at the cellular level.

COGNITIVE OBJECTIVES

At the end of this chapter the learner will demonstrate knowledge of assessment of the respiratory system by the ability to do the following:
• Apply the terms that are listed in the vocabulary section.
• Systematically list the elements included in inspection of the respiratory system.
• Correctly locate or diagram landmarks of the anterior thorax, including the following:
    1. Suprasternal notch

2. Second rib
3. Costochondral junctions
4. Manubrium of sternum
5. Costal angle
6. Sternal angle
7. Clavicle
8. Midsternal line
9. Midclavicular line
10. Anterior axillary line
• Correctly locate or diagram landmarks of the posterior thorax, including the following:
    1. C7
    2. T1
    3. Scapula
    4. Inferior angle of scapula, T6, and seventh rib
    5. Vertebral line
    6. Midscapular line
    7. Posterior axillary line

- Describe the qualities of the following breath sounds, and indicate the location in which they are normally heard in adults and children:
  1. Bronchial
  2. Bronchovesicular
  3. Vesicular
- Describe the significance of each of the breath sounds, just listed, when heard in areas other than their normal locations.
- Describe the normal respiratory rates for newborns, children, pregnant women, and adults.
- Describe the following respiratory patterns:
  1. Kussmaul respirations
  2. Cheyne-Stokes breathing
  3. Sighing respirations
  4. Biot breathing
  5. Tachypnea
  6. Bradypnea
  7. Air trapping
- Systematically list the elements included in palpating the thorax.
- Describe the techniques for palpating expansion of the thorax.
- Identify the following:
  1. One condition that increases lung expansion
  2. Four conditions that limit lung expansion
  3. One condition that results in asymmetrical expansion
- Describe identifying characteristics of the following adventitious sounds:
  1. Rales
  2. Rhonchi
  3. Wheeze
  4. Pleural friction rub
- Define the significance of and describe the procedures for eliciting:
  1. Tactile fremitus
  2. Bronchophony
  3. Egophony
  4. Whispered pectoriloquy
  5. Diaphragmatic excursion
- State a rationale for palpating for tenderness of the costovertebral angle.
- Describe a systematic method for percussing the thorax.
- Describe four percussion tones elicited throughout the body, and state their normal locations.
- Identify selected common variations with newborns, children, childbearing women, and older adults.

CLINICAL OUTLINE

At the end of this chapter the learner will perform systematic assessment of the thorax and lungs by demonstrating the ability to do the following:

- Obtain a pertinent health history from a client.
- Demonstrate inspection of the thorax and relate findings relevant to the following:
  1. General body build
  2. Thorax configuration
  3. Skin, nail, and lip color
  4. Chest movement
  5. Pattern of respiration, including type of breathing, rate, and depth
- Demonstrate palpation of the thorax and relate findings relevant to the following:
  1. Chest expansion
  2. Tenderness or pulsations
  3. Skin texture and lesions
  4. Subcutaneous structures or masses
  5. Tactile fremitus in symmetrical areas of the chest
  6. Position of the trachea
- Demonstrate percussion of the thorax and relate findings relevant to the following:
  1. Characteristics of percussion tones heard in various areas of the thorax
  2. Intensity, pitch, quality, and duration of tones heard
  3. Diaphragmatic excursion
- Demonstrate the ability to identify and differentiate lung sounds, including vesicular, bronchovesicular, and bronchial sounds, rales, rhonchi, and friction rub.
- Demonstrate systematic auscultation of the lungs and relate findings relevant to the following:
  1. Characteristics of auscultatory sounds heard throughout the lungs
  2. Checking abnormal findings by using tests for bronchophony, egophony, and whispered pectoriloquy
- Summarize results of the assessment with a written description of findings.

HISTORY

- Coughing is basically caused by either internal or external stimuli. Internal stimuli include allergic responses or response to an inflammatory process. External stimuli include irritants such as smoke, dust, or gas. When compiling history data from a client complaining of a cough, collect as much descriptive information as possible. The data should include the following:
  1. Duration of the coughing problem
  2. Frequency of the cough; related to time of day
  3. Type of cough: hacky, dry, bubbly, throaty, barky, hoarse, congested
  4. Sputum production versus nonproductive cough
  5. If sputum is produced, describe characteristics: mucoid versus purulent, color, odor, blood-tinged (note that some medications, such as those containing catecholamines, may cause pink-tinged sputum), amount

6. Circumstances related to cough, such as activity, time of day, client position (lying vs. sitting), anxiety, talking
7. Whether activity makes cough better or worse (sitting, walking, exercise)
8. History of allergies in client or others in family (see *data base allergy profile* in Chapter 1, p. 9)
9. Is client's cough currently being treated? By whom? With what: over-the-counter medications, prescription medications, other techniques, such as a vaporizer?
10. Client's concern about cough
11. Is cough tiring?

• If the client complains of shortness of breath or dyspnea on exertion:
1. Does cough or diaphoresis accompany dyspnea?
2. Onset of breathing problems (severity, duration, efforts to treat)
3. Is breathing problem associated with pain or discomfort?
4. How does different positioning affect the dyspnea (lying vs. sitting)?
5. Time of day when dyspnea is likely to occur
6. Does dyspnea interfere with, alter, or slow down any daily activities?
7. How much walking creates shortness of breath (number of steps, flights of stairs, or blocks)?
8. Are there stairs at home or work? How often must they be climbed each day? How does this affect breathing problem?
9. How much walking or other types of exertion must the client do each day? How does this affect breathing problem?

• If the client complains of difficulty breathing or breathlessness:
1. History of asthma, bronchitis, emphysema, or tuberculosis? (Have client describe what these mean personally and to the family.)
2. Does breathing problem cause lips or fingernails to become cyanotic?
3. During a "breathing attack," what does the client do (positioning, breathing aids, such as medications or oxyen)?
4. How does the breathing problem interfere with the client's activities of daily living or work?
5. Client's view of breathing problem
6. Does the client think the overall breathing problem is getting worse or staying about the same?

• Has the client had any previous respiratory illnesses, hospitalizations, or surgeries for lung or breathing problems? Describe what and when.
• When was the client's last chest x-ray examination, tuberculosis test, or pulmonary function test? What were the results?

• Is the client currently taking any medications for breathing or allergy problems? If so, describe.
• Is the client subject to work or environmental conditions that could irritate the respiratory system (e.g., chemical plants, dry-cleaning fumes, coal mines)? If so, what does the client do for protection or monitoring the exposure conditions (e.g., masks, frequent pulmonary function tests or chest x-ray examinations, or ventilatory systems in factory with chemical exposure analysis)?
• Certain "fumes" cause specific respiratory or systemic irritation. If the client reports a pollution exposure history, as well as these symptoms, the examiner must be alert to their interrelationship:
1. Carbon monoxide may cause dizziness, headache, or fatigue.
2. Sulphur oxide may cause irritation to the respiratory tract, resulting in a cough or congestion.
3. Nitrogen oxides may irritate the mucous membranes, resulting in a cough or congestion.

• If the client smokes:
1. What does he smoke?
2. How long has client smoked?
3. How much each day does client smoke?
4. Does client inhale?
5. Does client have cough related to smoking?
6. When did cough begin? Has cough gotten worse since that time?
7. Does client desire to quit smoking? If so, what techniques has client used in an attempt to stop?
8. If client has tried to quit smoking but has failed, what does he see as the reason for failure?

• If the client formerly smoked but has quit:
1. What had client been smoking?
2. How long did client smoke?
3. How much each day did client smoke?
4. Why did the client quit?

• • •

The following clinical guidelines have been developed to simulate the clinical setting. Total assessment of the thorax and lungs can be carried out with the client in a sitting position. The sequence of assessment techniques is inspection, palpation, percussion, and auscultation. A detailed discussion of the techniques of percussion and auscultation can be found in "Clinical Tips and Strategies," which follow.

Inspection of the anterior and posterior chest should be carried out first. After inspection, the examiner should perform palpation, percussion, and auscultation of the posterior chest; then the examiner palpates, percusses, and auscultates the anterior chest. This places the examiner in front of the client, where he can proceed to cardiovascular assessment.

Text continues on p. 245.

CLINICAL GUIDELINES

EVALUATION

ASSESSMENT PROCEDURE	NORMAL FINDINGS	DEVIATIONS FROM NORMAL

1. Secure equipment needed for assessment of thorax and lungs
  a. Stethoscope
  b. Ruler
  c. Marker
2. Instruct client to undress to waist so that thorax may be examined (Females will need anterior cover during posterior examination.)
 	
Inspection of anterior and posterior chest
1. Instruct client to sit on edge of examination table for general inspection of anterior and posterior chest (Gown should be removed.)
2. Observe:		

a. Skin color of thorax and lips	Pink, well oxygenated	Cyanosis, pallor Spider nevi
b. Nail beds and nail configuration	Smooth Flat surface	Clubbing of nails and distal portion of fingers
c. General appearance	Relaxed posture	Apprehensive Tense forward posture Restless Flaring nostrils Supraclavicular retractions Intercostal retractions Intercostal bulging with expiration Use of accessory muscles during breathing
d. Chest wall configuration (1) Imagine topographical landmarks of thorax (Fig. 8-6)	Symmetrical Equal muscular development	

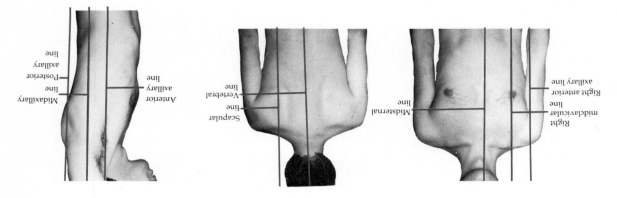

Fig. 8-6 Topographical landmarks of thorax.

Continued.

CLINICAL GUIDELINES—cont'd

	EVALUATION	
ASSESSMENT PROCEDURE	**NORMAL FINDINGS**	**DEVIATIONS FROM NORMAL**
Inspection of anterior and posterior chest—cont'd		

(2) Imagine underlying structures of thorax (Fig. 8-7)	*Posterior*
	   T4: angle of Louis
	Anterior
	   Second rib: angle of Louis, atria of heart	

(3) Anteroposterior (AP) diameter of chest	1:2 to 5:7 (AP:transverse diameter) flat connections of rib cartilage with sternum	Barrel chest (Fig. 8-8) Pectus carinatum Pectus excavatum

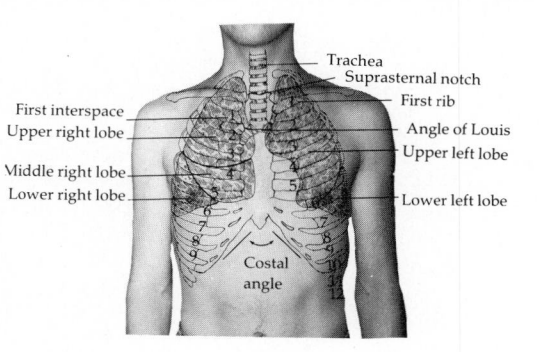

Fig. 8-7 Underlying structures of thorax.

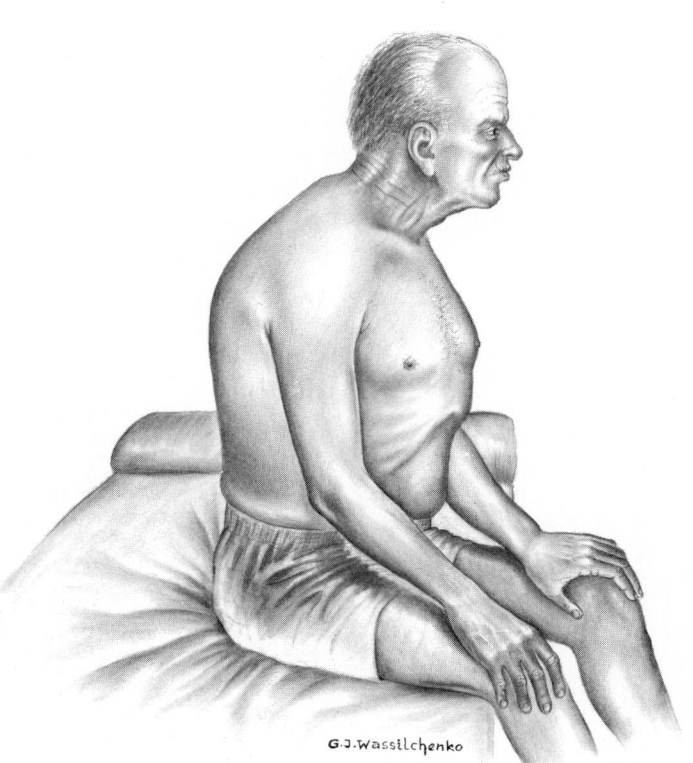

Fig. 8-8 Barrel chest. Note increased anteroposterior diameter.

Continued.

EVALUATION

ASSESSMENT PROCEDURE	NORMAL FINDINGS	DEVIATIONS FROM NORMAL
e. Symmetry of chest	Bilaterally equal musculature (may be slightly more muscle development on client's dominant side) Straight spinal processes (C7, T1 through T12) Symmetrical scapular placement Downward and equal slope of ribs Costal angle 90° or less	Asymmetry Atrophy, tremors Loss of or accentuated spinal curvature, scoliosis, kyphosis, deformities Asymmetrical scapular placement Horizontal ribs Costal angle greater than 90°
f. Breathing pattern	Diaphragmatic (male) Thoracic (female) Smooth, even breathing Passive breathing 12 to 20 per minute: ratio of respiratory to pulse rate 1:4 Even pattern 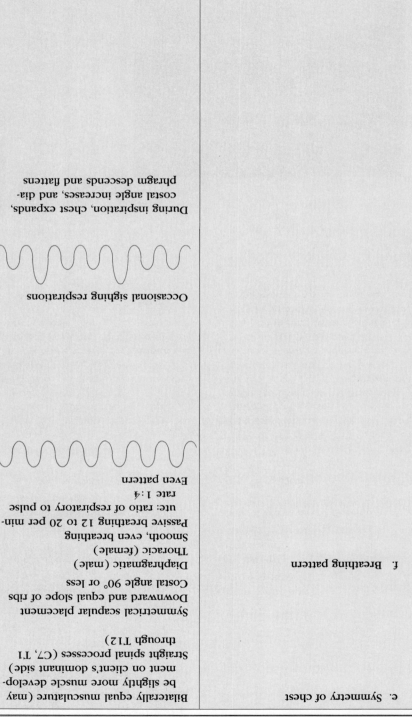 Occasional sighing respirations During inspiration, chest expands, costal angle increases, and diaphragm descends and flattens	Abnormal, irregular breathing Cheyne-Stokes breathing Increase in rate and depth Hyperpnea >20 per minute Decrease in rate Bradypnea <12 per minute Increase in rate and depth >20 per minute Kussmaul respirations Many sighing respirations accompanied by other characteristics of anxiety Biot breathing: shallow breathing followed by periods of apnea (may also be seen in some healthy persons) Air-trapping breathing in clients with pulmonary disease: because of obstructive process, air becomes trapped in lungs

CLINICAL GUIDELINES—cont'd

EVALUATION		
ASSESSMENT PROCEDURE	**NORMAL FINDINGS**	**DEVIATIONS FROM NORMAL**

Palpation of posterior chest

1. Use one or two hands to palpate skin and thorax of posterior chest; examiner should use palmar surface of hand, including palmar base of fingers (Fig. 8-9)

2. Evaluate and/or identify:
   a. Skin texture and temperature, spinal process
   b. C7 through T12
   c. Scapulae and surrounding musculature
   d. Chest wall

3. Use palmar surface of one hand to assess vocal fremitus; examiner should place hand over equal positions of right and left lung fields and instruct client to repeat "one, two, three" or "how now brown cow" (Fig. 8-10); technique should be continued down posterior and posterolateral chest wall, comparing response of one side with other; do not test over bone areas

---

Normal findings:

Smooth, warm skin

Straight spine, nontender

Symmetrical location with developed musculature
Stable ribs, nontender

Varies from person to person because of intensity and pitch of voice
Bilaterally equal mild vibratory sensation
Most intense area to feel vibration is upper posterior chest wall medial to scapulae

---

Deviations:

Dry or moist skin
Poor skin turgor
Crepitation
Curved spine
Scoliosis, kyphosis
Unequal musculature development
Unstable chest wall
Masses
Tenderness
Subcutaneous emphysema
Increased fremitus: increase in vibrations felt, caused by fluid or solid structures in the lung; may be felt when client has pneumonia or tumor of lung
Decreased fremitus: decrease in vibrations felt when extra air is trapped in lung or pleural space; may be noted when the client has emphysema or pneumothorax

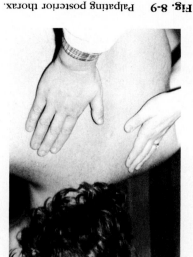

Fig. 8-9 Palpating posterior thorax.

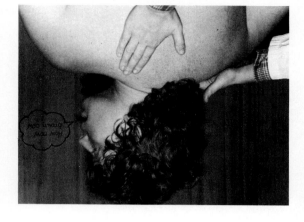

Fig. 8-10 Palpating for fremitus.

ASSESSMENT PROCEDURE	EVALUATION	
	NORMAL FINDINGS	DEVIATIONS FROM NORMAL
4. Palpate lateral chest wall excursion during deep respirations: examiner should place hands on lower posterior chest wall at about tenth rib level; examiner's thumbs should almost touch at spinal process; fingertips should wrap laterally around ribs (Fig. 8-11); instruct client to take several deep breaths; evaluate outward expansion	Bilaterally equal expansion of ribs during deep inspiration; thumbs move equally away from spine Nonpainful breathing No coughing	*Unequal fremitus* Unequal excursion or pain with deep inspiration
5. Percuss posterior chest: instruct client to sit and pull shoulders forward by crossing arms; this technique spreads scapulae and permits more lung area for evaluation (Fig. 8-12) (See "Clinical Tips and Strategies," p. 245, for percussion techniques.)	*Resonance* throughout lung fields Intensity: loud Pitch: low Duration: long Quality: hollow (Fig. 8-13)	*Hyperresonance* found over emphysematous lung Intensity: very loud Pitch: very low Duration: longer Quality: booming

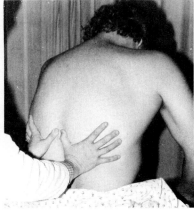

Fig. 8-11   Hand position for measuring respiratory excursion.

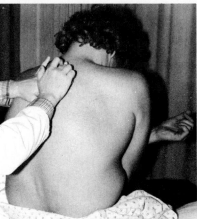

Fig. 8-12   Posture of posterior chest for percussion.

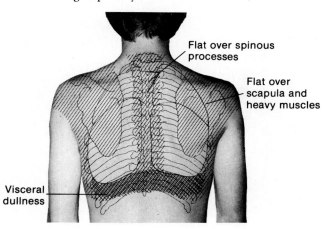

Flat over spinous processes

Flat over scapula and heavy muscles

Visceral dullness

Fig. 8-13   Percussion tones of the posterior chest.

Continued.

CLINICAL GUIDELINES—cont'd

	EVALUATION	
ASSESSMENT PROCEDURE	NORMAL FINDINGS	DEVIATIONS FROM NORMAL
Palpation of posterior chest— cont'd	*Flat sound* over bone or heavy muscle, such as shoulder or scapula, spinal processes Intensity: soft Pitch: high Duration: short Quality: extreme dullness	*Dullness* over lung field occurs when fluid or solid tissue replaces normal lung tissue or fluid in pleural space To identify consolidation, consolidated area must be at least 2 to 3 cm in diameter
6. Percuss down posterior chest, comparing one side with other; avoid percussing over bone surface (Fig. 8-14) a. During percussion, listen and feel for intensity, pitch, duration, and quality of each percussed sound	*Dull sound* over viscera and liver border Intensity: medium Pitch: medium high Duration: medium Quality: thudlike *Tympany sound* over stomach and gas bubble in intestine Intensity: loud Pitch: high Duration: medium Quality: drumlike *Hyperresonant* Intensity: very loud Pitch: very low Duration: longer Quality: booming	
7. Percuss diaphragmatic excursion of posterior lungs; client sits upright and breathes several times, then takes deep breath and holds it	Resonance should be heard first; this tone becomes *dull* at bottom of lungs Indicates level of diaphragm Should occur around tenth rib	Unusually high level may accompany pleural effusion or atelectasis

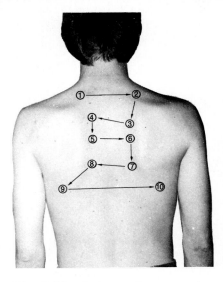

Fig. 8-14 Sequence for systematic percussion of the posterior thorax.

	EVALUATION	
ASSESSMENT PROCEDURE	**NORMAL FINDINGS**	**DEVIATIONS FROM NORMAL**
a. At this time percuss down posterior chest, starting at apex of scapulae	Higher diaphragm level may be present in pregnant women; may also have slightly narrower excursion volume	
b. Percussion continues downward until tone changes; mark that point with marker; then instruct client to breathe several times, exhale completely, and hold breath		
c. Again, percuss down line of apex of scapulae until tone changes; mark that point with marker		
d. Instruct client to breathe again		
8. Repeat procedure on other side of posterior chest	Equal response on both sides	Unequal responses
9. With ruler, measure and record distance between two lines (Fig. 8-15) (The purpose of this technique is to determine client's lung expansion capabilities.)	4 to 6 cm (1½ to 2½ inches) downward excursion	Less than 4 cm (1½ inches) downward excursion
Auscultation of posterior chest		
1. Auscultate posterior chest from apex to base; client should be seated; diaphragm of stethoscope should be used for breath sound auscultation (Fig. 8-16)	Vesicular breath sounds heard over almost all of posterior lung fields Low pitch, soft expirations	Bronchial breath sounds over peripheral lung High pitch, loud expirations

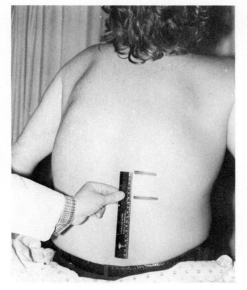

Fig. 8-15 Measurement of respiratory excursion.

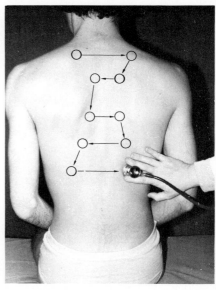

Fig. 8-16 Auscultatory pattern of posterior thorax with stethoscope.

Continued.

CLINICAL GUIDELINES—cont'd

ASSESSMENT PROCEDURE	EVALUATION	
	NORMAL FINDINGS	DEVIATIONS FROM NORMAL
Auscultation of posterior chest—cont'd 2. Instruct client to take slow, deep breaths in and out of mouth during auscultation; demonstrate breathing style for client	Bronchovesicular breath sounds over right upper posterior lung field *Medium pitch, medium expirations*	Bronchovesicular breath sounds over peripheral lung
3. Slowly move stethoscope from one spot to next; compare sounds of one side of posterior chest with other; make sure to remain in one spot long enough to clearly analyze both inspiratory and expiratory sounds (Fig. 8-17)		Adventitious sounds, including rales and fine rales, high-pitched crackling sound, heard toward end of inspiration; indicates inflammation or congestion

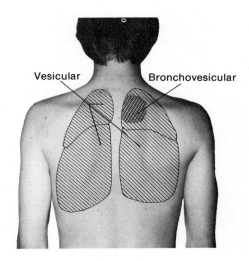

Fig. 8-17   Auscultatory sounds of the posterior chest.

ASSESSMENT PROCEDURE	EVALUATION	
	NORMAL FINDINGS	DEVIATIONS FROM NORMAL
a. If abnormal sound is heard, instruct client to cough, then reexamine to evaluate if adventitious sound has changed or disappeared (Table 8-1)		Medium rales: lower, more moist sound, heard about halfway through inspiration Found in clients with pneumonia or pulmonary edema (not cleared by cough) Coarse rales: loud, bubbly noise, heard during inspiration Found in clients with pneumonia (not cleared by coughing) Rhonchus: small airway noise Sibilant rhonchus (wheeze): musical noise like squeak May occur during inspiration or expiration, but usually louder during expiration

TABLE 8-1   Lung findings in common pathological conditions

CONDITION	PERCUSSION	BREATH SOUNDS	ADVENTITIOUS SOUNDS
Bronchitis	Resonance	Vesicular	Rales and/or rhonchi and/or wheezes, change or clear with cough
Pneumonia	Dull	Bronchial	Rales, do not clear with cough
CHF	Resonance	Vesicular	Rales, sometimes wheezes
Emphysema	Hyperresonance	Bronchovesicular	None or rales, rhonchi, wheezes
Asthma	Resonance or hyperresonance	Bronchial, or bronchovesicular	Rhonchi and wheezes
Atelectasis	Dull	Bronchial or none	None

Continued.

CLINICAL GUIDELINES—cont'd

ASSESSMENT PROCEDURE	EVALUATION	
	NORMAL FINDINGS	DEVIATIONS FROM NORMAL
Auscultation of posterior chest—cont'd		Sonorous rhonchus: low, loud, coarse sound like snore; may occur at any point of inspiration or expiration; usually means obstruction of trachea or large bronchi (coughing may clear sound)
		Pleural friction rub: dry, rubbing, or grating sound usually caused by inflammation of pleural surfaces; heard throughout inspiration and expiration; loudest over lower anterolateral surface; not cleared by cough
4. Evaluate vocal resonance of spoken voice if any abnormalities in tactile fremitus; use one of following techniques:		
a. Bronchophony: use stethoscope (diaphragm) to listen throughout posterior chest as client says "ninety-nine"	Muffled response: "nin-nin"	Sound increased in loudness and clarity: "ninety-nine" Found in consolidation or compression of lung
b. Whispered pectoriloquy: client instructed to whisper "one, two, three"; use stethoscope to listen throughout posterior chest	Muffled sounds: "one, two, three"	Clarity and loudness of sounds: "one, two, three" Found in consolidation or compression of lung
c. Egophony: use stethoscope to listen to posterior chest; ask client to say "e-e-e"	Muffled sound: "e-e-e"	Change in intensity and pitch of sound: "a-a-a" Caused by consolidation
Palpation of anterior chest		
1. Move anterior to client to evaluate anterior thorax and lungs		
2. Use one or two hands to palpate skin and thorax of anterior chest		
3. Evaluate:		
a. Skin texture and temperature, manubrium, suprasternal notch, sternal angle, second rib, body of sternum, costochondral junctions, costal angle, ribs, and chest wall stability	Smooth, warm skin Stable, nontender chest wall and landmarks Well-developed musculature	Dry or moist skin Poor skin turgor Crepitation Thorax deformities Pectus excavatum (funnel chest), characterized by depression defor-

	EVALUATION	
ASSESSMENT PROCEDURE	**NORMAL FINDINGS**	**DEVIATIONS FROM NORMAL**
		mity of lower sternum; may impair breathing or cause compression of heart Pectus carinatum (pigeon chest), characterized by outward deformity of sternum Increase in AP diameter Unequal muscle development, unstable chest wall, masses, tenderness
b. Tracheal position	Midline	Lateral tracheal deviation
4. Use palmar surface of one hand to assess vocal fremitus; examiner should place hand over equal positions of both lung fields of superior anterior chest and the anterolateral chest wall (Avoid areas with heavy breast tissue.)	Varies from person to person because of intensity and pitch of voice Bilaterally equal Mild vibratory sensation Most intense area of vibratory sensation should be upper medial chest area, lateral to sternum	Increased fremitus Decreased fremitus Unequal fremitus
5. Instruct client to repeat "one, two, three" or "how now brown cow"		
Percussion of anterior chest		
1. Instruct client to pull shoulders backward and to sit straight while anterior chest is percussed		
2. Percuss downward, comparing one side with other; avoid percussion over breast tissue or bony surface (Fig. 8-18) (If the examiner has difficulty percussing anterior chest while client is sitting, defer this part of examination until client is lying down.)	Resonance throughout lung fields Flat sounds over sternum or heavy breast tissue Dull sounds over heart or liver Tympany over stomach (Fig. 8-19)	Hyperresonance Dullness over lung field

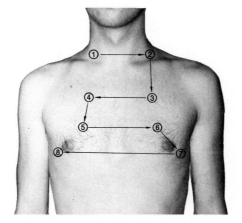

Fig. 8-18   Sequence for systematic percussion of the anterior thorax.

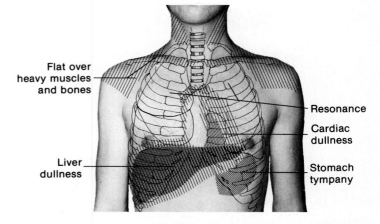

Flat over heavy muscles and bones

Liver dullness

Resonance

Cardiac dullness

Stomach tympany

Fig. 8-19   Percussion tones of the anterior chest.

Continued.

CLINICAL GUIDELINES—cont'd

ASSESSMENT PROCEDURE	EVALUATION	
	NORMAL FINDINGS	DEVIATIONS FROM NORMAL
Auscultation of anterior chest		
1. Auscultate anterior chest from apex to base; client may be sitting or lying; use same techniques as for posterior thorax auscultation	Vesicular breath sounds over anterior peripheral lung fields Bronchial breath sounds over trachea Bronchovesicular breath sounds over large bronchioles (Fig. 8-20)	Bronchial breath sounds over peripheral lung fields Bronchovesicular breath sounds over peripheral lung fields Adventitious sounds, including rales (fine, medium, coarse), rhonchi (sonorous, sibilant), and pleural friction rub
2. Evaluate anterior chest resonance of spoken voice if any abnormalities in tactile fremitus; use same techniques as for posterior chest		
a. Bronchophony: instruct client to say "ninety-nine"; evaluate with stethoscope	Muffled response: "nin-nin"	Sound increased in loudness and clarity: "ninety-nine"
b. Whispered pectoriloquy: instruct client to whisper "one, two, three"; evaluate with stethoscope	Muffled response: "one, two, three"	Clarity and loudness of sounds: "one, two, three"
c. Egophony: instruct client to say "e-e-e"	Muffled response: "e-e-e"	Change in intensity and pitch of sounds: "a-a-a"
Evaluation of lateral thorax and lungs		
1. Instruct client to abduct arm overhead so that lateral chest may be percussed and auscultated (Fig. 8-21)		
2. Percuss down each lateral thorax	Resonance over lung area Dull sound as percussion reaches liver (on right) and spleen (on left)	Hyperresonance or dullness over lung fields
3. Auscultate down each lateral thorax	Vesicular breath sounds	Bronchovesicular or bronchial breath sounds No breath sounds

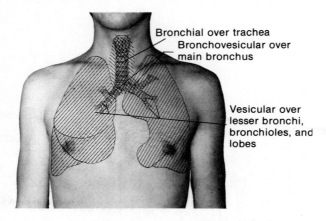

Fig. 8-20 Auscultatory sounds of the anterior chest.

Bronchial over trachea
Bronchovesicular over main bronchus

Vesicular over lesser bronchi, bronchioles, and lobes

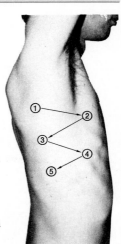

Fig. 8-21 Lateral percussion and auscultation position.

CLINICAL TIPS AND STRATEGIES

- **For evaluation of the thorax and lungs, the client must be undressed:** This means bra or undershirt should be off. During inspection of overall respiratory response, the client should be sitting with the gown dropped to the waist.

- **During inspection first stand back and observe the client:** It has been stated that once the examiner touches the client, the client's observable details are no longer seen. This is an essential concept and deserves foremost consideration. During observation, carefully analyze the client's posture, breathing difficulties, breathing style, audible sounds, and any other factors that reflect the client's breathing attempts. For example, a client with breathing difficulties may lean forward to breathe.

- **Inspection of the front and back is done together:** The other assessment techniques—palpation, percussion, and auscultation—are first done in the back and then in the front (or reverse, if you prefer).

- **When palpating, use both hands simultaneously:** One hand should be placed on the right chest wall and the other on the left chest wall. The purpose is to check symmetry, comparing the findings on one side with those on the other.

- **Abnormalities identified must be described and defined:** This is done by referring to intercostal space and distance from sternum, spine, axillary lines, etc.

- **Techniques of percussion are the same whether one is percussing the thorax, heart, liver, or abdomen:** However, the tones elicited in those areas are different. Percussion tones represent vibrations from 4 to 5 cm deep. As the beginning examiner learns the technique of percussion, considerable practice will be required until the five tones (resonance, hyperresonance, dullness, flatness, and tympany) are easily recognized. Only after the examiner has memorized the tones and their normal location is there hope of identifying abnormal findings. Following is a description of current percussion techniques:

1. Place the left hand flat on the posterior chest wall and slightly spread the fingers. The distal phalanx of the middle (pleximeter) finger should be firmly pressed on the chest wall. The other fingers should very gently rest on the thorax.

2. The middle finger of the right hand becomes the hammer (plexor), which taps the interphalangeal joint of the pleximeter.

3. The success of the technique of percussion depends on several elements, including the following (Fig. 8-22):

a. The downward snap of the plexor *must* be sharp and rapid.

b. The downward snap of the plexor *must* be a wrist action and *not* a forearm or shoulder motion.

c. The *tip* of the plexor finger *must* be used, not the finger pad.

d. Once the plexor has struck the pleximeter, quickly remove the plexor (this ensures pure quality of tone).

e. One location should be tapped several times to ensure clear interpretation of the tone elicited.

f. *Short* fingernails are essential. Otherwise the examiner is more likely to use the finger pad of the plexor and not the fingertip.

g. Loudness of the tone does not ensure good quality; the examiner should practice the percussion techniques until a light percussion tapping elicits an appropriate tone.

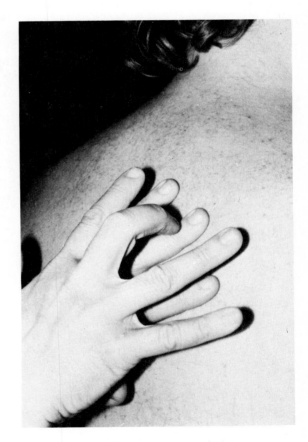

Fig. 8-22   Percussion technique.

- **When percussing the back, it is helpful to have clients sit with shoulders drooping slightly forward:** This pulls the scapulae laterally and allows increased access to the lung field.
- **When percussing the anterior chest wall, have clients sit with shoulders pulled back:** For women with large breasts, percuss the anterosuperior lung fields with the clients sitting, then have them recline to a 45-degree angle with hands up and behind the head. This position allows percussion access to the inferoanterior lung fields (Fig. 8-23).
- **When percussing for excursion on the posterior chest wall, the client should hold his breath:** It is also helpful for the examiner to hold his or her breath.
- **Auscultation requires the use of a stethoscope:** Because there are many different types of stethoscopes, the ability to accurately assess auscultatory sounds depends partially on the quality of the instrument. Following are characteristics of good stethoscopes and auscultatory techniques:
  1. Characteristics of high-quality stethoscopes:
     a. Use a diaphragm that will pick up high-pitched (breath) sounds and a bell that will pick up low-pitched sounds (heart murmurs).
     b. The diaphragm and bell should have enough weight to lay firmly on the chest wall when placed there.
     c. The diaphragm should be covered with a factory manufactured diaphragm cover, not a piece of x-ray film.
     d. The bell should have a small rubber or plastic ring around its tip to ensure a secure fit against the chest wall.
     e. The tubing may be in one or two pieces. The human ear cannot detect sound differences between one-tubing and two-tubing stethoscopes. Thick, stiff, and heavy tubing conducts sound better than thin, elastic or very flexible tubing. Do not use tubing intended for other uses in the hospital.
     f. Earpieces can make the difference between hearing or not hearing a sound. The examiner should choose the largest earpieces that will snugly fit into the ears. The ability of the earpieces to occlude outside noise is the important consideration.
  2. Auscultatory techniques:
     a. The earpieces should point toward the exam-

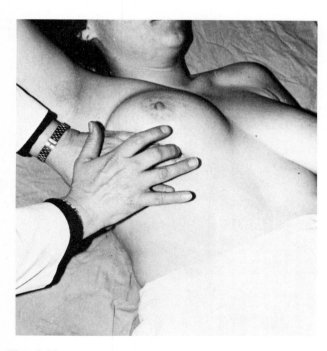

Fig. 8-23 Anterior thorax percussion technique for a large-breasted woman.

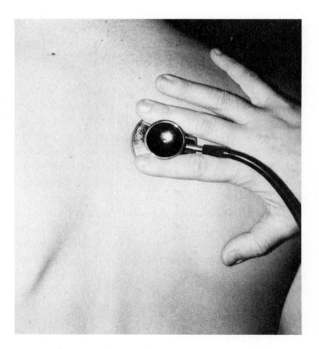

Fig. 8-24 Proper technique for holding the stethoscope.

iner's nose to snugly fit in the auditory canal.

b. The examiner should try not to touch or allow the tubing to touch rubbing surfaces during auscultation; this will cause extra noise.

c. The examiner should hold the head of the stethoscope between the index and middle fingers to stabilize it during auscultation (Fig. 8-24).

d. When using the diaphragm, exert firm pressure to ensure solid contact with the chest wall.

e. In using the bell, care must be taken not to flatten the underlying skin by pressing the bell too firmly. The bell must be lightly and evenly placed on the skin. There must be total skin contact around the bell edge. The bell functions by picking up vibratory sensations of the surface tissue in response to the visceral vibrations. If the tissue is stretched too much by firm pressure, vibrations are inhibited and the bell actually converts to a diaphragm.

- Before auscultating the breath sounds, it is appropriate to give instruction on how to breathe. The client should breathe deeply and slowly through the mouth. Stand in front and demonstrate. Nasal breathing is not encouraged because nasal turbulence interferes with clear auscultation of the thorax.

- When auscultating the posterior chest, again have the client sit with shoulders drooping slightly forward. When listening for breath sounds, move from apices to bases. Compare one side with the other as you move down the posterior wall. Avoid auscultation over bone. Be sure to listen to each spot for at least two inspirations and expirations. This will ensure a clearer interpretation of the sound heard.

- During auscultation of the anterior chest, the client should be sitting straight. Auscultation is begun above the clavicle and should again move down the chest wall while one side is compared with the other. For large-breasted women the breasts can be displaced upward and laterally for access to the lower anterior lung fields.

- When auscultating the chest, evaluate the quality of breath sound, compare inspiration length with expiration length, and listen for any abnormalities. Describe what you hear.

- If you hear adventitious sounds on auscultation, instruct the client to cough. See if the sounds are cleared by a cough.

- Do not forget to palpate, percuss, and auscultate the lateral chest walls. Compare one side with the other.

SAMPLE RECORDING: NORMAL FINDINGS

Respiration rate 14; regular rhythm without noted difficulty.

Diaphragmatic breathing.

Bilaterally equal excursion.

Client sitting erect, slight kyphosis noted.

Skin intact and warm; no bulging, retractions, tenderness, or asymmetry of chest wall noted.

Thorax oval; AP diameter < lateral diameter.

Tactile fremitus bilaterally equal.

Diaphragmatic excursion 4 cm (1½ inches) bilaterally.

Resonant percussion tone throughout.

Vesicular breath sounds bilaterally throughout.

Few fine basilar rales heard on right, which did not clear with cough.

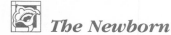 *The Newborn*

HISTORY AND CLINICAL STRATEGIES

- Newborn infants have irregular respiratory rates. A Cheyne-Stokes pattern may be observed until about 1 month of age. Respirations should be counted for an entire minute.
- The examination of the newborn's chest and lungs includes the assessment of soft and bony tissues and structures. Infants use their diaphragms for breathing. They are nose breathers except when crying.

- Environmental temperature should be noted and controlled, since cold and heat stress may result in apnea or tachypnea. Newborns are especially prone to cold stress, which may be reflected by their respiratory status.
- Abnormalities must be assessed and managed as needed. Asymmetry, "see-saw" breathing, any retractions, chest lag, nasal flaring (dilation), or expiratory grunting suggests respiratory problems. An infant breathing around 60 times per minute or more, except when crying, needs further evaluation.

CLINICAL VARIATIONS: THE NEWBORN

CHARACTERISTIC OR AREA EXAMINED	NORMAL FINDINGS	DEVIATIONS FROM NORMAL
1. Thoracic cage	Chest circumference over nipples about 30-36 cm (2 cm smaller than head) Thorax is cylindrical, round, symmetrical	Asymmetry (may be respiratory problem) Malformed chest: pectus carinatum (pigeon chest); pectus excavatum (funnel chest) Chest wall thrill movement (suggests heart murmur)
2. Bony structures	Clavicles intact, smooth, even Ribs and sternum symmetrical Hard, sharp, palpable xiphoid cartilage	Asymmetry, limited movement, lump (may be fracture) Masses, crepitance (may be pulmonary problem) Intercostal or xiphoid retractions (suggest respiratory problems; note any nasal flaring or grunting)
3. Lungs	Bilateral, irregular breath sounds, about 30-50 resp/min Infants born by cesarean section may have transient increased mucus and varied respiratory rates	Diminished breath sounds, apneic, tachypnea, labored or asynchronous breathing; asymmetric expansion (suggests diaphragmatic hernia or pneumothorax) Note any color changes (cyanotic) Audible bowel sounds in chest area (diaphragmatic hernia)
4. Crying	Spontaneous cry; higher pitch with pain Face may turn darker when crying and holding breath	Shrill, high-pitched cry (may be nervous system problem, drug withdrawal) Cri du chat cry (cat-type) (suggests chromosomal disorder) Dusky color, unless crying (may be nasal obstruction)

The Child

HISTORY AND CLINICAL STRATEGIES

- Because many childhood illnesses frequently involve the respiratory system, the thorax and respiratory function of children deserve thorough evaluation.
- The techniques of pediatric evaluation are the same as for the adult. The results of assessment will depend on cooperation from the child and the examiner's ability to gently assess the child.
- Coughs and colds seem to accompany the growing child. History data should be gathered about the same elements as discussed for the adult client. An allergic history should also be gathered. If the child is less than 2 years of age and is beginning to eat new foods, the examiner should gather a thorough nutritional history as well.
- Children with asthma or bronchitis histories should be questioned with regard to the overall progression of that condition. Data should be gathered regarding:
  1. Frequency and duration of the problem
  2. Current care techniques
  3. Precipitating factors
  4. Current medications
  5. Relationship of problem to activities and playing
  6. How child views the problem
  7. What child thinks is possible in terms of self-help
- Any child with a sudden onset of coughing or choking should be expected to have aspirated a foreign object until proved otherwise. The examiner should inquire about the child's playing activities before the current problem (e.g., was he playing with *toys* such as beads, a car with removable wheels, or pieces of a game that could have been put into his mouth). Great skill must be employed to gather the information needed without the child becoming frightened and answering "no" to every question asked.

  Food aspiration is another cause for sudden coughing or breathing problems. Commonly aspirated objects are peanuts, popcorn, carrot pieces, hot dogs, and peas. All these tend to block and not dissolve if accidentally aspirated. Although it is difficult to determine, some parents may admit that they were force feeding a child before the coughing episode or that the child had food and was playing or running around the house before the coughing period.
- The respiratory rate of children is obviously faster than that of the adult. Sometimes the parent may bring the child for evaluation because "he is breathing funny." If this occurs, the examiner must collect a detailed history, including a thorough evaluation of the possibility of poisoning or ingestion of a toxic substance.

Many times salicylate poisoning presents a child with rapid, panting respirations.

- For examination the child should be naked to the waist and sitting on the parent's lap or the examining table. Infants are laid on the examination table.
- The child must be breathing quietly for breath sounds to be evaluated. As soon as the child is old enough to cooperate, he should be instructed to breathe deeply through his mouth. One technique to facilitate this is to instruct the child to take a deep breath and "blow out" the examiner's penlight or otoscope (Fig. 8-25) while the examiner listens to the child's chest with the stethoscope in the other hand.
- There has been much written about stridor and retraction evaluation in children. We want to stress that the emphasis of this text is the clinical assessment of "normal" for both children and adults. If the examiner identifies retractions, wheezing, stridor, or persistent coughing, the child should be referred to a physician for further evaluation.

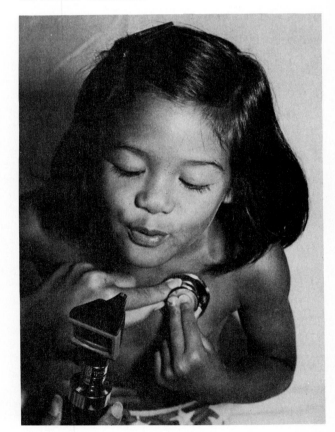

Fig. 8-25 Auscultating the lungs while child "blows out" otoscope light. (From Whaley LF, Wong DL: *Nursing care of infants and children,* ed 3, St Louis, 1987, Mosby–Year Book.)

CLINICAL VARIATIONS: THE CHILD

CHARACTERISTIC OR AREA EXAMINED	NORMAL FINDINGS	DEVIATIONS FROM NORMAL
1. Anterior and posterior chest		
a. Skin color, thorax, and lips	Pink, well oxygenated Infants' skin may become mottled if they are chilled	Cyanosis, pallor Spider nevi Dilated veins over lower thorax
b. Nail beds, nail configuration	Smooth Flat surface	Clubbing of nails and distal fingers
c. General appearance	Relaxed posture	Apprehensive Tense forward posture Restless Flaring nostrils Supraclavicular retractions Intercostal retractions Use of accessory muscles during breathing
d. Chest wall configuration	Symmetrical Equal muscular development	Asymmetry Asymmetry
e. AP diameter of chest	By age 6 years AP and lateral diameter ratio should approach adult normal of 1:2 or 5:7	Children with rounded rib cage after age 6 years (may be found in children with cystic fibrosis or asthma)
f. Chest wall configuration (1) Anterior	Symmetrical Flat sternum 45° costal angle Harrison groove may be normally found in some children: horizontal groove at level of diaphragm; with breathing there may be slight flaring below groove Bilaterally equal musculature Shoulders equal Clavicles equal	Pectus carinatum (pigeon chest) Pectus excavatum (funnel chest) Costal angle larger than 45° or 50° Harrison groove, with marked flaring below groove, should be considered abnormal Asymmetry Asymmetry Asymmetry
(2) Posterior	Straight spinal processes (C7, T1 through T12) Symmetrical scapulae Downward and equal slope of ribs	Spinal curvature Scoliosis Kyphosis (humpback) Asymmetry
2. Breathing pattern	Abdominal and nasal breathing during infancy Gradual change until age 6 or 7 years; then girls become mostly thoracic breathers and boys become abdominal breathers	Seesaw breathing where thorax and abdomen alternate during breathing Respiratory grunting Abnormal, irregular breathing pattern Cheyne-Stokes
3. Rate of respiration	Ratio of respirations to pulse 1:4 Newborn: 30 to 50 resp/min 6 months: 20 to 40 resp/min 1 year: 20 to 40 resp/min 3 years: 20 to 30 resp/min 6 years: 16 to 22 resp/min 10 years: 16 to 20 resp/min 17 years: 14 to 20 resp/min	Any respiration rates that fall short of or exceed stated normal rates

CHARACTERISTIC OR AREA EXAMINED	NORMAL FINDINGS	DEVIATIONS FROM NORMAL
4. Depth of respirations (This is an important quality to evaluate in children.)	Respiratory depth guide to be used when child is lying supine: examiner takes hand and holds it in front of child's nose; breathing normally felt at following distances*: Child's age — Depth of respiration 1 month — 2 inches 3 months — 3 inches 6 to 12 months — 4 inches 2 years — 6 inches 3 to 4 years — 8 inches 5 to 6 years — 9 inches 8 to 10 years — 10 inches	Breathing may become deeper and labored in cases of metabolic acidosis, such as Kussmaul respirations Breathing becomes labored during metabolic alkalosis as body conserves carbon dioxide Decreased depth could also be evidence of airway obstruction
5. Posterior chest palpation (may need to use one or two fingers instead of all fingers) a. Skin	Smooth, warm	Dry or moist skin Poor skin turgor
b. Bone, muscle structure	Symmetrical, straight spine, nontender	
c. Chest wall stability	Stable ribs, nontender	
6. Vocal fremitus: instruct child to speak as adult was instructed or evaluate when child is crying	Varies from person to person because of intensity and pitch of voice Bilaterally equal mild vibratory sensation Most intense area to feel vibration is upper posterior chest wall medial to scapulae	*Increased fremitus,* or increased vibratory sensation, as seen in pneumonia or consolidation of lung *Decreased fremitus,* or decreased vibratory sensation, when there is decreased production of sound (air blockage) or increase in space vibration must pass through before it reaches skin surface
7. Lateral chest wall excursion	Bilaterally equal expansion of ribs during deep inspiration; thumbs move equally away from spine Nonpainful breathing No coughing	Unequal excursion or pain with deep inspiration
8. Posterior chest wall percussion: requires lighter pressure than adult technique a. "Direct" single finger tapping percussion may elicit clearer tone in very small child	More resonant than adult Some children may display hyperresonant tone Older children: *resonance* Flat sound over bone or heavy muscle Dull sound over viscera or liver	Hyperresonant in older child Dullness over lung field
9. Diaphragmatic excursion: not routinely done in small child; when done in older child, use same technique as for adult	Resonance should be heard first; changes to a *dull* tone at bottom of lungs Indicates level of diaphragm Should occur around tenth rib Amount of downward excursion will depend on size of child	Unusually high diaphragmatic excursion level may be present in children with pleural effusion or atelectasis

*From Barness LA: Manual of pediatric physical diagnosis, *ed 5, Chicago, 1980, Mosby—Year Book.*

Continued.

CLINICAL VARIATIONS: THE CHILD—cont'd

CHARACTERISTIC OR AREA EXAMINED	NORMAL FINDINGS	DEVIATIONS FROM NORMAL
10. Posterior chest auscultation: use either *small* diaphragm or *small* rubber-edged bell stethoscope; all edges of either must have "good" contact with child's chest wall; use same technique as for adult	Louder than adult Bronchovesicular breath sounds normally heard in infant and small child because of thin chest wall with poorly developed musculature Vesicular breath sounds like adult's as child grows older	Bronchial breath sounds Bronchovesicular breath sounds in older child (over age 6 or 7 years) Adventitious sounds, such as fine rales, medium rales, coarse rales, sibilant rhonchi, sonorous rhonchi, and pleural friction rub
11. Vocal resonance: not routinely evaluated in children; when evaluation is desired, use same technique as for adult		
12. Anterior chest palpation		
a. Skin	Smooth warm skin	Dry or moist skin Poor skin turgor Cold or hot skin
b. Bone, muscle structure		Crepitation
c. Chest wall stability	Stable, nontender chest wall and landmarks Well-developed musculature	Thorax deformities: pectus excavatum (funnel chest) characterized by depression deformity of lower sternum; may impair breathing or cause compression of heart Pectus carinatum (pigeon chest) characterized by outward deformity of sternum
d. Tracheal position	Midline	Lateral tracheal deviation
13. Vocal fremitus palpation	Varies from person to person because of intensity and pitch of voice Bilaterally equal Mild vibratory sensation Most intense area of vibratory sensation should be upper medial chest area, lateral to sternum	Increased fremitus Decreased fremitus Unequal fremitus
14. Anterior chest percussion: may use direct or indirect palpation technique	More resonant than in adult; some small children may demonstrate hyperresonant tone Dull sound over heart and liver; liver starts at approximately fifth interspace on right at midclavicular line Tympany over stomach	Hyperresonance in older children or dullness over lung fields
15. Anterior chest auscultation	Bronchovesicular breath sounds normally heard throughout peripheral lungs of smaller child Vesicular breath sounds throughout peripheral lungs of older child Bronchial breath sounds heard over trachea Bronchovesicular breath sounds heard over large bronchioles	Bronchial breath sounds over peripheral lung Bronchovesicular breath sounds over peripheral lung fields in older child Adventitious sounds, such as fine, medium, and coarse rales, sibilant and sonorous rhonchi, and pleural friction rub

CHARACTERISTIC OR AREA EXAMINED	NORMAL FINDINGS	DEVIATIONS FROM NORMAL
16. Vocal resonance of anterior chest (not normally evaluated in children); when evaluation is desired, use same techniques as for adult		
17. Lateral thorax and lungs	Resonance over lung area Dull sound as percussion reaches liver (on right) and spleen (on left) Vesicular breath sounds	Hyperresonance or dullness over lung fields Bronchovesicular breath sounds No breath sounds

The Childbearing Woman

HISTORY AND CLINICAL STRATEGIES

- Pregnant women may notice an increased respiratory rate with shortness of breath. Women with nasal stuffiness may have more difficulty breathing. Education about usual respiratory physiology of pregnancy may help alleviate anxiety associated with dyspnea.

- Women with a history of asthma, tuberculosis, or respiratory tract infections require ongoing assessment and management. During pregnancy there is an increase in tidal volume, respiratory rate, plasma pH and PO_2. There is a decrease in residual volume, plasma PCO_2, and expiratory reserve.

CLINICAL VARIATIONS: THE CHILDBEARING WOMAN

CHARACTERISTIC OR AREA EXAMINED	NORMAL FINDINGS	DEVIATIONS FROM NORMAL
1. Characteristics	Shortness of breath from upward diaphragm and pressure on lungs from enlarged uterus Breathing more thoracic than abdominal Thoracic cage widens, costal angle increases from 68° to 103° Diminished diaphragmatic excursion Increased respiratory tract vascularity Increased breathing rate 15% for oxygenation and compensation for structural changes (stimulated by progesterone) Breathing more difficult until fetus moves into pelvis (lightening)	Chest wall pain, air hunger, tachypnea, apprehension (pulmonary embolism may occur from venous thrombosis)
2. After delivery	Chest wall may not return to prepregnant state; thoracic cage may remain wider Respiratory characteristics return to prepregnant state	

The Older Adult

HISTORY AND CLINICAL STRATEGIES

- The examiner should not assume that aging is automatically accompanied by respiratory disease. The literature reports that physical changes occur with aging; however, the "normal," healthy elderly individual is usually free of chronic respiratory symptoms. Many of the changes that occur may not be clinically remarkable or may not alter or interfere with the client's lifestyle. Following are some major changes that occur:
  1. Decrease in muscular strength of the chest wall muscles
  2. Possible stiffening and decreased expansion of chest wall (calcification at the rib articulation points may be involved)
  3. Decrease in vital capacity and increase in residual volume
  4. Decrease in elastic lung recoil and increased lung distensibility; alveoli and bronchioles stretched (enlarged)
  5. Loss of some of the interalveolar septa (folds), resulting in a decrease in alveolar surface available for gas exchange
  6. Underventilation of the alveoli in the lower lung fields
  7. Increase in the mucus production cells in the bronchioles

     As with all other changes, these alterations take place at different rates with different individuals. Physical conditioning and general physical health are two very important variables that affect the efficiency of respiratory function. Obese, sedentary, or immobilized individuals have less opportunity to maintain physical fitness and are more vulnerable to respiratory disability.

     In summary, it often takes more energy for the older individual to expand the chest wall to carry through the function of respiration. Many elderly clients do not experience dyspnea unless they exceed the ordinary mild to moderate exertion demands that they are accustomed to. Sudden intense activity can result in shortness of breath. Heavy or unusually demanding exercise can create problems. With aging changes a diminished functional reserve occurs, creating a higher vulnerability to respiratory distress or infection. Elderly people should be cautious about exposure to colds, flu, or other infections.

- The symptoms of cough, dyspnea on exertion, and breathlessness were covered on pp. 231-232.
- Chest pain may be diminished in an older client. Pleuritic pain may not be reported or sensed as intensely as it would be in a younger person. If chest pain does exist, be certain to examine the client for fractured ribs (sustained from a fall or coughing), as well as arthritic changes in the rib cage.
- The examiner should inquire about the effects of weather on the client. Some people have an increase in respiratory infections in cold, damp weather.
- Ask about the incidence of colds and flu and whether the number and/or severity of the episodes has been increasing.
- The incidence of chronic respiratory disease is higher among the elderly population. Chronic bronchitis, emphysema, lung cancer, and tuberculosis are four of the major health problems. (Pulmonary edema associated with heart disease is covered in Chapter 9.) In addition to cough, dyspnea on exertion, chest pain, and breathlessness, chronic health problems can include:
  1. History of smoking (see p. 232 for specific questions)
  2. Periodic bouts of low-grade fever
  3. Night sweats
  4. Remarkable weight change in last 6 to 12 months
  5. New problems with fatigue
  6. Any sensations in the chest other than pain (e.g., feeling of heaviness)
  7. Family history of any respiratory problems
  8. Daily activities altered or decreased because of problems with fatigue, shortness of breath, or discomfort
- *Note:* It may be difficult for some clients to breathe deeply or to hold breath on command during the physical assessment.

RISK FACTORS FOR RESPIRATORY DISABILITY WITH ELDERLY INDIVIDUALS

- History of smoking
- History of frequent respiratory infections
- Immobilization or marked sedentary habits
- History of chronic exposure to environmental pollutants
- Difficulty swallowing
- Indication of weakened chest muscles (e.g., general physical disability, inability to cough or breathe deeply)
- Evidence of spinal structural deformity (e.g., scoliosis, kyphosis)
- Family history of respiratory disability

CLINICAL VARIATIONS: THE OLDER ADULT

CHARACTERISTIC OR AREA EXAMINED	NORMAL FINDINGS	DEVIATIONS FROM NORMAL
1. Anterior and posterior chest a. Color of skin, lips, and nail beds	Pink, well oxygenated Dark-skinned clients' mucous membranes and nail beds appear pink and well oxygenated	Cyanosis, pallor Spider nevi
b. Nail configuration	106° angle at nail bed	Clubbing (angle disappears)
c. General appearance	Relaxed posture (Note elderly client's general condition of physical fitness: muscle weakness associated with general physical disability or sedentary life-style may affect client's ability to use respiratory muscles and to expand the chest.)	Apprehensive Tense, forward posture Restless Nostrils flaring Supraclavicular retractions Intercostal retractions Use of accessory muscles during breathing (*Note:* Pursed-lip breathing—chiefly expiration—is compensatory pattern associated with chronic obstructive pulmonary disease.)
d. Chest wall configuration	Symmetrical landmarks Downward and equal slope of ribs Bilaterally equal muscular development (may be slightly more muscle development on client's dominant side) Subcutaneous fat is often decreased, and bony prominences are more marked Costal angle less than 90° (*Note:* Kyphosis [Fig. 8-26, next page] is a fairly common problem with elderly clients. Dorsal scoliosis may exist, accompanied by tracheal deviation. Loss of normal spinal curvature in the dorsal and lumbar regions may occur with arthritis.)	Asymmetry of landmarks Horizontal ribs Costal angle greater than 90° (*Note:* Chronic marked stooping or bending forward may diminish lung expansion in localized areas.)
e. Anteroposterior diameter of chest in relation to lateral diameter	1:2 to 5:7 ratio Kyphosis is often accompanied by increased anteroposterior diameter	Barrel chest (see Fig. 8-8)
2. Breathing pattern	Client is able to close mouth and breathe through nose Diaphragmatic (male) Thoracic (female)	Mouth breathing

Continued.

CLINICAL VARIATIONS: THE OLDER ADULT—cont'd

CHARACTERISTIC OR AREA EXAMINED	NORMAL FINDINGS	DEVIATIONS FROM NORMAL
3. Rate of respiration	Quiet, smooth, even breathing, relatively passive in nature During inspiration chest expands, costal angle increases, and diaphragm descends and flattens (*Note:* With elderly clients the vital capacity is reduced, and general chest expansion may be somewhat reduced. Calcification at rib articulation points may contribute to decreased chest expansion. These alterations may not be clinically evident.) 12 to 20 respirations per minute (*Note:* Anxiety or exertion will increase rate.)	Noisy breathing Breathing appears labored or painful; accompanied by grunting noises; inspiration interrupted by pain Irregular breathing patterns, such as Cheyne-Stokes: periods of deep, rapid breaths alternating with periods of apnea Obstructive breathing pattern: expiration period prolonged and labored; may alternate with periods of shallow breathing Hyperpnea: increase in rate and depth Tachypnea: increased and relatively shallow respirations Bradypnea: decrease in rate Many heavy sighing respirations may occur in depressed or disturbed emotional states

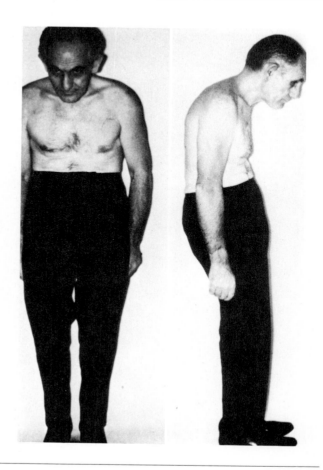

Fig. 8-26 Kyphosis. (*Note:* Increased thoracic curvature is accompanied by loss of normal lumbar curvature.) (From Prior JA, Silberstein JS, Stang JM: *Physical diagnosis: the history and examination of the patient,* ed 6, St Louis, 1981, Mosby–Year Book.)

CHARACTERISTIC OR AREA EXAMINED	NORMAL FINDINGS	DEVIATIONS FROM NORMAL
		(*Note:* Some elderly clients with a chronic respiratory disturbance may present a general uncoordinated breathing pattern, varying in rate, depth, and chest expansion. The exertion of moving from chair to examining table, undressing, or sitting up from a lying position may disrupt a breathing pattern. Monitor the client's response to mild exertion.)
4. Posterior chest palpation a. General surface characteristics	Skin feels warm, smooth (*Note:* Elderly clients chill easily in a cool environment.)	Excessively dry or moist skin Poor skin turgor Cold or hot skin Crepitation
b. C7 through T12 spinal processes	May be quite prominent Kyphosis may be present Spine straight, nontender	Curved spine, tender on palpation
c. Scapulae and surrounding musculature	Symmetrical location	Asymmetry Asymmetrical muscle atrophy
d. General chest wall	Stable ribs, nontender	Tenderness Masses Crepitation
5. Respiratory excursion	Bilaterally equal expansion of ribs during inspiration (thumbs move equally away from the spine) (*Note:* Elderly client may have some difficulty breathing as deeply as a younger individual.)	Unequal excursion
6. Vocal fremitus response	Response varies among individuals because of intensity and pitch of voice Bilaterally equal mild vibratory sensation Most intense vibrations at upper posterior chest wall medial to scapulae	Increased fremitus: increased vibratory sense accompanies consolidation of lung or portion of lung Decreased fremitus: occurs with decreased production of sound (air blockage) or increase in air space or muscle/tissue space between client's lung and examiner's hands (e.g., emphysema)
7. Entire posterior chest percussion	Resonance throughout lung fields	Hyperresonance found over emphysematous lung
a. Intensity	Moderately loud	Very loud
b. Pitch	Low	Very low pitch
c. Duration	Long	Longer
d. Quality	Hollow (*Note:* Some elderly clients manifest an increased distensibility of lungs and may respond with normal hyperresonance on percussion. However, all beginning examiners should refer hyperresonant responses to a physician.)	Booming Dullness over lung: occurs when fluid or solid tissue replaces normal lung tissue or when fluid is in the pleural space To identify consolidation, consolidated area must be at least 2 to 3 cm in diameter

Continued.

CLINICAL VARIATIONS: THE OLDER ADULT—cont'd

CHARACTERISTIC OR AREA EXAMINED	NORMAL FINDINGS	DEVIATIONS FROM NORMAL
8. Diaphragmatic excursion percussion	Diaphragmatic dullness to percussion usually occurs at about tenth rib; level may be slightly higher on right Downward excursion (bilateral) should measure approximately 3 to 5 cm (1 to 2 inches), depending on size, age, and general physical condition of client	Asymmetrical response Diaphragm lower than usual in severe emphysema Diaphragm higher than usual if there is increase (of any form) of intraabdominal pressure Severe limited excursion of diaphragm

9. Posterior chest auscultation (*Note:* Elderly client may have difficulty breathing deeply and holding breath on command.)	Vesicular breath sounds heard over almost all of posterior lung fields
	Bronchovesicular breath sounds over right upper posterior lung field
		Bronchial breath sounds over peripheral lung
		Bronchovesicular breath sounds over peripheral lung
		Adventitious sounds, including:
		Rales: discrete, noncontinuous sounds produced by secretions in tracheobronchial tree, usually heard in inspiration
		  Fine rales: high-pitched crackling noise heard toward end of inspiration; sound originates in alveoli
		  Medium: lower, more moist sound, occurring earlier in inspiration and originating in bronchioles and small bronchi
		  Coarse: loud, bubbling sound occurring in larger air passages; can sometimes be cleared with cough
		Rhonchi (wheezes): continuous sounds produced in narrowed air passages may be more prominent on expiration
		Sibilant: high-pitched musical sound occurring on inspiration or expiration, originating in smaller air passages
		Sonorous: low, loud, coarse sound originating in trachea or large bronchi; coughing may alter sound
		Pleural friction rub: dry, rubbing or grating sound usually caused by inflammation of pleural surfaces

10. Vocal resonance bronchophony: client instructed to say "ninety-nine"	Auscultation sounds muffled: "nin-nin"	Sound increased in loudness and clarity: "ninety-nine"

CHARACTERISTIC OR AREA EXAMINED	NORMAL FINDINGS	DEVIATIONS FROM NORMAL

11. Anterior chest palpation:
   a. Skin texture and temperature, manubrium, suprasternal notch, sternal angle, second rib, body of sternum, costochondral junctions, costal angle, ribs, and chest wall stability
	Smooth, warm skin
	Stable, nontender chest wall and landmarks
	Symmetrical musculature
	Decreased subcutaneous fat
		Dry or moist skin
		Poor skin turgor
		Cold or hot skin
		Crepitation
		Thorax deformities:
		   Pectus excavatum (funnel chest): characterized by depression deformity of lower sternum; may impair breathing or cause compression of heart
		   Pectus carinatum (pigeon chest): characterized by outward deformity of sternum; increase in AP diameter
		Unequal muscle development, unstable chest wall, masses
		Tenderness on palpation (fairly common with arthritic clients at rib articulation points)

b. Tracheal position	Midline (position may be altered in scoliosis)	Lateral tracheal deviation
12. Vocal fremitus response	Varies from person to person because of intensity and pitch of voice Bilaterally equal mild vibratory sensation Most intense area of vibratory sensation is upper medial chest area, lateral to sternum	Increased fremitus Decreased fremitus Unequal fremitus
13. Anterior chest percussion	Resonance throughout lung fields Flat sounds over sternum or heavy breast tissue Dull sounds over heart or liver Tympany over stomach	Hyperresonance Dullness over lung field
14. Anterior chest auscultation	Vesicular breath sounds over anterior peripheral lung fields Bronchial breath sounds over trachea Bronchovesicular breath sounds over large bronchioles	Bronchial breath sounds over peripheral lung fields Bronchovesicular breath sounds over peripheral lung fields Adventitious sounds, such as rales (fine, medium, coarse), rhonchi (sonorous, sibilant), and pleural friction rub
15. Anterior chest vocal resonance a. Bronchophony	Muffled response: "nin-nin"	Sound increased in loudness and clarity: "ninety-nine"
16. Lateral thorax percussion	Resonance over lung area Dull sound as percussion reaches liver (on right) and spleen (on left)	Hyperresonance or dullness over lung fields
17. Lateral thorax auscultation	Vesicular breath sounds	Bronchovesicular breath sounds No breath sounds

Study Questions

General

Mark each statement as either "T" for true or "F" for false.

1. _____ The right lung comprises two lobes, and the left lung comprises three lobes.

2. _____ During inspiration the diaphragm descends and flattens.

3. _____ Biot breathing may be seen in healthy persons.

4. _____ The ratio of respiratory rate to pulse rate normally is 1:6

5. _____ The nipple line is the common landmark for identifying the midclavicular line for all patients, with the exception of large-breasted women.

6. _____ In palpating for rib identification, the initial rib felt below the clavicle is the first rib.

7. The trachea bifurcates at about the level of the:
   - ☐ a. Cricoid cartilage
   - ☐ b. Manubrium
   - ☐ c. Costal angle
   - ☐ d. Sternal angle
   - ☐ e. Sternum

8. Tactile fremitus will be *decreased* with:
   - ☐ a. Pneumonia (consolidation of lung)
   - ☐ b. Chronic obstructive diseases
   - ☐ c. Area of atelectasis
   - ☐ d. Pneumothorax
   - ☐ e. Large airway obstruction
   - ☐ f. All of the above
   - ☐ g. All except e
   - ☐ h. a, c, and d
   - ☐ i. All except b
   - ☐ j. All except a

9. A client with increased density of the lung caused by pneumonia would be expected to have the following lung percussion tones:
   - ☐ a. Resonance
   - ☐ b. Hyperresonance
   - ☐ c. Tympany
   - ☐ d. Dullness
   - ☐ e. Flatness

10. Bronchial breath sounds are normal when heard:
    - ☐ a. Over the posterior lateral chest at the level of the scapulae
    - ☐ b. Between the scapulae
    - ☐ c. Over the trachea
    - ☐ d. In the anterior chest upper lateral areas
    - ☐ e. Nowhere throughout the chest

The Newborn

11. A newborn's chest circumference is approximately:
    - ☐ a. 2 cm smaller than the head
    - ☐ b. 2 cm larger than the head
    - ☐ c. 4 cm larger than the head
    - ☐ d. the same size as the head

12. A newborn's respirations are usually about:
    - ☐ a. 15 to 30 per minute
    - ☐ b. 30 to 50 per minute
    - ☐ c. 50 to 70 per minute
    - ☐ d. 70 to 85 per minute

The Child

13. When examining a 6-month-old child, the nurse must evaluate respiratory rate and depth, as well as breath sound and percussion quality. Which of the following would indicate a *normal* response:

		Respiration rate	Expiratory distance	Breath sound	Percussion tone
☐	a.	52	3 inches	Vesicular	Hyperresonant
☐	b.	18	2 inches	Bronchovesicular	Resonant
☐	c.	22	5 inches	Vesicular	Hyperresonant
☐	d.	32	4 inches	Bronchovesicular	Hyperresonant
☐	e.	36	6 inches	Bronchovesicular	Resonant

The Childbearing Woman

14. Respiratory changes during pregnancy include:
    - ☐ a. Decreased respiratory tract vascularity
    - ☐ b. Increased diaphragmatic excursion
    - ☐ c. Decreased breathing rate by 15%
    - ☐ d. More thoracic than abdominal breathing

15. During pregnancy, the thoracic cage:
    - ☐ a. Remains unchanged
    - ☐ b. Lengthens
    - ☐ c. Shortens
    - ☐ d. Widens

The Older Adult

16. The aging process of the lungs usually involves:
    - ☐ a. Decreased residual volume
    - ☐ b. Decreased vital capacity
    - ☐ c. Decreased chest wall compliance
    - ☐ d. Decreased force of elastic recoil of the lungs
    - ☐ e. Decreased anteroposterior chest diameter
    - ☐ f. All of the above
    - ☐ g. a, c, and e
    - ☐ h. a and d
    - ☐ i. b, c, and d
    - ☐ j. None of the above

17. Some of the risk factors for respiratory disability in elderly people include:
    - ☐ a. Smoking
    - ☐ b. Difficulty swallowing
    - ☐ c. History of frequent respiratory infections
    - ☐ d. Immobility
    - ☐ e. Decreased physical fitness
    - ☐ f. All of the above
    - ☐ g. All except b
    - ☐ h. a, c, and e
    - ☐ i. a and d

18. In the older adult total lung capacity:
    - ☐ a. Is markedly diminished by 80 years of age
    - ☐ b. Increases significantly
    - ☐ c. Does not change significantly

SUGGESTED READINGS
General

Appenheimer L: The thoracic patient, *AORN J* 40(5):732, 1984.

Bates B: *A guide to physical examination,* ed 4, Philadelphia, 1987, JB Lippincott.

DeGowin E, DeGowin R: *Bedside diagnostic examination,* ed 4, New York, 1981, Macmillan.

Leverenz CJ, Skelly AH: Assessment of thorax and lungs, *Occup Health Nurs* 31(6):9, 1983.

Malasanos L, Barkauskas V, Stoltenberg-Allen K: *Health assessment,* ed 4, St Louis, 1990, Mosby—Year Book.

Mitchell RS, Petty TL, editors: *Synopsis of clinical pulmonary disease,* ed 3, St Louis, 1982, Mosby—Year Book.

Phipps WJ, Long BC, Woods NF, Cassmeyer VL: *Medical-surgical nursing: concepts and clinical practice,* ed 4, St Louis, 1991, Mosby—Year Book.

Seidel HM, Ball JW, Dains JE, Benedict GW: *Mosby's guide to physical examination,* ed 2, St Louis 1991, Mosby—Year Book.

Smith C: Breath sounds, *NursingLife* 4(6):33, 1986.

Stevens SA, Becker KL: How to perform picture perfect respiratory assessment, *Nurs '88* 1:57, 1988.

Taylor DL: Clinical applications: assessing breath sounds, *Nurs '85,* 15(3):60, 1985.

Thompson JM, McFarland GK, Hirsch JE, and others: *Clinical nursing,* ed 2, St Louis, 1989, Mosby—Year Book.

The newborn

Auvenshine MA, Enriquez MG: *Maternity nursing: dimensions of change,* ed 2, Belmont, Calif, 1985, Wadsworth.

Beischer NA, MacKay EV: *Obstetrics and the newborn: an illustrated textbook,* ed 2, Philadelphia, 1986, WB Saunders.

Bobak IM, Jensen MD: *Essentials of maternity nursing,* ed 3, St Louis, 1991, Mosby—Year Book.

Judd JM: Assessing the newborn from head to toe, *Nurs '85,* 15(12):34, 1985.

Kiernan BS, Scoloveno MA: Assessment of the neonate, *Top Clin Nurs* 8(1):1, 1986.

The Organization for Obstetrical, Gynecological and Neonatal Nurses (NAACOG): *Physical assessment of the neonate,* OGN Nursing Practice Resource, Oct. 1986, The Association.

Pillitteri A: *Maternal-newborn nursing: care of the growing family,* ed 3, Boston, 1985, Little, Brown.

Scanlon JW and others: *A system of newborn physical examination,* Baltimore, 1979, University Park Press.

Scharping EM: Physiological measurements of the newborn, *Matern Child Nurs J* 8:70, 1983.

Seidel HM, Ball JW, Dains JE, Benedict GW: *Mosby's guide to physical examination,* ed 2, St Louis, 1991, Mosby—Year Book.

Whaley LF, Wong DL: *Nursing care of infants and children,* ed 4, St Louis, 1991, Mosby—Year Book.

The child

Alexander M, Brown MS: Physical examination. XII. Chest and lungs, *Nurs '75* 5(1):44, 1975.

Barness L: *Manual of pediatric physical diagnosis,* ed 5, Chicago, 1981, Mosby—Year Book.

Prior JA, Silberstein JS, Stang JM: *Physical diagnosis: the history and examination of the patient,* ed 6, St Louis, 1981, Mosby—Year Book.

Whaley LF, Wong DL: *Essentials of pediatric nursing,* ed 3, St Louis, 1989, Mosby—Year Book.

The childbearing woman

Auvenshine MA, Enriquez MG: *Maternity nursing: dimensions of change,* Belmont, Calif, 1985, Wadsworth.

Beischer NA, MacKay EV: *Obstetrics and the newborn: an illustrated textbook,* ed 2, Philadelphia, 1986, WB Saunders.

Bobak IM, Jensen MD: *Essentials of maternity nursing,* ed 3, St Louis, 1991, Mosby—Year Book.

Gilbert ES, Harmon JS: *High-risk pregnancy and delivery: nursing perspectives,* St Louis, 1986, Mosby—Year Book.

Pillitteri A: *Maternal-newborn nursing: care of the growing family,* ed 3, Boston, 1985, Little, Brown.

Pritchard JA, MacDonald PC: *William's obstetrics,* ed 17, New York, 1985, Appleton-Century-Crofts.

Seidel HM, Ball JW, Dains JE, Benedict GW: *Mosby's guide to physical examination,* ed 2, St Louis, 1991, Mosby—Year Book.

The older adult

Burnside IM, editor: *Nursing and the aged,* ed 3, New York, 1988, McGraw-Hill.

Campbell EJ, LeFrak S: How aging affects the structure and function of the respiratory system, *Geriatrics* 33(6):68, 1978.

Carotenuto R, Bullock J: *Physical assessment of the gerontologic client,* Philadelphia, 1980, FA Davis.

Ebersole P, Hess P: *Toward healthy aging: human needs and nursing response,* ed 3, St Louis, 1990, Mosby—Year Book.

Steinberg FU, editor: *Care of the geriatric patient,* ed 6, St Louis, 1983, Mosby—Year Book.

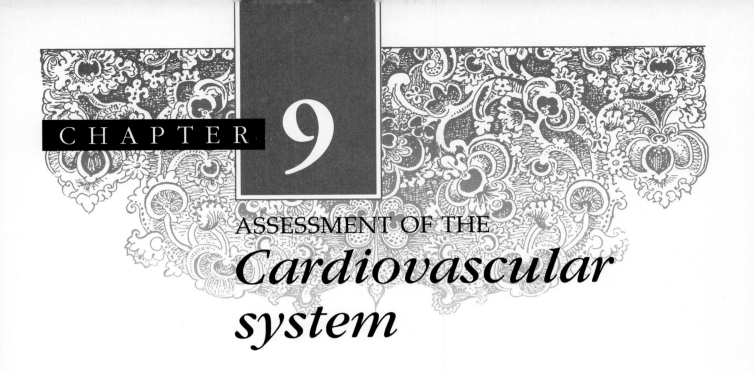

CHAPTER 9

ASSESSMENT OF THE
Cardiovascular system

VOCABULARY

angina pectoris Paroxysmal pain in chest, often associated with myocardial ischemia; pain patterns and severity vary among individuals; pain sometimes radiates to neck, jaw, or left arm; may be accompanied by choking or smothering sensations.

arteriosclerosis General term denoting hardening and thickening of the arterial walls; atherosclerosis is one type of arteriosclerosis.

atherosclerosis The formation of plaques within arterial walls resulting in thickening of the walls and narrowing of the lumen; end organs supplied by these vessels receive diminished circulation.

atrial fibrillation Rapid, involuntary, random atrial contractions that cause rapid, irregular ventricular contractions and diminished cardiac output; this arrhythmia results from chaotic electrical impulses within the atrial myocardium.

atrial flutter Rapid atrial rhythm (approximately 300 per minute) that may or may not cause ventricular tachycardia, depending on the degree of A-V (atrioventricular) blocking.

auscultatory gap A phenomenon sometimes noted by an examiner listening for blood pressure sounds; temporary silent interval between systolic and diastolic sounds that may cover a range of 40 mm Hg.; commonly occurs with hypertensive clients with a wide pulse pressure.

bigeminal pulse Abnormal pulse characterized by a strong beat and a weaker one in close succession, followed by a pause when no beat is felt; pulse is irregular in rhythm; associated with premature contractions, digitalis toxicity, or a partial heart block.

bisferiens pulse Abnormal pulse characterized by two main peaks; occurs with aortic stenosis and/or regurgitation.

bradycardia An abnormally slowed heart rate, usually under 50 beats per minute. *Note:* Conditioned athletes often manifest a normally slowed rate of 50 beats, or slightly less, per minute.

bruit Audible murmur (a blowing sound) heard in auscultating over a peripheral vessel or an organ.

coarctation Stricture or narrowing of the wall of a vessel.

diastole Period of time within the cardiac cycle in which ventricles are relaxed and filling with blood.

ectopic Describes an event that occurs in an unusual manner or form; in reference to the heart, it could pertain to an extra beat or contraction.

embolus A foreign object (composed of air, fat, or clustered cellular elements) that circulates through the blood and usually lodges in a vessel, causing some degree of occlusion.

gallop rhythm Audible extra heart sound in the diastolic interval. A *proto-*

diastolic sound, or *ventricular* gallop, is heard shortly after S_2. A late diastolic sound is called a *presystolic,* or *atrial,* gallop. A *summation* gallop is a combination of four sounds within a cycle and includes both protodiastolic and presystolic sounds.

heave Palpable, diffuse, sustained lift of the chest wall or a portion of the wall.

hepatojugular reflux A phenomenon indicating right heart failure, in which venous pressure rises when the upper abdomen is compressed for 30 to 45 seconds; upon upper right quadrant compression, increased prominence of the jugular vein is noted.

holosystolic (pansystolic) Pertaining to the entire systolic interval; usually refers to an audible murmur.

Homans sign Calf pain associated with rapid dorsiflexion of the foot, often indicative of thrombophlebitis.

hyperkinetic Hyperactive.

hypovolemic Pertaining to decreased blood volume; usually refers to a state of shock resulting from massive blood loss and inadequate tissue perfusion.

"inching" Recommended method for moving the stethoscope over the precordium while listening for heart sounds; small, sliding movements (versus lifting and lowering stethoscope from side to side) may enable the listener to hear more sounds.

infarct Localized area of tissue necrosis caused by prolonged anoxia.

intermittent claudication   Condition characterized by symptoms of pain, aching, cramping, and localized fatigue of the legs that occur while walking but can be quickly relieved by rest (2 to 5 minutes); discomfort occurs most often in the calf but may arise in the foot, thigh, hip, or buttock; caused by prolonged ischemia.

ischemia   Diminished blood supply to an organ or body part.

Korotkoff sounds   Sounds heard during the taking of blood pressure; an inflated cuff encircles a limb and obstructs normal blood flow through the arteries; as the cuff is released, turbulent blood flow creates a series of sounds that enable the listener to determine systolic and diastolic pressures.

NSR (normal sinus rhythm)   The heart rate that originates within sino-atrial (S-A) node in right atrium; the average adult heart beats 72 to 78 times per minute while at rest.

orthopnea   Shortness of breath aggravated by lying flat; caused by redistribution of body fluid and pressure from abdominal contents; relieved by sitting upright or propping upper body with pillows.

palpitation   Sensation of pounding, fluttering, or racing of the heart; can be a normal phenomenon or caused by a disorder of the heart.

paradoxical pulse   Diminished pulse amplitude on inspiration and increased amplitude on expiration; an exaggeration of a normal response to respiration; often associated with obstructive lung disease.

paroxysmal nocturnal dyspnea (PND)   Periodic acute attacks of shortness of breath while recumbent; relieved by sitting or standing.

PMI (point of maximum impulse)   Specific area of the chest where the heartbeat is palpated most clearly; usually the apical impulse, a brief systolic beat in the fourth or fifth intercostal space, 7 to 9 cm left of the midsternal line.

precordium   Area of the chest that overlies the heart and adjacent great vessels.

pulse deficit   A discrepancy between the ventricular rate auscultated over the heart and the arterial rate palpated over the radial artery; caused by a ventricle that contracts with a partially filled chamber and is unable to produce a palpable pulse with each beat.

pulse pressure   The difference between systolic and diastolic pressures, usually within the range of 30 to 40 mm Hg; tends to increase as systolic pressure rises with arteriosclerosis of the large vessels (specifically the aorta); can be altered with vigorous exercise, fever, or other disease states.

pulsus alternans   Alternating pulse; abnormal pulse characterized by a regular rhythm in which a strong beat alternates with a weaker one; sometimes differences in amplitude are subtle and more easily distinguished during taking of blood pressure; associated with severe hypertension, coronary artery disease, and left ventricular failure.

sinus arrhythmia   Normal pulse pattern commonly occurring in some children and young adults; characterized by speeding up of the pulse rate on inspiration and slowing down on expiration.

systole   Period of time within the cardiac cycle in which the ventricles are contracted and ejecting blood into the aorta and pulmonary artery.

tachycardia   Rapid heart rate (usually more than 100 beats per minute); normally occurs with exercise, excitement, anxiety, or fever, but can also indicate abnormal states, such as anemia, heart failure, or shock.

thrill   Palpable murmur described as feeling like the throat of a purring cat.

thrombophlebitis   An inflammation of a vein often associated with clot formation; can be induced by trauma, prolonged immobility, postoperative venous stasis, infection, or blood hyper-coagulation disorder.

thrombus   Blood clot attached to the inner wall of a vessel; usually causes some degree of occlusion.

ANATOMY AND PHYSIOLOGY REVIEW

The cardiovascular system, composed of the heart and a complexity of blood vessels, supplies oxygen, nutrients, and other substances to all of the body's organs and tissues. It also disposes of metabolic waste products through the kidneys and exhalation from the lungs. The heart is about the size of a fist and beats 60 to 100 times a minute without rest for a lifetime. The healthy heart muscle does not become fatigued, and it can respond instantly to external and internal demands, such as exercise, temperature changes, and stress, by increasing rate and cardiac output to blood vessels, which constrict or dilate and redistribute blood flow to meet these demands. The nervous and endocrine systems contribute to the regulation and responses of the heart and vessels to stimuli that continuously assault the body.

The heart is situated in the thoracic cavity, behind the sternum and above the diaphragm in the mediastinum (Fig. 9-1). It lies at an angle so that the right ventricle makes up most of the anterior surface and the left ventricle extends to the left and posteriorly. The upper part of the heart is called the *base,* and the lower left ventricle is referred to as the *apex* (or the apical area). The chest surface overlying the heart is called the *precordium.*

The movement of the left ventricle creates the apical impulse (or the point of maximum impulse) in the fourth or fifth intercostal space, 7 to 9 cm from the midsternal line. The right atrium forms the right border of the heart, and the left atrium lies posteriorly. The aorta curves upward out of the left ventricle and bends posteriorly and downward just above the sternal angle. The pulmonary artery emerges from the superior aspect of the right ventricle near the third intercostal space.

The heart is encased in a tough, fibrous sac called the *pericardium,* which contains fluid within its layers that reduces friction with cardiac movement. Beneath the

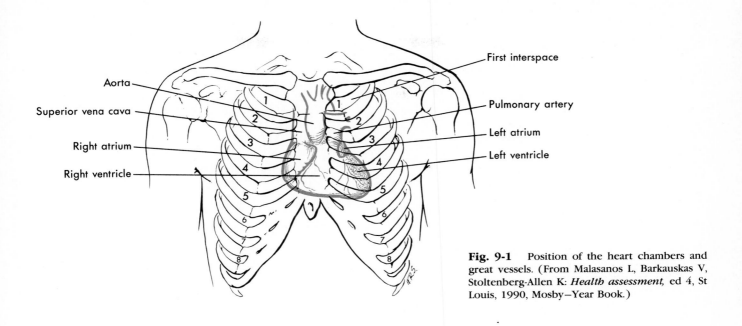

Aorta

Superior vena cava

Right atrium

Right ventricle

First interspace

Pulmonary artery

Left atrium

Left ventricle

Fig. 9-1 Position of the heart chambers and great vessels. (From Malasanos L, Barkauskas V, Stoltenberg-Allen K: *Health assessment,* ed 4, St Louis, 1990, Mosby—Year Book.)

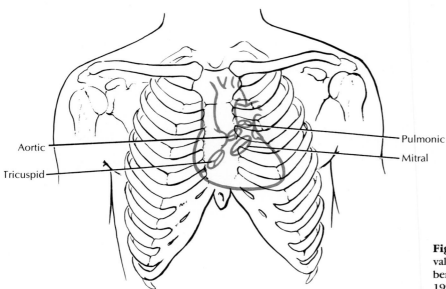

Aortic

Tricuspid

Pulmonic

Mitral

Fig. 9-2 Anatomical location of the heart valves. (From Malasanos L, Barkauskas V, Stoltenberg-Allen K: *Health assessment,* ed 4, St Louis, 1990, Mosby—Year Book.)

pericardium lies the cardiac muscle, which is composed of three layers. The outer layer, the epicardium, covers the heart surface; the middle layer, the myocardium, is thick, muscular tissue that controls the pumping action; and the endocardium lines the inner chambers and valves.

The tricuspid and mitral valves (known as *atrioventricular* valves, or *AV* valves) separate the right atrium and ventricle and the left atrium and ventricle respec-

tively (Fig. 9-2). The aortic valve emerges from the left ventricle into the aorta, and the pulmonic valve opens into the pulmonary artery from the right ventricle. The aortic and pulmonic valves are called *semilunar* valves because of their half-moon shape. The blood flows through each atrium, empties into the ventricles through the AV valves, is then pumped out of the ventricles through the semilunar valves into the pulmonary artery into the lungs, and into the aorta (Fig. 9-3).

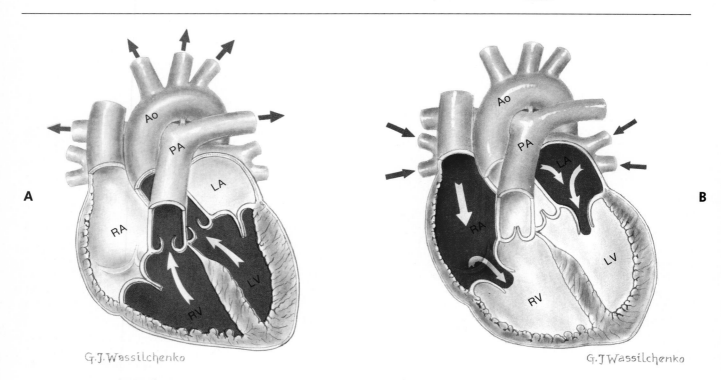

Fig. 9-3   The route of blood flow through the chambers of the heart and the great vessels. (From Malasanos L, Barkauskas V, Stoltenberg-Allen K: *Health assessment,* ed 4, St Louis, 1990, Mosby—Year Book.)

Fig. 9-4   **A,** Blood flow during systole. **B,** Blood flow during diastole. (From Canobbio MM: *Mosby's clinical nursing series,* vol 1, *Cardiovascular disorders,* St Louis, 1990, Mosby—Year Book.)

The Cardiac Cycle

The cardiac cycle includes the sequence of blood flow through the chambers, the action of the valves, the varying pressures within the heart chambers and vessels, and the alternating contractions of the atria and ventricles. The overall accomplishment of this cycle is (1) the routing of deoxygenated blood from the body to the lungs for oxygenation and (2) the transporting of oxygenated blood from the lungs to the body (Fig. 9-4).

Systemic blood enters the right atrium through the vena cava, and oxygenated blood flows into the left atrium. The AV valves (tricuspid and mitral) snap shut because of increased pressure in the ventricles, which are filled with blood and beginning to contract. As the atria relax and fill, ventricular pressure forces the opening of the semilunar valves so that blood can leave the ventricles. The *systolic phase* begins with the first heart sound (S_1) (which is the closure of the AV valves), con-

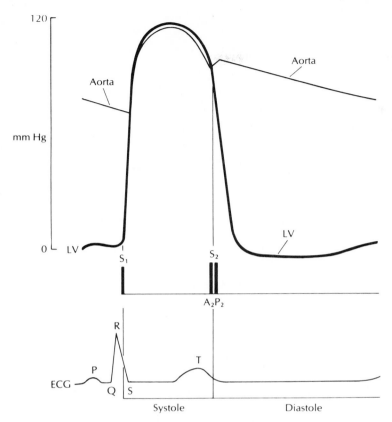

Fig. 9-5 Pressure curves of the left ventricle and aorta, S_1 and S_2 and the ECG. (From Malasanos L, Barkauskas V, Stoltenberg-Allen K: *Health assessment,* ed 4, St Louis, 1990, Mosby–Year Book.)

tinues with pressure building in the ventricles that forces the opening of the semilunar valves, and ventricular squeezing, which ejects the blood and empties the ventricles. In the *diastolic phase* the semilunar valves snap shut (S_2) because aortic and pulmonic pressures exceed the diminished pressure in the empty ventricles. The AV valves open from pressure in the filled atria to allow emptying of the blood into the relaxed ventricles.

The heart is stimulated by an electrical discharge that originates in the sinoatrial (SA) node in the superior aspect of the right atrium. This node, called the *cardiac pacemaker,* discharges about 60 to 100 impulses per minute. The electrical discharge stimulates contraction of both atria and then flows to the AV node in the inferior aspect of the right atrium. The impulses are then transmitted through a series of branches (the bundle of His) and fibers in the myocardium which results in ventricular stimulation and contraction. The AV node prevents excessive atrial impulses from reaching the ventricles. If the SA node fails, the remaining electrical system can generate heart contraction at a slower rate (20 to 60 beats per minute). The sequence of electrical impulses slightly precedes cardiac cycle events. The electrical discharges are measured in an electrocardiogram (ECG) (Fig. 9-5). The p wave designates atrial depolarization

(stimulation), and the QRS complex indicates ventrical stimulation. The P-R interval shows the duration of the passage of the impulse from the SA node to the AV node and the myocardial fibers. The t wave designates ventricular repolarization (recovery). Fig. 9-5 correlates electrical events with the left cardiac cycle. The QRS complex slightly precedes ventricular contraction, which forces closure of the mitral valve (S_1) and creates ventricular pressure. When ventricular pressure exceeds aortic pressure, the valve opens and ventricular pressure peaks and falls as blood is ejected. When ventricular pressure falls below aortic pressure, the aortic valve closes (S_2). Ventricular pressure continues to fall as the atrium fills and eventually contracts through SA stimulation (p wave).

Heart Sounds

The sounds generated by valve closure are best heard where blood flows away from the valve instead of directly over the valve area (Fig. 9-6). The designated auscultatory sites indicate that the aortic valve closure is best heard in the second right interspace, pulmonic closure in the second left interspace, mitral closure in the fifth left interspace, and tricuspid closure in the fourth or fifth interspace near the midline. The left side of the

Fig. 9-6 Transmission of closure sounds from the heart valves. (From Malasanos L, Barkauskas V, Stoltenberg-Allen K: *Health assessment,* ed 4, St Louis, 1990, Mosby—Year Book.)

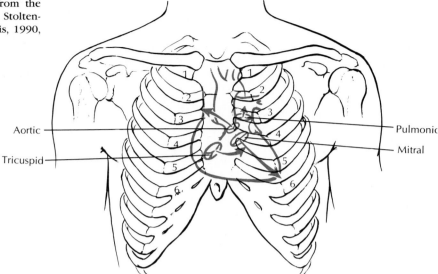

Aortic

Tricuspid

Pulmonic

Mitral

heart slightly precedes the right side in the cardiac cycle, and two closely adjacent sounds of the tricuspid and the mitral valves may sometimes be heard in the tricuspid listening area (called a *split S_1*). A normal split S_2 may be heard in the pulmonary area, because pulmonary closure lags behind aortic closure. Inhaling air creates a negative thoracic pressure, increases venous return to the right heart, delays pulmonic valve closure, and exaggerates the split S_2.

The quality of heart sounds is affected by many factors. Sounds are louder and more distinct in small, thin people, because there is less adipose tissue to filter noise. A person who exhales and leans forward for the listener positions the heart closer to the chest wall for improved listening. If the client turns to the left side, often the heart is closer to the left chest wall and may improve the palpation of the apical impulse or the auscultatory sound of the mitral valve. States of anxiety, fever, or immediate postexercise shorten the P-R interval and cause a faster beat with rapid intense closure of the AV valves, resulting in a louder S_1. S_1 and S_2 sounds can be diminished or exaggerated by normal physiological events or alterations in the circulatory system, the electrical system, or the configuration of the valves, cardiac chambers, musculature, or layers. The listener must be aware of the location, intensity, and pitch of each sound; the duration of the sound; and the duration and quality of the silence between sounds. The specific characteristics of S_1 and S_2 are listed in the "Clinical Guidelines," p. 279. A third heart sound (S_3) can sometimes be heard at the apex. This occurs early in diastole and is caused by rapid filling and distention of the ventricles. It may be a normal phenomenon in children and young adults but is indicative of heart disease in older adults. S_4, a

sound heard in late diastole (right before S_1), is also caused by blood rushing against the ventricular wall and is associated with hypertension or other cardiac disorders. Another abnormal diastolic sound is the opening snap, caused by the opening of the mitral valve when it is thickened or deformed. The sound is high pitched and occurs early in the diastolic phase. In systole, ejection clicks may be heard if either the pulmonic or aortic valves are deformed or if either of the great vessels is dilated. A pulmonic ejection click is best heard at the second or third left interspace, and the aortic click is heard over the apex or the base of the heart. Pericardial friction rubs are caused by inflammation of the layers of the pericardial sac. A rubbing sound is usually present in both systole and diastole and is best heard over the apical area.

The sounds of heart murmurs are usually caused by turbulent blood flow within heart chambers or vessel walls or vibrations of heart valves. A murmur may be a normal physiological phenomenon or indicative of valve deformity or heart disease. Murmurs are prolonged sounds and can occur early, midway, or throughout systole or diastole. Sometimes S_1 or S_2 seems to sound blurred or muffled, which could be a slight prolongation of a normal sound indicative of a murmur. In other instances the murmur is so loud and prolonged that it obscures S_1 and/or S_2 with a dramatic swishing noise. "Innocent" murmurs, those that are physiological, usually occur in children and young adults and in states of pregnancy, anxiety, or fever. Turbulent flow arises from intense ventricular contraction, and systolic murmurs are audible, especially in thin, small people. Diastolic murmurs are almost always pathological. Table 9-1 shows a method used by some for classifying or grading sounds.

TABLE 9-1   Grading of cardiac murmurs

CLASSIFICATION	DESCRIPTION
Grade I	Soft, barely audible in quiet room
Grade II	Quiet, but clearly audible
Grade III	Moderately loud, without thrill
Grade IV	Loud, associated with thrill
Grade V	Very loud, thrill easily palpable
Grade VI	Very loud, audible with stethoscope off the chest, thrill palpable and visible

From Canobbio MM: Mosby's clinical nursing series, *vol 1,* Cardiovascular disorders, *St Louis, 1990, Mosby—Year Book.*

The Circulatory System and Blood Pressure

The circulatory system is composed of arteries, veins, and capillaries. Arteries carry oxygenated blood to all organs, tissues, and cells. Veins deliver waste materials and deoxygenated blood back to the lungs for disposal and reoxygenation. Arteries and veins are gradually reduced to microscopic vessels (capillaries), which permit the exchange of oxygen, nutrients, and waste products between body cells and blood (Fig. 9-7). Arteries have tough, elastic walls that constrict and dilate in response to parasympathetic and sympathetic, chemical, and temperature stimuli. Arterioles (smaller artery branches) also dilate and constrict and are responsible for the maintenance of blood pressure. Veins are more distensible than arteries, which enables them to store blood in reserve. Veins also contain valves that assist with forward blood flow to the heart. The circulatory system also responds to mechanical stimuli, such as exercise, by speeding blood flow and redistributing blood to muscles instead of to internal organs.

The arterial system is evaluated through examination and palpation of pulses (Fig. 9-8). Palpable pulses are evaluated by observing the rate, rhythm, pulse amplitude and contour, and amplitude pattern.

- **Rate** The resting cardiac rate is 60 to 90 beats per minute (bpm), with the exception of conditioned athletes, who may exhibit rates of about 50 bpm. A rapid rate (tachycardia) can occur with exercise, fever, anxiety, or anemia. A slow rate (bradycardia) may indicate electrical conduction blockage or chemical influence.
- **Rhythm** The rhythm is normally regular, with the exception of a physiological increase of rate on inspiration, which occurs with children and young adults (sinus arrhythmia). Abnormal rhythms may occur in patterns with extra beats that might indicate premature ventricular contractions or digitalis toxicity (bigeminal pulse). Atrial fibrillation causes an ir-

regular rhythm with no pattern. An irregular, rapid, or slow pulse should be palpated simultaneously with auscultation of the apical pulse. Any difference between peripheral and apical pulse rates should be noted; premature and extra heartbeats may not be detected with palpation (pulse deficit). If the pulse irregularity is patterned, note if it occurs during (1) inspiration or expiration and (2) systole or diastole.

- **Amplitude and Contour** Pulse amplitude is the strength of the beat as felt by the fingerpads. Amplitude is dictated by the volume of blood rushing through the artery and the force of ventricular contraction. During exercise, the cardiac output increases as the heart rate speeds up, and the pulse feels strong and bounds under the fingerpads. A bounding pulse cannot be obliterated by pressure. Bounding pulses also occur with pathological conditions, such as systolic hypertension; the arterial walls are rigid, and the rush of blood creates a bounding effect. Weak or "thready" pulses can be obliterated with finger pressure. A low blood volume (hypovolemia), aortic stenosis, or diminished ventricular contraction can create a weak pulse. Pulse contour also relates to the "feel" of the stroke and the surface of the vessel. Sclerotic vessels feel rigid and sometimes knotted or irregular on the surface, in contrast to a normal vessel, which is smooth and resilient.
- **Amplitude Patterns** In some pathological conditions the pulse strokes may vary without affecting the rhythm. Pulsus alternans is characterized by a regular rhythm with a strong beat alternating with a weaker one. This may occur in severe hypertension, coronary artery disease, or left ventricular failure. Pulsus paradoxus, associated with pulmonary emphysema, manifests an increase in amplitude on expiration.

Arterial sufficiency can also be appraised by examining extremities and posing questions about symptoms related to exercise or other body functions that place a demand on arterial flow. The "end organs" for arterial supply include muscles and skin (periphery), as well as all internal organs. Diminished arterial supply, existing with diabetes, atherosclerosis, Buerger disease, and aneurysms or mechanical vessel blockages, creates symptoms. Angina pectoris results from diminished coronary artery supply. Confusion may indicate arterial insufficiency or blockage of flow to a portion of the brain. Diminished flow can occur in larger vessels, such as the carotid arteries, with resultant localized effects; or diminished flow may be systemic, with decreased flow throughout the artery branches and arterioles. Systemic arterial insufficiency may cause such symptoms as generalized fatigue or intermittent claudication (extremity pain or cramping accompanying exercise and quickly relieved with rest). Arterial insufficiency is exhibited in

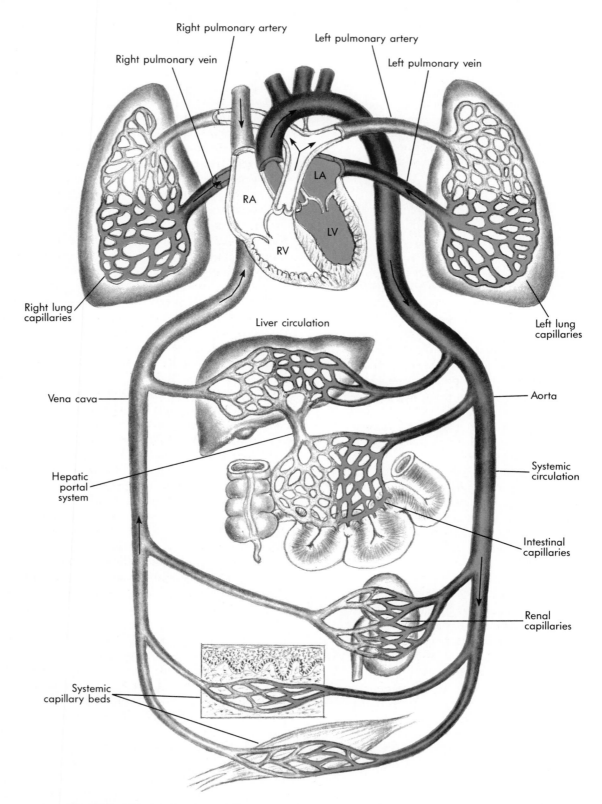

Fig. 9-7   Diagram showing serially connected pulmonary and systemic circulatory systems. Right heart chambers propel unoxygenated blood through pulmonary circulation, and left heart propels oxygenated blood through systemic circulation. (From McCance KL, Huether SE: *Pathophysiology: the biological basis for disease in adults and children,* St Louis, 1990, Mosby—Year Book.)

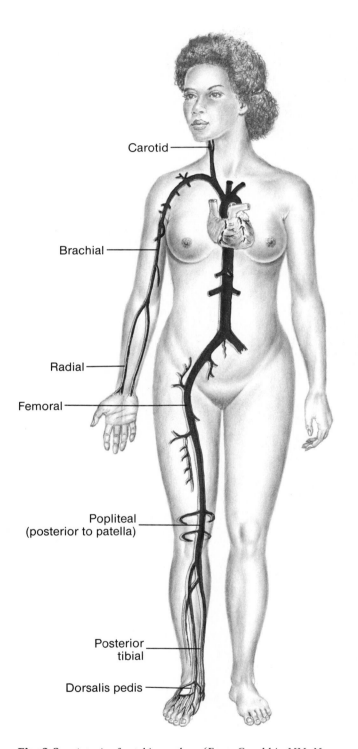

Carotid

Brachial

Radial

Femoral

Popliteal
(posterior to patella)

Posterior
tibial

Dorsalis pedis

Fig. 9-8   Arteries for taking pulses. (From Canobbio MM: *Mosby's clinical nursing series,* vol 1, *Cardiovascular disorders,* St Louis, 1990, Mosby—Year Book.)

varying degrees, depending on the cause or the longevity of the insufficiency. Tissue death (gangrene) occurs with sustained absence of oxygenated blood. Ischemia, a diminished blood supply, may appear as marked pallor or mottling, accompanied by coolness of an extremity. Arterial insufficiency may only occur if extra demands, such as exercise or anxiety, call for increased arterial response. Fig. 9-9 illustrates the complex arterial network in the body.

Blood pressure is created by the volume of blood that resides in arterioles and the degree of resistance (capacity for volume) existing in the vessels; in other words, arteriole constriction reduces the capacity for a given volume and pressure rises. This occurs as a normal response with exercise or anxiety as cardiac output increases. Elevated pressure is also indicative of disease, commonly hypertension, if arterioles remain chronically constricted. Systolic pressure occurs and is measured during ventricular contraction, and diastolic pressure occurs during ventricular relaxation. Pulse pressure is the difference between systolic and diastolic pressures. A normal pulse pressure is usually within the range of 30 to 40 mm Hg but can widen in normal states of exercise or anxiety. Sclerosis of large vessels (specifically the aorta) can increase systolic pressure and widen the pulse pressure. Table 9-2 describes blood pressure norms for children and adults. Methods for measuring blood pressure are described on pp. 290-291.

Venous system efficiency is evaluated through examination of the extremities and observation of the jugular vein. Veins carry deoxygenated blood back to the heart. Venous return depends on an adequate blood volume and, ultimately, arterial pressure, because venous pressure is much lower than arterial pressure. The valves within the veins assist with the pumping, and skeletal muscle contraction also stimulates return. Venous return is slowed when the right heart is not receiving blood adequately or when the pulmonary vascular system is failing. The jugular vein is like a manometer with a level of blood in its column that indicates the pressure in the right heart. Both the external and internal veins may be observed (Fig. 9-10). The external vein is quite visible and slowly fills when one is lying flat; however, the internal vein is more difficult to observe because it lies behind the sternocleidomastoid muscle. It can often be seen emerging toward the surface just under the mandible. Abnormal jugular venous pressure (JVP) is greater than 3 cm above the sternal angle when one lies at a 30- to 45-degree elevation. An elevated JVP is commonly associated with right heart failure, congestive heart failure, or obstruction of the superior vena cava. The method for inspection of the jugular vein is described on pp. 282-283. The extremities demonstrate insufficient venous return as veins pool blood and become

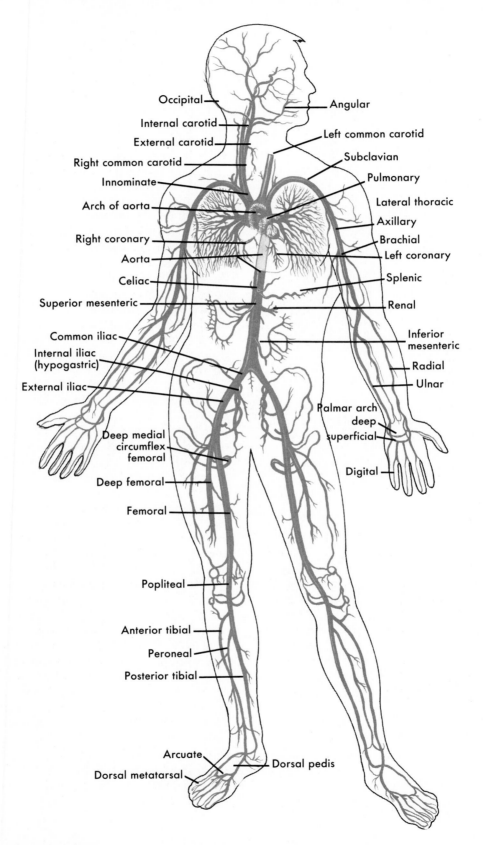

Fig. 9-9 Circulatory system. Main arteries of body. (From McCance KL, Huether SE: *Pathophysiology: the biological basis for disease in adults and children,* St Louis, 1990, Mosby–Year Book.)

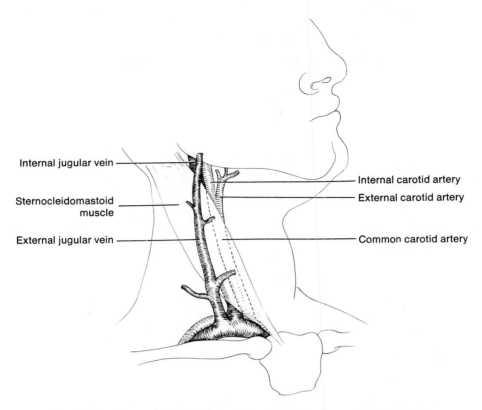

Fig. 9-10   Anatomical placement of carotid and jugular vessels in the neck.

TABLE 9-2   Normal blood pressures

	SYSTOLIC	DIASTOLIC
Infants	60-96 mm Hg	30-62 mm Hg
Age 2	78-112 mm Hg	48-78 mm Hg
Age 8	85-114 mm Hg	52-85 mm Hg
Age 12	95-135 mm Hg	58-88 mm Hg
Adult	100-140 mm Hg	60-90 mm Hg

From Canobbio MM: Mosby's clinical nursing series, *vol 1,* Cardiovascular disorders, *St Louis, 1990, Mosby–Year Book.*
Systolic pressure in the thigh can be higher by 10 to 40 mm Hg as compared with brachial artery pressure. Diastolic pressure remains the same.

engorged and visible as bulges, which sometimes are nodular and twisted. The saphenous vein is one of the most common to distend (Fig. 9-11), but smaller branches twist and bulge over the lower legs. The ankles and lower legs may also be edematous (fluid filled), because interstitial fluid accumulates when vessels are engorged and pooled with blood. Venous incompetence can result in a chronic inflammation of the lower legs and ankles (stasis dermatitis), which appears as brown, patchy, sometimes thickened skin that flakes and itches. The chronic inflammation may advance to ulcers that weep, granulose, heal, and break down again. Redness and tenderness over a superficial vein may indicate thrombophlebitis. Note that both arterial and venous systems can be viewed on the retinal surface (see Chapter 7 for descriptions).

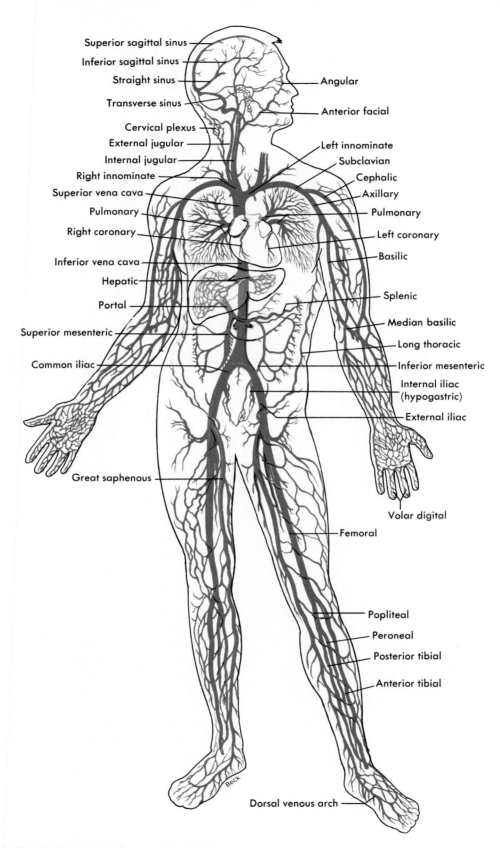

Superior sagittal sinus
Inferior sagittal sinus
Straight sinus
Transverse sinus
Cervical plexus
External jugular
Internal jugular
Right innominate
Superior vena cava
Pulmonary
Right coronary
Inferior vena cava
Hepatic
Portal
Superior mesenteric
Common iliac
Great saphenous

Angular
Anterior facial
Left innominate
Subclavian
Cephalic
Axillary
Pulmonary
Left coronary
Basilic
Splenic
Median basilic
Long thoracic
Inferior mesenteric
Internal iliac (hypogastric)
External iliac
Volar digital
Femoral
Popliteal
Peroneal
Posterior tibial
Anterior tibial
Dorsal venous arch

Beck

Fig. 9-11 Principal veins of body. Only superficial veins are shown on forearms and hands. (From Thibodeau GA: *Anatomy and physiology,* St Louis, 1987, Mosby–Year Book.)

COGNITIVE OBJECTIVES

At the end of this chapter the learner will demonstrate knowledge of assessment of the cardiovascular system by the ability to do the following:

- Apply the terms that are listed in the vocabulary section.
- Record a blood pressure, identifying the variables of auscultatory gap, first and second diastolic pressures, and pulse pressure.
- Point out the common variables that alter blood pressure in healthy individuals.
- Identify the characteristics of arterial pulse that an examiner notes with inspection and palpation.
- Name the causes attributed to selected variations of arterial pulse characteristics.
- State the major differences between observable signs of chronic venous insufficiency and chronic arterial insufficiency.
- Identify the major differences between carotid and jugular pulsation.
- Point out some major characteristics of the normal jugular veins and jugular venous pressure.
- Describe the major characteristics and causes of leg varicosities.
- Identify and locate the anatomical positions of the heart, the major components of the heart, and adjacent great vessels.
- Describe the events and mechanisms of the cardiac cycle.
- Identify some major characteristics of normal signs elicited during inspection and palpation of the precordium.
- Explain the appropriate purpose and use of the bell and diaphragm of the stethoscope.
- Identify the origin of the first and second heart sounds.
- Describe the major auscultatory characteristics of the first and second heart sounds in terms of the following:
  1. Location
  2. Intensity
  3. Frequency
  4. Timing
  5. Splitting
- Identify the origin and major characteristics of the third and fourth heart sounds.
- Recognize the following precordial auscultatory areas and identify selected auscultatory events in each area:
  1. Aortic area
  2. Pulmonary area
  3. Third left interspace
  4. Tricuspid area
  5. Apical area
- Point out the following six characteristics of cardiac murmurs that must be described during their assessment:
  1. Timing: systole, diastole, continuous

2. Location: using precordial landmarks and/or distance in centimeters from a landmark
3. Radiation: described in centimeters, landmarks
4. Intensity: grades 1 through 6, or loud, medium, soft
5. Pitch: high, medium, low
6. Quality: blowing, harsh, rumbling, crescendo, decrescendo

- Identify the origin and selected major characteristics of systolic and diastolic murmurs.
- Recognize selected major characteristics of "innocent" murmurs.
- Identify selected common cardiovascular variations in the newborn, the child, the childbearing woman, and the older adult.

CLINICAL OUTLINE

At the end of this chapter the learner will perform a systematic assessment of the cardiovascular system, demonstrating the ability to do the following:

- Obtain a pertinent health history from a client.
- Palpate and auscultate arterial blood pressure.
- Assess carotid, radial, femoral, popliteal, dorsalis pedis, and posterior tibial pulses through inspection and palpation for the following:
  1. Rate
  2. Rhythm
  3. Amplitude
  4. Variations in amplitude
  5. Contour
  6. Symmetry
- Conduct a predesignated maneuver to test for arterial sufficiency in extremities.
- Evaluate and describe jugular venous pressure.
- Inspect and describe jugular pulsation quality.
- Inspect, palpate, and describe the appearance of superficial veins and surface characteristics of the legs.
- Maneuver the foot and describe the results of an assessment for calf pain.
- Inspect and palpate the extremities for arterial and venous sufficiency.
- Observe and describe the client's general condition (at rest) in terms of the following:
  1. Positioning and comfort
  2. Ease of respirations (in supine or 30- to 45-degree position)
  3. General skin color
- Inspect and palpate the anterior chest precordium, sternoclavicular, aortic, pulmonary, right ventricular, apical, epigastric, and ectopic areas for the following:
  1. Contour
  2. General movement
  3. Pulsations
  4. Heaves or lifts
- Palpate and describe the results of assessment of the apical impulse for the following:

1. Amplitude
2. Duration
3. Location
4. Diameter

- Locate and auscultate the following sites with a stethoscope bell and diaphragm:
  1. Aortic area
  2. Pulmonary area
  3. Third left interspace
  4. Tricuspid area
  5. Apical area
- Describe the results of cardiac auscultation in terms of the following:
  1. Rate
  2. Rhythm
  3. S_1: location, intensity, frequency, timing, and splitting
  4. S_2: location, intensity, frequency, timing, and splitting
  5. Systole: relative duration
  6. Diastole: relative duration
- Identify additional systolic or diastolic sounds in terms of the following:
  1. Timing
  2. Location
  3. Radiation
  4. Intensity
  5. Pitch
  6. Quality
- Auscultate and describe cardiac sounds while the client is supine, turned to left decubitus position, and sitting up.
- Summarize the results of the assessment with a written description of the findings.

HISTORY

- If the client complains of leg pains (cramps), inquire about specific situations or activities that worsen or relieve the problem.
  1. *Arterial insufficiency* results in pain that worsens with activity, particularly prolonged exercise (e.g., walking). The pain is usually quickly relieved (within 2 minutes) with cessation of movement (standing). Pain may occasionally occur when limbs are elevated and be relieved with dangling of feet. Claudication distance should be specified. Determine how many average city blocks (or yards, numbers of stairs, etc.) a client walks before pain occurs. Remember that variables such as a hilly terrain, walking in start-stop heavy traffic areas, environmental temperature, and pace of walking affect exertion intensity. Signs and symptoms indicating a severe problem are the following:
     a. Sudden decrease in claudication distance

b. Diminished or absent pulses or cold, mottled, or blue extremities
c. Cutaneous changes, such as reddened pressure areas, ulcers, or taut, shiny skin
d. Pain not relieved by rest
   Pain is most commonly located in the calf but may be in the lower leg or dorsum of the foot. Hip, buttock, or thigh pain may be present. The client should provide a clear description of the pain (e.g., numbness, feeling of cold, burning, tingling, sharp cramp, aching). Risk factors include family history of diabetes, vascular disease, or heart disease, hyperlipidemia, hypertension, and smoking.

2. *Venous insufficiency* pain intensifies with prolonged standing or sitting in one position. Relief often occurs by elevating the leg, lying down, or exercise (walking). Edema often accompanies the problem. Varicosities may be present. Discomfort may be increased at the end of the day. Pain is commonly located in the calf and lower leg. It may be described as an aching, tiredness, or feeling of fullness.

RISK FACTORS FOR VENOUS INSUFFICIENCY

- Occupations that involve prolonged sitting or standing
- Family or client history of varicosities
- Obesity
- Constrictive clothing (e.g., garter, girdles)
- Pregnancy
- History of thrombophlebitis
- Chronic systemic disease (e.g., heart disease, cirrhosis, hypertension)

---

3. Neurologically caused pain exhibits fewer predictable patterns. The pain often occurs at night and awakens the client. The pain may be associated with exercise or movement, but nothing in particular relieves it. There is usually no edema, cyanosis, cold extremities, or marked cutaneous changes associated with it. The pain may locate in the calf. A family or client history of diabetes mellitus should always be explored.
4. There may be other causes for leg pain, such as the following:
   a. New type of shoe (e.g., very high heels, "negative heel" shoes)
   b. Foot problems (with inadequate shoe support)

   c. Participation in new type of exercise or increased exercise

   d. Problems with back and pain radiating to legs (see Chapter 14 for further information)

   e. Recent injury

5. Clients who complain of leg pain at night should clarify what specifically relieves it (e.g., rubbing leg, walking, dangling) and the duration of pain.

6. All leg pain complaints should be treated with a full symptom analysis. The preceding descriptions may help the examiner to categorize a profile.

• The following questions concern heart disease and hypertension:

  1. Have you experienced any visual changes? Loss of consciousness? Headaches? Marked weakness or fatigue?

  2. Are there any new or marked stress factors in your life (home, work, family, friends)?

  3. Have you noticed a weight change in the last 6 months?

  4. Do you feel dizzy? Does your body position affect the dizziness? (Postural hypotension might affect the client's safety in the home.) Have you ever fallen down?

  5. If orthopnea and paroxysmal nocturnal dyspnea are present, inquire about sleep habits.

RISK FACTORS FOR CARDIOVASCULAR DISEASE

• Age (increasing incidence after 30 years of age)
• Sex (males at higher risk, also postmenopausal women)
• Elevated blood pressure (systolic higher than 180 mm Hg; diastolic higher than 90 mm Hg)*
• Diabetes, especially juvenile onset type
• Obesity (more than 10% overweight)
• High fat diet (more than 30% of total intake per day)
• Elevated cholesterol level
• Elevated triglyceride levels
• Sedentary life-style/occupation
• Cigarette smoking
• Stressful life-style (*Note*: the degree and type of stress must be carefully reviewed by client and examiner; some individuals tolerate or enjoy a moderate to high amount of stress.)
• Environmental pollution
• Use of oral contraceptives (especially if more than 40 years of age)
• Family history of diabetes mellitus
• Family history of cardiovascular disease

Elevation risk varies with individual age and general health status.

EXERTION/EXERCISE PROFILE (SAMPLE FORM)

	Sleeping	Lying down	Sitting	Light exercise*	Moderate exercise†	Moderately heavy exercise‡	Others§
Hr/day	8	3 to 4	4	3	2 to 3		Twenty-eight stairs (climbs BID)
Hr/wk					5 to 6 (short walks to shopping center)	5 to 6 (heavy housework; occasional long walks)	
Hr/mo							
Symptoms and problems	None	Feels tired if unable to take AM and PM naps	None	None	None (but carries out daily routines at slow pace)	Occasional SOB; must rest after heavy housework	Feels "winded" midway at landing; rests 2 min

*Walking from one room to another, fixing small meals, etc.
†Light housework, making bed, sweeping floor, dusting, office work, short walks (flat surface), etc.
‡Scrubbing floors, sexual intercourse, long walks (specify amount), stair climbing (specify flights), lifting, construction work, etc.
§Long periods of standing, exercise programs, jogging, stair climbing (may be recorded as unusual activity if many flights are climbed frequently).

6. If edema is present, inquire about the times of day when it is most apparent (e.g., first thing in the morning vs. late afternoon or evening).
7. Inquire closely about medications being consumed. (If nitroglycerin or other "prn" preparations are being taken, determine how often per day.) Review over-the-counter medications carefully. Some antacid medications contain large amounts of sodium. Many cold preparations (antitussives, decongestants), nose drops, nasal sprays, and weight control preparations contain sympathomimetic amines.
8. Inquire closely about dietary habits; consider caloric, cholesterol, and salt intakes.
9. For clients with a history of heart disease, severe hypertension, or vascular disease, it may be helpful to establish an exertion/exercise profile. Definitions of light, moderate, or heavy exercise can be established in advance by the examiner or agency or can be defined for individual clients. The profile can be renewed periodically to follow the client's progress. (See sample form on p. 277.)
10. Chronic pain, shortness of breath, fatigue, or other symptoms must be related to reduction or change in functions of daily living. For example, dyspnea increases with stair climbing, and a client might live four flights up in an apartment building. Many people have to walk to the grocery store every day. Interference with sleep, work environment, physical demands, and family relationships should be explored.
• Information should be obtained from the client to provide an accurate chest pain profile. Table 9-3 is not intended to be a complete guide to differential diagnosis. Gastrointestinal and musculoskeletal problems can mimic angina. It will, however, provide some ideas about specific questions to pose.

Text continues on p. 290.

TABLE 9-3 Chest pain profile*

	ANGINA PECTORIS	ESOPHAGITIS	MUSCULOSKELETAL PROBLEMS
Precipitated by	Effort (usually emotion, exercise, eating)	Eating, Nervousness	Motion, especially neck movement, Hyperventilation, Coughing
Duration	10 to 15 min	Variable (up to several hours)	Variable
Alleviated by	Stopping activity or rest (often in 2 to 3 min), Nitroglycerin	Eructation, Sitting upright, Eating, Antacids	Heat, Analgesic, Change of position
Worsening of pain	Soon after rising (AM), After heavy meal	Any time (especially at night)	Bedtime or after day of exertion
Onset	Often remembers date (pain seldom continues over 5 years without developing abnormal exercise ECG)	Uncertain	Uncertain
Disease	Myocardial infarction, diabetes, hypertension, rheumatic heart disease, obesity, indigestion	Indigestion	Trauma

*Data from Warner-Chilcott Laboratory, AEGIS Production: Differential diagnosis of chest pain, New York, 1967, American Heart Association. Wasson J, Walsh BT, Tompkins R, Sox H: The common symptom guide, New York, 1975, McGraw-Hill.

CLINICAL GUIDELINES

*If pressure is elevated, especially if accompanied by rapid pulse, repeat in 30 minutes.

Continued.

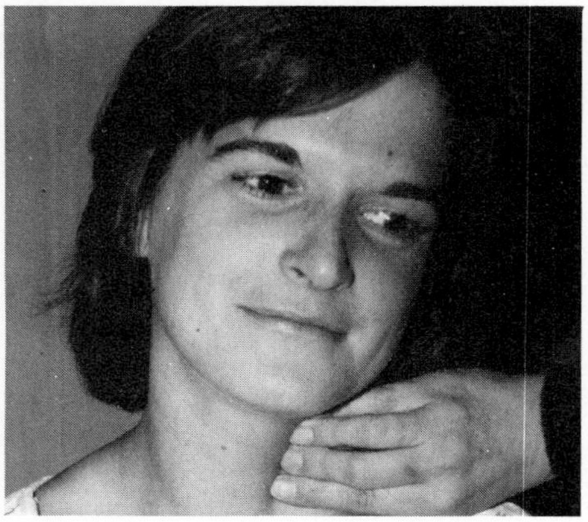

Fig. 9-12 Palpating for carotid pulse.

EVALUATION		
ASSESSMENT PROCEDURE	NORMAL FINDINGS	DEVIATIONS FROM NORMAL

1. Assemble equipment
  a. Stethoscope
  b. Sphygmomanometer
2. Palpate, then auscultate brachial artery to determine arterial blood pressure in both arms (See "Clinical Tips and Strategies," p. 290, for description of procedure for measuring blood pressure.)
3. Measure blood pressure while client is standing (as well as lying) if client offers history or complaint of syncope or dizziness or is taking antihypertensive medications
4. Measure blood pressure in both legs if pedal, popliteal, and femoral pulses are weak or absent (See "Clinical Tips and Strategies," pp. 291-292 for technique.)
5. Palpate both carotid arteries
  a. Use flat surface of first three fingerpads
  b. Place fingers between trachea and sternocleidomastoid muscle under mandible
  c. Client should flex neck and rotate head slightly toward side being examined (Fig. 9-12)
	Upper limits (adult):
	140 mm Hg systolic
	90 mm Hg diastolic
	30 to 40 mm Hg pulse pressure
	
	Varies with sex, body weight, time of day
	Other variables that can be somewhat controlled by examiner are listed in *Clinical Tips and Strategies*
	
	Pressure in both arms is same or does not vary more than 5 to 10 mm Hg systolic
	On standing, client may manifest drop of maximum of 10 to 15 mm Hg (systolic) and 5 mm Hg (diastolic)
	
	Popliteal artery auscultation reveals systolic pressure 5 to 15 mm Hg higher than brachial artery measurement; diastolic reading is same or slightly lower
		Elevated systolic (↑ 140)*
		Elevated diastolic (↑ 90)*
		Widened pulse pressure
		Narrow pulse pressure
		Low systolic (↓ 90)
		Low diastolic (↓ 60)
		Significant (↑ 5 to 10 mm Hg) discrepancy in pressure readings between upper extremities
		
		Significant decrease of systolic (more than 15 mm Hg) or diastolic (more than 5 mm Hg) and/or symptoms of dizziness
		
		Systolic pressure is lower in leg(s) than in arms

CLINICAL GUIDELINES—cont'd

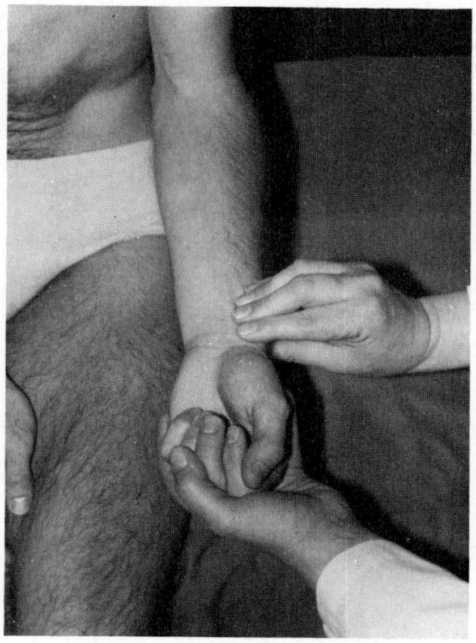

Fig. 9-13   Radial artery palpation.

ASSESSMENT PROCEDURE	EVALUATION	
	NORMAL FINDINGS	DEVIATIONS FROM NORMAL
d. Palpate one artery at a time for:		
(1) Rate	60 to 90 beats/min (conditioned athletes may be as low as 50/min)	↓ 90/min (tachycardia) (*Note:* Recent exertion, smoking, or anxiety will elevate pulse.) ↑ 60/min (bradycardia)
(2) Rhythm	Regular (*Note:* Slight transient increase in rate during inspiration, especially in clients under 40 years.)	Irregular, without any pattern (e.g., atrial fibrillation) Regularity with occasional pauses or extra beats (e.g., premature contraction) Coupled beats (e.g., bigeminal pulse)
(3) Pulse amplitude and contour	Upstroke smooth, rounded, prompt	Upstroke exaggerated or bounding Pulse weak, small, or thready; peak prolonged
(4) Amplitude pattern	Series of pulse strokes unvaried in amplitude or contour	Upstrokes vary (e.g., strong and weaker beats alternate [pulsus alternans]) Force of beat reduced during inspiration (paradoxical pulse)
(5) Symmetry	Symmetrical response (i.e., both carotid pulses manifest same rate, rhythm, amplitude, and contour)	Asymmetrical response
(6) Arterial wall contour and consistency	Soft and pliable	Increased resistance to compression; beaded or tortuous
6. Using fingerpads of first three fingers, palpate: a. Both radial pulses at medial aspect of wrist (Fig. 9-13)		

ASSESSMENT PROCEDURE	EVALUATION	
	NORMAL FINDINGS	**DEVIATIONS FROM NORMAL**
b. Both femoral pulses, immediately inferior to inguinal ligament, midway between anterior superior iliac spine and pubic tubercle (*Note:* Firmer compression may be necessary for accurate palpation of obese clients.) (Fig. 9-14) c. Both popliteal pulses: press fingers firmly into popliteal fossae (Fig. 9-15) d. Both dorsalis pedis pulses: press lightly over dorsum of foot; foot should be moderately dorsiflexed (Fig. 9-16)	(*Note:* Dorsalis pedis pulses may be difficult to find or absent in some normal individuals.)	

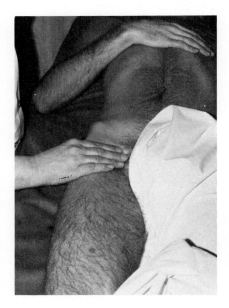

Fig. 9-14   Femoral artery palpation.

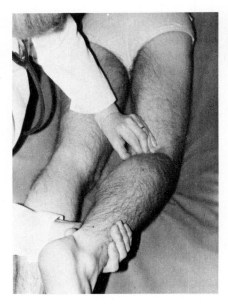

Fig. 9-15   Popliteal artery palpation.

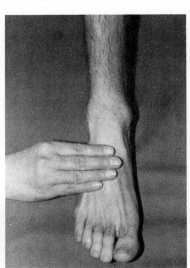

Fig. 9-16   Dorsalis pedis artery palpation.

Continued.

CLINICAL GUIDELINES—cont'd

	EVALUATION	
ASSESSMENT PROCEDURE	**NORMAL FINDINGS**	**DEVIATIONS FROM NORMAL**
e. Both posterior tibial pulses: curve fingers behind and slightly inferior to medial malleolus of ankle (Fig. 9-17)	(*Note:* Posterior tibial pulses may also be absent in some normal individuals.)	
7. Palpate all pulses for: a. Symmetrical response	All pulses should be full, strong, and symmetrical	Any asymmetry in force or pulse contour
b. Arterial wall contour and consistency	Soft and pliable	Increased resistance to compression; beaded or tortuous
8. Conduct the following maneuver if arterial insufficiency is suspected: a. With client lying down, elevate client's legs 30 cm (12 inches) above heart level		
b. Ask client to move feet up and down at ankles for 60 seconds	Extremities (feet) exhibit mild pallor	Marked pallor of one or both feet
c. Have client sit up and dangle legs (This maneuver can also be conducted with arms and hands.)	Original color returns in about 10 seconds Veins in feet fill in about 15 seconds	Delayed color return or mottled appearance (Fig. 9-18) Delayed venous filling Marked redness of dependent feet
9. Evaluate venous pressure by inspecting both sides of client's neck as he lies at 30° to 45° angle; elevate chin slightly and tilt away from side being examined		

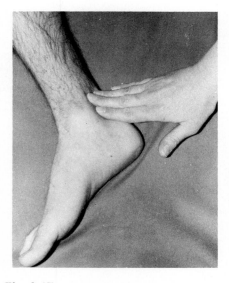

Fig. 9-17   Posterior tibial artery palpation.

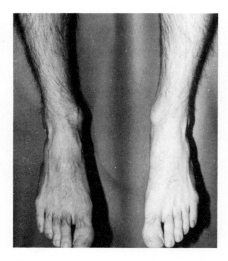

Fig. 9-18   Arterial insufficiency with contrasting pallor of foot in dependent position. Note increased venous filling on normal foot.

ASSESSMENT PROCEDURE	EVALUATION	
	NORMAL FINDINGS	DEVIATIONS FROM NORMAL
10. Identify highest point at which jugular vein blood level or pulsations can be seen, using sternal angle as reference point for "zero" level; estimate jugular venous pressure (JVP) in centimeters	JVP should not rise more than 3 cm (1 inch) above level of sternal angle* (Fig. 9-19)	JVP exceeds 3 cm above level of manubrium† (Fig. 9-20) Note if other veins in neck, shoulder, and upper chest are distended
11. Inspect jugular pulsations for quality	Regular Soft and undulating Level of pulsation decreases with inspiration Pulsation increases in recumbent position	Fluttering or oscillating Irregular rhythm Unusually prominent waves

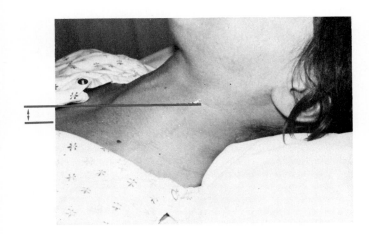

Fig. 9-19   Normal jugular venous pressure in external jugular vein. Blood level is less than 3 cm above the sternal angle.

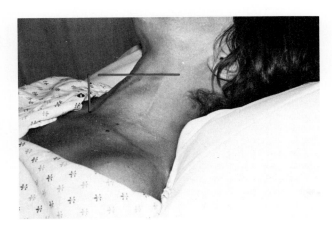

Fig. 9-20   Distended external jugular vein.

If jugular vein is difficult to locate, ask client to lie flat for a few minutes. Neck vein (particularly external jugular) should distend with client in this position.

†*If venous pressure is elevated (vein is distended up to neck), raise client's head until highest jugular pulsation can be detected. Record distance in centimeters above sternal angle* and *angle at which client is reclining.*   Continued.

CLINICAL GUIDELINES—cont'd

| | EVALUATION | |
ASSESSMENT PROCEDURE	NORMAL FINDINGS	DEVIATIONS FROM NORMAL
12. Inspect and palpate legs for presence and/or appearance of superficial veins	Distention in dependent position Venous valves may appear as nodular bulges Veins collapse with elevation of limbs	Distended veins in anteromedial aspect of thigh and lower leg or on posterolateral aspect of calf from knee to ankle (Fig. 9-21)
13. Inspect and palpate thigh and calf for surface characteristics	Legs symmetrical Nontender No excess warmth	Swelling (or one leg, especially calf, appears larger than other)* Tenderness on palpation Warmth Redness
14. Sharply dorsiflex client's foot (with knee slightly flexed) to assess calf pain response	No pain	Pain (Homans sign)
15. Inspect and palpate extremities for evidence of adequate arterial supply	Absence of hair over digits or dorsum of hands and feet may be normal Skin pink and warm, nonedematous	Reduced or absent peripheral hair (over digits and dorsum of hands and feet) Thin, shiny, taut skin Cold extremities (in warm environment) Mild edema

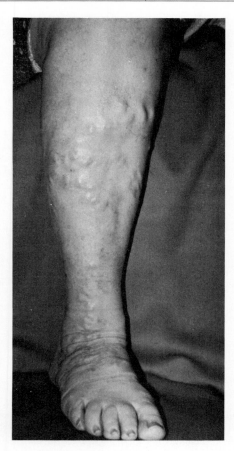

Fig. 9-21 Distended veins on lower leg with nodular bulges.

*If swelling is suspected, both thighs and calves should be measured with a tape to ensure accuracy.

ASSESSMENT PROCEDURE	EVALUATION	
	NORMAL FINDINGS	DEVIATIONS FROM NORMAL
16. Inspect and palpate extremities for evidence of venous sufficiency		Marked pallor or mottling when extremity is elevated Digit tips ulcerated Stocking anesthesia Tenderness on palpation Peripheral cyanosis Edema (pits on pressure), bilateral or unilateral* Pigmentation around ankles (See Fig. 3-3.) Thickening skin Ulceration (especially around ankles)
17. Observe client's general condition while lying supine or at elevation of 30° to 45°		

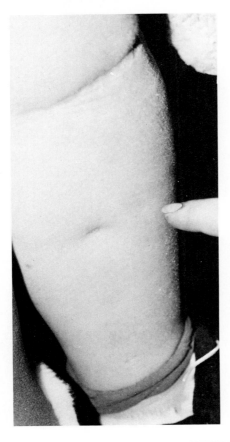

Fig. 9-22   Moderate pitting edema at midcalf. Note indentation at top of calf caused by constrictive stocking.

Edema should be measured against a bony prominence (over ankle or tibia). Record the following:

1. Type
  a. Pitting (Fig. 9-22)
  b. Nonpitting

2. Extent and location
  a. Ankle and foot
  b. Ankle only
  c. Foot to knee, etc.
  d. Hands and fingers

3. Degree of pitting
  a. 0 to 0.6 cm (0 to ¼ inch)—mild
  b. 0.6 to 1.3 cm (¼ to ½ inch)—moderate
  c. 1.3 to 2.5 cm (½ to 1 inch)—severe

4. Symmetrical or unilateral response

Continued.

CLINICAL GUIDELINES—cont'd

| | EVALUATION | |
ASSESSMENT PROCEDURE	NORMAL FINDINGS	DEVIATIONS FROM NORMAL
a. Positioning, comfort	Relaxed posture, without discomfort	Pain, coughing, or choking; "smothering" feeling; inability to lie flat for extended period
b. Respirations	Even and deep	Respirations uneven, shallow, gasping; inadequate exchange
c. Skin color	Pink/brown	Cyanosis, gray pallor Mottling Note color around lips, neck, upper chest
d. Nail color and configuration	Pink 106° angle at nail bed	Cyanotic Clubbing (angle disappears)
18. Inspect and palpate anterior chest a. Precordium (1) Contour	Rounded, symmetrical	Kyphosis Sternal depression Any asymmetry
(2) General movement: use palmar surface of hand and fingerpads (Fig. 9-23)	Even respiratory movements (precordium may lift slightly in thin people)	Entire chest heaving or lifting with heartbeat
19. Inspect and palpate the following specific areas (Fig. 9-24): a. Sternoclavicular area for pulsations	Slight or absent	Bounding
b. Aortic area (right second intercostal space adjacent to sternum) for pulsations	None	Pulsation, thrill (*Note:* Low-frequency vibrations can often be more easily felt than heard.)

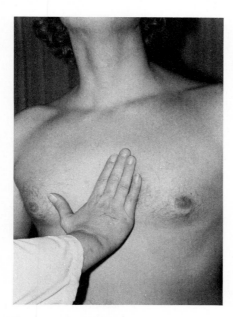

Fig. 9-23 Palpation over precordium. Note use of palmar surface of hand and finger pads.

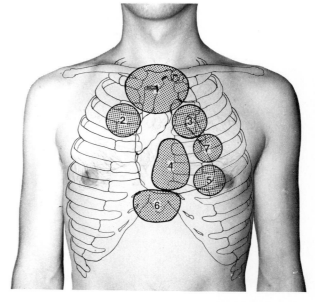

Fig. 9-24 Palpation areas for cardiac examination: *1,* sternoclavicular; *2,* aortic; *3,* pulmonary; *4,* anterior pericardium (right ventricular); *5,* apical; *6,* epigastric; *7,* ectopic.

ASSESSMENT PROCEDURE	EVALUATION	
	NORMAL FINDINGS	DEVIATIONS FROM NORMAL
c. Pulmonary area (left second intercostal space adjacent to sternum) for pulsations	None	Pulsation, thrill
d. Right ventricular area (left and right fifth intercostal space close to sternum) for heave or lift	May be present in hyperkinetic, thin, or pregnant adults	Diffuse lift or heave, pulsations e. Apical area (fifth intercostal space, 5 to 7 cm [2 to 3 inches] from midsternal line) (Fig. 9-25) for:
(1) Pulsation	May be present	
(2) Amplitude	Tapping	Thrusting
(3) Duration	First third to half systole	Sustained throughout systole
(4) Location	Fourth or fifth intercostal space, 5 to 7 cm from midsternal line*	Displaced left lateral or down
(5) Diameter	1 to 2 cm ($\frac{1}{3}$ to $\frac{1}{2}$ inch)	Over 2 cm ($\frac{1}{2}$ inch)
f. Epigastric area for pulsations: slide fingers up under rib cage	Aortic pulsation with forward thrust Right ventricular pulsation with downward thrust	Bounding pulsation
g. Ectopic area (midway between pulmonary and apical areas) for pulsations	None	Outward pulsation
20. Auscultate the following specific areas (Fig. 9-26) (*Note:* Even though auscultation areas are pictured as separate locations, examiner should "inch" from one area to next); use both diaphragm and bell to listen to all areas		

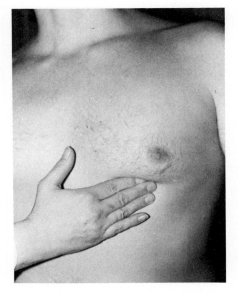

Fig. 9-25   Palpation for pulse at apical area. Finger pads are more sensitive to light pulsations.

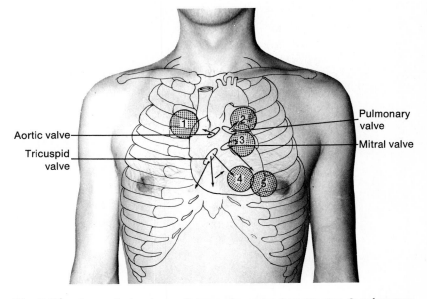

Fig. 9-26   Anatomical and auscultatory valve areas: *1,* aortic area; *2,* pulmonary area; *3,* third left interspace; *4,* tricuspid area; *5,* mitral area.

Note: Apical pulse location may displace slightly laterally if client turns to the left side.

Continued.

CLINICAL GUIDELINES—cont'd

ASSESSMENT PROCEDURE	EVALUATION	
	NORMAL FINDINGS	DEVIATIONS FROM NORMAL
a. Aortic area (second right interspace)		
b. Pulmonary area (second left interspace		
c. Third left interspace		
d. Tricuspid area (fifth left interspace near sternum)		
e. Apical area (fifth left interspace medial to midclavicular line)		
(1) Rate	60 to 90 beats/min (conditioned athletes or "seasoned" joggers may have normally slower rate)	Over 90 Under 60
(2) Rhythm	Regular	Irregular (without any pattern) Sporadic extra beats or pauses
(3) S_1 sound (mitral and tricuspid valve closure)		
(a) Location	Usually heard at all sites	
(b) Intensity	Often louder at apex (muscle, fat tissue, and air will diminish sound; rapid rate will accentuate sound)	Accented Diminished (muffled) Varying intensity with different beats (e.g., complete heart block)
(c) Frequency	Usually lower in pitch than S_2	Frequency (pitch) becomes higher with accented intensity
(d) Timing	Almost synchronous with carotid impulse Slightly longer in duration than S_2	
(e) Splitting	May be heard occasionally in tricuspid area Normal S_1 splitting sound usually varies from beat to beat: occasionally single sound, occasionally narrow split	S_4 sound sometimes mistaken for S_1 splitting
(4) S_2 sound (aortic and pulmonic valve closure)		
(a) Location	Usually heard at all sites	
(b) Intensity	Often louder at base (intensity diminished with fat, muscle, or air)	Increased intensity, usually in aortic (e.g., arterial hypertension) or pulmonary area (e.g., pulmonary hypertension)
(c) Frequency	Usually higher in pitch than S_1	Decreased intensity
(d) Timing	Sound shorter in duration than S_1	
(e) Splitting	Commonly heard in pulmonary area (on inspiration) in young adults	Wide splitting (e.g., right bundle branch block) Fixed splitting Paradoxical splitting (e.g., left bundle branch block)
(5) Systole		
(a) Duration	Shorter than diastole at normal heart rate (60 to 90 beats/min)	
(b) Sounds	S_1 sound duration brief; silent interval	Early systolic ejection click: Aortic—heard at base and apex Pulmonary—heard in pulmonary area

	EVALUATION	
ASSESSMENT PROCEDURE	**NORMAL FINDINGS**	**DEVIATIONS FROM NORMAL**
		Middle and late systolic clicks (e.g., mitral valve deformity) heard at left sternal border Clicks high pitched and sharp in sound
(6) Diastole		
(a) Duration	Longer than systole at normal rate (60 to 100 beats/min) Shortens in duration as rate increases	
(b) Sounds	S₂ duration brief Silent interval	
— S₃	S₃ normal in young adults	S₃ abnormal in older adults
— Location	Apex	Apex (may signify heart failure)
— Intensity	Dull, low pitched	Dull, low pitched
— Timing	Early in diastole (normal S₃ sounds often disappear when client sits up)	Early in diastole
— S₄		
— Location		Medial to apex
— Intensity	Rarely heard in normal client	Higher pitch
— Timing		Late diastole (may be confused with split S₁)
— Other sounds		Opening snap At apex Higher pitch Very early in diastole
(7) Murmurs	("Innocent" murmurs in children and young adults)	
(a) Timing	Usually early systolic, but characteristics are hard to differentiate from pathological sounds	Systolic: early, middle, late; continuous Diastolic: early, middle, late; continuous
(b) Location	Usually at pulmonary area, apex, or medial to apex	Area where sound is heard may be small and confined or may cover most of precordium Describe in terms of precordial landmarks and distance in centimeters from landmarks
(c) Radiation		Describe in relation to landmarks and centimeters distance
(d) Intensity	Soft, usually below grade 3 Varies with position and respiration	Grades 1 to 6, or loud, medium, soft Stable, or varies with respiration and position
(e) Pitch		High, medium, low
(f) Quality		Blowing, harsh, rumbling Crescendo Decrescendo
(8) Other sounds		Pericardial friction rub (to-and-fro rubbing sound, usually heard during systole and diastole; sound usually is increased when client sits up and leans forward)

Continued.

CLINICAL GUIDELINES—cont'd

		EVALUATION	
ASSESSMENT PROCEDURE	**NORMAL FINDINGS**	**DEVIATIONS FROM NORMAL**	
21. Auscultate over each carotid artery with bell of stethoscope (Fig. 9-27) to listen for possible bruits	Faint heart sounds are heard	Unilateral blowing or swishing sound (localized obstruction of carotid artery) Bilateral blowing or swishing sound (referred murmur sound from heart, or hyperkinetic state)	
22. Repeat palpation and auscultation maneuvers with client a. Lying in left decubitus position		Left decubitus position may enable examiner to pick up S_3 and S_4 sounds not heard in prone position	
b. Sitting		Sitting and leaning forward may highlight aortic murmurs not heard in prone position	

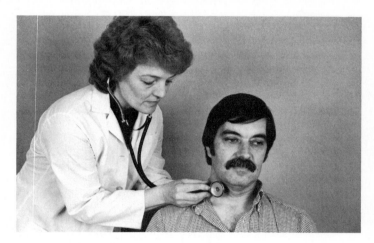

Fig. 9-27   Auscultation over the carotid arteries. Examiner lightly places stethoscope bell over area.

CLINICAL TIPS AND STRATEGIES

- **Measuring arterial blood pressure (arm):**
  1. Client should be comfortably seated, in a partially raised position, or lying down.
  2. Arm should be stabilized at heart level with the elbow slightly flexed.
  3. Arm should be uncovered; shirt sleeves should be removed, not rolled up, if they are at all constrictive.
  4. Cuff:
     a. Contains an inflatable bladder; width of this bladder should be 40% of circumference of arm (measure at midpoint between elbow and shoulder).
     b. Bladder should be centered over the artery.
     c. Lower edge should be placed 2 to 5 cm (1 to 2 inches) above the antecubital space.
     d. Should be completely deflated when applied.
     e. Should be snugly and smoothly wrapped around the arm.
     f. Tubing will rest at the medial aspect of the arm (Fig. 9-28).
  5. Examiner should be positioned comfortably so that:
     a. Aneroid or mercury gauge can be viewed at close range (closer than 90 cm [3 feet]).
     b. Aneroid gauge can be viewed straight on (avoiding an oblique view) (Fig. 9-29).
     c. Mercury column top is viewed at eye level.
  6. If a mercury manometer is used, it should be placed on a flat surface.
  7. Examiner should palpate the brachial or radial

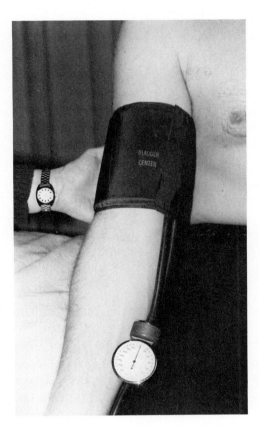

Fig. 9-28 Arterial blood pressure measurement. Note the following: (1) bladder is centered over artery; (2) lower edge of cuff is 3 cm above antecubital space: (3) deflated cuff is wrapped snugly and smoothly around arm; (4) tubing rests at medial aspect of arm.

artery and inflate the cuff 30 mm Hg above the point where the pulse is no longer palpated (Fig. 9-29).

8. Deflate the cuff slowly (2 to 3 mm Hg per heartbeat), and note onset of pulse.

9. Apply the stethoscope bell to the previously palpated brachial artery. The bell should be applied as lightly as possible but with no space between the skin and stethoscope. The stethoscope should not be in contact with the cuff or clothing.

10. Inflate the cuff 30 mm Hg above the point where the previously palpated pulse was obliterated. Deflate slowly (2 to 3 mm Hg per heartbeat).

11. Note (1) onset of first sound, (2) muffling (or change in character) of sound, and (3) disappearance of sound. (*Note:* In 1980 the Postgraduate Education Committee for the American Heart Association recommended that the diastolic reading be interpreted and recorded at the disappearance of sound for adults.)

12. If the blood pressure procedure must be repeated to clarify results, wait a minimum of 60 seconds to repeat. (Deflate cuff completely.)

13. Note variables that can alter client's blood pressure: eating, drinking, or smoking within 30 minutes before measurement is taken, exercise, anxiety, cold environment, pain or discomfort, exertion, bladder distention.

• **Measuring arterial blood pressure (thigh):**
1. Client should be lying prone.
2. Leg should be stabilized and uncovered (no re-

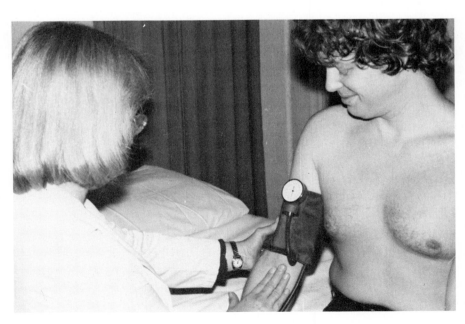

Fig. 9-29 Blood pressure measurement. Examiner views gauge "straight on" within a 90 cm range. Examiner palpates brachial artery before auscultation maneuver.

strictive clothing bunched or rolled at upper thigh).

3. Cuff:
   a. Should be wider and longer than that used for client's arm (e.g., an 18 to 20 cm bag).
   b. Should be applied over midthigh so that the bladder is centered over the posterior aspect.
4. Examiner must be positioned so that the aneroid or mercury guage can be viewed at close distance. The mercury column should be at eye level.
5. Examiner should palpate the popliteal fossa and locate the pulsation.
6. Place the stethoscope over the artery and proceed as with brachial pressure maneuvers.
7. *Note:* Examiner can anticipate that popliteal systolic arterial pressure will register higher (5 to 15 mm Hg) than brachial systolic pressure.
8. Diastolic pressure is usually the same or slightly lower.

- **If jugular pulsations are difficult to find have the client lie flat for maximum venous distention:** It is recommended that the internal jugular vein be viewed for registering venous pressure. However, it is often difficult to locate because of its anatomical placement. Be certain not to confuse the arterial with the venous pulsations. Venous pulsations (1) are less vigorous (of an undulating quality), (2) can be eliminated by pressing over the clavicle, (3) increase in intensity when the client is recumbent, and (4) are rarely palpable.

- **Inspect and palpate the extremities carefully:** Foot pulses (dorsalis pedis) are sometimes difficult or impossible to find. *Note:* A cold environment may alter the appearance and temperature of extremities.

- **Inspect the client carefully before proceeding with palpation and auscultation:** Stand back and view the entire person. Establish a general picture of posture, comfort, character of respiration, tension, and general skin color.

- **Inspect the precordium** *carefully:* Beginners

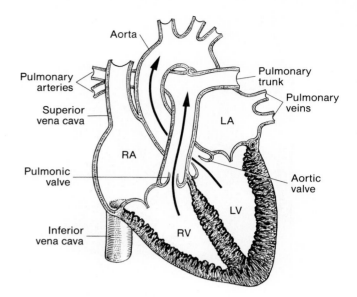

Fig. 9-30   Ventricular systole; contraction of ventricles.

sometimes tend to miss the obvious because they are anxious to auscultate. View the entire anterior chest. It is possible that the whole chest could be heaving. Then let your eyes focus on each inspection site described in the guidelines.

- **Ensure good lighting:** It is necessary for good inspection.

- **Develop a careful routine for cardiac auscultation:** First, one should have a clear mental image of the cardiac cycle as one differentiates sounds and identifies silences. S_1 (the closure of the mitral and tricuspid valves) occurs early in systole as the ventricles contract and force blood into the aorta and the pulmonary artery (Fig. 9-30). In diastole, the ventricles relax, the mitral and tricuspid valves open to receive blood, and the pulmonic and aortic valves close (S_2) (Fig. 9-31).

Next, one should develop a system for listening and

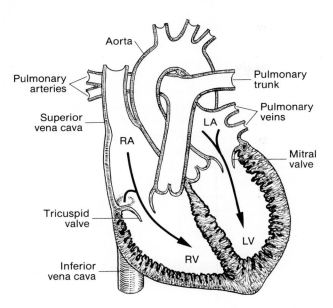

Fig. 9-31   Ventricular diastole; relaxation of ventricles.

concentration. Differentiate S_1 from S_2. Differentiate systole from diastole. Note the timing and characteristics of the silences, as well as the sounds. All of these details are described in the guidelines. Practice them carefully. For the beginner, each entity must be evaluated separately. It is impossible to hear everything initially.

In addition, create an auscultation routine that becomes consistent with each examination. There are a number of choices: moving from base to apex or apex to base, having the client sit first or lie down first, alternating diaphragm with bell, or completing the use of one before beginning the other, etc. Establish a systematic approach that is comfortable for you.

Finally, *take your time* and listen until you are secure with each characteristic. One cannot accurately identify abnormalities until one is confident with identifying what is normal. One laboratory exercise that is helpful is to ask your partner to run in place for a minute, then listen carefully for the changes in intensity, pitch, and timing of sounds. Also, listen for the differences in the timing of the silences. This listening exercise develops sensitivity to the subtle changes of sound.

- **When auscultating, "inch" the endpiece along the route (avoid "jumping" from one site to another):** This maneuver helps avoid missing important sounds.
- **Stabilize the endpiece on the chest:** Let your fourth and fifth fingers, or your wrist, rest on the adjacent chest wall. This will prevent sliding and extraneous noise. Use light pressure with the bell and a firmer pressure with the diaphragm.
- **Heart sounds are better heard if the client breathes out and holds the expiration:** Asking the client to breathe out and to lean forward while in a sitting position is helpful.
- **For women with large breasts displace the breast upward with one hand and palpate or auscultate with the other:** Some clients can assist in displacement.
- **Place a hand on the client's shoulder:** This will steady him while he is sitting.

SAMPLE RECORDING: NORMAL FINDINGS

Pulses, pressures: Carotid, radial, femoral, dorsalis pedis, and posterior tibial pulses symmetrical, strong, and regular. No bruits. Jugular venous pressure at the level of the sternal angle while client elevated at 30°.

Extremities: Warm, without pallor, cyanosis, edema. No varicosities or calf tenderness. Homans sign negative.

Precordium/heart: No thrills, heaves, or pulsations other than PMI barely palpable at fifth left ICS, 8 cm from midsternal line. AP = RP. S_1 and S_2 are brief and clear. No extra sounds or murmurs.

The Newborn

HISTORY AND CLINICAL STRATEGIES

- General skin color is an important aspect of cardio-vascular assessment of the newborn. Cyanosis (blue), pallor (white), plethora (purple), and jaundice (yellow) tones need investigation and management of underlying causes.
- Capillary filling time is assessed by blanching a central and peripheral area. A time of greater than 3 seconds suggests abnormality. Capillary filling time is difficult to assess in a foot or hand that still shows acrocyanosis (blueness of hands and feet soon after delivery).

- Pulses should be strong and equal. Systemic blood pressures should be measured when infants are quiet. Normal pressures depend on birth weights, but range between 55 and 80 mm Hg systolic and 30 and 55 mm Hg diastolic. Palpation of the precordium determines the point of maximum impulse (PMI). It is usually located to the left of the fourth intercostal space.
- Heartbeats in newborns are irregular and should be counted for an entire minute. A murmur may be present while the ductus arteriosus is closing soon after birth. Bradycardia and tachycardia are not normal and should be evaluated.

CLINICAL VARIATIONS: THE NEWBORN

CHARACTERISTIC OR AREA EXAMINED	NORMAL FINDINGS	DEVIATIONS FROM NORMAL
1. Position and sounds	Point of maximum impulse (PMI), heart pulsation, at 4th or 5th intercostal space to left, medial of midclavicular line "Toc-tip" sound of 1st and 2nd heart sounds Transient murmur (may be closing patent ductus arteriosus (PDA)	Epigastric pulsations (suggests enlarged heart) Shifted PMI (may be pneumothorax, diaphragmatic hernia, dextrocardia Persistent murmur extending into diastole Dysrhythmias Pallor, cyanosis (may be heart condition) More cyanosis with crying, bradycardia, tachycardia, tachypnea, poor feeding, foot and face edema (suggests heart problem) Pedal edema (may be Turner syndrome)
2. Pulses and pressure	Equal and full femoral and brachial pulses without bounding Pronounced jugular pulse disappears a few hours after birth Capillary filling time 3 seconds or less for skin color return after blanching peripheral area Blood pressure (BP) varies with birth weight and gestational age Usual heart rate 120-160 beats per minute Heart rate variability not more than 6-10 beats per minute (BPM)	Weak femoral, strong brachial pulses (suggests coarctation of aorta) Bounding pulses (may be PDA, aortic valve insufficiency) Hypotension (may be respiratory, cardiac, circulatory, or other disease, problem) Hypertension (suggests renal disease)

The Child

HISTORY AND CLINICAL STRATEGIES

- There are basically two types of cardiovascular disease in children. The first is a *congenital* problem with the heart itself or its pumping mechanisms. The second type, called *acquired,* occurs as the result of a systemic disease, such as rheumatic fever.
- The examiner must use every sense available to evaluate the child's cardiovascular system. The obvious decompensating characteristics, such as cyanosis, peripheral edema, and dyspnea, will be recognized early and easily. But it is the subtle, early signs and symptoms that the examiner must continuously watch for. Early warning symptoms of a *potential* cardiovascular problem *may be:*
  1. Infant who becomes tired of sucking and must rest periodically before able to finish
  2. Infant who has tachycardia and tachypnea while eating
  3. Child who is reported to tire frequently during playing (In this case it is important to clarify how much and what kinds of activities cause fatigue: an hour of playing tag vs. a short walk.)
  4. Child who is reported to "turn blue" with prolonged crying episodes
  5. Child who requires several rest/sleep periods during the day beyond what is normal for the age
  6. Child who repeatedly complains that he does not want to go out and play because he cannot keep up with the others or because he becomes short of breath or tired when he plays
  7. Child who assumes a knee-chest position during sleeping; or squats instead of sits when playing or watching television
  8. Child who complains of leg pains with running (inquire as to how much running causes pains and what pains actually feel like)
  9. Excessively labored breathing in an infant during defecation
  10. Child who is falling behind the normal growth and development schedule
  11. Child with a history of frequent headaches or nosebleeds accompanying a rise in blood pressure and/or leg cramping

  Although any single symptom listed above may not be caused by cardiovascular dysfunction, it warrants full investigation of additional subjective and objective data.
- Cardiovascular evaluation of the child extends far beyond examination of the heart. The evaluation should begin as the examiner first sees the child. The overall health, nutritional state, color, ease of respirations, and general overt qualities of the child should communicate information about the child's cardiovascular function.

- The blood pressure of children under the age of 1 year may be difficult to obtain because of improper cuff size or excessive baby fat or simply because the child is extremely wiggly. The examiner can be assured that if the infant is screaming and pink, the blood pressure is substantial. It is the lethargic or ill-appearing infant whose blood pressure must be measured and recorded. If the examiner has difficulty obtaining an audible blood pressure, a Doppler may be used.
- Following are general guidelines for obtaining blood pressure readings in children:
  1. Every child 18 months and older should be screened for hypertension. This means that the child's blood pressure should be evaluated during every well-child examination.
  2. Equipment for obtaining pediatric blood pressures is the same as for the adult. The cuff should not be larger than two thirds or smaller than half of the length of the child's arm between the elbow and shoulder. Proper size of cuffs is mandatory for adequate evaluation of children. Pediatric cuffs are available in 2½ and 5 inch sizes. (Table 9-4.)
  3. The American Heart Association states that the muffling of the blood pressure tone in children should actually be considered the diastolic reading.
  4. Crying or sudden jerking may alter the child's blood pressure between 5 and 10 mm Hg. The child should be evaluated during a quiet period.
  5. Every child should have at least one or two thigh screening blood pressure measurements during early childhood to rule out a vast difference between upper and lower extremity pressure (a sign of coarctation of the aorta).
- Fever in a child will normally increase the child's pulse. For every degree of fever, the pulse may increase 8 to 10 beats/min.
- In physically examining the child's cardiovascular system, the techniques of inspection, palpation, and auscultation are normally used. Percussion may be used by the experienced examiner with the older child, but generally small patients poorly tolerate the procedure.

TABLE 9-4 Guidelines for choosing correct width of blood pressure cuff for children

AGE (yr)	CUFF WIDTH (cm)
Less than 1½	4.5
1½ to 2	8
2 to 10	9.5
Older than 10	12

Data from Waring WW, Jeansonne LO: Practical manual of pediatrics: a pocket reference for those who treat children, ed 2, St Louis, 1982, Mosby–Year Book.

- All techniques require that the child be undressed to the underwear and sitting on the table (infants may be held). It is helpful for cooperative children to recline to a 45-degree angle during examination. If that is impossible, a supine position is preferable to an upright position because more cardiovascular "sounds" are generally heard with the child lying down.
- Auscultating the hearts of infants and toddlers is a true feat. The child must be quiet during the examination. Crying, talking, or pulling at the stethoscope tubing will defeat the process. The examiner is encouraged to examine the cardiovascular system early during the examination before the child becomes frightened, bored, or cold.
- As will be discussed in subsequent clinical guidelines, a child's chest should be auscultated in the same spots as an adult's heart. Because of the rapidity of a child's heart rate, the examiner may need to listen to each selected area for a fairly long time to feel comfortable in describing the findings. Some parents may become concerned because of the long listening time; therefore it is suggested that the examiner explain to the parent that a long listening time is not a cause for concern.
- If the examiner identifies any unusual findings, suggestive history, extra noises, or murmurs, it is recommended that the child be referred to a physician for further verification. The beginning examiner should *not* attempt to define a murmur as "functional" or an extra odd heart sound as insignificant. It is the examiner's duty at this time to identify normal findings and to recognize and refer abnormal or suggestive findings. The cardiovascular health of a young child is too valuable to provide an experimental opportunity for the examiner.

Text continues on p. 302.

CLINICAL VARIATIONS: THE CHILD

CHARACTERISTIC OR AREA EXAMINED	NORMAL FINDINGS		DEVIATIONS FROM NORMAL	
Assessment of pressures, pulses, and the peripheral vascular system				
1. Blood pressure: technique described under "Clinical Tips and Strategies," p. 290			Elevated blood pressures are those that exceed the following readings†	
	*Mean systolic** (± 2 S.D.)	*Mean diastolic** (± 2 S.D.)		
a. Sitting or lying, depending on age	Newborn 80 ± 16	46 ± 16	3 to 6 yr‡	>110/70
	2 mo to 1 yr 89 ± 29	60 ± 10	6 to 9 yr‡	>120/75
	1 yr 96 ± 30	66 ± 25	10 to 13 yr‡	>130/80
	2 yr 99 ± 25	64 ± 25	14 yr‡	
	3 yr 100 ± 25	67 ± 23	M	>133/82
	4 yr 99 ± 20	65 ± 20	F	>128/84
	5 to 6 yr 94 ± 14	55 ± 9	15 yr§	
	6 to 7 yr 100 ± 15	56 ± 8	M	>137/85
	7 to 8 yr 102 ± 15	56 ± 8	F	>128/84
	8 to 9 yr 105 ± 16	57 ± 9	16 to 19 yr§	
	9 to 10 yr 107 ± 17	57 ± 9	M	>140/85
	10 to 11 yr 111 ± 17	58 ± 10	F	>128/84
	11 to 12 yr 113 ± 18	59 ± 10		
	12 to 13 yr 115 ± 19	59 ± 10		
	13 to 14 yr 118 ± 19	60 ± 10		
	Pressure in both arms is same or does not vary more than 5 to 10 mm Hg		Significant (>5 to 10 mm Hg) discrepancy in pressure readings between upper extremities	

Data from Haggerty RJ, Maroney MW, Nadas AS: Am J Dis Child 92:536, 1956, Copyright 1973, American Medical Association.
†Data from Londe S, Goldring D: Am J Cardiol 37:650, 1976.
‡Supine reading
§Seated reading.

CLINICAL VARIATIONS: THE CHILD—cont'd

CHARACTERISTIC OR AREA EXAMINED	NORMAL FINDINGS	DEVIATIONS FROM NORMAL
b. Standing	(Not routinely done with children. If problem is suspected, have child stand up. Follow adult guidelines.)	
	Pulse pressure between 20 and 50 mm Hg throughout childhood	Narrowing of pulse pressure seen with aortic stenosis
		Widening of pulse pressure may be seen in children with patent ductus arteriosus or aortic regurgitation
c. Thigh measurement: technique same as adult	In child less than 1 year, systolic pressure in thigh should equal that of arm	Systolic pressure in thigh measurement is *lower* than systolic arm measurement (sign of coarctation of aorta)
	In child over 1 year, systolic pressure in thigh greater than that in arm by 10 to 40 mm Hg; diastolic pressure in thigh equals that in arm	
2. Carotid artery palpation a. Rate		Any findings beyond limits stated

Age*	Rate/min*
Newborn	100 to 180
12 mo	80 to 160
2 yr	80 to 130
3 yr	80 to 120
4 yr	80 to 120
6 yr	75 to 115
Beyond 6 yr	70 to 110

CHARACTERISTIC OR AREA EXAMINED	NORMAL FINDINGS	DEVIATIONS FROM NORMAL
		Increases may be caused by factors such as toxicity, fever, excitement, and respiratory distress
		Decreases may be caused by heart block, digitalis poisoning, sepsis, *Salmonella* infection
b. Rhythm	Regular	Irregular pulse unrelated to breathing†
	Sinus arrhythmia: pulse rate will speed up with inspiration and slow down with expiration; makes pulse seem irregular in rhythm; to further evaluate, instruct child to hold breath while you continue to feel pulse; rate should become regular	
	Carefully watch respirations in infant to evaluate if pulse rhythm fluctuates with breathing	
	Common in children over age 3 years and especially prominent at puberty	
	Especially prominent at puberty	
	Extrasystoles or premature ventricular contractions (PVC) *may* be normal in healthy child; will feel like skipped beat; emotional factors may trigger; exercise will usually cause disappearance	Extrasystoles or PVCs heard for first time in ill child; child with known cardiac disease; or child with suggestive or questionable history
c. Pulse amplitude	Pulse upstroke smooth, rounded, and prompt	Upstroke exaggerated, bounding, weak, thready

*Gillette PC: Dysrhythmias. In Adams FH, and others: Moss' heart disease in infants, children, and adolescents, ed 3, Baltimore, 1983, Williams & Wilkins.

†An irregular (rapid or slow) pulse should be palpated simultaneously with auscultation of the apical pulse. Any difference between apical and peripheral pulse rate should be noted. If pulse irregularity is patterned (occurs in repeated sequences), note whether irregularity occurs during (1) inspiration or expiration and (2) systole or diastole.

Continued.

CLINICAL VARIATIONS: THE CHILD—cont'd

CHARACTERISTIC OR AREA EXAMINED	NORMAL FINDINGS	DEVIATIONS FROM NORMAL
Assessment of pressures, pulses, and the peripheral vascular system—cont'd		
d. Amplitude pattern	Series of pulse strokes unvaried in amplitude or contour	Upstrokes vary; for example, strong and weaker beats alternate (pulsus alternans)
e. Symmetry	Symmetrical response (i.e., both carotid pulses manifest same rate, rhythm, amplitude, and contour)	Asymmetrical response
f. Arterial wall contour	Soft and pliable	Increased resistance to compression, beaded or tortuous
3. Radial artery palpation 4. Popliteal pulse palpation 5. Dorsalis pedis pulse palpation 6. Posterior tibial pulse palpation 7. Femoral pulse palpation	(Pulses in nos. 4 to 6 may or may not be evaluated, depending on the age and overall health of the child. Any child with known cardiovascular disease or suggestive symptomatology should receive a thorough evaluation. Other children are normally screened by evaluating carotid, femoral, radial, and apical pulses. Criteria for evaluation have been listed previously.)	Significant difference between radial and femoral pulses Weak or absent femoral pulses may indicate coarctation of aorta
8. Evaluation of venous pressures (Not routinely done in well children.)	Jugular veins may be visible but should not pulsate or appear engorged	Noted pulsations of neck or engorgement
9. Evidence of adequate arterial supply	Warm, pink, nonedematous extremities Mottling (if infant is in cool environment and has been uncovered for some time)	Thin, shiny, taut skin Cold or mottled extremities in warm environment Edema* Marked pallor Tenderness of skin
10. Evidence of adequate venous sufficiency		Peripheral cyanosis Edema* Thickening of skin
Assessment of the heart and precordium		
1. General appearance a. Positioning, comfort	Playing Relaxed posture, without discomfort	Client experiencing pain, coughing or choking, "smothering" feeling (unable to lie flat for extended period)
b. Respirations	Even and deep	Respirations uneven, shallow, gasping Inadequate exchange
c. Skin color	Pink/brown	Cyanosis, gray pallor Mottling Variation of color around lips, neck, upper chest

Often one associates heart failure with peripheral edema. In children, however, the signs of heart failure are quite different. Signs may include a rapid respiratory rate in the supine position followed by slight dyspnea, liver enlargement, venous engorgement, orthopnea, pulsus alternans, and a gallop rhythm. Only very late in its course are signs of pulmonary or peripheral edema noticeable (Barness, 1990).

CHARACTERISTIC OR AREA EXAMINED	NORMAL FINDINGS	DEVIATIONS FROM NORMAL
d. Nail color and configuration	Pink 160° angle at nail bed	Cyanotic Clubbing (angle disappears)
2. Anterior chest precordium		
a. Contour	Rounded, symmetrical	Kyphosis Sternal depression Any asymmetry
b. General movement	Even respiratory movements (precordium may lift slightly in thin children)	Areas of bulging, or entire chest heaving or lifting with heartbeat Appearance of thrill across chest wall
3. Inspection and palpation (Child should be sitting and leaning forward.)		
a. Sternoclavicular area pulsations	Slight or absent	Bounding
b. Aortic area (second right intercostal space beside sternum) pulsations	None	Pulsation, thrill (*Note:* Low-frequency vibrations can often be more easily felt than heard.)
c. Pulmonary area (second and third left intercostal spaces near sternum) pulsations	May feel some slight pulsations after physical activity	Thrill or strong pulsations that continue even when patient is at rest
d. Right ventricular area (third, fourth, and fifth intercostal spaces to right and left over sternum); note difference from adult	Very thin children may feel slight palpations	Systolic thrill, strong pulsations Heaves
e. Apical area (PMI) (infants and small children: fourth intercostal space to left of midclavicular line; after age 7 years, fifth intercostal space to right of the midclavicular line)		
(1) Pulsation	May be present May be difficult to palpate in children under 2 years	
(2) Amplitude	Tapping	Thrusting
(3) Duration	First third to half systole	Sustained throughout systole
(4) Location	As described	Displaced lateral left or down
(5) Diameter	1 to 1.5 cm (⅓ inch)	More than 2 cm (¾ inch)
f. Epigastric area (at sternal angle) pulsations	Aortic pulsations with forward thrust Right ventricular pulsation with downward thrust	Bounding pulsation
g. Ectopic area (space between pulmonary and aortic area) pulsations	None	Outward pulsations
4. Auscultation (child sitting)		
a. Aortic area (location as discussed)		

Continued.

CLINICAL VARIATIONS: THE CHILD—cont'd

CHARACTERISTIC OR AREA EXAMINED	NORMAL FINDINGS	DEVIATIONS FROM NORMAL
Assessment of the heart and precordium—cont'd		
b. Pulmonary area (location as discussed)		
c. Third left intercostal space (Erb's point)		
d. Tricuspid area (fifth interspace near sternum to right in young children; to left in older children)		
e. Apical area (location as discussed)		
(1) Rate	As previously discussed	As previously discussed
(2) Rhythm	Described under *pulses*	Described under *pulses*
(3) Pitch	Higher pitch/shorter duration than in adult	
(4) S_1 sound		
(a) Location	Usually heard at all sites	
(b) Intensity	Often louder at apex (Muscle, fat tissue, and air will diminish sound; rapid rate will accentuate sound.)	Accented Diminished (muffled) Varying intensity with different beats (e.g., complete heart block)
(c) Frequency	Usually lower in pitch than S_2	Frequency (pitch) becomes higher with accented intensity
(d) Timing	Almost synchronous with carotid impulse Slightly longer in duration than S_2	
(e) Splitting	May be heard occasionally in tricuspid area	
	Normal S_1 splitting sound usually varies from beat to beat, occasionally a single sound, occasionally a narrow split	S_4 sometimes mistaken for S_1 splitting
(5) S_2 sound		
(a) Location	Usually heard at all sites May be loudest in pulmonary area	
(b) Intensity	Often louder at base Intensity diminished with fat, muscle, or air	Increased intensity, usually in aortic area (e.g., arterial hypertension) or pulmonary area (e.g., pulmonary hypertension) Decreased intensity
(c) Frequency	Usually higher in pitch than S_1	
(d) Timing	Sound shorter in duration than S_1	
(e) Splitting	Commonly heard in pulmonary area (on inspiration) in child Equal quality and intensity of sound	Wide splitting (e.g., right bundle branch block) Fixed splitting Paradoxical splitting (e.g., left bundle branch block) Area of apex

CHARACTERISTIC OR AREA EXAMINED	NORMAL FINDINGS	DEVIATIONS FROM NORMAL
(6) Systole		
(a) Duration	Shorter than diastole at normal heart rate	
(b) Sounds	S_1 sound duration brief; silent interval	Early systolic ejection click: aortic—heard at base and apex; pulmonary—heard in pulmonary area
		Middle and late systolic clicks (e.g., mitral valve deformity) heard at left sternal border
		Clicks high pitched and sharp in sound
(7) Diastole		
(a) Duration	Longer than systole at normal rate	
	Shortens in duration as rate increases	
(b) Sounds	S_2 duration brief	
	Silent interval	
(8) S_3 sound	May be normal in children and young adults (may occur in as many as 30% of all children)	
(a) Location	Apex	
(b) Intensity	Different intensity from second sound, dull, low in pitch	
(c) Timing	Early in diastole	
(9) S_4 sound	Never normal	
(a) Location		Medial to apex
(b) Intensity		Higher pitch
(c) Timing		Late diastole (may be confused with split S_1)
		Opening snap: at apex; higher pitch; very early in diastole
(10) Other sounds		Pericardial friction rub: scratchy, high pitched, grating sound, unaffected by change in respirations
f. Murmurs	"Innocent" murmurs	"Organic" or "functional" murmurs
(1) Timing	Usually early systolic	Systolic or diastolic at any point during or continuous
(2) Location	Second or third intercostal space along left sternal border	
(3) Position in which heard	Usually supine	Heard in all positions
(4) Duration	Short	Longer
(5) Quality	Soft and musical	Louder, blowing, harsh, rumbling
(6) Intensity	Soft (grades 1, 2)	Loud (grades 3, 4, 5)
(7) Affected by exercise	Yes	Constant
5. Repeat palpation and auscultation with child lying and in left decubitus position		

The Childbearing Woman

HISTORY AND CLINICAL STRATEGIES

- Heart auscultation may be difficult in women with pendulous breasts. Ask the patient to hold her left breast upward and to the left.
- Changes in murmurs and heart sounds normally occur in pregnancy around the 12th to 20th week of gestation, and they subside near the end of the first week after delivery.
- Blood pressure should be assessed throughout pregnancy, because pregnancy-induced hypertension may occur. Pregnancy may promote feelings of dyspnea, orthopnea, fatigue, and palpitations. These symptoms should be evaluated.

CLINICAL VARIATIONS: THE CHILDBEARING WOMAN

CHARACTERISTIC OR AREA EXAMINED	NORMAL FINDINGS	DEVIATIONS FROM NORMAL
1. Heart	Increased heart rate to 10-15 beats per minute, from adjustment to increased blood volume Heart is shifted transversely (caused by uterus and diaphragm positions) Audible murmurs may occur (from changed heart position about 12-20 weeks) Increased S_1 split (from early closure of mitral valve) Heart palpitations (from sympathetic nervous system or thoracic pressure)	Patients with preexisting cardiac conditions may have pronounced symptoms (from pregnancy-induced increased volume)
2. Blood pressure (BP) and vascular changes	BP may decrease in 2nd trimester (from decreased peripheral resistance) BP rises to usual level during 3rd trimester Supine hypotension syndrome may occur; faintness, palpitations, sweating, pallor, when lying on back (from uterus pressure on vessels) Edema of legs and increased varicosities (from increased blood volume, decreased venous tone, pressure on inferior vena cava)	Pregnancy-induced hypertension (140/90 mm Hg or higher) Chronic hypertension, occurring before 20th week, may worsen, especially during 3rd trimester (there is risk of cerebral hemorrhage)
3. Postdelivery	After delivery, heart begins shifting back into place Supine hypotension ceases Prepregnant levels occur within days after delivery When uterus empties, pressure is removed from vena cava Bradycardia, pulse 40-50, may occur early in postpartum period	Leg pain, red and warm areas, edema (may be thrombophlebitis; trauma) Increasing edema (may be toxemia, cellulitis, renal problems, trauma) Signs of heart failure (cardiac patients at most risk 1-3 days postdelivery from increased cardiac output) Low BP (may be sign of toxemia) Tachycardia (may be anemia, hypotension)

The Older Adult

HISTORY AND CLINICAL STRATEGIES

The incidence of cardiovascular disease is higher in elderly individuals than in younger adults. However, the examiner should not assume that all elderly people are suffering from hypertension, cardiac or coronary artery disease, or vascular impairment.

The heart size of an older client who is not hypertensive or manifesting a heart disease often becomes smaller. Cardiac enlargement is usually associated with hypertension or other disease within the heart or vessels.

At rest, cardiac output decreases by 30% to 40% by 65 to 70 years of age. However, general organ atrophy and reduced exertion decrease the need for blood flow. Several authors have stated that the aging heart functions well under *normal* conditions but may not be able to respond efficiently to increased circulatory needs associated with extreme stress, blood loss, tachycardia, unusual exertion, or fever.

Although the process of arteriosclerosis advances with age, the amount of circulatory inadequacy at any given age is not predictable. This process may not cause symptoms or signs in many individuals.

Signs or symptoms associated with cardiovascular disease in the elderly are often the same as those manifested in younger adults. (Refer to the history portion of the adult cardiovascular section, pp. 276-278, for related questions.)

Following are special needs, concerns, and responses of older adults in relation to cardiovascular problems.

- Angina pectoris. In some instances the elderly individual may not experience chest pain to the extent that a younger person does. Dyspnea or palpitation on exertion may be reported as an initial symptom. Chest pain radiation may be reported as a "tightness" in the chest, neck, or shoulder. The pain radiation pattern is usually the same as with younger adults.
- Confusion or slowed mental function may be an early sign of low cardiac output. Note that confusion (even in mild form) alters the client's ability to provide an accurate account of symptoms.
- Other early symptoms of cardiac distress are fatigue, light-headedness, or weakness.
- Explore complaints such as "fatigue," "out of breath," and "tired" carefully. They are sometimes used interchangeably to indicate dyspnea. The precise amount of exertion that precedes the symptom should be described. Note that shortness of breath may indicate many problems other than heart disease. Sedentary elderly people with limited cardiac reserve may complain of breathlessness. Clarify whether shortness of breath interferes with sleep. If insomnia or wakefulness coexists with the dyspnea, clarify the number of times the client awakens each night and exactly what is done to deal with the symptom.
- Coughing and wheezing may be indicative of heart disease, particularly if the onset is sudden or recent.
- Dizziness, syncope, palpitations, or transient ischemial attacks may be associated with arrhythmias. Chest pain may accompany these symptoms.
- Transient ischemial attacks are usually of limited duration (15 to 20 minutes) and are indicated by a variety of symptoms or signs. Dizziness, confusion, unilateral weakness or numbness, and aphasia are some of the complaints. These episodes often leave little or no aftereffects and frequently precede a stroke. Carotid arterial atherosclerosis can contribute to these "attacks." A history of "spells" or "attacks" should be a signal for immediate referral to a physician.
- A complaint of hemoptysis may be associated with congestive heart failure or a pulmonary embolism.
- Edema of both legs is often associated with heart disease. Clarify the pattern of swelling with the client in terms of frequency and time of day when it is most pronounced.
- Weakness, bradycardia, hypotension, and confusion may indicate an excess of potassium, which sometimes occurs in conjunction with therapeutic measures for heart disease.
- Weakness, fatigue, muscle cramps, and a variety of arrhythmias may indicate a low potassium level.
- Digitalis toxicity may be indicated by anorexia, nausea, vomiting, diarrhea, headache, yellow vision, arrhythmias, or mental confusion
- Hypertension. Some authors state that the systolic pressure may normally rise gradually as an individual ages. Other authorities feel that the average systolic pressure is not altered by age. Most authors agree that the diastolic pressure does not change markedly with aging. The Joint National Committee on Detection, Evaluation, and Treatment of High Blood Pressure recommended in 1976 that blood pressures of individuals over 50 years of age in the range of 140/90 to 160/95 be rechecked in 6 to 9 months. The final diagnosis of hypertension is usually based on a number of blood pressure readings taken over a period of weeks or months. An elderly individual's blood pressure may fluctuate widely from one assessment to another (particularly the systolic pressure).

Most of the time, hypertension is asymptomatic. Severe hypertension may produce symptoms of headache (dull, in the morning), memory impairment, visual changes, epistaxis, angina pectoris, and dyspnea on exertion.

One of the major problems associated with hypertension is maintaining client compliancy with prescribed therapy. The following questions might be helpful in assessing the hypertensive client:

1. How much of a problem is hypertension for you in terms of:
   a. Symptoms
   b. Interference with activities of daily living
   c. Taking medications
2. Do you feel the prescribed therapy is effective?
3. Do you have any difficulty with the therapy (e.g., fear of addiction to drugs, side effects of drugs, false hope that drugs will "cure" the problem, wishing to take medication only when hypertensive symptoms occur)?
4. Have you had any experience with other family members (or close friends) who had hypertension?

- If the examiner is assessing a client who offers a history of chronic heart or vascular disease, the effects of disability or symptoms, the client's coping skills, and state of "chronicity" should be explored. (Review questions in Chapter 1 under *Activities of Daily Living Assessment* (in box on p. 26) and "Psychosocial History" on p. 30.) The overall concerns to be covered are:
   1. The client's understanding of his health state
   2. The client's comprehension of his therapy
   3. The client's overall *feelings* about his state of health and the success of the therapy
   4. Interference with activities of daily living
   5. The client's self-assessment of his and his family's coping ability
- *Note:* Some elderly clients have difficulty complying with examiner requests for body position or breathing patterns during the physical assessment. It may be impossible for an individual to lie flat for any extended period. It may be difficult to fully exhale and to hold the exhalation for the required period of listening time. The examination may have to proceed more slowly, and the practitioner should be aware of variables contributing to and indicators of client discomfort (e.g., arthritis, emphysema, pulmonary congestion, kyphosis).

Risk Factors for Borderline Hypertensive Clients (Indicating More Rigorous Monitoring or Treatment)

- Left ventricular hypertrophy
- Other target organ damage (e.g., kidneys, eyes, brain)
- High serum cholesterol
- Diabetes mellitus
- Smoking
- Family history of hypertension with complications
- Being a male

Risk Factors for Diagnosed Coronary Atherosclerosis Clients

- Hypertension
- Obesity (an excess of 30% over ideal weight)
- Smoking
- Diabetes mellitus
- Marked stress factors in life-style
- Cardiotoxic drugs (e.g., antidepressants, phenothiazines)
- Inactivity
- Erratic strenuous exercise

CLINICAL VARIATIONS: THE OLDER ADULT

CHARACTERISTIC OR AREA EXAMINED	NORMAL FINDINGS	DEVIATIONS FROM NORMAL
Assessment of pressures, pulses, and the peripheral vascular system		
1. Blood pressure (*Note:* For an initial examination the examiner should record blood pressure.)	Normal (adult) upper limits: Systolic—140 mm Hg Diastolic—90 mm Hg Pulse pressure—30 to 40 mm Hg	Low systolic (↓ 90) Systolic pressure over 160 mm Hg
a. In both arms while client is lying down	Some authorities state that maximum systolic pressure of 160 mm Hg may be within normal limits if:	Systolic pressure between 140 and 160 mm Hg with accompanying risk factors:
b. Client standing up during measurement	1. It remains stable over period of time 2. Client has no symptoms or evidence of end organ damage	1. Left ventricular hypertrophy 2. Evidence of other end organ damage (e.g., kidneys, eyes, brain)

CLINICAL VARIATIONS: THE OLDER ADULT—cont'd

CHARACTERISTIC OR AREA EXAMINED	NORMAL FINDINGS	DEVIATIONS FROM NORMAL
	3. Client is checked regularly (every 6 to 9 months)*	3. High serum cholesterol 4. Diabetes mellitus 5. Smoking 6. Family history of hypertension with complications 7. Male sex
	Most authorities agree that maximum diastolic pressure level is 90 to 95 mm Hg†	Diastolic pressure exceeding 90 mm Hg Low diastolic pressure ($\downarrow$ 60) Widened pulse pressure (*Note:* Widened pulse pressure is fairly common because of decreased elasticity of aorta.) Narrow pulse pressure
	Pressures in both arms same or do not vary more than 5 to 10 mm Hg systolic On standing, client may manifest drop of maximum of 10 to 15 mm Hg systolic and 5 mm Hg diastolic	Significant ($\uparrow$ 5 to 10 mm Hg) discrepancy in pressure readings between upper extremities Significant decrease of systolic (more than 15 mm Hg) or diastolic (more than 5 mm Hg) pressure and/or symptoms of dizziness
c. Measurement of blood pressure in both legs if pedal, popliteal, and femoral pulses are weak or absent	Popliteal artery auscultation reveals systolic pressure 5 to 15 mm Hg higher than brachial artery measurement Diastolic reading same or slightly lower	Systolic pressure lower in leg(s) than in arms
2. Palpation of carotid, radial, femoral, popliteal, dorsalis pedis, and posterior tibial pulses for: a. Rate	60 to 90 beats/min (*Note:* The heart normally slows in rate with aging because of increase in vagal tone. Some individuals may normally manifest a rate of 50 beats/min; however, patients with slow heart rates should be referred for further evaluation.)	$\uparrow$ 90 beats/min (tachycardia) (*Note:* Recent exertion, smoking, anxiety will elevate pulse.) $\downarrow$ 60 beats/min (bradycardia) (*Note:* Bradycardia and atrial fibrillation are two of the most common irregularities encountered; associated with "sick sinus syndrome." Often dizziness, syncope, or transient ischemia attacks accompany above signs.)
b. Rhythm	Regular (*Note:* Infrequent ectopic beats are fairly common. However, all patients with irregularities should be referred for further evaluation.)	Irregular (without any pattern, e.g., atrial fibrillation) Regularity with occasional pauses or extra beats (e.g., premature contractions) Coupled beats (e.g., bigeminal pulse)

If pressure is elevated (especially if accompanied by rapid pulse), repeat in 30 minutes.
†*A nurse, physician, or agency protocol should be established to determine systolic and diastolic pressures warranting referral.* Note: *Systolic pressure may show a wide variation at different times. Several measurements should be taken (over a period of weeks) to determine accuracy.*
Continued.

CLINICAL VARIATIONS: THE OLDER ADULT—cont'd

CHARACTERISTIC OR AREA EXAMINED	NORMAL FINDINGS	DEVIATIONS FROM NORMAL
Assessment of pressures, pulses, and the peripheral vascular system—cont'd		
c. Amplitude and contour	Pulse upstroke is often more rapid in older adults	Upstroke exaggerated or bounding
	Should be smooth and rounded	Pulse weak, small, or thready; peak prolonged
d. Amplitude pattern	Series of pulse strokes is unvaried in amplitude or contour	
e. Symmetry	All pulses are symmetrical (i.e., manifest same rate, rhythm, amplitude, and contour)	Asymmetrical response
(*Note:* If client has a history of hypertension, palpate femoral and brachial arteries at the same time.)	Femoral and brachial pulses occur at approximately same time with equal amplitude	Delayed, diminished femoral pulse (in comparison with brachial pulse)
3. Arterial wall contour and consistency	Arterial wall thickens; loses elasticity with aging, resulting in some increased resistance to compression	
	(*Note:* Dorsalis pedis pulses may be difficult to find or absent in some normal individuals.)	
	(*Note:* Posterior tibial pulses may also be absent or decreased in some normal individuals.)	
a. Conduct following maneuver if arterial insufficiency is suspected:		
(1) With client lying down, elevate legs 30 cm (12 inches) above his heart level		
(2) Ask client to move feet up and down at ankles for 60 seconds	Extremities (feet) exhibit mild pallor	Marked pallor of (one or both) feet
(3) Have client sit up and dangle legs (This maneuver can also be conducted with arms and hands.)	Original color returns in about 10 seconds	Delayed color return or mottled appearance
	Veins in feet fill in about 15 seconds	Delayed venous filling
		Marked redness of dependent feet
4. Jugular venous pressure (JVP) (client sitting at 30° to 45° angle)	JVP should not rise more than 3 cm above level of sternal angle	JVP exceeds 3 cm above level of manubrium*
		Note whether other veins in neck, shoulder, and upper chest are distended
a. Inspection of jugular pulsations for quality	Regular	Fluttering or oscillating
	Soft and undulating	Irregular rhythm
	Level of pulsation decreases with inspiration	Unusually prominent waves
	Pulsation increases in recumbent position	

*If venous pressure is elevated (vein is distended up to neck), raise client's head until highest jugular pulsation can be detected. Record distance in centimeters above sternal angle and angle at which client is reclining.

CHARACTERISTIC OR AREA EXAMINED	NORMAL FINDINGS	DEVIATIONS FROM NORMAL
5. Inspection and palpation of arms and legs for presence and/or appearance of superficial veins	Distention in dependent position Venous valves may appear as nodular bulges Veins collapse with elevation of limbs (*Note:* Vessels may appear tortuous or distended in elderly clients.)	Distended veins in anteromedial aspect of thigh and lower leg or on posterolateral aspect of calf from knee to ankle
6. Inspection and palpation of thigh and calf for surface characteristics	Leg symmetrical Nontender No excess warmth	Swelling (or one leg, especially calf, appears larger than other) Tenderness on palpation Warmth Redness (*Note:* If swelling is suspected, both thighs and calves should be measured with tape for accuracy.)
a. Sharp dorsiflexion of client's foot (with client's knee slightly flexed) to assess calf pain response	No pain	Pain elicited (Homans sign)
7. Inspection and palpation of extremities for evidence of adequate arterial supply	Absence of hair over digits or dorsum of hands and feet may be normal Skin pink and warm, nonedematous (*Note:* Extremities may feel cool to touch in a cool environment. Loss of subcutaneous fat contributes to increased response to cool environment.)	Reduced or absent peripheral hair (over digits and dorsum of hands and feet) Thin, shiny, taut skin Cold extremities (in warm environment) Mild edema Marked pallor or mottling on elevating extremity Digit tips ulcerated Stocking anesthesia Tenderness on palpation
8. Inspection and palpation of extremities for evidence of venous sufficiency		Peripheral cyanosis Edema (pits on pressure), bilateral or unilateral* Pigmentation around ankles (see Fig. 3-3) Thickening skin Ulceration (especially around ankles)

Edema should be measured against a bony prominence (over ankle or tibia). Record the following:

1. Type	*2. Extent and location*	*3. Degree of pitting*
a. Pitting	*a. Ankle and foot*	*a. 0 to 0.6 cm (0 to ¼ inch) — mild*
b. Nonpitting	*b. Ankle only*	*b. 0.6 to 1.3 cm (¼ to ½ inch) — moderate*
	c. Foot to knee, etc.	*c. 1.3 to 2.5 cm (½ to 1 inch) — severe*
	d. Hands, fingers	

Continued.

CLINICAL VARIATIONS: THE OLDER ADULT—cont'd

CHARACTERISTIC OR AREA EXAMINED	NORMAL FINDINGS	DEVIATIONS FROM NORMAL
Assessment of the heart and precordium		
1. Observation of general condition while client is lying supine or at elevation of 30° to 45°		
a. Positioning, comfort	Relaxed posture, without discomfort	Client experiencing pain, coughing or choking, "smothering" feeling (unable to lie flat for extended period)
b. Respirations	Even and deep	Respirations uneven, shallow, gasping Inadequate exchange
c. Skin color	Pink/brown	Cyanosis, gray pallor Mottling Blue-gray color around lips, neck, upper chest
d. Nail color and configuration	Pink 160° angle at nail bed	Cyanotic Clubbing (angle disappears)
2. Inspection and palpation of anterior chest		
a. Precordium		
(1) Contour	Kyphosis and scoliosis are fairly common in elderly people; may distort normal rounded symmetrical contour and contribute to heart displacement	All asymmetry should be noted in summary
(2) General movement	Even respiratory movements (precordium may lift slightly in thin people)	Entire chest heaving or lifting with heartbeat
3. Inspection and palpation of following areas:		
a. Sternoclavicular area pulsations	Slight or absent	Bounding
b. Aortic area (right second intercostal space adjacent to sternum) pulsations	None	Pulsation, thrill (*Note:* Low-frequency vibrations can often be more easily felt than heard.)
c. Pulmonary area (left second intercostal space adjacent to sternum) pulsations	None	Pulsation, thrill
d. Right ventricular area (left and right fifth intercostal space close to sternum) heave or lift	May be present in hyperkinetic, thin adults	Diffuse lift or heave, pulsations
e. Apical area (left fifth intercostal space 5 to 7 cm [2 to 2¾ inches] from midsternal line) for:		
(1) Pulsation	May be present	
(2) Amplitude	Tapping	Thrusting
(3) Duration	First third to half systole	Sustained throughout systole
(4) Location	Fourth or fifth intercostal space, 5 to 7 cm from midclavicular line*	Displaced left lateral or down
(5) Diameter	1 to 2 cm	More than 2 cm

*Note: Apical pulse location may displace slightly laterally if client turns to left side.

CHARACTERISTIC OR AREA EXAMINED	NORMAL FINDINGS	DEVIATIONS FROM NORMAL
f. Epigastric area (slide fingers up under rib cage) pulsations	Aortic pulsation with forward thrust Right ventricular pulsation with downward thrust	Bounding pulsation
g. Ectopic area (midway between pulmonary and apical areas) pulsations	None	Outward pulsation
4. Auscultation of following specific areas: a. Aortic area (second right interspace) b. Pulmonary area (second left interspace) c. Third left interspace d. Tricuspid area (fifth left interspace near sternum) e. Apical area (fifth left interspace medial to midclavicular line) for:		
(1) Rate	60 to 90 beats/min (*Note:* The heart normally slows in rate with aging because of increase in vagal tone.) Some individuals may normally manifest rate of 50 beats/min; however, patients with slow heart rates should be referred for further evaluation	More than 90 beats/min Less than 60 beats/min
(2) Rhythm	Regular (*Note:* Infrequent ectopic beats are fairly common with aging. However, all patients with irregularities should be referred.)	Irregular (without any pattern) Sporadic extra beats or pauses
(3) S_1 sound (a) Location	Usually heard at all sites	
(b) Intensity	Often louder at apex (muscle, fat tissue, and air will diminish sound; rapid rate will accentuate sound)	Accented Diminished (muffled) Varying intensity with different beats (e.g., complete heart block)
(c) Frequency	Usually lower in pitch than S_2	Frequency (pitch) becomes higher with accented intensity
(d) Timing	Almost synchronous with carotid impulse Slightly longer in duration than S_2	
(e) Splitting	May be heard in tricuspid area (normal S_1 splitting sound usually varies from beat to beat: occasionally single sound, occasionally narrow split)	S_4 sometimes mistaken for S_1 splitting
(4) S_2 sound (a) Location	Usually heard at all sites	
(b) Intensity	Often louder at base (intensity diminished with fat, muscle, or air)	Increased intensity, usually in aortic area (e.g., arterial hypertension) or pulmonary area (e.g., pulmonary hypertension) Decreased intensity

Continued.

CLINICAL VARIATIONS: THE OLDER ADULT—cont'd

CHARACTERISTIC OR AREA EXAMINED	NORMAL FINDINGS	DEVIATIONS FROM NORMAL
Assessment of the heart and precordium—cont'd		
(c) Frequency	Usually higher in pitch than S_1	
(d) Timing	Sound shorter in duration than S_1	
(e) Splitting	Occasionally heard in pulmonary area (on inspiration)	Wide splitting (e.g., right bundle branch block) Fixed splitting Paradoxical splitting (e.g., left bundle branch block)
(5) Systole		
(a) Duration	Shorter than diastole at normal heart rate (60 to 90 beats/min)	
(b) Sounds	S_1 sound duration brief, silent interval	Early systolic ejection click: aortic—heard at base and apex; pulmonary—heard in pulmonary area Middle and late systolic clicks (e.g., mitral valve deformity) heard at left sternal border Clicks high pitched and sharp in sound
(6) Diastole		
(a) Duration	Longer than systole at normal rate (60 to 90 beats/min) Shortens in duration as rate increases	
(b) Sounds	S_2 duration brief Silent interval	
— S_3	Absent	May signify heart failure
— Location		At apex
— Intensity		Dull, low pitched
— Timing		Early in diastole (best heard when client is in left lateral decubitus position, with bell of stethoscope)
— S_4	Absent (*Note:* Some authorities state that S_4 sounds are fairly common in the elderly and may just indicate decreased left ventricular compliance. However, all patients with extra sounds should be referred for evaluation.)	May indicate left ventricular hypertrophy or myocardial ischemia
— Location		Usually at apex or medial to apex
— Intensity		Slightly higher in pitch than S_3
— Timing		Late diastole (may be confused with split S_1) Best heard when client is in left lateral decubitus position, with bell
(c) Other sounds	None	Opening snap: at apex or left sternal border; higher pitch; very early in diastole

CHARACTERISTIC OR AREA EXAMINED	NORMAL FINDINGS	DEVIATIONS FROM NORMAL
(7) Murmurs (a) Systolic	Most authorities agree that soft, early systolic murmurs may be "functional" in elderly clients; commonly found, and caused by aortic lengthening, tortuosity, and sclerotic changes Best heard in aortic area or at base of heart; however, all clients with murmurs should be referred for further evaluation	Loud aortic (ejection) murmurs that radiate into the neck may indicate obstructive aortic disease Systolic murmurs heard at apex may indicate mitral calcification
(b) Diastolic	Diastolic murmurs are always abnormal	
(c) Timing		Systolic—early, middle, late, continuous Diastolic—early, middle, late, continuous
(d) Location		Area where sound is heard may be small and confined or may cover most of precordium (Describe in terms of precordial landmarks and distance in centimeters from landmarks.)
(e) Radiation of sound		(Describe in terms of landmarks and distance in centimeters.)
(f) Intensity		Loud, medium, soft, or grades 1 through 6 Stable, or varies with respiration or position
(g) Pitch		High, medium, low
(h) Quality		Blowing, harsh, rumbling Crescendo Decrescendo
(8) Other sounds		Pericardial friction rub: to-and-fro rubbing sound, usually heard during systole and diastole; sound usually increased when client sits up and leans forward
5. Auscultation over carotid arteries	Faint heart sounds	Unilateral bruit (swishing sound) caused by obstruction or partial obstruction of carotid artery Bilateral bruit resulting from referred heart murmur sound (particularly aortic systolic) or hyperkinesis
6. Repeat palpation and auscultation maneuvers with client (a) lying in left decubitus position and (b) sitting		

Study Questions

General

1. Which of the following statements are true about arterial blood pressure:
   - ☐ a. A difference of 5 to 10 mm Hg systolic pressure between arms is within normal limits
   - ☐ b. The systolic pressure in the upper extremities is usually about 10 mm Hg higher than in the lower extremities
   - ☐ c. A narrow cuff on an obese arm will yield a false low value
   - ☐ d. Standing might lower the systolic pressure by 10 to 15 mm Hg in a healthy individual
   - ☐ e. A wide cuff on a very small arm will yield a false low value
   - ☐ f. a, b, and e
   - ☐ g. a, c, and d
   - ☐ h. All except c
   - ☐ i. a, d, and e
   - ☐ j. a, b, and c

2. Identify the variables that might alter a healthy client's blood pressure:
   - ☐ a. Age, sex, and weight
   - ☐ b. Circadian rhythm
   - ☐ c. Stress or anxiety
   - ☐ d. Food intake
   - ☐ e. Cuff/arm ratio
   - ☐ f. a, c, and e
   - ☐ g. All of the above
   - ☐ h. All except b
   - ☐ i. All except d

3. Identify the *true* statements about the following types of arterial pulses:
   - ☐ a. Anxiety can create a bounding pulse
   - ☐ b. Aortic rigidity and atherosclerosis can create a bounding pulse
   - ☐ c. Obstructive lung disease can cause a paradoxical pulse
   - ☐ d. Pulsus alternans is evidence of left-sided heart failure
   - ☐ e. The normal pulse contour is smooth and rounded
   - ☐ f. a and d
   - ☐ g. a, c, and e
   - ☐ h. b and c
   - ☐ i. All of the above
   - ☐ j. a, b, and e

4. Which statement(s) is/are true about the jugular veins and jugular venous pressure:
   - ☐ a. The internal jugular vein connects to the right atrium
   - ☐ b. Jugular pulsation can usually be obliterated by moderate pressure at the scapular base of the neck
   - ☐ c. Neck veins frequently distend when a healthy client is in a supine position
   - ☐ d. The sternal angle is the common reference point for measuring jugular venous pressure
   - ☐ e. Pregnancy usually increases jugular venous pressure
   - ☐ f. All of the above
   - ☐ g. All except e
   - ☐ h. b and d
   - ☐ i. a, b, and c

5. Mr. Jones's feet are cool to touch. You have asked him to elevate both legs about 30 cm (12 inches) above his body for approximately 60 seconds. Both feet manifest a mild pallor. Then you ask him to sit up and dangle his legs. His normal (pink) skin color returns to his toes in about 15 seconds. Which statement(s) is/are true about what you have observed:
   - ☐ a. Venous insufficiency should be suspected
   - ☐ b. Arterial insufficiency should be suspected
   - ☐ c. The results are within normal limits
   - ☐ d. The leg-raising drained the feet of most of the venous blood
   - ☐ e. The leg-raising drained the feet of most of the arterial blood
   - ☐ f. c and d
   - ☐ g. a and d
   - ☐ h. b and d
   - ☐ i. c and e
   - ☐ j. None of the above

6. Which of the following statements is/are true about the heart:
   - ☐ a. The heart lies within the mediastinum
   - ☐ b. The base of the heart is normally found in the fifth intercostal space
   - ☐ c. Most of the anterior cardiac surface consists of the right ventricle
   - ☐ d. The left ventricle makes up a small portion of the anterior cardiac surface
   - ☐ e. In a normal, average individual, two thirds of the heart lies to the right of the midsternal line
   - ☐ f. All of the above
   - ☐ g. All except b and e
   - ☐ h. All except c

7. Which of the following statement(s) is/are true:
   - [ ] a. Heart murmurs are of longer duration than heart sounds
   - [ ] b. Heart murmurs originate within the heart itself
   - [ ] c. Heart murmurs originate within the great vessels
   - [ ] d. Most "innocent" murmurs are faint or under grade 3 intensity
   - [ ] e. "Innocent" murmurs are usually systolic murmurs
   - [ ] f. a, b, and d
   - [ ] g. All except e
   - [ ] h. All of the above
   - [ ] i. a, c, and d

8. A systolic ejection murmur occurs:
   - [ ] a. At the mitral or tricuspid valves
   - [ ] b. At the pulmonary or aortic valves

9. A systolic regurgitant murmur occurs:
   - [ ] a. At the mitral or tricuspid valves
   - [ ] b. At the pulmonary or aortic valves

Identify the characteristics of an arterial pulse that an examiner notes when palpating (as identified in the *Clinical Guidelines*), beginning with:
   Rate
   Rhythm

10. _____
11. _____
12. _____

13. Label the cardiac chambers, valves, and vessels as shown in the accompanying illustration.

   a. _____   h. _____
   b. _____   i. _____
   c. _____   j. _____
   d. _____   k. _____
   e. _____   l. _____
   f. _____   m. _____
   g. _____

14. The first sound is caused by closure of _____ and _____ valves. It occurs at the beginning of: Systole? Diastole?

15. The second sound results from _____ and _____ valve closure. It occurs at the beginning of: Systole? Diastole?

The following statements describe characteristics of the first heart sound (S_1) or the second heart sound (S_2). Assign "a" (S_1) or "b" (S_2) to each statement.

16. _____ Usually sounds louder at the apex of the heart

17. _____ Splitting heard near the pulmonary area

18. _____ Slightly higher frequency than the other sound

19. _____ Almost synchronous with carotid impulse

The following statements describe characteristics of the third heart sound (S_3) or the fourth heart sound (S_4). Assign "a" (S_3) or "b" (S_4) to each statement.

20. _____ The sound originates in early diastolic rapid ventricular filling and wall vibration

21. _____ The sound originates in late diastolic rapid ventricular filling

22. _____ Very commonly heard in normal children and young adults

23. _____ Often signifies myocardial failure in older adults

The Newborn

24. The point of maximum impulse in a newborn should be near the:
   - [ ] a. Left 2nd to 3rd intercostal space
   - [ ] b. Right 2nd to 3rd intercostal space
   - [ ] c. Left 4th to 5th intercostal space
   - [ ] d. Right 4th to 5th intercostal space

25. Capillary filling time should be:
   - [ ] a. 1 second or less
   - [ ] b. 2 seconds or less
   - [ ] c. 3 seconds or less
   - [ ] d. 4 seconds or less

The Child

26. When examining 5-year-old John M., the examiner identifies the following findings:

    History: healthy child

    Pulse: 88 regular

    BP: 102/52

    Peripheral circulation: good

    Heart sounds: S_1, S_2 regular

    Extra sound consistently heard just following S_2 sound (split? S_3?)

    Murmur identified in systole; child was sitting; had soft, short sound; remained audible after 30-second jumping exercise

    The examiner should:

    ☐ a. Record the finding as a probable functional murmur and recheck the child in 8 weeks

    ☐ b. Consider the cardiovascular examination normal; reevaluate child at next regularly scheduled well-child visit

    ☐ c. Send the child *immediately* to the physician for further evaluation

    ☐ d. Schedule the child for an ECG and stress test

    ☐ e. Send the child for physician evaluation fairly soon, at a time convenient for both parties

27. Steven is a 7-year-old black boy. During his examination the nurse evaluated his pulse and blood pressure, which were normal. Which of the following readings would it have been:

    ☐ a. BP 94/40; pulse 88

    ☐ b. BP 128/72; pulse 84

    ☐ c. BP 112/78; pulse 74

    ☐ d. BP 102/48; pulse 102

    ☐ e. BP 120/62; pulse 94

The Childbearing Woman

28. Audible murmurs may occur from a changed heart position around the:

    ☐ a. 8th to 10th week of gestation

    ☐ b. 12th to 20th week of gestation

    ☐ c. 21st to 28th week of gestation

    ☐ d. 30th to 40th week of gestation

29. A sign of thrombophlebitis is:

    ☐ a. Leg pain

    ☐ b. Hypotension

    ☐ c. Bradycardia

    ☐ d. Breast pain

The Older Adult

30. In elderly people, cardiac output:

    ☐ a. Decreases by 30% to 40% over a 40- to 50-year span

    ☐ b. Is the same as in younger adults unless there is disease present

    ☐ c. May not respond adequately during severe stress

    ☐ d. May not respond adequately to tachycardia

    ☐ e. Increases because of normal left ventricular enlargement and increasing peripheral resistance

    ☐ f. None of the above

    ☐ g. d and e

    ☐ h. a, c, and d

31. Pulses in geriatric clients:

    ☐ a. May normally be slower than the average pulse of adults

    ☐ b. Are normally irregular and rapid

    ☐ c. Are normally irregular and slow

    ☐ d. Are less symmetrical in timing and amplitude than younger adult pulses

32. The systolic pressure in an older individual:

    ☐ a. May be slightly higher because elderly people are often more excitable

    ☐ b. May be slightly higher than the young adult because of elasticity changes in the large arteries

    ☐ c. May be slightly lower than in the young adult because of loss of subcutaneous fat

    ☐ d. Is within 5 to 10 mm Hg of 120 range unless the client is hypertensive

SUGGESTED READINGS
General

Bates B: *A guide to physical examination,* ed 4, Philadelphia, 1987, JB Lippincott.

Canobbio MM: *Mosby's clinical nursing* series, vol 1, *Cardiovascular disorders,* St Louis, 1990, Mosby–Year Book.

Corman LC: Strokes and the carotid: myths and realities, *Geriatrics* 45(7):28, 1990.

Erickson BA: Detecting abnormal sounds, *Nurs '86,* Jan, p 58, 1986.

Kirkendall WM, and others: *Recommendations for human blood pressure determination by sphygmomanometers,* Dallas, 1980, Communication Division, American Heart Association.

Malasanos L, Barkauskas V, Stoltenberg-Allen K: *Health assessment,* ed 4, St Louis 1990, Mosby–Year Book.

McCance KL, Huether SE: *Pathophysiology: the biological basis for disease in adults and children,* St Louis, 1990, Mosby–Year Book.

McMahan BE: Why deep vein thrombosis is so dangerous, *RN* Jan, p 20, 1987.

Miracle VA: Anatomy of a murmur, *Nurs '86,* 16(7):26, 1986.

Pender NJ: *Health promotion in nursing practice,* ed 2, Norwalk, Conn, 1987, Appleton & Lange.

Prior JA, Silberstein JS, Stang JM: *Physical diagnosis: the history and examination of the patient,* ed 6, St Louis, 1981, Mosby–Year Book.

Seidel HM, Ball JW, Dains JE, Benedict GW: *Mosby's guide to physical examination,* ed 2, St Louis, 1991, Mosby–Year Book.

Thompson JM, McFarland GK, Hirsch JE, and others: *Mosby's manual of clinical nursing,* ed 2, St Louis, 1989, Mosby–Year Book.

Warner-Chilcott Laboratory, AEGIS Production: *Differential diagnosis of chest pain,* New York, 1967, American Heart Association.

The newborn

Auvenshine MA, Enriquez MG: *Maternity nursing: dimensions of change,* Belmont, Calif, 1985, Wadsworth.

Bobak IM, Jensen MD: *Essentials of maternity nursing,* ed 3, St Louis, 1991, Mosby–Year Book.

Judd JM: Assessing the newborn from head to toe, *Nurs '85,* 15(12):34, 1985.

Kiernan BS, Scoloveno MA: Assessment of the neonate, *Top Clin Nurs* 8(1):1, 1986.

The Organization for Obstetrical, Gynecological and Neonatal Nurses (NAACOG): *Physical assessment of the neonate,* OGN Nursing practice resource, Oct. 1986, The Association.

Pillitteri A: *Maternal-newborn nursing: care of the growing family,* ed 3, Boston, 1985, Little, Brown.

Scanlon JW, and others: *A system of newborn physical examination,* Baltimore, 1979, University Park Press.

Scharping EM: Physiological measurements of the newborn, *Matern Child Nurs J* 8:70, 1983.

Seidel HM, Ball JW, Dains JE, Benedict GW: *Mosby's guide to physical examination,* ed 2, St Louis, 1991, Mosby–Year Book.

Whaley LF, Wong DL: *Nursing care of infants and children,* ed 4, St Louis, 1991, Mosby–Year Book.

The child

Alexander M, Brown MS: *Pediatric history taking and physical diagnosis for nurses,* ed 2, New York, 1979, McGraw-Hill.

Barness L: *Manual of pediatric physical diagnosis,* ed 6, St Louis, 1990, Mosby–Year Book.

DeAngelis C: Pediatric primary care, ed 3, Boston, 1984, Little, Brown.

Haggerty RJ, Maroney MW, Nadas AS: Essential hypertension in infancy and childhood, *Am J Dis Child* 92:536, 1956.

Seidel HM, Ball JW, Dains JE, Benedict GW: *Mosby's guide to physical examination,* ed 2, St Louis, 1991, Mosby–Year Book.

Taylor DL: Clinical applications: assessing heart sounds, *Nurs '85* 15:51, 1985.

Waring WW, Jeansonne LO: *Practical manual of pediatrics: a pocket reference for those who treat children,* ed 2, St Louis, 1982, Mosby–Year Book.

Whaley LF, Wong DL: *Nursing care of infants and children,* ed 4, St Louis, 1991, Mosby–Year Book.

Whaley LF, Wong DL: *Essentials of pediatric nursing,* ed 3, St Louis, 1989, Mosby–Year Book.

The childbearing woman

Auvenshine MA, Enriquez MG: *Maternity nursing: dimensions of change,* Belmont, Calif, 1985, Wadsworth.

Beischer NA, MacKay EV: *Obstetrics and the newborn, an illustrated textbook,* ed 2, Philadelphia, 1986, WB Saunders.

Bobak IM, Jensen MD: *Essentials of maternity nursing,* ed 3, St Louis, 1991, Mosby–Year Book.

Gilbert ES, Harmon JS: *High-risk pregnancy and delivery: nursing perspectives,* St Louis, 1986, Mosby–Year Book.

Pillitteri A: *Maternal-newborn nursing: care of the growing family,* ed 3, Boston, 1985, Little, Brown.

Pritchard JA, MacDonald PC: *Williams' obstetrics,* ed 17, New York, 1985, Appleton-Century-Crofts.

Whitley N: *A manual of clinical obstetrics,* Philadelphia, 1985, JB Lippincott.

The older adult

Babu TN, and others: What is "normal" blood pressure in the aged? *Geriatrics* 32(1):73, 1977.

Carotenuto R, Bullock J: *Physical assessment of the gerontologic client,* Philadelphia, 1980, FA Davis.

Eliopoulos C: *Gerontological nursing,* ed 2, Philadelphia, 1987, JB Lippincott.

Mead WF: The aging heart, *Am Fam Physician* 18(2):73, 1978.

Nachtigall L, Nachtigall L: "Protecting older women from their growing risk of cardiac disease, *Geriatrics* 45(5):24, 1990.

Shock NW, and others: *Normal human aging: the Baltimore longitudinal study of aging,* Baltimore, 1984, US Department of Health and Human Services, NIH Pub No 84-2450, p 117.

Steinberg FU, editor: *Care of the geriatric patient,* ed 6, St Louis, 1983, Mosby–Year Book.

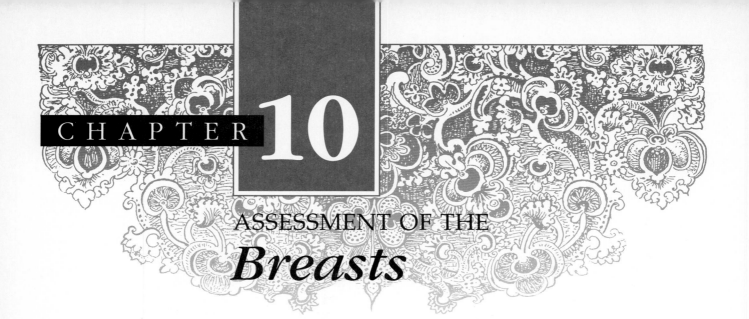

CHAPTER 10

ASSESSMENT OF THE
Breasts

VOCABULARY

areola A circular, darkly pigmented area around the nipple of the breast.
Cooper ligaments Suspensory ligaments of the breast.
gynecomastia Condition characterized by abnormally large mammary glands in the male.
inverted nipple Nipple that is turned inward.
mastitis An inflammation of the breast
Montgomery tubercles Small seba-

ceous glands located on the areola of the breast.
Paget disease Condition characterized by an excoriating or scaling lesion of the nipple, extending from an intraductal carcinoma of the breast.
peau d'orange Dimpling of the skin that resembles the skin of an orange.
pectoralis major muscle One of the four muscles of the anterior upper portion of the chest.

retraction Shortening or drawing backward of the skin.
sebaceous gland An oil-secreting gland of the skin.
striae Colorless lines caused by mechanical stretching of the skin.
supernumerary nipple Extra nipple.
tail of Spence Upper outer tail of the breast that extends into the axillary region.

ANATOMY AND PHYSIOLOGY REVIEW

The breasts are mammary glands that lie on the ventral surface of the thorax, within the superficial fascia of the chest wall. They extend vertically from the second rib to the sixth or seventh intercostal space, and laterally from the side of the sternum to the midaxillary line. Breast tissue extending up into the axilla is called the *tail of Spence.* The majority of breast tumors are located in the upper lateral breast quadrant and in the tail of Spence.

The breast is composed of 15 to 20 pyramid-shaped lobes, which are separated and supported by Cooper ligaments (Fig. 10-1). Each lobe contains 20 to 40 alveoli, which subdivide into many functional units, called *acini.* Each acinus is lined with a layer of epithelial cells capable of contracting to express milk from it. The acini empty into a network of lobular collecting ducts, which empty into interlobular collecting and ejecting ducts. The ducts reach the skin through openings (pores) in the nipple.

Lymphatic drainage of the breast occurs largely through axillary nodes (Fig. 10-2). The three types of

lymphatic drainage of the breast are as follows:

- Cutaneous lymphatic drainage is of lymph from the skin of the breast excluding the areolar and nipple area; this lymph flows into the ipsilateral axillary nodes. Lymph from the medial cutaneous breast area may flow to the opposite breast. Lymph from the inferior portion of the breast can reach the lymphatic plexus of the epigastric region and subsequently the liver and other abdominal regions and organs.
- Areolar lymphatic drainage is of lymph formed in the areolar and nipple areas of the breast; this lymph flows into the anterior axillary group of nodes (the mammary nodes)
- Deep lymphatic drainage is of lymph from the deep mammary tissues; this lymph flows into the anterior axillary nodes. Some of this lymph also flows into the apical, subclavian, infraclavicular, and supraclavicular nodes. Also, lymph from the retroareolar areas and medial glandular breast tissue areas communicates with lymphatic systems draining into the thorax and abdomen.

The nipple is a pigmented, cylindrical structure that

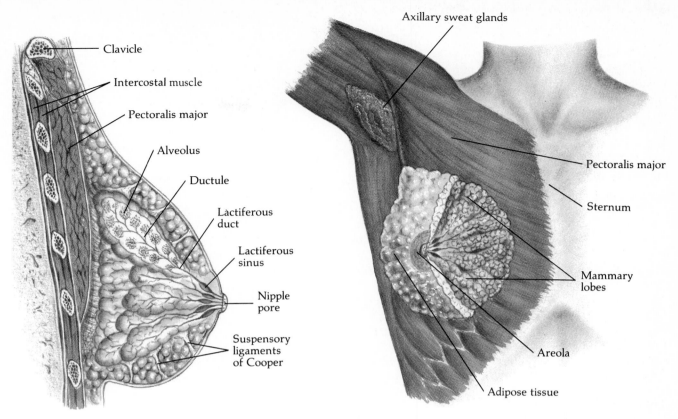

Fig. 10-1   Anatomy of breast. (From Thompson JM, McFarland GK, Hirsch JE, and others: *Mosby's manual of clinical nursing,* ed 2, St Louis, 1989, Mosby—Year Book.)

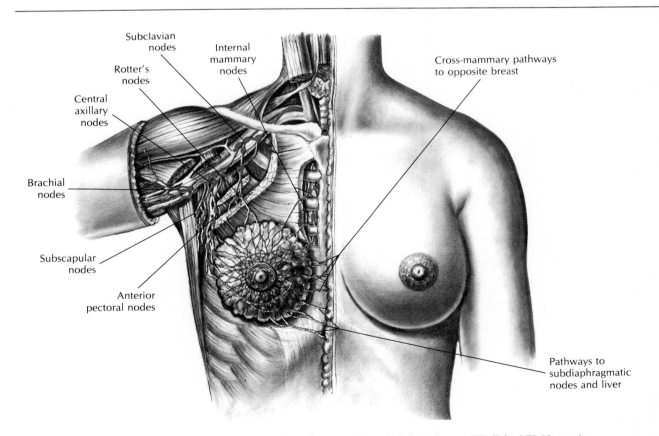

Fig. 10-2   Mammary gland: lymphatic drainage. (From Bobak IM, Jensen MD, Zalar MK: *Maternity and gynecologic care: the nurse and the family,* ed 4, St Louis, 1989, Mosby—Year Book.)

is usually located at the fourth or fifth intercostal space. It is approximately 10 to 20 mm in height when erect. On its surface lie multiple openings, one from each lobe. The areola is the pigmented, circular area around the nipple. It may be from 15 to 60 mm in diameter. A number of sebaceous glands, the glands of Montgomery, are located within the areola and aid in lubrication of the nipple during lactation.

COGNITIVE OBJECTIVES

At the end of this chapter the learner will demonstrate knowledge of assessment of the breasts by the ability to do the following:

- Apply the terms that are listed in the vocabulary section.
- Identify the lymphatic system associated with the breasts, and discuss lymphatic drainage patterns.
- List inspection criteria associated with examination of the breasts.
- List palpation criteria associated with examination of the breasts.
- Identify client positions for examination of the breasts.
- Describe selected signs and/or symptoms that would warrant physician referral or further investigation.
- List instruction techniques associated with breast self-examination.
- Identify the appropriate times of the month for women to perform breast self-examination.
- Point out maturational variations associated with the breasts and their assessment.
- Identify selected variations for the newborn, the child, the childbearing woman, and the older adult.

CLINICAL OUTLINE

At the end of this chapter the learner will perform a systematic assessment of the breasts, demonstrating the ability to do the following:

- Obtain a pertinent health history from the client.
- Demonstrate and record results of inspection of the breasts while the client is seated and lying down. This assessment should include:
  1. General breast assessment
     a. Size
     b. Symmetry
     c. Contour
     d. Appearance of skin (color, texture, venous patterns)
     e. Moles (nevi)
  2. Areolar area
     a. Size
     b. Shape
     c. Surface characteristics
  3. Nipples
     a. Direction

     b. Size and shape
     c. Color
     d. Surface characteristics
     e. Discharge
- Demonstrate and record results of palpation of the breasts while the client is seated and lying down, including:
  1. General breast assessment
     a. Firmness
     b. Tissue qualities
  2. Nipples
     a. Elasticity
     b. Tissue qualities
     c. Discharge
  3. Lymphatic assessment
     a. Supraclavicular and infraclavicular nodes
     b. Central and lateral axillary nodes
     c. Pectoral, scapular, and subscapular nodes
     d. Brachial, intermediate, and internal mammary nodal chains
- Demonstrate and record appropriate inspection and palpation of the male breasts.
- Demonstrate instructional techniques and rationale in teaching self-examination of the breasts.

HISTORY

- By synthesizing historical data, genetic factors, and information about exposure to carcinogenic agents, compile a risk profile for the client. Table 10-1 shows the assessment criteria that will help to develop a breast cancer risk profile for women living in the United States. Use these data to develop a profile for *every* female client assessed. If the examiner determines that the client has a basically high-risk profile, thorough examination, breast self-examination instruction techniques, and regular reevaluation periods become vitally important.
- If the client has a symptomatic complaint of the breasts (e.g., pain, tenderness, lump, nipple discharge, skin rashes, or changes in size or shape of the breasts), a thorough investigation must be made. In addition to the steps stated in the Symptom Analysis (Chapter 1, p. 11), the following questions should be asked:
  1. How long has the lump or thickening been present?
  2. Have there been recent changes in breast characteristics, such as pain, tenderness, size, shape, overlying skin characteristics? Describe.
  3. If there is pain, is it described as stinging, pulling, burning, or drawing?
  4. Is the pain unilateral or bilateral?
  5. Is the pain or discomfort localized, or does it spread?
  6. Does the lump or discomfort change in size or character with menses?

TABLE 10-1 Assessment criteria for development of a breast cancer risk profile

QUESTIONS FOR CLIENT	HIGH-RISK CRITERIA	LOW-RISK CRITERIA
Age	Women over 40 years of age	Women under 25 years of age
Ethnic ancestry	Northern European, Jewish ancestry	Latin or Mediterranean ancestry; American Indians, Orientals
Hemisphere	Western	Eastern
Climate	Cold	Warm
Income (high, medium, low)	High and middle income	Lower incomes
Home location past 10 years (city, town, rural community)	Large cities, industrial cities, especially in Northeast	Medium cities, small towns, rural areas
Breast cancer in family that occurred before menopause (inquire about mother, sisters, maternal grandmother, maternal aunts, maternal first cousins)	Positive response to any of these if it occurred before menopause	Negative response to any of these; positive response if it occurred after menopause
Menarche and menopause history: early, late	Early menstruation, late menopause	Late menstruation, early menopause
Chronic psychological stress	Yes	No
Obesity	Yes	No
Obesity-diabetes-hypertension triad	Yes	No
High-dietary-fat intake	Yes	No
History of breast abnormalities (may include fibrocystic disease, adenomas, mastitis, breast abscesses, or breast injury)	Positive response to any items listed; other abnormalities	Negative response to any items listed
Diet history: whether it is high in animal proteins and fats or high in vegetable consumption and low in animal proteins and fats; caffeine	Diet high in animal proteins and/or animal fats High consumption of caffeine	Diet mostly vegetarian or low in animal proteins and/or animal fats Low consumption of caffeine
Reproductive and sexual histories	Late beginning of sexual activity No history of sexual activity	Early beginning of sexual activity
Children	No children	Has had children
Breast-fed children	No breast-feeding	Has breast-fed children
Age when children were born	Delivered first child after age 35 years	Delivered first child before age 20 years

Data from Leis HP Jr: Epidemiology of breast cancer: identification of the high-risk woman. In Gallagher HS, and others, editors: The breast, *St Louis, 1978, Mosby—Year Book; Kushner R: Breast cancer risks for U.S. women. In Martin LL:* Health care of women, *Philadelphia, 1978, JB Lippincott.*

7. Has the client been involved in any strenuous activity that could contribute to the breast discomfort?
8. Does the client complain of nipple discharge? If so, inquire about:
   a. Duration of problem
   b. Drainage characteristics, including color, consistency, odor, amount
   c. Times present (always, before menses, other)
   d. Drug therapy, such as oral contraceptives, phenothiazines, digitalis, diuretics, or steroids

9. Continued questioning should include items from the risk profile assessment criteria in Table 10-1.
- Does the client examine her own breasts regularly? Has she been taught the breast self-examination? At what part of the month does she examine her breasts? Have client explain the technique she uses. The box on p. 320 contains the American Cancer Society evaluation guidelines for detection of breast cancer in asymptomatic women.
- Once a breast mass is determined, the data in Table 10-2 may be used to classify the lesion.

Text continues on p. 328.

EVALUATION GUIDELINES FOR DETECTION OF BREAST CANCER IN ASYMPTOMATIC WOMEN

- Women 20 years of age and older should perform breast self-examination every month.
- Women 20 to 40 should have a physical examination of the breasts every 3 years, and women over 40 should have a physical examination of the breasts every year.
- Women between the ages of 35 and 40 should have a baseline mammogram.
- Women under 40 should consult their personal health care provider about the need for mammography.
- Women over 40 should have a mammogram every 1 to 2 years when feasible.
- Women over 50 should have a mammogram every year when feasible.
- Women with personal or family histories of breast cancer should consult their health care provider about the need for more frequent examinations or about beginning periodic mammography before the age of 40.

From American Cancer Society: 1990 Cancer facts and figures.

TABLE 10-2   Staging and tumor node metastasis (TNM) classification of breast malignancy

Stage 1	T_1 (Tumor 2 cm or less)
	N_0 (No palpable axillary nodes)
	M_0 (No evident metastasis)
Stage 2	T_0 (No palpable tumor)
	T_1 (Tumor 2 cm or less)
	T_2 (Tumor less than 5 cm)
	N_1 (Palpable axillary nodes with histologic evidence of breast malignancy)
	M_0
Stage 3	T_3 (Tumor more than 5 cm; may be fixed to muscle or fascia)
	N_1 or N_2 (Fixed nodes)
	M_0
Stage 4	T_4 (Tumor any size with fixation to chest wall or skin; presence of edema, including peau d'orange; ulceration; skin nodules; inflammatory carcinoma)
	N_3 (Supraclavicular or infraclavicular nodes or arm edema)
	M_1 (Distant metastasis present or suspected)

Data from American Cancer Society and American Society of Plastic and Reconstructive Surgery, The Association, 1979.

CLINICAL GUIDELINES

ASSESSMENT PROCEDURE	EVALUATION	
	NORMAL FINDINGS	DEVIATIONS FROM NORMAL
Assessment of the female breasts 1. Instruct client to *sit* comfortably and erect on side of bed; *arms should be at side*; gown should be around waist so that breasts may be fully evaluated (Fig. 10-3)		

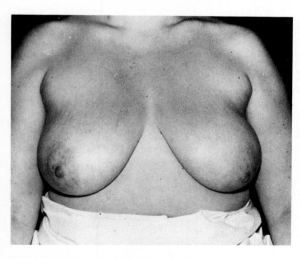

Fig. 10-3   Breasts ready for visual examination.

CLINICAL GUIDELINES—cont'd

ASSESSMENT PROCEDURE	EVALUATION	
	NORMAL FINDINGS	DEVIATIONS FROM NORMAL
2. Inspect and bilaterally compare:		
a. Breasts		
(1) Size	Varies	
(2) Symmetry	Bilaterally equal Slight asymmetry (Fig. 10-4)	Recent unilateral increase in size Marked asymmetry
(3) Contour	Smooth, convex, even pattern	Dimpling, retraction Interruption of convex pattern Fixation
(4) Skin color	Even throughout	Hyperpigmentation Erythema
(5) Skin texture	Smooth, elastic, movable, striae	Thickened, rough Lesions or thickening Edema (peau d'orange) (Fig. 10-5)
(6) Venous patterns	Bilaterally similar	Localized, unilateral increase in vascular pattern
(7) Moles (nevi)	Long history of presence Nonchanging Nontender	Newly developed or changed Tender
b. Areolar area		
(1) Size	Bilaterally equal	Unequal
(2) Shape	Round or oval	Other than round or oval

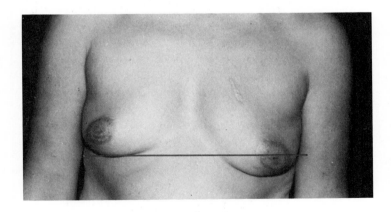

Fig. 10-4   Breast asymmetry.

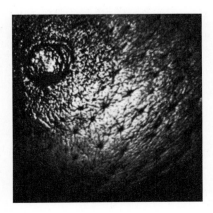

Fig. 10-5   Peau d'orange. (From Gallagher HS, and others, editors: *The breast,* St Louis, 1978, Mosby–Year Book.)

Continued.

CLINICAL GUIDELINES—cont'd

	EVALUATION	
ASSESSMENT PROCEDURE	**NORMAL FINDINGS**	**DEVIATIONS FROM NORMAL**
Assessment of the female breasts—cont'd		
(3) Surface characteristics	Smooth, bilaterally similar, Montgomery tubercles (Fig. 10-6)	Masses, lesions Color pigment changes Unilateral pigment change
c. Nipples		
(1) Direction	Bilaterally equal in pointing direction (Fig. 10-7, *A*) Supernumerary nipples	Asymmetrical deviations (Fig. 10-7, *B*)

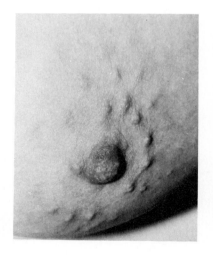

Fig. 10-6   Montgomery tubercles.

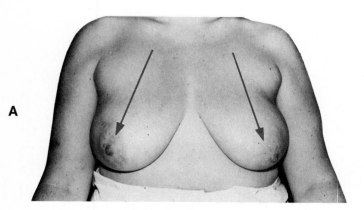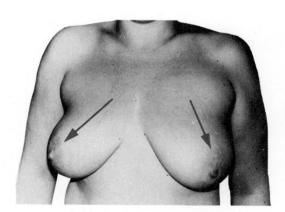

A   B

Fig. 10-7   **A,** Symmetrical breasts (note nipple position). **B,** Lateral deviation of right breast (note nipple position).

ASSESSMENT PROCEDURE	EVALUATION	
	NORMAL FINDINGS	DEVIATIONS FROM NORMAL
(2) Size, shape	Bilaterally equal Long-standing inversion (unilateral or bilateral) (Fig. 10-8, *A*)	Asymmetrical Recent inversion or retraction (unilateral or bilateral) (Fig. 10-8, *B*)
(3) Color	Homogeneous	Edema, redness Bilaterally unequal Pigment changes
(4) Surface characteristics	Smooth, may be slightly wrinkled Skin intact	Ulceration, crusting Erosion, scaling Wrinkled, dry, cracking, with lesions
(5) Discharge (if present, describe odor, color, amount, consistency)	Absent	Serous, bloody, purulent discharges (Fig. 10-9)

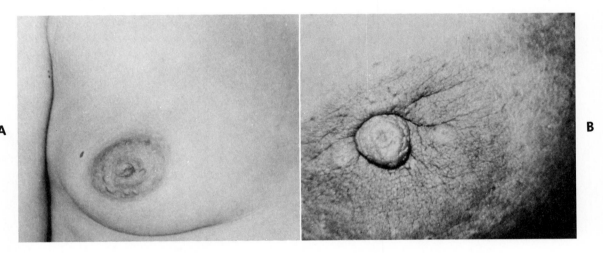

A **B**

Fig. 10-8 **A,** Simple inversion of the nipple. **B,** Nipple retraction. (**B** from Gallagher HS, and others, editors: *The breast,* St Louis, 1978, Mosby–Year Book.)

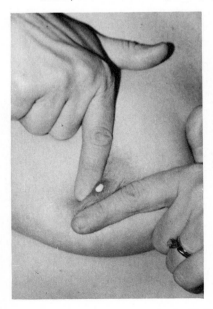

Fig. 10-9 Nipple discharge.

Continued.

CLINICAL GUIDELINES—cont'd

	EVALUATION	
ASSESSMENT PROCEDURE	**NORMAL FINDINGS**	**DEVIATIONS FROM NORMAL**
Assessment of the female breasts—cont'd 3. Inspect breasts while client is *seated with arms extended overhead* (Fig. 10-10), to observe and bilaterally compare all items previously listed, as well as: a. Bilateral pull on suspensory ligaments	 Equal; breasts bilaterally symmetrical	 Asymmetry Shortening or appearance of attachment of either breast (fixation)
4. Inspect breasts while client is *seated and leaning over* (Fig. 10-11), to observe and bilaterally compare: a. Symmetry	 Breasts hang equally Smooth skin contour	 Asymmetry Bulging retraction
b. Bilateral pull on suspensory ligaments	Equal; breasts bilaterally symmetrical	Shortening or appearance of attachment of either breast (fixation)

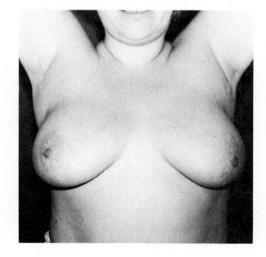

Fig. 10-10   Inspect breasts with client's arms extended overhead.

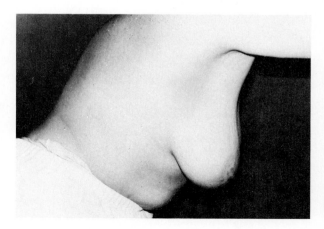

Fig. 10-11   Inspect breasts with client leaning forward.

	EVALUATION	
ASSESSMENT PROCEDURE	**NORMAL FINDINGS**	**DEVIATIONS FROM NORMAL**

5. Inspect breasts while client is *seated and pushing hands onto hips or pushing palms together* and contracting pectoral muscles (Fig. 10-12), to observe and bilaterally compare all items as previously listed
6. Palpate each breast in a systematic clockwise direction; client is seated with arms at sides (Fig. 10-13)
7. Palpate and bilaterally compare:
  a. Four quadrants, tail of breast, and areolar area for:
    (1) Firmness
	Bilaterally equal
	With aging or poor bra support, sagging of breast tissue may occur
		Asymmetry

(2) Tissue qualities (see "Clinical Tips and Strategies," p. 328, for further description)	Smooth, diffuse tissue bilaterally Nodular, bilateral granular consistency Premenstrual engorgement Elastic, nontender Firm mammary ridge found along each breast at approximately 4 to 8 o'clock position	Tenderness unrelated to menstrual cycle Unilateral pain or tenderness, unilateral mass Heat of tissue
b. Nipple (1) Elasticity and tissue characteristics	Bilaterally equal, nontender Smooth, skin intact	Tender, friable tissue, cracks, bleeding Lesions, dryness, crusting, erosion
(2) Discharge (note color, odor, consistency, amount)	Absent	Present; serous, bloody, purulent

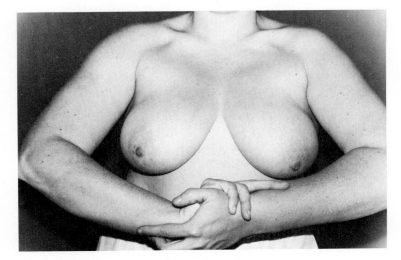

Fig. 10-12   Inspect breasts while client flexes pectoral muscles.

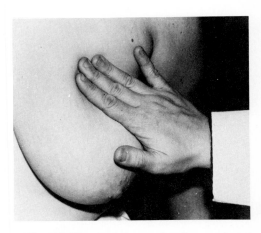

Fig. 10-13   Examiner using fingerpads to examine breasts.

Continued.

CLINICAL GUIDELINES—cont'd

	EVALUATION	
ASSESSMENT PROCEDURE	**NORMAL FINDINGS**	**DEVIATIONS FROM NORMAL**
Assessment of the female breasts— cont'd		
c. Lymph nodes associated with lymphatic drainage system (Fig. 10-14); location and characteristics of lymph nodes, including supraclavicular and infraclavicular, central and lateral axillary, pectoral, subscapular, scapular, brachial, intermediate, and internal mammary chains (Fig. 10-15)	Nonpalpable	Palpable *Note:* 1. Location 2. Size 3. Contour 4. Consistency 5. Discreteness 6. Mobility 7. Tenderness

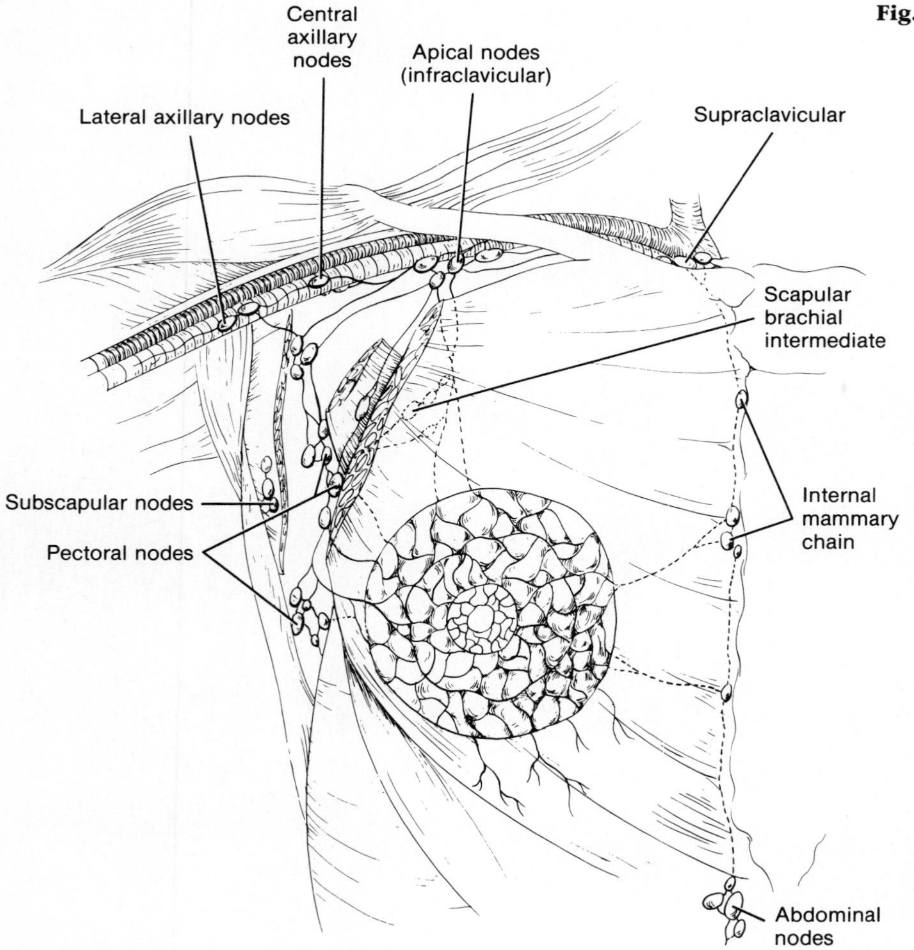

Central axillary nodes

Apical nodes (infraclavicular)

Lateral axillary nodes

Supraclavicular

Fig. 10-14   Lymphatic drainage of the breast.

Scapular brachial intermediate

Subscapular nodes

Pectoral nodes

Internal mammary chain

Abdominal nodes

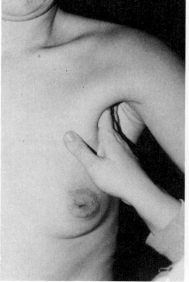

Fig. 10-15   Palpating axillary lymph nodes.

ASSESSMENT PROCEDURE	EVALUATION	
	NORMAL FINDINGS	DEVIATIONS FROM NORMAL
Assessment of the female breasts—cont'd		
8. Instruct client to remain *sitting* and *raise both arms over head;* may be most comfortable for client to grasp hands and rest them on top of head; repeat and compare bilaterally the palpation of:		
a. Four quadrants of each breast	Criteria as previously described	Criteria as previously described
b. Tail of each breast		
c. Areolar area		
d. Nipple		
e. Lymph nodes		
9. Instruct client to lie supine with arm that is on side of breast to be examined resting over head (Fig. 10-16); place small towel under shoulder and back of breast to be examined (this displaces breast tissue more diffusely over chest wall)		
10. Inspect:		
a. Breasts, noting:	Criteria as previously described	Criteria as previously described
(1) Symmetry		
(2) Contour		
(3) Skin color		
(4) Skin texture		
(5) Venous patterns		
(6) Moles (nevi)		
b. Areolar area surface characteristics		
c. Nipple characteristics		
11. Palpate each breast in systematic clockwise direction; carefully evaluate:		
a. Four quadrants of each breast	Criteria as previously described	Criteria as previously described
b. Tail of each breast		
c. Areolar area		
d. Nipple		
e. Lymph nodes		

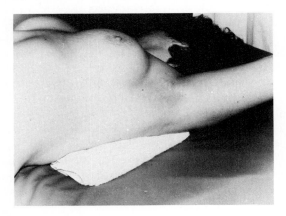

Fig. 10-16   Positioning for breast examination. Note placement of towel.

Continued.

CLINICAL GUIDELINES—cont'd

ASSESSMENT PROCEDURE	EVALUATION	
	NORMAL FINDINGS	DEVIATIONS FROM NORMAL
Assessment of the male breasts		
1. Inspect male client's breasts while he is seated, arms resting at sides		
2. Inspect nipple and areolar area; compare bilaterally	Intact, smooth Bilaterally equal color	Ulcerated Masses, swelling
3. Palpate client's breasts and areolar area while he is seated, arms resting at sides; note skin texture, tissue consistency; compare bilaterally	Smooth, nontender Skin intact, nontender	Tenderness Unilateral or unequal swelling or masses (Fig. 10-17)
4. Palpate lymphatic system associated with the breast (similar to female breast assessment)		

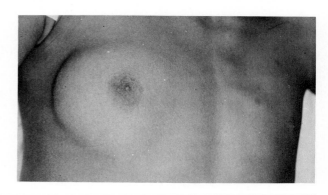

Fig. 10-17 Adult gynecomastia in male (diffuse type). (From Gallagher HS, and others, editors: *The breast*, St Louis, 1978, Mosby–Year Book.)

CLINICAL TIPS AND STRATEGIES

- **Complete breast examination requires that the breast be evaluated in numerous positions:** This facilitates pull on the suspensory ligaments that will most likely demonstrate retraction or dimpling of an affected breast. To summarize the previous clinical guidelines; the evaluation positions include:
  1. Inspection: client sitting, arms at side; sitting, arms above head; sitting or standing, leaning over; sitting, hands pressed onto hips
  2. Palpation: client sitting, arms at side; sitting, arms above head
  3. Palpation: client lying, arm above head
  The total time required to completely evaluate the breasts should be between 5 and 10 minutes.
- **Symmetry is a key consideration in the assessment of the breasts:** There should be a comparison of one side with the other throughout the assessment process.
- **For proper breast assessment, the client must be undressed to the waist:** She must be encouraged to uncover both breasts at once so that they may be viewed together and compared. The examiner is not doing the client a favor by allowing her to uncover only one breast at a time.
- **Room lighting for examination of the breast is very important:** The illumination should be overhead and adequate to shed an even light over all breast surfaces. Recognizing subtle coloring or surface characteristic changes of the breasts may depend on the lighting of the examination room.
- **The male client must be evaluated with the same sensitivity as the female client:** Male breast cancer accounts for about 1% of all cancer of the breast. Beyond that, there are numerous other disease or inflammatory processes that can cause gynecomastia or areolar inflammation (see Fig. 10-17).
- **When palpating the breast, the examiner must learn to use the sensitive fingerpads of the palmar surface of the hand (see Fig. 10-13):** The examiner must inch along the breast surface, using a rotating exploratory manner. Try *not to lift* the fingers

off the breast when moving from one point to the next. The examination technique should smoothly and continually move forward.

- **It is most beneficial to first do a complete light palpation and then repeat the procedure, changing to a deeper, heavier palpation:** Most authorities state that the light exploratory palpation will yield more information than the deeper palpation.
- **Examining women with very large breasts requires special considerations:** The palpation component of the seated examination is best performed when the examiner immobilizes the breast underneath with one hand while examining the above surface when the other hand. This bimanual palpation technique may assist in the detection of small mobile masses not picked up by other techniques.
- **If a client is examined immediately before her menstrual period, her breasts may be tender and engorged:** Make arrangements for the client to return after the end of her period for a thorough breast assessment.
- **During the examination of the nipples, the examiner should gently express the nipple with the index fingers of both hands and slowly strip the nipple between the fingers as they slide from the areola to the tip of the nipple:** Palpation of the nipple should also include an exploration for small masses or duct thickening. If nipple discharge is present, note if it is coming from a single duct opening or multiple ones.
- **Although it is relatively simple to palpate the areas where the lymph nodes are located, it is another issue to relate the lymph nodes with their drainage significance:** Following is an outline of the patterns for breast lymphatic drainage. (See Fig. 10-14.)
  1. Lymphatic drainage of superficial breast tissue
     a. Mammary chain (located along medial and superior borders of breast tissue; drainage occurs toward opposite breast)
     b. Scapular ⎫
     c. Brachial ⎬ All located in upper outer quadrant of breast; drainage occurs toward axillary nodes
     c. Intermediate ⎭
  2. Lymphatic drainage of deep breast tissue
     a. Supraclavicular
     b. Apical nodes or subclavicular or infraclavicular
     c. Central axillary
     d. Lateral axillary
     e. Pectoral (anterior)
     f. Subscapular (posterior)

  All these lymph nodes drain the breast. The most common drainage patterns are toward the *lateral axillary* (drains arm), *subscapular,* and *supraclavicular chains.* The medial and inferior deep breast

tissue may also drain into the abdominal region.
  3. Areolar lymphatic drainage (areolar and nipple areas)
     a. Central axillary
     b. Apical nodes or subclavicular or infraclavicular
     c. Superior mammary chain

Drainage of the areolar area involves an upward movement, toward the subclavicular and supraclavicular regions.

- **If a client presents with a symptomatic breast problem, the examiner should examine the unaffected breast first.**
- **If the examiner identifies a lump or mass in the client's breast, it should be evaluated according to the following criteria:**
  1. Location according to clock orientation and distance from the nipple
  2. Size
  3. Contour and shape—margin regularity versus irregularity
  4. Consistency (soft, firm, rough)
  5. Discreteness (difficulty determining borders)
  6. Mobility
  7. Tenderness (marked or absent)
  8. Erythema of overlying skin
  9. Tissue characteristics over mass (bulging, dimpling)
- **In compiling the data associated with a breast mass or breast problem, the examiner must determine the urgency of the client's problem:** Table 10-3 presents the physical findings related to benign and malignant breast masses and thus will help the examiner evaluate the data collected during the physical assessment.
- **Develop a systematic assessment method:** As with all of the body systems, a patterned assessment process reduces the likelihood of missing a significant finding.

  The following are recommendations from the American Cancer Society and the National Cancer Institute:
- Annual or other periodic mammography for asymptomatic women 50 years of age and older
- Annual or periodic mammography for women between 40 and 49 years of age if they are at high risk, that is, have a history of breast cancer, have had prior breast biopsy results of lobular carcinoma in situ or an atypical proliferative process, or have been successfully treated for carcinoma of the ovary or endometrium
- Annual or other periodic mammography in women younger than 40 years of age if they have a history of breast cancer or a premenopausal mother or sister with breast cancer, especially if bilateral
- Baseline mammogram for women 35 to 50 years of age.

TABLE 10-3   Physical findings helpful in the differential diagnosis of a breast lump

PHYSICAL FINDINGS	FAVORS MALIGNANCY	FAVORS BENIGNANCY
Hard, dominant lump	Single, definite	Multiple, indistinct
Firm, palpable, radiating ducts	No help	Indicates cystic disease
Venous engorgement	Unilateral	Bilateral
Nipple deviation	Unilateral	Bilateral, symmetrical
Nipple excoriation	Unilateral	Bilateral
Skin dimpling	Present	Absent
Chest wall fixation	Present	Absent
Peau d'orange	Present	Absent
Bloody discharge	Present	Absent
Axillary or supraclavicular nodes	Present	Absent
Freely movable mass	No help	Typical of fibroadenoma
Tenderness	No help	May indicate cystic mass
Inflammation, heat	Ominous in nonlactating or nonpostpartum breast	Abscess in lactating or postpartum breast

From Nance F: Clin Obstet Gynecol *18(2):188, 1975.*

TECHNIQUES AND STRATEGIES FOR TEACHING BREAST SELF-EXAMINATION

Although it is impossible to prevent cancer of the breast, every health care provider must assume the position that it is possible to detect a breast mass early and to initiate prompt treatment. Each examiner must incorporate teaching breast self-examination techniques into the examination procedures because most breast masses will be detected by the women themselves. The American Cancer Society states that 91% of all women who are treated promptly for early breast cancer do recover.

The examiner can facilitate client education and health maintenance by (1) developing a risk profile for the client and sharing the data collected and by (2) teaching breast self-examination techniques.

The teaching program should include both an informal and a structured presentation. The informal component will take place as the examiner is actually checking the client's breasts. Each step should be explained as it is being done. Involve the client in the process. If the client understands what is being done and why, compliance is likely to increase.

The formal component involves scheduling 10 to 15 minutes with the client to systematically discuss the anatomy of the breast, the sequence of the examination techniques, the anticipated findings, the appropriate times of the month to examine the breasts, and what the client should do about abnormal or questionable findings.

The following sequence of information provides the examiner with an instructional overview of breast self-examination*:

1. Breast cancer facts
   a. The estimate for the number of new cases of breast cancer diagnosed in 1991 is more than 175,000.
   b. More than 44,800 women die from breast cancer each year.
   c. Up to 91% of women who receive prompt treatment for early breast cancer recover.
   d. Breast cancer is the second leading cause of death from cancer in women. (Lung cancer is the leading cause.)
   e. Breast cancer usually begins as a lump or thickening in the breast.
   f. About 90% of all breast lumps are found by the women themselves.
   g. About 80% of all breast lumps are benign.
2. Age of women who should examine breasts: *all* women from menarche through old age.
3. Best time of month to examine breasts
   a. Menstruating women: sixth to seventh day of menstrual period; at this time the breasts are least engorged or tender.
   b. Pregnant women: pick single day of each month; the birthdate is generally used.
   c. Postmenopausal women: pick a single day of each month; again, the birthdate is usually a convenient number to remember.

*Data from American Cancer Society.

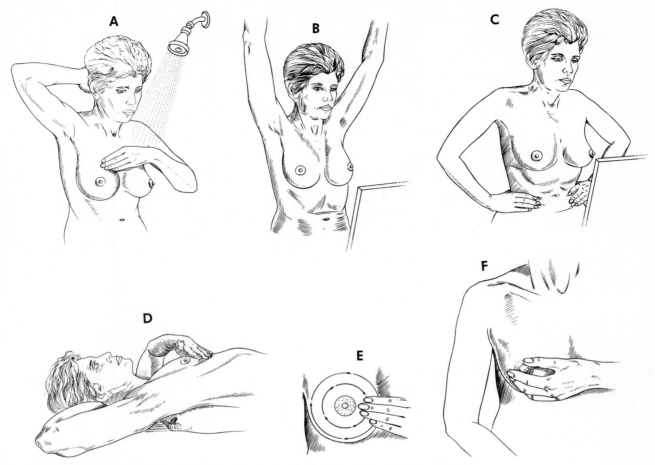

Fig. 10-18 Breast self-examination. **A,** Examine breasts during bath or shower, since flat fingers glide easily over wet skin. Use right hand to examine left breast and vice versa. **B,** Sit or stand before a mirror. Inspect breasts with hands at sides, then raised overhead. Look for changes in contour or dimpling of skin. **C,** Place hands on hips and press down firmly to flex chest muscles. **D,** Lie down with one hand under head and pillow or folded towel under the scapula. **E,** Palpate that breast with other hand using concentric circle method. It usually takes three circles to cover all breast tissue. Include the tail of the breast and the axilla. Repeat with other breast. **F,** End in a sitting position. Palpate the areola areas of both breasts, and inspect and squeeze nipples to check for discharge. (From Phipps WJ, Long BC, Woods NF: *Medical-surgical nursing: concepts and clinical practice,* ed 3, St Louis, 1987, Mosby–Year Book.)

4. Breast anatomy the client must know
   a. Lymph nodes and locations associated with breast self-examination
   b. The four quadrants, the tail, the mammary ridge
   c. Areolar area
   d. Nipple
   e. Tissue characteristics: tenderness, nodular
5. Steps in teaching breast self-examination (Fig. 10-18); instructions for client
6. What to do if lump or abnormality is identified
   a. Note time of month in relation to menses.
   b. Assist client to make appointment with physician for further evaluation.

SAMPLE RECORDING: NORMAL FINDINGS

Breasts moderate size.

Left slightly larger than right.

Firm, smooth texture bilaterally, without masses, retractions, bulges, or skin lesions.

Silver striae noted bilaterally.

Nipples erect; no discharge.

Areolar area intact and smooth bilaterally; pigmentation bilaterally equal.

No nodes palpated: axillary, supraclavicular, or infra-clavicular.

Instructed on breast self-examination; return demonstration completed.

The Newborn

HISTORY AND CLINICAL STRATEGIES

- Breast areola is one indicator of gestational age. A small areola is a sign of prematurity, irrespective of a newborn's birth weight. A full-term infant will have a full, raised areola bud, between 5 and 10 mm across.

- Parents may need education about the nonproblematic nature of supernumerary nipples, breast engorgement, and watery nipple discharge seen in some newborns.

CLINICAL VARIATIONS: THE NEWBORN

CHARACTERISTIC OR AREA EXAMINED	NORMAL FINDINGS	DEVIATIONS FROM NORMAL
1. Breast	Engorgement, watery discharge (witch's milk) may be caused by maternal hormones	Mastitis, infected newborn breasts
2. Nipples	Breast areola (about 5-10 mm)	Smaller areola in preterm, larger in postterm infants
	Supernumerary nipples may be present	Full-term infant has nipple about 0.75 cm

 ## The Child

HISTORY AND CLINICAL STRATEGIES

Although the breasts should be inspected during each well-child visit as part of the chest examination, there are basically two time periods when the examiner systematically evaluates the breasts: (1) during the newborn period; and (2) as a girl reaches puberty and her breasts begin to develop. Because the clinical guidelines for inspection and palpation remain the same for both the child and the adult, this section of the chapter has been developed to provide information about breast development and clinical strategies when approaching the pediatric client.

Often the neonate's breast may be enlarged for 1 to 2 months. This is a simple hypertrophic breast, which is normal. Characteristics include flat nipple, small areola, and a small amount of milky discharge. Deviations requiring referral include hypertrophy extending beyond 3 months, redness, heat, or firmness around the nipple, and increased pigmentation around the areola.

Boys who are stocky or heavy may experience some hypertrophy of breast tissue. This may be a normal finding but many times is of great concern to the boy. He should be assured that, as he grows and thins, the hypertrophy will disappear. The examiner should assess the breast to rule out actual breast development, tenderness, masses, redness, or inflammation. At puberty, true gynecomastia is normal for some boys, but for others it may be a symptom of a systemic disease process. Refer these boys for further evaluation.

As breast tissue in girls begins to develop, there will usually be protrusion of the nipple first. Breasts in girls normally develop between the ages 10 years 8 months and 13 years 6 months. Menarche occurs in most girls at about 12 years 3 months (Fig. 10-19). Table 10-4 summarizes the physical development of girls. If there

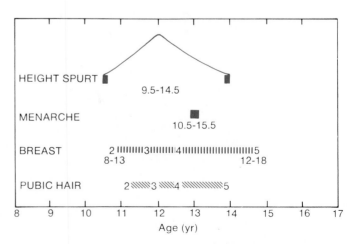

Fig. 10-19 Summary of maturational development of girls. For explanation of numbers 2 through 5, see Table 10-4; summary numbers on table (e.g., 9.5-14.5) indicate average or common range for development characteristic. (From Marshall WA, Tanner JM: *Arch Dis Child* 44:291, 1969.)

is no evidence of breast or other puberty development by age 13 years, the girl should be referred to a physician. Once menarche has begun, the examiner should employ the same breast examination techniques as for the adult client. The young client will need much reassurance and assistance to feel comfortable during the breast examination.

Following are educational factors that may help the client feel more comfortable during examination of the breasts:

1. Breasts may develop at different ages, this is based on hereditary and hormonal characteristics and has nothing to do with the client's femininity.
2. The right and left breasts may not develop at the same rate.
3. Assess the client's understanding of breast development and menarche.
4. Begin educational instruction regarding care of the breasts, qualities of a supportive bra, and breast self-examination techniques.

TABLE 10-4   Maturational sequence in girls

STAGE	BREAST DEVELOPMENT	DEVELOPMENT DESCRIPTION
1		Preadolescent
2		Breast and papilla elevated as small mound; areolar diameter increased
3		Breast and areola enlarged; no contour separation
4		Areola and papilla form secondary mound
5		Mature; nipple projects areolar part of general breast contour

From Tanner JM: Growth at adolescence, ed 2, Oxford, England, 1962, Blackwell Scientific Publications.

The Childbearing Woman

HISTORY AND CLINICAL STRATEGIES

- Prenatal visits may be ideal times to assess and teach clients about monthly breast self-examinations. Although breast cancer is rare in childbearing women, it does occur. Pregnancy can mask the signs of breast cancer.
- Bilateral flat or inverted nipples may present a challenge to breast-feeding women. Women should be educated during physical assessment to be prepared for lactation or lactation suppression.

CLINICAL VARIATIONS: THE CHILDBEARING WOMAN

CHARACTERISTIC OR AREA EXAMINED	NORMAL FINDINGS	DEVIATIONS FROM NORMAL
1. Breasts	Breasts have early signs of pregnancy: enlargement, feelings of increased fullness, heaviness, tenderness, tingling, stretching, and perhaps throbbing Breast blood supply and vessels enlarge; venous patterns may be visible Breast changes less noticeable in multiparous women	Pregnancy-induced breast hypertrophy Redness, pain, hot skin areas, discharge, excoriation, palpable nodule requires investigation
2. Nipples	Nipples elevate; tingling feeling Areola pigment darkens, may widen 5-6 cm, sebaceous glands grow; more prominent Montgomery tubercles Nipples soften Secondary areola may develop Colostrum; thin, yellow fluid develops	
3. Postdelivery	Engorgement may occur about 3rd day after delivery from milk production Pigment fades, but doesn't disappear	Inverted, sore, or cracked nipples require treatment Severe engorgement may occur, especially if not breast-feeding Mastitis, inflammation (usually from cracked nipples and engorgement; *Staphylococcus* is usual causative organism) Abscess (usually from untreated mastitis)

The Older Adult

HISTORY AND CLINICAL STRATEGIES

The elderly client is subject to the same risk factors and physical change parameters as the younger client. The incidence of breast cancer (among women) rises steadily after the age of 40 and continues throughout the aging process. Breast self-examination remains an important consideration for older women.

The physical changes in the breasts that accompany aging follow:

1. Adipose tissue often increases (even if subcutaneous fat decreases over extremities).

2. In some women subcutaneous fat may decrease in the breasts.
3. Breast glandular tissue atrophies.
4. Suspensory ligaments relax, and the breasts appear elongated or pendulous.
5. Chronic cystic disease diminishes after menopause.

In summary, breast palpation is often easier to accomplish because the nodular, glandular palpatory sensation associated with the breast glandular tissue in younger women is diminished. Breast lumps become even more significant in older clients. Refer to pp. 320-328 for assessment guidelines.

Study Questions

General

1. All the following inspection findings are *normal except one.* Identify the *abnormal* finding:
   - ☐ a. Slight breast asymmetry
   - ☐ b. Deviated nipple
   - ☐ c. Venous pattern seen on both breasts
   - ☐ d. Inverted nipples (bilateral)
   - ☐ e. Montgomery tubercles

2. All the following palpation criteria are *normal except one.* Identify the *abnormal* finding:
   - ☐ a. Diffuse nodularity
   - ☐ b. Mammary ridge
   - ☐ c. Palpable supraclavicular lymph node
   - ☐ d. Bilateral tenderness
   - ☐ e. Soft tissue bilaterally

3. Which of the following women should be referred to a physician for further examination:
   - ☐ a. A 26-year-old with multiple nodules palpated in each breast
   - ☐ b. A 48-year-old who has a 6-month history of reddened and sore left nipple and areolar area
   - ☐ c. A 35-year-old with asymmetrical breasts and inversion of nipples since birth of second child 8 years ago
   - ☐ d. A 15-year-old with minimal breast development
   - ☐ e. A 64-year-old with very slight ulcerated area at tip of right nipple; no masses, tenderness, or lymph nodes palpated
   - ☐ f. All except c
   - ☐ g. a, c, and d
   - ☐ h. b, d, and e
   - ☐ i. a and c
   - ☐ j. b and e

4. When palpating lymph nodes associated with drainage of the breasts, the examiner must palpate:
   - ☐ a. Along the sternum
   - ☐ b. Supraclavicular and subclavicular area
   - ☐ c. Pectoral area
   - ☐ d. Axillary area
   - ☐ e. Lower thoracic area under breast
   - ☐ f. All of the above
   - ☐ g. All except a
   - ☐ h. All except c and e
   - ☐ i. All except c
   - ☐ j. All except a and e

The Newborn

5. Full-term breast areola is about:
   - ☐ a. 1 to 2 mm
   - ☐ b. 2 to 3 mm
   - ☐ c. 3 to 4 mm
   - ☐ d. 5 to 10 mm

The Child

6. Of the following children, *one* has an abnormal finding during the breast examination and should be referred. Identify the child with the abnormal finding:
   - ☐ a. John is a 9-day-old boy who has bilateral hypertrophy of the breast; a slight amount of milky-colored nipple discharge is observed
   - ☐ b. Bonnie is a 1-month-old girl who has bilateral hypertrophy of the breast; there is no nipple discharge
   - ☐ c. Amy is a 3-month-old female who has bilateral hypertrophy of the breast; there is no nipple discharge
   - ☐ d. Michael is a 12-year-old husky boy who has recently developed bilateral hypertrophy of the breast; there is no nipple discharge
   - ☐ e. Marilyn is a 13-year-old girl who is concerned because, unlike all her friends, she has had no breast development

7. Which of the following 15-year-old girls should receive breast self-examination instructions:
   - ☐ a. Nancy: well developed; negative family history for breast cancer
   - ☐ b. Cindy: just beginning breast development; negative family history for breast cancer
   - ☐ c. Judy: has small breasts; both her aunt and grandmother have had breast cancer
   - ☐ d. Lynn: average breast development appropriate for age; has just started menstruating; mother has fibrocystic disease
   - ☐ e. Karen: very large breasted; started menstruating at age 12 years; negative family history for breast cancer
   - ☐ f. a, b, and e
   - ☐ g. All except d
   - ☐ h. b, c, and e
   - ☐ i. All of the above
   - ☐ j. None of the above

The Childbearing Woman

8. Colostrum is thin:
   - ☐ a. Yellow fluid
   - ☐ b. Clear fluid
   - ☐ c. White fluid
   - ☐ d. Pink fluid

9. Breast engorgement usually occurs in postpartum around the:
   - ☐ a. 1st day
   - ☐ b. 2nd day
   - ☐ c. 3rd day
   - ☐ d. 4th day

The Older Adult

10. With aging, breasts have more:
    - ☐ a. Adipose tissue
    - ☐ b. Subcutaneous fat
    - ☐ c. Ligament support
    - ☐ d. Glandular tissue

SUGGESTED READINGS
General

American Cancer Society: *1986 cancer facts and figures,* New York, New York, 1986.

American Cancer Society: *Mammography 1982: a statement of the American Cancer Society, CA* 32(4):226, 1982.

American Cancer Society: *Teaching breast self-examination,* Instructional material no 77-1R-50M-6/77; no 2015-LE.

American Cancer Society and American Society of Plastic and Reconstructive Surgeons: *Breast reconstruction following mastectomy for cancer: questions and answers,* New York, 1979.

Bates B: *A guide to physical examination,* ed 4, Philadelphia, 1987, JB Lippincott.

Bonadonna G, editor: *Cancer investigation and management,* vol 1, *Breast cancer: diagnosis and management,* New York, 1984, John Wiley & Sons.

Goodson WA, and others: What do breast symptoms mean? *Am J Surg* 150(2):271, 1985.

Grump FE: Premalignant diseases of the breast, *Surg Clin North Am* 64(6):1051, 1984.

Malasanos L, Barkauskas V, Stoltenberg-Allen K: *Health assessment,* ed 4, St Louis, 1990, Mosby–Year Book.

Mammography guidelines 1983: background statement and update of cancer-related check-up guidelines for breast cancer detection in asymptomatic women age 40 to 49, *CA* 33:225, 1983.

Phipps WJ, Long BC, Woods NF, Cassmeyer VL: *Medical-surgical nursing: concepts and clinical practice,* ed 4, St Louis, 1991, Mosby–Year Book.

Prior JA, Silberstein JS, Stang JM: *Physical diagnosis: the history and examination of the patient,* ed 6, St Louis, 1981, Mosby–Year Book.

Richardson JD: Imaging of the breast, *Med Clin North Am* 68(6):1481, 1984.

Seidel HM, Ball JW, Dains JE, Benedict GW: *Mosby's guide to physical examination,* ed 2, St Louis, 1991, Mosby–Year Book.

Silverberg E, Lubera JA: A review of American Cancer Society estimates of cancer cases and deaths, *CA* 33(1):2, 1983.

Thompson JM, McFarland GK, Hirsch JE, and others: *Clinical nursing,* ed 2, St Louis, 1989, Mosby–Year Book.

The newborn

Auvenshine MA, Enriquez MG: *Maternity nursing: dimensions of change,* Belmont, Calif, 1985, Wadsworth.

Judd JM: Assessing the newborn from head to toe, *Nurs '85* 15(12):34, 1985.

Kiernan BS, Scoloveno MA: Assessment of the neonate, *Top Clin Nurs* 8(1):1, 1985.

The Organization for Obstetrical, Gynelogical and Neonatal Nurses (NAACOG): *Physical assessment of the neonate,* OGN Nursing Practice Resource, Oct. 1986, The Association.

Whaley LF: Wong DL: *Nursing care of infants and children,* ed 4, St Louis, 1991, Mosby–Year Book.

The child

Barness L: *Manual of pediatric physical diagnosis,* ed 6, St Louis, 1991, Mosby–Year Book.

Marshall WA, Tanner JM: Variations in the pattern of pubertal changes in boys, *Arch Dis Child* 45:22, 1970.

Pillitteri A: *Nursing care of the growing family: a child health text,* Boston, 1977, Little, Brown.

Tanner JM: *Growth at adolescence,* ed 2, Oxford, England, 1962, Blackwell Scientific Publications.

Whaley LF, Wong DL: *Essentials of pediatric nursing,* ed 3, St Louis, 1989, Mosby–Year Book.

The childbearing woman

Auvenshine MA, Enriquez MG: *Maternity nursing: dimensions of change,* Belmont, Calif, 1985, Wadsworth.

Bobak IM, Jensen MD: *Essentials of maternity nursing,* ed 3, St Louis, 1991, Mosby–Year Book.

Pillitteri A: *Maternal-newborn nursing: care of the growing family,* ed 3, Boston, 1985, Little, Brown.

Pritchard JA, MacDonald PC: *Williams' obstetrics,* ed 17, New York, 1985, Appleton-Century-Crofts.

Seidel HM, Ball JW, Dains JE, Benedict GW: *Mosby's guide to physical examination,* ed 2, St Louis, 1991, Mosby–Year Book.

Whitley N: *A manual of clinical obstetrics,* Philadelphia, 1985, JB Lippincott.

The older adult

Carotenuto R, Bullock J: *Physical assessment of the gerontologic client,* Philadelphia, 1980, FA Davis.

Malasanos L, Barkauskas V, Stoltenberg-Allen K: *Health assessment,* ed 4, St Louis, 1990, Mosby–Year Book.

Seidel HM, Ball JW, Dains JE, Benedict GW: *Mosby's guide to physical examination,* ed 2, St Louis, 1991, Mosby–Year Book.

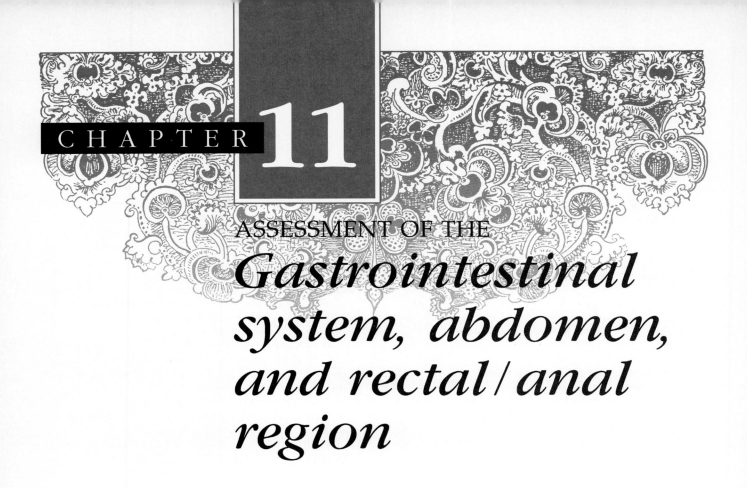

CHAPTER 11

ASSESSMENT OF THE
Gastrointestinal system, abdomen, and rectal/anal region

VOCABULARY

ascites Accumulation of serous fluid in the perintoneal cavity.

ballottement Technique of palpating a floating structure by bouncing it gently and feeling it rebound.

borborygmi Abdominal sounds produced by hyperactive intestinal peristalsis, audible at a distance.

diastasis recti Lateral separation of the two halves of the rectus abdominis muscle.

flank Part of the body between the bottom of the ribs and the upper border of the ilium.

flatulence Presence of excessive amounts of gases in the stomach or intestine.

guarding Protective withdrawal or positioning of a body part.

linea alba White line of connective tissue in the abdomen extending from sternum to pubis.

McBurney point Point of specialized tenderness in acute appendicitis, situated on a line between the umbilicus and the right anterosuperior iliac spine, about 1 or 2 inches above the latter.

Murphy sign Sign of gallbladder disease consisting of pain on taking a deep breath when the examiner's fingers are pressing on the approximate location of the gallbladder.

pilonidal fistula (or sinus) Abnormal channel containing a tuft of hair, situated most frequently over or close to the tip of the coccyx but also occurring in other regions of the body.

Poupart ligament Inguinal ligament.

pyrosis Burning sensation in the epigastric and sternal region with the raising of acid liquid from the stomach; also called *heartburn*.

rebound tenderness Sign of inflammation in the peritoneum in which pain is elicited by sudden withdrawal of a hand pressing on the abdomen.

Riedel lobe Tongue-shaped mass of tissue projecting from the right lobe of the liver.

shifting dullness Change in the dull sounds heard with palpation; at first the dull sound is heard in one location, then in a different location.

striae Streaks of linear scars that often result from rapidly developing tension in the skin; also called *stretch marks*.

tenesmus Spasmodic contraction of the anal or vesical sphincter with pain and a persistent desire to empty the bowel or bladder; involves involuntary, ineffective straining efforts.

tympanites Distention of the abdomen caused by pressure of gas in the intestine or the abdominal cavity.

verge (anal) External ring opening of the anus.

ANATOMY AND PHYSIOLOGY REVIEW

The abdominal cavity is the largest cavity in the human body. It contains the stomach, small intestine, colon, liver, pancreas, spleen, kidneys, adrenal glands, uterus in women, and major vessels. The abdomen is bordered anteriorly by the abdominal and iliac muscles, posteriorly by the vertebral column and lumbar muscles, inferiorly by the plane of the superior aperture of the lesser pelvis, and superiorly by the diaphragm (Fig. 11-1).

Stomach

The stomach is a hollow, muscular organ that stores food during eating, secretes digestive juices, mixes food with the digestive juices, and propels partially digested food into the duodenum of the small intestine.

Small Intestine

In the small intestine, ingested food is mixed, digested, and absorbed. The small intestine is divided into three segments: the duodenum, jejunum, and ileum. The first portion, the duodenum, is the shortest segment, measuring 20 to 30 cm in length. The ligament of Treitz is the dividing point between the duodenum and jejunum, although histological changes cannot be demonstrated. The jejunum is 2.5 meters long, and the ileum is 3.5 meters (Fig. 11-2).

Large Intestine (Colon) and Rectum

The large intestine is about 1.5 meters long. It consists of the cecum, appendix, colon, rectum, and anal canal. The cecum is a pouch that receives chyme from the ileum. Attached to the cecum is the appendix (Fig. 11-3).

Liver, Gallbladder, and Pancreas

The liver, gallbladder, and pancreas all secrete substances necessary for the digestion of chyme. The liver produces bile, which contains salts necessary for fat digestion and absorption. Between meals bile is stored in the gallbladder. The pancreas produces enzymes

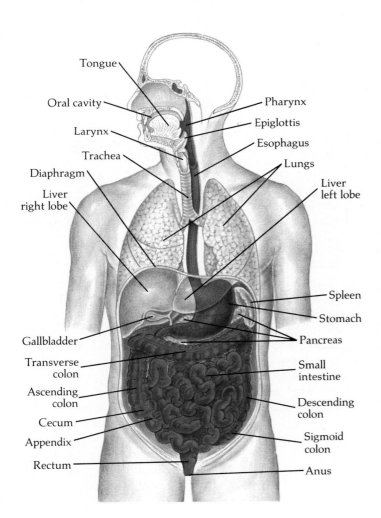

Tongue
Oral cavity
Larynx
Trachea
Diaphragm
Liver right lobe
Pharynx
Epiglottis
Esophagus
Lungs
Liver left lobe
Gallbladder
Transverse colon
Ascending colon
Cecum
Appendix
Rectum
Spleen
Stomach
Pancreas
Small intestine
Descending colon
Sigmoid colon
Anus

Fig. 11-1 Anatomy of gastrointestinal system. (From Thompson JM, McFarland GK, Hirsch JE, and others: *Mosby's manual of clinical nursing,* ed 2, St Louis, 1989, Mosby–Year Book.)

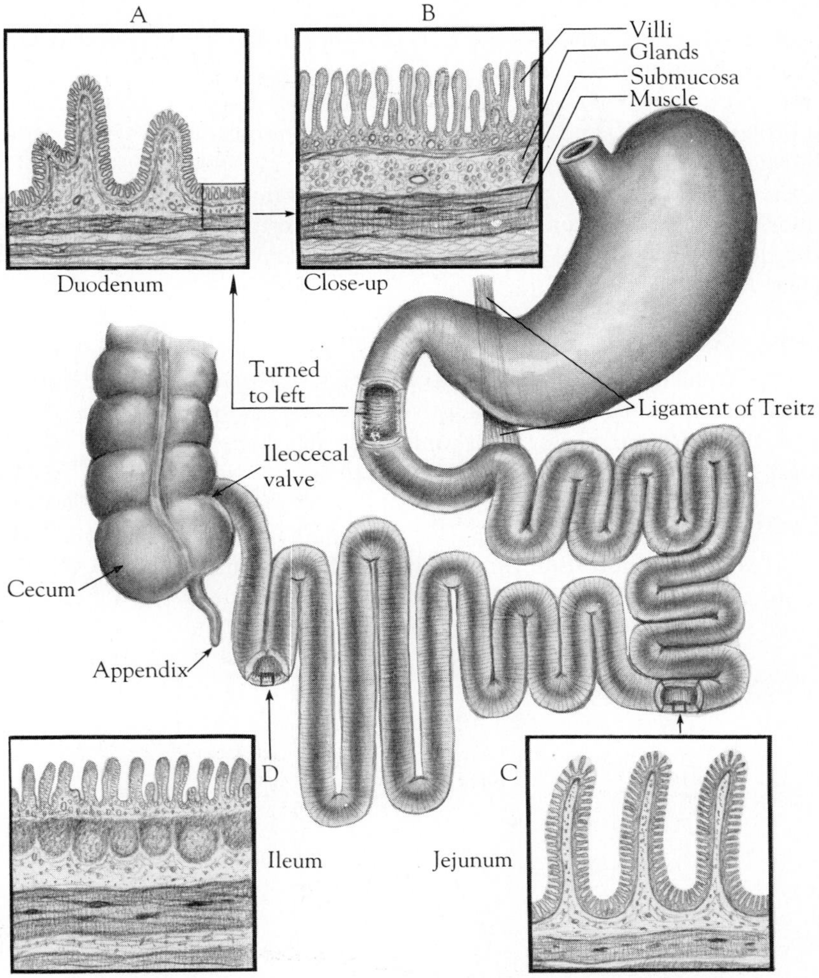

Fig. 11-2 Clinical anatomy of small intestine. (From Thompson JM, McFarland GK, Hirsch JE, and others: *Mosby's manual of clinical nursing,* ed 2, St Louis, 1989, Mosby—Year Book.)

needed for the complete digestion of carbohydrates, proteins, and fats.

The liver is the largest organ in the body, weighing 3 to 4 pounds. It is a complex organ with many functions, including bile production, protein metabolism, carbohydrate metabolism, fat metabolism, coagulation, detoxification, and storage of certain minerals and vitamins. The liver is located under the right diaphragm and is divided into right and left lobes. The larger, right lobe is further divided into the caudate and quadrate lobes.

The gallbladder is a pear-shaped sac 6 to 8 cm long and attached to the inferior surface of the liver. Its purpose is to store bile, which is produced by the liver.

The pancreas lies in the upper abdominal cavity behind the stomach. It has a long tail that extends over to the spleen. It functions as an exocrine gland in that it produces digestive juices containing inactive enzymes used to break down proteins, fats, and carbohydrates. The pancreatic duct empties into the duodenum. Once

in the common bile duct, the hormones *insulin* and *glucagon* are secreted directly into the blood, to regulate the body's level of glucose.

Spleen

The spleen is a concave, encapsulated organ that weighs about 150 g and is about the size of a fist. It is located in the upper left abdominal cavity. Blood that circulates through the spleen comes from the splenic artery. The portion of arterial blood that enters the spleen first encounters the white splenic pulp, which consists of masses of lymphoid tissue containing lymphocytes and macrophages. The white pulp forms clumps around the splenic arterioles and is the chief site of immune and phagocytic function within the spleen.

The red pulp of the spleen contains a capillary network and venous sinus system that allow for the storage and release of blood, permitting the spleen to accommodate up to several hundred milliliters of blood at one time.

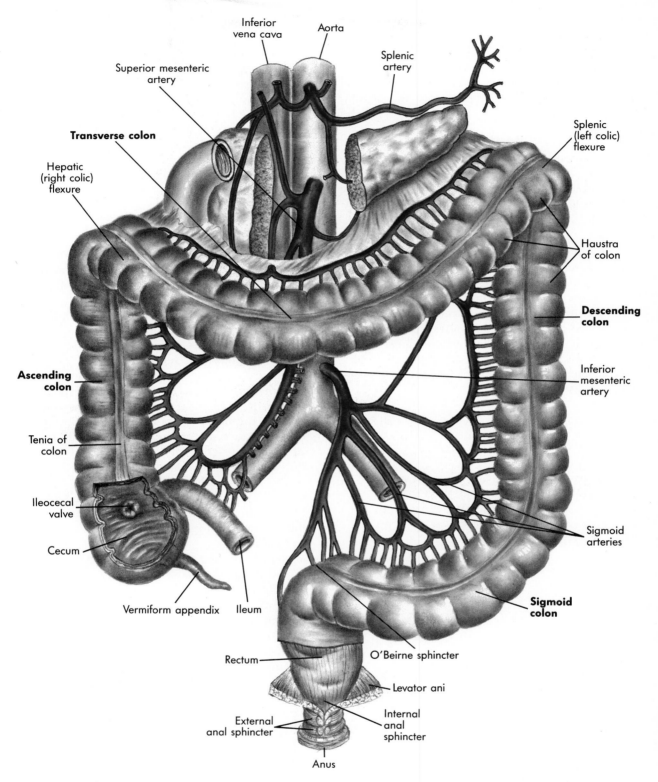

Fig. 11-3 Divisions of the large intestine. *Clockwise from lower left:* The cecum, ascending colon, transverse colon, descending colon, sigmoid colon, rectum, and anal canal. Unlike the small intestine, the large intestine contains teniae coli, three bands of longitudinal muscle that are shorter than the intestinal wall. The teniae coli gather the large intestine lengthwise, forming outpouchings called *haustra.* (From McCance KL, Huether SE: *Pathophysiology: the biological basis for disease in adults and children,* St Louis, 1990, Mosby—Year Book.)

The spleen is not necessary for life or for hematological function. However, splenic absence causes leukocytosis. This suggests that the spleen exerts some control over the rate of proliferation of leukocyte stem cells in the bone marrow or their release into the bloodstream.

Kidneys, Ureters, and Bladder

The kidneys are located in the posterior abdominal cavity (Fig. 11-4). Each kidney is covered by a tough capsule, surrounded by a cushion of fat, and supported by fascia. Each kidney is partially protected by the ribs. The lower end of each kidney extends below the ribs; the right kidney is lower than the left one. One kidney lies on each side of the vetebral column with its upper and lower pole extending from the twelfth thoracic to the third lumbar vertebra. Each kidney contains more than one million nephrons—the structural and functional units of the kidneys.

The urine formed by the nephrons flows from the distal tubules and collecting ducts through the ducts of the renal pelvis and is funneled into the ureters. Each ureter is approximately 30 cm long and is composed of long, intertwining muscle bundles.

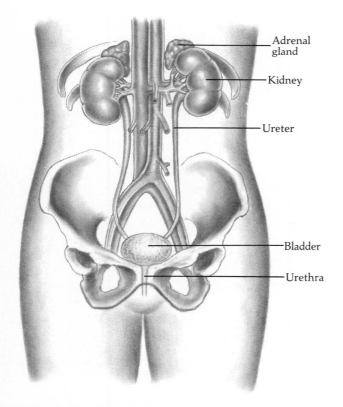

Adrenal gland

Kidney

Ureter

Bladder

Urethra

Fig. 11-4 Components of the urinary system. (From Thompson JM, McFarland GK, Hirsch JE, and others: *Mosby's manual of clinical nursing,* ed 2, St Louis, 1989, Mosby—Year Book.

The bladder is a sac composed of smooth muscle fibers that form the detrusor muscle and the bladder's smooth epithelial lining.

• • •

Examination of the gastrointestinal system is quite complex. The examiner must know the underlying anatomy, as well as the parameters of normal findings. The examiner is encouraged to conduct the assessment carefully and thoroughly so as not to overlook any clinical findings.

COGNITIVE OBJECTIVES

At the end of this chapter the learner will demonstrate knowledge of assessment of the gastrointestinal system and the abdomen by the ability to do the following:

- Apply the terms that are listed in the vocabulary section.
- Describe eight variables that might alter a client's capacity for adequate nutrition.
- Describe five activities or conditions that contribute to client comfort and relaxation in preparation for an abdominal examination.
- Describe the location of the major abdominal organs in terms of abdominal quadrants.
- Identify the major abdominal organs in terms of location, relative size, and relationship to adjacent structures by completing an illustration.
- Recognize normal findings associated with inspection of the abdominal surface, configuration, and pulsations.
- Identify the rationale for performing auscultation of the abdomen before performing percussion and palpation.
- Recognize normal findings associated with auscultation of the abdomen.
- Identify normal findings associated with percussion of the abdomen.
- Recognize the major characteristics of a normal liver span and location.
- Identify the major characteristics of a normal spleen location and accessibility through percussion and palpation.
- Describe the method for effective percussion and palpation of liver and spleen borders.
- Give three reasons for performing light palpation of the abdomen.
- Describe three reasons for performing deep palpation of the abdomen.
- Recognize the major palpable characteristics of liver, kidney, small bowel, and pancreatic masses.
- Identify abdominal areas that might be normally tender during deep palpation.
- Recognize normal drainage patterns of the superficial inguinal nodes.

- Identify specific examiner behaviors that will minimize client discomfort and enhance efficiency of the rectal examination.
- Point out major characteristics of structures within the anal and rectal canals.
- Identify selected common variations for the newborn, the child, the childbearing woman, and the older adult.

CLINICAL OUTLINE

At the end of this chapter the learner will perform a systematic assessment of the abdomen and the inguinal area, demonstrating the ability to do the following:
- Obtain a pertinent health history from a client.
- Inspect the abdominal surface for the following:
  1. Skin color
  2. Surface characteristics
  3. Presence of scars
  4. Venous network pattern
  5. Umbilicus contour, placement, and surface characteristics
  6. Abdominal contour and symmetry
  7. Surface motion: peristalsis and pulsations
  8. General movement with respirations
- Auscultate all four quadrants and the epigastrium for the following:
  1. Presence and timing of bowel sounds
  2. Presence and creation of vascular sounds
- Percuss all four quadrants of the abdomen and describe the tone(s) elicited in specific areas.
- Percuss the upper and lower liver borders and estimate the midclavicular liver span and descent during inspiration.
- Percuss in the left midaxillary line for splenic dullness or absence of dullness.
- Percuss the gastric bubble and estimate its size.
- Lightly palpate all four quadrants for the following:
  1. Tenderness
  2. Guarding
  3. Surface characteristics
  4. Masses
- Deeply palpate all four quadrants for normal and abnormal tenderness and masses.
- Deeply palpate at the right costal margin for the following:
  1. Liver border
  2. Contour
  3. Tenderness
- Deeply palpate at the left costal margin for the splenic border.
- Deeply palpate the abdomen for the right and left kidneys.
- Deeply palpate the midline epigastric area for aortic pulsation.
- Lightly palpate the inguinal regions for the following:
  1. Horizontal and vertical lymph nodes
  2. Contour
  3. Consistency
  4. Delimitation
  5. Tenderness
  6. Redness
  7. Size
- Inspect and palpate the sacrococcygeal and perianal areas for surface characteristics and tenderness.
- Inspect and palpate the anus for the following:
  1. Sphincter tone
  2. Tenderness
  3. Surface characteristics
- Palpate the distal rectal walls for surface characteristics.
- Summarize results of the assessment with a written description of findings.

HISTORY

- Nutritional assessment screening questions, outlined in the original data base (Chapter 1, p. 7), provide the examiner with basic information about the client's food intake (through the use of a 24-hour recall chart), the client's weight measurement and stability, and major variables that might alter intake pattern. These data can be analyzed to assure the client and examiner that daily nutritional needs are being met in terms of the basic four good groups.

  If food consumption or weight problems exist, further assessment is warranted.
  1. The 24-hour recall intake record can be extended to cover a week's intake (to give an overview of day-to-day *and weekend* variations).
  2. The final data can be analyzed in terms of recommended daily dietary allowances for calories, proteins, fats, carbohydrates, vitamins, and minerals.
  3. Further variables that might affect food intake should be explored:
     a. A survey of food preferences and dislikes
     b. Family routines and values (e.g., food portions, eating times, control of food purchase and service, insistence on having a "clean place," family values regarding ideal weight or appearance)
     c. Cultural and religious values (e.g., forbidden foods, foods that are served frequently)
     d. Psychological variables (e.g., depression, anxiety, compulsive eating habits, alteration in coping capacity caused by multiple life-style changes)
     e. Physical status (e.g., ill health, allergies or food idiosyncracies, mouth or dental problems, alterations in physical activity)
     f. Access to food (e.g., transportation, type and availability of grocery store)
     g. Personal habits of life-style (e.g., use of convenience foods because of limited time or interest

in cooking, frequent dining out, night occupation and unusual eating schedule, dormitory or rooming house controls, disorganized life-style with no regular eating or shopping patterns, constant use of "fast food" restaurants for lunch or dinner, frequent entertaining or feasting on weekends and holidays, sedentary life-style with frequent snacks, or high-caloric expenditure with very active life-style)

   h. Eating behaviors (e.g., rapid eating, nibbling food all day, skipping meals, late-night snacks)

   i. Self-imposed dietary additions or restrictions (e.g., vitamin/mineral supplements, food supplements, vegetarian diet, low-calorie diet, low-carbohydrate diet, other diet forms)

   j. Body image profile (self-assessment of satisfaction with present weight, weight distribution, and recall of peer reaction to client's appearance)

   k. Medication profile (to evaluate drug interference with appetite, absorption)

   l. General knowledge of basic four food requirements, shopping within a budget, and content of fat, sugar, and proteins in basic foods

- Anorexia nervosa and bulimia have been recognized as increasingly common and serious eating disorders. Although it is beyond the scope of this text to offer any in-depth explanation of these illnesses, the following list of their possible characteristics may alert the examiner to pursue further investigation:

   1. Female (a very small percentage is male)

   2. Twelve to 22 years of age (the disorder may include clients 30 to 40 years of age)

   3. Perfectionism (related to appearance, work, scholastic or other achievements)

   4. Weight loss of 20% of body weight (or more)

   5. Erratic food-intake history (client may be preoccupied, anxious, or secretive about the subject)

   6. History of mood lability; irritability

   7. History of amenorrhea

   8. History of sleep disturbances

   9. Integumentary changes (e.g., dry skin, loss of hair)

   10. Gastrointestinal complaints (e.g., diarrhea, constipation, abdominal pains)

   11. Emaciated appearance (may exhibit delayed skeletal maturation)

- Abdominal pain may be reported as "indigestion," "heartburn," "stomachache," or other vague descriptions that need clarification and a full symptom analysis by the examiner. The client may experience pain that is diffuse and may be unable to specifically locate the discomfort. The pain may be precisely located, and/or it may radiate to adjacent or remote areas. The discomfort may feel superficial or very deep. Referred pain often occurs as the pain intensifies. The following referral patterns may be helpful in eliciting information from the client (Fig. 11-5).

- Various interpretations of indigestion might include a feeling of fullness, heartburn, mild diffuse discomfort, excessive belching, flatulence, nausea, a bad taste, loss of appetite, or severe pain. The client must clarify the following:

   1. Location of feeling or pain (if possible); radiation of pain (to arms, shoulders)

   2. Symptoms associated with food intake (e.g., immediately before? immediately after? delayed response?)

   3. Amount and type of food associated with discomfort

   4. Associated symptoms (e.g., vomiting, headache, diarrhea)

   5. Associated problems (e.g., anxiety, sleeplessness)

   6. Time of day or night that symptom most often occurs

   7. Body position or activity that causes or relieves pain

- Nausea might be described as an upset stomach, queasy stomach, a need to vomit, a fullness or tightness in the throat. Associated symptoms, such as dizziness, increased salivation, headache, and weakness, should be explored. Again, onset, duration, and patterns should be clarified. Are there any notable stimuli (e.g., particular foods, odors, times of day, activity)? Does it occur with a certain meal? Does it occur before or after food intake? Is it associated with vomiting? If so, how?

- To what extent is vomiting associated with abdominal pain, nausea, retching? Are there other associated symptoms (e.g., fever, headache, diarrhea)? Clarify the timing between food intake and a vomiting episode. Once the symptom has been fully analyzed, the estimated quantity, color, consistency, odor, and taste should be established. If vomiting has occurred repeatedly, find out if the appearance of the vomitus has changed. Ask if there has been a weight loss. Determine whether fluid intake has been maintained, increased, or decreased. Specify which solids or liquids can be retained.

- The location of heartburn is usually substernal. Ask if pain radiates to other areas (e.g., chest, neck, shoulders, back, or arms). Ask if body movement or position change alters the pain (e.g., bending over, sitting up, or lying down). Ask about specific food irritants (e.g., spices, coffee, alcohol). Establish the time of day or night when discomfort is most noticeable.

- Appetite changes (loss or gain) should be explored in terms of particular foods that have been eliminated or added, as well as an estimate of the quantity of food

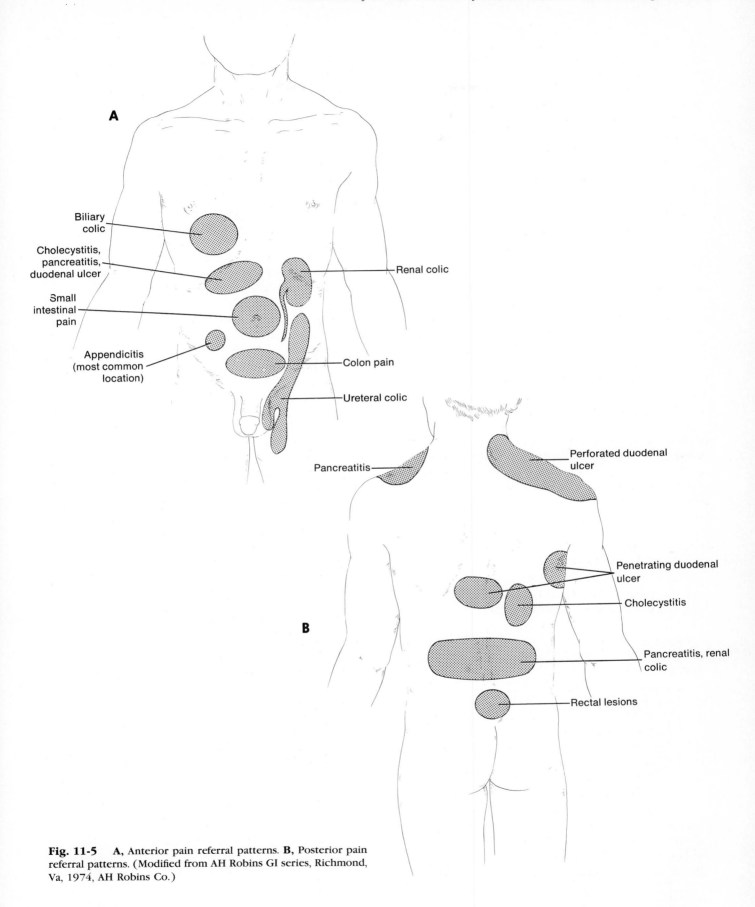

Fig. 11-5   **A,** Anterior pain referral patterns. **B,** Posterior pain referral patterns. (Modified from AH Robins GI series, Richmond, Va, 1974, AH Robins Co.)

that has been changed. Careful inquiry about average weight and recent (past 3 to 9 months) loss or gain is important. Inquire about associated symptoms or situations that might interfere with appetite (e.g., increased stress, abdominal pain, bowel habit changes, other illnesses, or deliberate attempts to reduce caloric intake). Comparing a sample of a previous "normal" 24-hour intake with a present 24-hour intake might be helpful. (*Note:* Recent oral or dental problems can affect appetite.)

- If diarrhea is present, the number of stools per day (24-hour period) or week should be established. Clarify whether this present pattern represents a change in bowel habits. If so, note the onset. Associated symptoms, such as fever, nausea, vomiting, abdominal pain, abdominal distention, flatus, intermittent cramping, marked peristalsis, explosive diarrhea, or urgency to evacuate, should be explored. The consistency, color, quantity, and odor of each stool should be noted. Does the client notice accompanying mucus, blood, or food particles with the stool? Is there nocturnal diarrhea? Has the client been taking antibiotics? Has there been a weight loss? Has the diarrhea interfered with activities of daily living?

- Constipation is usually defined as decreased number of stools, marked difficulty or pain with passage of stools, and/or excessive dryness or hardness of stools. Again the number of stools per day or week must be established. The date and time of the most recent stool should be noted. Establish whether this is a *change* of bowel habit. If so, was the onset sudden or gradual? Have the stools changed in size (smaller, thinner, larger)? Does the client feel that there is stool re-

maining in the rectum? Have there been any food intake changes recently (quantity or type of foods)? Has fluid intake been altered? Other associated abdominal or general symptoms should be inquired about. For example, has the client been depressed?

- Anal discomfort may be described in terms of itching, pain on defecation, a painful lump, or a stinging or burning sensation. Clarify whether body position (e.g., lying down or standing erect) alters the pain. Ask about the color, form, size, and consistency of stools. Ask if the client has noticed mucus or blood (streaks over stool, droplets on toilet paper, discoloration of water in the toilet bowl) at the time of bowel movement. Itching often interferes with sleep. Clarification of duration and daily patterns of itching is important.

- General considerations for gastrointestinal symptom analysis are as follows:

1. It is very important to list all medications that the client is taking and to carefully explore medicines, enemas, or any self-help treatments that the client has been using.
2. Severity of the symptom is often best determined by the client's account of symptom interference with activities of daily living (e.g., loss of sleep, marked eating habit change, loss of time at work, or alteration of daily tasks).
3. The final accuracy of the description of the severity, duration, rhythmicity, and patterns of the pain depend greatly on the client's ability to articulate subjective sensations and a personal pain threshold and the examiner's ability to maintain a balance between nondirective and selective probing approaches.

Text continues on p. 359.

CLINICAL GUIDELINES

ASSESSMENT PROCEDURE	NORMAL FINDINGS	EVALUATION
		DEVIATIONS FROM NORMAL
Abdomen		
1. Assemble necessary equipment a. Stethoscope b. Small ruler c. Marking pencil 2. Position client comfortably in a supine position, making sure: a. Client's bladder recently emptied b. Arms on chest or at sides c. Small pillow under head d. Client's knees slightly flexed, supported by small pillow e. Client draped over breasts and at pubis		

CLINICAL GUIDELINES—cont'd

ASSESSMENT PROCEDURE	EVALUATION	
	NORMAL FINDINGS	DEVIATIONS FROM NORMAL

3. Take additional measures to ensure client comfort:
  a. Make sure room is warm
  b. Have warm hands, short fingernails, warm stethoscope
  c. Instruct client to breathe slowly through mouth if he appears anxious
  d. Offer explanations of examiner activity as assessment progresses		

4. Observe general behavior and appearance of client	Appears relaxed Facial muscles relaxed Lying quietly Respirations even and slow	Emaciated Obese Marked restlessness Marked immobility or rigid posture Knees drawn up Facial grimacing Respirations rapid, uneven, or grunting
5. Inspect the abdominal surface for: a. Skin color	May be paler than other parts because of lack of exposure	Jaundice Redness (inflammation) Lesions, bruises, discoloration, cyanosis (localized by umbilicus or generalized)
b. Surface characteristics	Smooth, soft Silver-white striae (usually lower abdomen) (see Fig. 3-6)	Rashes, lesions Glistening, taut appearance Pink, red striae Purple striae
c. Scars (configuration, location, length)		
d. Venous network	Very faint fine network may be visible	Prominent venous pattern Engorgement of veins around umbilicus
e. Umbilicus (1) Placement	Centrally located	Displaced upward, downward, or laterally
(2) Contour	Usually sunken, may protrude slightly	Visible hernia around or slightly above umbilicus
(3) Surface characteristics	Smooth, noninflamed	Inflamed
f. Contour	Flat	Distended

Continued.

CLINICAL GUIDELINES—cont'd

ASSESSMENT PROCEDURE	EVALUATION	
	NORMAL FINDINGS	DEVIATIONS FROM NORMAL
Abdomen—cont'd	Rounded (Fig. 11-6) Scaphoid (concave profile) (Fig. 11-7)	Marked concavity associated with general wasting signs or antero-posterior rib expansion (Fig. 11-8)
g. Symmetry (*Note:* Examiner must view abdomen at eye level from the side, as well as from behind client's head.)	Evenly rounded with maximum height of convexity at umbilicus	Distention of upper or lower half Visible masses or bulges in any area of abdominal surface
h. Surface motion		
(1) Peristalsis	Usually not visible	Visible
(2) Pulsation	Upper midline pulsation may be visible in thin people	Marked pulsation
i. General movement with respirations	Smooth, even movements Female exhibits chiefly costal movement Male exhibits chiefly abdominal movement	Grunting, labored Respirations accompanied by restricted abdominal movement
6. Instruct client to take a deep breath and hold it	Contour remains smooth and symmetrical	Bulges or masses appear
7. Instruct client to raise head without using arms for support	Rectus abdominis muscles prominent Midline bulge may appear (Fig. 11-9)	Appearance of bulges through muscle layer

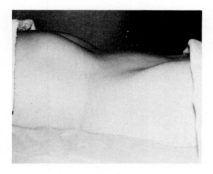

Fig. 11-6   Rounded abdominal contour.

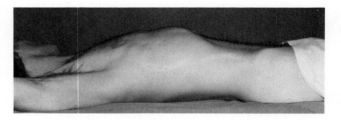

Fig. 11-7   Scaphoid abdominal contour.

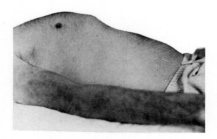

Fig. 11-8   Marked concavity below margin associated with increased anteroposterior chest diameter.

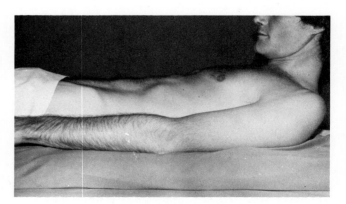

Fig. 11-9   Rectus abdominis muscles become prominent when head and neck are raised. Note that superficial masses will rise with muscles.

ASSESSMENT PROCEDURE	EVALUATION	
	NORMAL FINDINGS	DEVIATIONS FROM NORMAL
8. Auscultate all four abdominal quadrants and the epigastrium, using diaphragm of stethoscope and pressing lightly		
a. Presence and timing of bowel sounds	Usually 5 to 34/min Irregular in timing	Absence of sound established after 5 minutes of listening Note sounds that are infrequent
b. Quality of sounds	Gurgles, clicks Quality of sound varies greatly	High-pitched, tinkling noises
c. Arterial vascular sounds concentrated in epigastric area, in area surrounding umbilicus, over liver, and at posterior flank		Bruits (usually high-pitched, soft "swishing" sound, and systolic in timing) (*Note:* Bruit will continue as client is moved into various positions.)
d. Bell of stethoscope will pick up lower (venous) sounds		Venous hum (lower in pitch, softer, and continuous sound)
e. Friction rub		Infrequently heard sound, associated with respirations (soft, and may be confused with normal breath sounds) Rubs most often heard over spleen or liver
9. Percuss lightly in all four quadrants; note tone (*Note:* Develop a system or route for percussion process, as shown in Fig. 11-10.)	General distribution of tympany (depending on amount of air and solid material in bowel) Suprapubic dullness heard over distended bladder	Marked dullness in local area

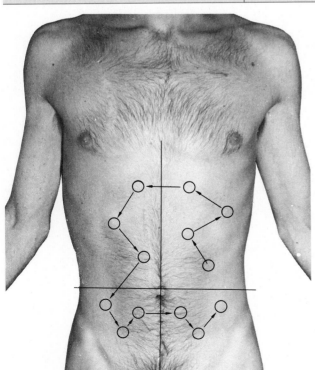

Fig. 11-10 Suggested percussion route for the abdomen.

CLINICAL GUIDELINES—cont'd

ASSESSMENT PROCEDURE	EVALUATION	
	NORMAL FINDINGS	DEVIATIONS FROM NORMAL
Abdomen—cont'd		
a. Liver percussion		
(1) Percuss upward at right midclavicular line, beginning below level of umbilicus; continue percussing over tympanic area until dull percussion rate indicates liver border; note location of lower liver border with marker	Lower border of liver usually at costal margin or slightly below	Lower border of liver exceeds 2 to 3 cm (¾ to 1 inch) below costal margin
(2) Percuss downward at right midclavicular line, beginning from area of lung resonance, and continue until dull percussion rate indicates upper liver border; note location of upper liver border with marker (Fig. 11-11)	Upper border of liver usually begins in fifth to seventh intercostal space	Upper border lowered Dullness extending above fifth intercostal space
(3) Estimate midclavicular liver span	6 to 12 cm (2½ to 4½ inches) Normal liver span usually greater in men than women and in taller individuals	Span exceeds 12 cm (4½ inches)
(4) Additional liver percussion maneuvers		

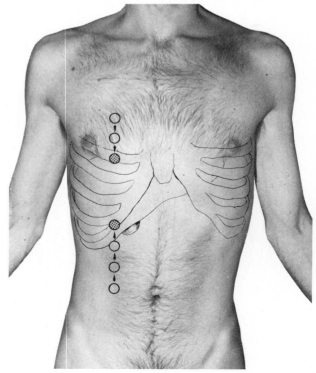

Fig. 11-11 Liver percussion route.

| | EVALUATION | |
ASSESSMENT PROCEDURE	NORMAL FINDINGS	DEVIATIONS FROM NORMAL
(a) Percuss upward, then in downward direction over right midaxillary line	Liver dullness may be felt in fifth to seventh intercostal space	Dull percussion exceeds limits of fifth to seventh intercostal space
(b) Percuss upward, then in downward direction over midsternal line and estimate midsternal liver span	Normal midsternal liver span ranges from 4 to 8 cm (1½ to 3 inches)	Span exceeds 8 cm (3 inches)
(c) Instruct client to take a deep breath and hold it; then percuss upward in right midclavicular line again; estimate liver descent	Lower border of liver should move inferiorly by 2 to 3 cm	Liver does not move with inspiration, or movement is less than 2 cm
b. Spleen percussion		
(1) Percuss down lower left thoracic wall in posterior midaxillary region beginning from an area of lung resonance to costal margin (Fig. 11-12)	Small area of splenic dullness may be heard at sixth to tenth rib, or tone may be tympanic (colonic)	Dullness extends above sixth rib or covers large area between sixth rib and costal margin
(2) Percuss lowest intercostal space in left anterior axillary line before and after client takes a deep breath (Fig. 11-13)	Area usually tympanic	Tympany changes to dullness on inspiration Enlarged spleen is brought forward on inspiration to produce dull percussion note
(3) Percuss over left lower rib cage	Gastric "bubble" tympanic and varies in size	

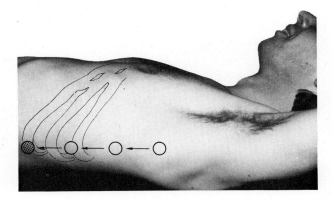

Fig. 11-12   Spleen percussion route.

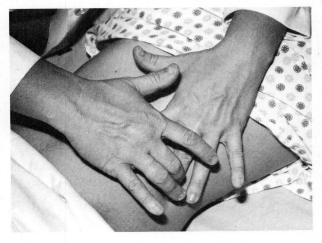

Fig. 11-13   Percussion at lowest intercostal space in left anterior axillary line before and after client takes a deep breath.

Continued.

CLINICAL GUIDELINES—cont'd

ASSESSMENT PROCEDURE	EVALUATION	
	NORMAL FINDINGS	DEVIATIONS FROM NORMAL
Abdomen—cont'd		
10. Abdominal palpation		
a. Lightly palpate all four quadrants with pads of fingertips (Fig. 11-14, *A*)		
(1) Tenderness	Not present	Cutaneous (superficial areas of hypersensitivity)
(2) Muscle tone	Abdomen relaxed Muscular resistance may be seen in anxious client	Involuntary resistance (muscles cannot be relaxed by voluntary effort)
(3) Surface characteristics	Smooth; consistent tension felt by examiner	Masses (superficial) Localized areas of rigidity or increased tension
b. Continue palpation of all four quadrants using moderate pressure with flat and sides of hand (Fig. 11-14, *B*) (*Note:* This intermediate maneuver is performed as a method of gradually approaching deep palpation without alarming client and stimulating muscular resistance. If onset of resistance is noted, use a lighter touch and proceed again.)		
(1) Tenderness	None	Present
(2) Masses	None	Present
(3) General tone and location of major structures	Abdominal surface feels smooth, and tension under palpating hand feels consistent throughout	Localized areas of rigidity or increased tension

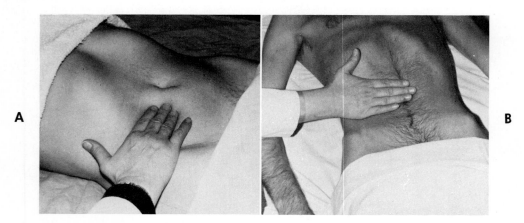

Fig. 11-14   **A,** Light abdominal palpation with distal pads of fingers. **B,** Abdominal palpation with moderate pressure; examiner uses flat and side of hand.

| | EVALUATION | |
ASSESSMENT PROCEDURE	NORMAL FINDINGS	DEVIATIONS FROM NORMAL
c. Deeply palpate all four quadrants; one of two methods may be used (1) Distal flat portions of fingers (fingerpads) are pressed gradually and deeply into palpation areas (Fig. 11-14, *C*) (2) Bimanual: lower hand rests lightly on surface and upper hand exerts pressure for deep palpation (Fig. 11-14, *D*) 　(a) Tenderness	Often present in midline near xiphoid process Often present over cecum May be present over sigmoid colon	Present in local or generalized areas Client response to pain may be muscle guarding and/or facial grimace, pulling away from examiner
(b) Masses	Aorta often palpable at epigastrium and pulsates in forward direction Borders of rectus abdominis muscles Feces in ascending or descending colon Sacral promontory	Masses that descend during inspiration Pulsatile masses Laterally mobile masses Fixed masses
(3) Palpate with fingertips around umbilicus for: 　(a) Bulges 　(b) Nodules 　(c) Umbilical ring	Umbilical ring round with no irregularities or bulges Umbilicus may be inverted or slightly everted	Masses, bulges Umbilical ring may be incomplete or may feel soft in center
11. Specific organ identification 　a. Liver palpation		

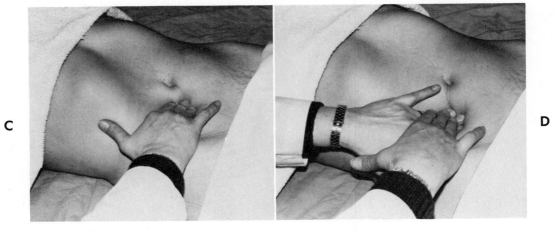

C　　　　　　　　　　　　　　　　　　　　　　　　　　**D**

Fig. 11-14, cont'd.　**C,** Deep abdominal palpation; examiner uses flat surface of distal pads of fingers. **D,** Deep abdominal palpation using bimanual technique.

Continued.

CLINICAL GUIDELINES—cont'd

	EVALUATION	
ASSESSMENT PROCEDURE	NORMAL FINDINGS	DEVIATIONS FROM NORMAL
Abdomen—cont'd		
(1) Deeply palpate at right costal margin before and during deep inspiration and after complete expiration; left hand is placed under eleventh and twelfth ribs; right hand is parallel to right costal margin (Fig. 11-15)		
(a) Liver border and contour (*Note:* If border is felt, repeat palpation/inspiration maneuver at medial and lateral sites of costal border for better estimate of contour.)	Liver often not palpable Liver often "bumps" against fingers during inspiration (especially in thin clients)	(*Note:* Very enlarged liver may lie under examiner's hand as it extends downward into abdominal cavity.)
(b) Liver border surface	Border feels smooth	Irregular surface or edge
(c) Liver tenderness (*Note:* Both hands can be "hooked" over right costal margin as examiner faces client's feet to palpate liver border on deep inspiration.)	None	Tenderness elicited (*Note:* Client's inspiration may be abruptly halted if pain exists.)
b. Spleen palpation		
(1) While standing at client's right side, palpate the spleen by placing left hand over client's left costovertebral angle and exerting pressure to move the spleen anteriorly; right hand is pressed gently under left anterior costal margin (Fig. 11-16)		

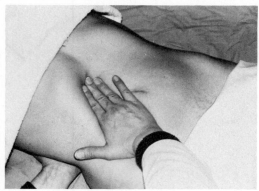

Fig. 11-15 Liver palpation with left hand under eleventh and twelfth ribs and right hand parallel to right costal margin.

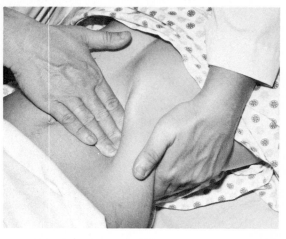

Fig. 11-16 Palpation of the spleen. Note that examiner's left hand is pressing spleen anteriorly.

	EVALUATION	
ASSESSMENT PROCEDURE	**NORMAL FINDINGS**	**DEVIATIONS FROM NORMAL**

(2) Instruct client to take a deep breath and then to exhale; as client exhales, examiner's hand should follow tissue contour under border of ribs in an attempt to palpate the spleen edge
(3) Repeat procedure with client lying on right side with legs and knees somewhat flexed; stand to client's right and place left hand over client's left costovertebral angle; right hand is pressed under left anterior costal margin (Fig. 11-17)
c. Kidney palpation
  (1) Left kidney
    (a) Examiner stands to client's right; client returns to supine position
    (b) Examiner's left hand is placed at left posterior costal angle; right hand is placed at client's left anterior costal margin
	Spleen not normally palpable	Spleen palpated (as firm mass that bumps against examiner's fingers)

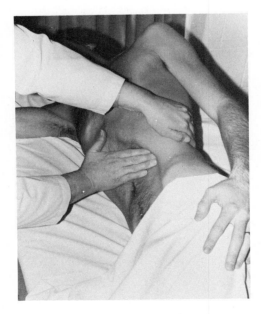

Fig. 11-17 Spleen palpation.

CLINICAL GUIDELINES—cont'd

	EVALUATION	
ASSESSMENT PROCEDURE	**NORMAL FINDINGS**	**DEVIATIONS FROM NORMAL**
Abdomen—cont'd		
(c) Client is instructed to take a deep breath and to exhale completely. As the client exhales, the examiner elevates client's left flank with left hand and palpates deeply with right hand (Fig. 11-18)	Occasionally lower pole of the kidney can be felt in thin clients Contour smooth and no tenderness on palpation	
(2) Right kidney		
(a) Same maneuver is repeated on client's right side; examiner remains at client's right, elevates posterior costal margin with left hand, and palpates deeply at anterior margin with right hand	Lower pole of right kidney may be palpated (during inspiration) as smooth, firm, and nontender	

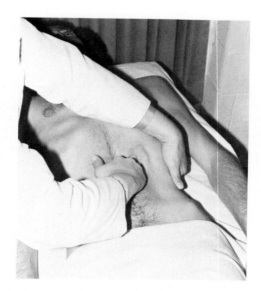

Fig. 11-18   Left kidney palpation.

	EVALUATION	
ASSESSMENT PROCEDURE	**NORMAL FINDINGS**	**DEVIATIONS FROM NORMAL**

d. Inguinal nodes
  (1) Lightly palpate (with finger-pads) inguinal areas just below inguinal ligament and inner aspect of upper thigh at the groin (Fig. 11-19) for horizontal and vertical inguinal nodes
    (a) Presence
	Small, mobile
	Nontender nodes often present
		Enlarged, tender

(b) Contour	Smooth or nonpalpable	
(c) Consistency	Soft or nonpalpable	Hard
(*Note:* Femoral pulses can also be palpated at this time. Techniques and palpable qualities are discussed in Chapter 9.)		
12. Jar kidneys to evaluate tenderness a. Approach from behind as client is seated; identify right and left costovertebral angles		
b. Strike each angle with ulnar surface of right fist (Fig. 11-20)	Client perceives jar or thud	Tenderness elicited

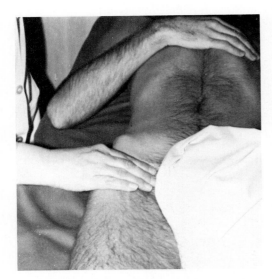

Fig. 11-19 Palpation of inguinal area; finger-pads applied just below inguinal ligament.

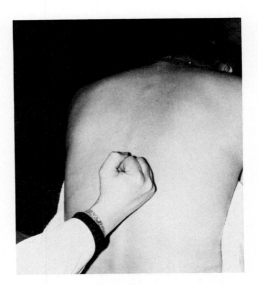

Fig. 11-20 First percussion over costovertebral angle.

Continued.

CLINICAL GUIDELINES—cont'd

	EVALUATION	
ASSESSMENT PROCEDURE	NORMAL FINDINGS	DEVIATIONS FROM NORMAL

Abdomen—cont'd

Special maneuvers

1. If fluid within the abdomen is suspected:
   a. As the client remains in a supine position, fluid associated with ascites will pool in the lateral (flank) areas. Lines can be drawn on the abdomen to indicate the midline tympany percussion area in contrast to lateral dullness.
   b. If the client turns to the right side, the tympanic sound will shift toward the upper (left) side. As the fluid pools in the right side, the area of dullness will rise toward the midline.
   c. As the client turns to the left lateral position, the fluid will migrate to the left side, and the left dullness will rise toward the midline.
2. Small amounts of free fluids can be identified if the client assumes an elbow-knee position. The fluid will pool in the periumbilical region, and the area of dullness can be identified through percussion.
3. If the client is experiencing pain, the examiner should test for rebound tenderness: press firmly over an area of the abdomen that is remote from the area of discomfort, and release the hand suddenly. If the client experiences a sharp, stabbing pain at the site of original discomfort, this can be interpreted as rebound tenderness.

Rectal/anal region

1. Evaluate anal and rectal region		
a. Inspect sacrococcygeal and perianal areas, especially skin and surface characteristics, while client is lying on left side with right hip and knee flexed	Surface smooth and clear	Lumps, rash, inflammation, scars, pilonidal area
b. Palpate coccygeal area for tenderness	No tenderness	Tender
c. Spread buttocks with both hands; inspect anus for surface characteristics (penlight can be used)	Increased pigmentation Coarse skin	Inflammation Lesions Scars Skin tags Fissures Lumps Swelling Excoriation Hemorrhoids Mucosal bulging
d. Ask client to strain down; place gloved and lubricated finger at anal opening; as sphincter relaxes, slowly insert finger pointing toward client's umbilicus		
e. Ask client to tighten sphincter around finger to assess sphincter tone	Sphincter tightens evenly around finger with minimum discomfort to client	Hypotonic sphincter Hypertonic sphincter, with marked tenderness
f. Rotate finger to examine anal muscular ring for surface characteristics	Smooth, even pressure on finger	Nodules Irregularities
g. Insert finger farther to palpate all four rectal walls (*Note:* Prostate examination is discussed in Chapter 12.)	Continuous, smooth surface with minimal discomfort to client	Nodules Masses (*Note:* The cervix is sometimes palpable on the anterior wall; do not mistake for a mass.) Tenderness
h. As finger is extracted, note characteristics of any stool		
(1) Color	Brown	Presence of blood, pus Black, tarry stool Pale or yellow; light tan or gray
(2) Consistency	Soft	

CLINICAL TIPS AND STRATEGIES

- **Help the client to feel comfortable before an abdominal examination:** It is extremely difficult to complete an assessment if the abdominal muscles are not relaxed. The basic comfort measures described in the "Clinical Guidelines" are essential; however, the examiner must be sensitive to the client's state of anxiety and should be prepared to be flexible with examination procedures if the client remains tense.

  1. If palpation stimulates muscle tension, it might be helpful to lighten the touch and to proceed more slowly.
  2. The abdominal examination can be delayed until later in the assessment when the client might feel more comfortable.
  3. Drape the client as fully as possible.
  4. It is sometimes difficult to examine the abdomen while the client is talking; clients tend to lift and bob their heads as they converse. However, it is often soothing to have the examiner talking quietly, describing the procedures and perhaps reviewing the client's history.

- **Look before you touch:** Once an individual begins using other senses, the impact of the visual sense diminishes. It is helpful to circle around the examining table and to view the abdomen carefully from all angles for surface and contour characteristics.

- **Visualize organs or major structures within the abdominal cavity during inspection, auscultation, percussion, and palpation of the abdomen** (Fig. 11-21 and the box on the right): This mental picture heightens the tactile sense.

- **Inquire about a history of pain or discomfort *before* beginning palpation:** If discomfort is described and located, begin the palpation in another region of the abdomen.

- **The beginning examiner must establish early and consistent routines for carrying out the mechanics of the assessment:** Most individuals examine the abdomen from the client's right side. Making this decision early in the learning period is extremely helpful in expediting assessment skills.

- **Draw a picture of lesions, scars, masses, or fluid levels (lines) if identified:** It is often easier and clearer to draw a picture of the finding and indicate dimensions and location rather than to attempt a description of it.

STRUCTURES OF THE ABDOMINAL CAVITY

Right upper quadrant

Liver
Gallbladder
Duodenum
Head of pancreas
Right kidney
Hepatic flexure of colon
Pylorus
Right adrenal gland
Portions of ascending and transverse colon

Left upper quadrant

Stomach
Spleen
Left kidney
Tail of pancreas
Splenic flexure of colon
Left lobe of liver
Left adrenal gland
Portions of transverse and descending colon

Right lower quadrant

Cecum
Appendix
Right ovary and tube
Portion of ascending colon
Right spermatic cord
Right ureter

Left lower quadrant

Sigmoid colon
Left ovary and tube
Portion of descending colon
Left spermatic cord
Left ureter

Superpubic midline

Bladder
Uterus

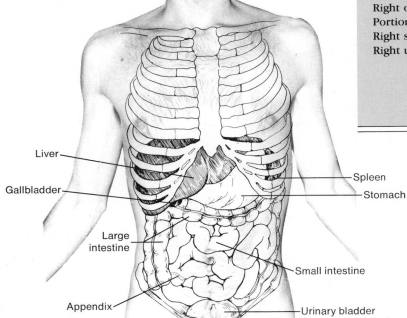

Fig. 11-21 Major structures of abdominal cavity.

SAMPLE RECORDING: NORMAL FINDINGS

Abdomen: Rounded and symmetrical with centrally placed umbilicus. No lesions, rashes, discolorations, scars, inflammation, or visible peristalsis. Normal bowel sounds; no bruits or venous hums. Tympanic percussion tones throughout. Abdomen relaxed and without tenderness or masses. Liver 10 cm in right midclavicular line. Spleen and kidneys not palpated. No CVA tenderness.

Rectal and anal region: Sacrococcygeal, perianal, and anal surfaces present no lesions, rash, inflammation, masses, or hemorrhoids. Good sphincter tone. Anal and distal rectal mucosa smooth and without masses.

 The Newborn

HISTORY AND CLINICAL STRATEGIES

- The newborn's abdomen should be rounded and prominent. Diaphragmatic respirations should be observed. The umbilical stump becomes dry within hours after birth.
- Examiners should note any retractions, fractured clavicles, or asymmetry of chest expansion or nipple placement. A scaphoid abdomen is not normal and requires investigation. Further examination is also needed if there are any abnormalities in organ position or characteristics.

CLINICAL VARIATIONS: THE NEWBORN

CHARACTERISTIC OR AREA EXAMINED	NORMAL FINDINGS	DEVIATIONS FROM NORMAL
1. Abdomen	Symmetric, soft and round, slightly protruding, no masses Diastasis swelling and gap between rectus muscles may be felt during crying Bowel sounds present	Distention, masses, concaved, sunken, or flat (possible organ abnormality, "prunebelly" syndrome) Scaphoid, turnip-shaped (suggests diaphragmatic hernia) Distention, vomiting (suggests intestinal obstruction)
2. Organs	Liver edge 1 to 2 cm below right rib cage (costal margin) Spleen not usually palpable; tip may be felt in left upper quadrant—far left costal margin Left kidney detected with deep palpation; kidneys usually 1 to 2 cm above umbilicus Bladder ballottement above symphysis pubis	Enlarged liver 3 cm or more below margin (liver may be low or enlarged because of disease, problem) Palpable spleen (suggests sepsis, blood incompatibility) Masses near kidneys (possible Wilms tumor, hydronephrosis, neuroblastoma) Enlarged kidneys (possible renal vein thrombosis, polycystic kidneys, obstruction)
3. Umbilicus	No hernia, signs of infection, or protrusion Vessels: two arteries, one vein Cord white-to-black as it dries Cord spontaneously falls off 7 to 14 days after birth; should be dry within 5 days and off by 2 weeks	Cord discharge, odor, redness, blueness, umbilical polyp (suggests infection) Protrusion or nodular appearance (possible hernia, omphalocele) One artery (possible congenital heart or urinary defect) Thick Wharton's jelly (suggests large for gestation period) Thin cord (suggests small for gestation period) Green cord (intrauterine meconium)

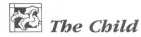 *The Child*

HISTORY AND CLINICAL STRATEGIES

- Nutritional assessment requires that a basic list of nutritional questions is asked (presented in Chapter 1). In addition, the examiner must be alert to common nutritional concerns associated with the child.

  1. *Obesity.* This is a common problem for children. Questions about a child's overweight situation should include those presented in the adult nutritional assessment section, p. 343, as well as those that follow:

     a. Family history regarding obesity problems

     b. Age of the child when overweight problems began

     c. Whether the child is concerned about his overweight state

     d. Whether the child understands the relationship between foods consumed and weight gained (e.g., a story is told about one teenage girl who consumed three cases of liquid diet supplement every day to cancel the 1000 calories she consumed by eating three meals.)

  2. *Toddler nutrition.* Many parents of toddlers will express concern that their child's eating patterns have changed. The examiner must gather a food consumption profile from the past week, as well as assess the child physically. If the child shows normal progression of height, weight, and maturational development, the examiner should try to decrease parental anxiety by sharing growth and development progression facts, as well as normal development eating changes, of the toddler.

  3. *Adolescent nutrition.* Studies have shown that less than 50% of all teenagers in the United States eat breakfast every day. This usually arouses concern among parents who state that their teenager is not eating correctly. Although the examiner should develop a profile of the adolescent's nutritional style and food consumption, unless a problem arises, such as overweight, underweight, anemia, fatigue, or systemic disease, there may be little the examiner can do to change the adolescent's style of food consumption. It is important to assess the adolescent's knowledge of good nutrition and to supply educational facts where necessary.

  4. *Anorexia nervosa.* This disease, referred to as a "socially acceptable" form of suicide, is becoming more common in the United States. Its assessment is included at this point because of the close correlation with adolescent nutrition. A hypothetical profile of a child affected by anorexia nervosa follows:

The individual is usually a female teenager from an upper middle class family. Her parents, who may be perfectionists, are successful and view themselves as being well adjusted and supportive. Both her mother and father have made many personal sacrifices for the child. The girl is popular and successful. Throughout her life she has conformed to the wishes of her parents. Hardly ever has she expressed her own wishes or translated her own desires into actions.

Anorexia nervosa is such a serious situation that the examiner must explore its potential with all very thin teenagers, especially those whose parents express a concern that the teenager has lost too much weight or will not eat. Although there is usually some significant event that triggers the situation, typically the first symptom to appear will be weight loss. As the anorexia nervosa cycle continues, the examiner will find the parent and the teenager in battle about eating, food, and weight loss. The more the parent harps, the more serious the situation becomes.

The examiner should use the following questions to gather data. Any teenager who appears at risk should be referred immediately.

a. Is the client less than 25 years of age?

b. Has there been a weight loss of more than 25% of the client's original weight?

c. Does the client express an intractable or negative attitude about gaining weight or eating?

d. Are there any other physical problems present?

e. Are any of the following factors pertinent (a cluster of at least four is considered high risk)?

   (1) Distorted body image

   (2) Periods of amenorrhea

   (3) Periods of hyperactivity

   (4) History of being overweight

   (5) Denial of hunger

   (6) Denial of fatigue

   (7) History of self-induced vomiting to stay thin

   (8) Morbid fear of obesity

   (9) Preoccupation with food

- Abdominal pain in the child is extremely difficult to assess. If the examiner asks the child if the palpation hurts or to point to the spot where it hurts, the child will usually comply and provide a response indicating discomfort or pain. More important, the examiner should rely on objective findings to assist in assessing the pain. Such factors as different pitch in a cry, a grimace or change in facial expression, or sudden protective movement by arms and legs are helpful indications.

- A history of abdominal pain in the older child may

have many causes. Some of the most common are anxiety, constipation, urinary tract infections, parasite invasion, or irritated bowel. The examiner should carefully question the child or parent about each of them.

- Pinworms may be common in children, especially those who frequently have dirty hands and have their hands in their mouths. The child may complain of abdominal pain or nighttime rectal itching. The parent should be encouraged to observe the child's rectal area with a flashlight at night as the child sleeps. The worms are most likely to be seen at that time. If the parents suspect pinworms, a specimen should be obtained for analysis. The best technique for this is to put cellophane tape, sticky side up, on the end of a tongue blade and gather the specimen as close to the anal opening as possible.
- For crawling infants and toddlers the examiner should inquire about pica. Common items eaten are plaster, dirt, paint chips, grass, and blanket fuzz. Although it is normal for children to put nonfood items into their mouths, most learn by age 2 years what is and is not edible.
- Constipation is a common problem during childhood, expecially during the toilet-training period. If this is a problem, the examiner should inquire about the following:
  1. How long the problem has existed
  2. Family history of similar problems or diseases affecting bowels
  3. Whether toilet training has been associated with the problem
  4. How many stools per day and week the child usually has (and within the past week)
  5. Current family or home stresses (describe)
  6. Food, juice, and water consumption during the past 48 hours
  7. What parent has done about problem
  8. How parent feels about problem
- Symptoms such as indigestion, nausea, vomiting, and diarrhea should be explored as detailed on p. 344.
- The approach to the child is extremely important in attempting to assess the abdomen. The abdomen may be the place to start the entire physical examination of the child, but if the examiner moves in with both hands to palpate the abdomen of an 18-month-old, this is bound to fail. The following approach may be helpful for assessing the young infant and child. By age 5 years the child should be ready to cooperate more fully.
  1. Undress the infant or child to diaper and have him on the parent's lap. Do not attempt to examine the small child's abdomen by placing him on the examination table. The child may tense, fight, or cry.

2. Observe the child's abdomen as he sits or lies on the parent's lap.
3. Instruct the parent to stand the child up for observation of the abdominal contour and "pot belly" appearance. This is also a time to observe for umbilical bulging or hernia.
4. For auscultation, percussion, and palpation, the child may be laid in the parent's lap with the child's legs extending onto the examiner's lap.
5. There is some disagreement as to the sequence of pediatric abdominal assessment elements. Should it be: (1) inspection, (2) auscultation, (3) percussion, and (4) palpation; or (1) inspection, (2) auscultation, (3) palpation, and (4) percussion? Some authorities suggest that percussion is a frightening procedure and should be done last. Try it both ways and then decide for yourself.
6. Even for a small infant the position that facilitates a soft abdomen is one in which both the knees and the neck are flexed. This is easy to achieve as the parent holds the child.
7. Because of the soft examination surface during palpation, it is helpful in both young and older children for the examiner to place the left hand under the child's back and palpate downward with the right hand directly over the same surface. This facilitates a ballottement approach to assessing the abdominal contents. Be gentle but firm during palpation.
8. An internal rectal examination is not routinely performed for the well child because of the invasiveness of the technique. If there is an obvious problem, such as constipation, that requires an internal rectal examination, the examiner should proceed with the same guidelines as for the adult. An ill child with an abdominal complaint should be referred for further evaluation.
9. It will be most helpful to undress the child and make some introductory attempts to touch the child during the history session. Another technique involves letting the child play with the examiner's stethoscope while the initial history and physical assessment are occurring.
10. If the examiner has a question about a finding but because of the parent's soft lap, cannot assess adequately, a last choice is to move both the parent and the child to the examination table. The child should be placed on the examination table, and the parent should assist in holding the child.
11. For the most part the abdomen is easy to assess early during the examination process before the child becomes upset. If, however, the child is crying during the initial part of the examination,

delay the assessment. Crying tenses the abdominal muscles and interferes with accurate assessment.

12. Giving the infant a bottle during the abdominal examination is fine and will, in fact, assist in quieting the child and relaxing the abdominal muscle wall. Caution should be taken to avoid vigorous deep palpation in a child who has just consumed a large bottle of milk, juice, or formula.

13. Older children are generally eager to cooperate but may pose two new problems: ticklishness and firm abdominal muscles.
    a. Ticklishness may be overcome by gentle, continued contact with the child's skin. The sensation should decrease. If not, the examiner may place the child's hand under the examiner's hand.

b. A firm abdomen will be a problem in older children and especially in teenage boys. A pillow under the head and flexion of the knees may help to relax the abdominal muscles.

14. Tenseness of the abdominal wall in all children may be a problem, especially if the child is afraid. The examiner should attempt to engage the child in small talk to take the child's mind off the examination. Although it is important for the examiner to observe the child's facial response during palpation of the abdomen, the examiner should try to avoid direct eye contact with the child continuously. It alone may increase tenseness of the child, as well as of the abdomen.

Text continues on p. 368.

CLINICAL VARIATIONS: THE CHILD

CHARACTERISTIC OR AREA EXAMINED	NORMAL FINDINGS	DEVIATIONS FROM NORMAL
Abdomen		
1. Inspection		
a. Skin color	May be paler than other parts because of lack of exposure	Jaundice Redness (inflammation) Lesions, bruises, discoloration, cyanosis (localized at umbilicus or generalized)
b. Surface characteristics	Smooth, soft Note scars, striae	Rashes, lesions Glistening, taut appearance Pink or red striae Purple striae
c. Venous network	Very faint fine network may be visible, mostly during infancy	Prominent venous pattern Engorgement of veins around umbilicus

d. Umbilicus
    Note: Is hernia present during crying only or also at quiet times?
    Note how size changes.
	Surface smooth, noninflamed
	Umbilical hernia common, especially in blacks
	Considered normal in white children until 2 years of age, in black children until 7 years of age (by 1 month of age hernia should attain its maximum size)
	Hernia may vary from few millimeters to 3 cm (1 inch)
		Umbilical hernia extending beyond 2 years of age in white children, beyond 7 years of age in black children
		
		Child with hernia over 2 cm (¾ inch) should be referred for further assessment
		Hernia that continues to grow after 1 month of age requires referral

Continued.

CLINICAL VARIATIONS: THE CHILD—cont'd

CHARACTERISTIC OR AREA EXAMINED	NORMAL FINDINGS	DEVIATIONS FROM NORMAL
Abdomen—cont'd		
e. Contour	Infant, toddler: rounded "pot belly" both standing and lying (Fig. 11-22)	Scaphoid abdomen in infant or toddler
	School age: may show some pot belly (lordotic stance) until age 13 years when standing; when child is lying, abdomen should appear scaphoid (Fig. 11-23)	Generalized distention
f. Symmetry	Evenly rounded with maximum height of convexity at umbilicus	Distention of upper or lower half
		Visible masses or bulges in any area of abdominal surface
g. Surface motion		
(1) Peristalsis	Usually not visible	Marked peristalsis
(2) Pulsations	Upper-midline pulsation may be visible in thin children	Marked pulsation
h. Movement with respirations	Until approximately age 7 years, children are abdominal breathers; after age 7 years, boys exhibit chiefly abdominal movement, girls exhibit chiefly costal movement	Grunting, labored respirations accompanied by restricted abdominal movement

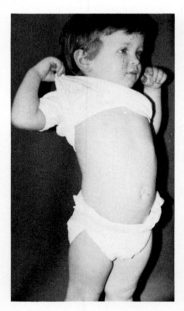

Fig. 11-22   Toddler displaying "pot belly" profile.

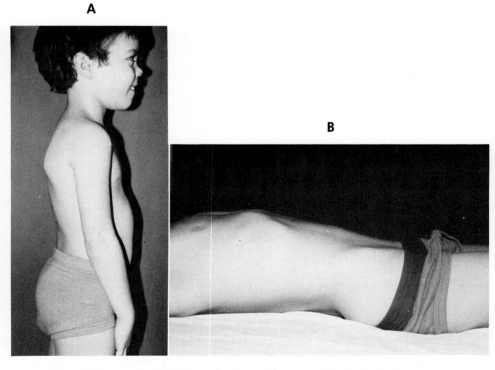

Fig. 11-23   **A,** "Pot belly" stance of preschool-age child. **B,** Scaphoid contour of school-age child.

CHARACTERISTIC OR AREA EXAMINED	NORMAL FINDINGS	DEVIATIONS FROM NORMAL
i. Tenseness of abdominal muscles	Diastasis recti abdominis condition in which two recti muscles do not approximate each other; common in black children; should disappear during preschool years May be 1 to 5 cm (½ to 2 inches) wide	Same condition with evidence of accompanying hernia Problem continues in school-age child
2. Auscultation a. Bowel sounds; quality	Usually 5 to 34/min Irregular in timing Gurgles, clicks (quality of sound varies greatly)	Absence of sound established after 5 minutes of listening; note sounds that are infrequent High-pitched, tinkling noises May sound like metallic tinkling
b. Vascular sounds		Bruits (usually high-pitched, soft "swishing" sound, and systolic in timing) (*Note:* Bruit will continue as client is moved into various positions.) Murmur near umbilical area Venous hum (lower in pitch, softer, and a continuous sound)
c. Friction rub		Infrequently heard sound, associated with respirations (soft and may be confused with normal breath sounds) Rubs most often heard over spleen or liver
3. Percussion a. General tone	General distribution of tympany (depending on amount of air and solid material in bowel) Suprapubic dullness heard over distended bladder Children's abdomens frequently sound louder in tympany tones than those of adults, primarily because children often swallow more air during drinking and eating	Marked dullness in local area
b. Liver tone and span	Upper liver border usually percussed at approximately sixth rib or interspace anteriorly and at ninth rib posteriorly Lower liver border usually percussed at approximately costal margin or 2 to 3 cm (¾ to 1 inch) lower Average: 5 years of age—7 cm (2¾ inches); 12 years of age—9 cm (3½ inches)	Upper border lower Dullness extending above fifth intercostal space Lower border of liver exceeds 2 to 3 cm below costal margin Span that exceeds these limits

Continued.

CLINICAL VARIATIONS: THE CHILD—cont'd

CHARACTERISTIC OR AREA EXAMINED	NORMAL FINDINGS	DEVIATIONS FROM NORMAL
Abdomen—cont'd		
c. Spleen tone and span	May hear small area of dullness above ninth interspace along left midaxillary line In young infants and children: may extend to 1 to 2 cm below costal margin	Dullness extends above sixth rib or covers large area between sixth rib and costal margin Spleen in any ill-appearing child that extends below costal margin Spleen in children over 1 year of age that extends below costal margin
4. Palpation		
a. Light and moderate palpation		
(1) Tenderness	Not present	Cutaneous (superficial areas of hypersensitivity)
(2) Muscle tone	Abdomen relaxed Muscular resistance may accompany anxious child	Involuntary resistance (muscles cannot be relaxed by voluntary effort)
(3) Surface characteristics	Smooth; consistent tension felt by examiner	Masses (superficial) Localized areas of rigidity or increased tension
(4) Umbilical area	Note size of umbilical hernia if present	Tenderness
b. Deep palpation (be gentle, use one hand):		
(1) Tenderness	Often present in midline near xiphoid process Often present over cecum May be present over sigmoid colon	Present in local or generalized areas Client response to pain may be muscle guarding and/or facial grimace, pulling away from examiner
(2) Masses	Aorta often palpable at epigastrium and pulsates in forward direction Borders of rectus abdominis muscles Feces in ascending or descending colon	Masses that descend on inspiration Pulsatile masses Laterally mobile masses Fixed masses Wilms tumor located adjacent to vertebral column; does not extend across midline
(3) Umbilical ring	Umbilicus may be inverted or slightly everted Umbilical ring round, with no irregularities or bulges	Umbilical ring may be incomplete or may feel soft in center Masses, bulges
c. Organ identification		
(1) Liver palpation		
(a) Border location	0 to 6 months: palpable 0 to 3 cm below costal margin 6 months to 4 years: palpable 1 to 2 cm below costal margin Over 6 years: palpable 1 to 2 cm or not palpable below right costal margin	Greater than 2 cm below right costal margin
(b) Tenderness	None	Tenderness elicited (*Note:* Client's inspiration may be abruptly halted if pain exists.)

CHARACTERISTIC OR AREA EXAMINED	NORMAL FINDINGS	DEVIATIONS FROM NORMAL
(2) Spleen palpation	May feel at costal margin or slightly under ribs in small children Only tip (feeling like tongue) should be palpable	Able to palpate more than tip Palpable spleen in older child who also appears ill or has multiple other symptoms
(3) Kidney palpation	Palpated periodically, not always Lies adjacent to vertebral column Descends slightly with inspiration Most likely able to palpate lower pole of right kidney; smooth contour	
(4) Bladder palpation	Frequently palpated as smooth mass extending midline, somewhere between pubis and umbilical area Ability to palpate should disappear after urination	Bladder distention after voiding
(5) Inguinal area (a) Nodes — Presence	Small, mobile Nontender nodes often present	Enlarged, tender
— Contour	Smooth or nonpalpable	
— Consistency	Soft or nonpalpable	Hard
(b) Hernia evaluation	No bulging felt in inguinal ring area	Bulging palpable as finger is placed in inguinal ring Evaluation performed as client increases intraabdominal pressure
(6) Kidney jarring to evaluate costovertebral angle tenderness	Client perceives jar or thud No tenderness elicited	Tenderness elicited

Anal/rectal region

1. Inspection: skin surface characteristics	Surface smooth and clear	Lumps, rash, inflammation, scars, pilonidal dimpling, tuft of hair at pilonidal area
2. Palpation of coccygeal area for tenderness	No tenderness	Tender
3. Inspection of anus: surface characteristics	Increased pigmentation Coarse skin	Inflammation Lesions Scars Skin tags Fissures Lumps Swelling Excoriation
4. Internal rectal examination not routinely done in children unless ill or specific problem exists; when performed, follow same guidelines as for adult client		

The Childbearing Woman

HISTORY AND CLINICAL STRATEGIES

- It may be difficult to assess the abdomen because of the client's pregnancy and the discomfort women may have in a supine position. Physical examination depends on the stage of gestation and the safety and comfort of the pregnant person.
- Several unique assessment skills are needed for examining the pregnant woman. For example, using Leopold's maneuvers can help determine fetal presentation and position. When auscultating the abdomen, fetal heart beats should be counted for an entire minute. The uterine or placental souffle may be heard. Fundal height measurements are obtained to evaluate appropriate uterine growth during pregnancy.
- The uterus becomes an abdominal organ around the twelfth week of gestation. It percusses dull above the symphysis pubis. A dull sound may be heard also over a full bladder.

CLINICAL VARIATIONS: THE CHILDBEARING WOMAN

CHARACTERISTIC OR AREA EXAMINED	NORMAL FINDINGS	DEVIATIONS FROM NORMAL
1. Characteristics	Morning sickness: first trimester, nausea and vomiting may occur Constipation, heartburn, flatus may occur later in pregnancy (from less gastrointestinal tract tone and more uterine pressure) Hemorrhoids (from vascularity and pressure)	Hyperemesis gravidarum: pernicious vomiting after first trimester (may be from hormonal or psychological influence) Vomiting in second or third trimester (may be reflux from hiatal hernia)
2. Abdomen and uterus	Diastasis recti: enlarged uterus separates muscles Venous patterns may be seen over abdomen Fundus (top of uterus) in midline or slightly to right (from pressure of sigmoid colon on left) (See Chapter 13 for uterine characteristics) Quickening: fetal movement felt by pregnant woman, at end of fifth month (16 to 20 weeks) Fetal movement felt by another when placing hand over abdomen occurs around 20 weeks Ballottement: when tapped, fetus rebounds in amniotic fluid in fourth to fifth months Outline of fetus seen after sixth month	Diarrhea, anorexia, weight loss, constipation (may relate to inflammatory bowel disease) Jaundice (may be cholestasis of pregnancy, hepatitis, liver disease) Gallstone pain (stones formed by increased bile from hormonal influence)
3. Sounds and characteristics	Fetal heart tones heard by Doppler about 8 to 10 weeks, heard with stethoscope about 17 to 19 weeks Funic souffle: blood through umbilical cord Uterine souffle: blood through uterine vessels Lightening: fetal head into maternal pelvis before delivery	Fetal heart sounds not appropriate (possibly miscalculated dates or fetal problem)

CLINICAL VARIATIONS: THE CHILDBEARING WOMAN—cont'd

CHARACTERISTIC OR AREA EXAMINED	NORMAL FINDINGS	DEVIATIONS FROM NORMAL
4. Postdelivery	Decreased bowel sounds (from smooth muscle relaxation caused by progesterone)	
	Constipation may occur during pregnancy and postpartum	
	Abdominal muscle tone restored in a few weeks	
	Rectus muscles may remain separated	
	Hemorrhoids usually resolved in 1 to 3 weeks	
	Constipation common during first 3 to 4 days (from perineal pain, lack of tone, or dehydration)	
	Thirst during early puerperium (may be caused by dehydration during labor or postpartum diuresis)	

The Older Adult

HISTORY AND CLINICAL STRATEGIES

- Maintaining adequate nutritional intake may be a major problem for the older adult. This problem is not confined to chronically ill individuals or to low-income persons. Following are risk factors for poor nutritional intake patterns.
  1. Living alone
  2. Physical disability (e.g., diminished vision, neurological deficits, decreased mobility, arthritic changes, diminished strength, general symptoms of fatigue, dyspnea, or pain)
  3. Depression; anxiety
  4. Mouth or dental problems
  5. Swallowing or choking problems
  6. Sedentary life-style (particularly if associated with boredom, depression, or obesity)
  7. Obesity (usually accompanied by long-standing overeating habits)
  8. Limited access to markets (especially if client is unable to drive, if stores are within walking distance and require daily trips, or if client must rely on driving services of others)
  9. Limited cooking facilities or capability (often results in increased use of convenience foods or "empty" calories)
  10. Limited income (this problem exists in all income ranges; fixed incomes do not reflect inflation trends)
  11. Numerous food idiosyncrasies or general loss of senses of taste and smell
  12. Confusion (even mild, transient states of confusion will interrupt eating patterns)
  13. Misconceptions about nutritional requirements (e.g., belief that fewer nutrients are required for the elderly)
  14. Special diets prescribed (especially if difficult to purchase or to prepare or if taste is less desirable)
  15. Medications (prescribed or over-the-counter drugs may cause gastrointestinal side effects, such as dry mouth, anorexia, nausea, sedation, "heartburn") (*Note:* Aspirin is frequently the source of gastrointestinal symptoms.)
  16. Alcohol or drug abuse

The questions described in the original data base, Chapter 1, will help the examiner to elicit information related to the variables that alter food and fluid intake.

The actual *amounts* or *types* of food that are routinely consumed are sometimes difficult to assess because many older adults eat erratically (numerous meals are taken in smaller amounts scattered over a 24-hour period, or eating habits vary widely from day to day). A

24-hour recall may not reflect true eating patterns. A diary of a week or a month's food consumption may be helpful if the client is sufficiently motivated to follow through with recording. Several appointments devoted to nutritional assessment may be necessary if the examiner suspects intake is inadequate.

- Elderly clients frequently express numerous problems associated with elimination, and individuals may be preoccupied with bowel movement regularity to the extent that it can alter daily living functions. Problems may be described as a "spastic" or "irritable" colon, colitis, "gas on the stomach," constipation, or diarrhea. Clarification of symptoms is necessary. Constipation and diarrhea are discussed on p. 346. If long-standing problems exist, inquire carefully about the client's effort to treat himself. Risk factors associated with bowel elimination problems follow:
  1. Hemorrhoids
  2. Taking of laxatives (clarify whether this is a long-standing or recent habit)
  3. Recent dietary changes: reduced intake; elimination of certain foods
  4. Dietary intake with insufficient bulk
  5. Limited fluid intake
  6. Depression (often associated with constipation)
  7. Anxiety
  8. Physical immobility
  9. Weakened abdominal muscles
  10. Medication side effects or abuse (prescribed or over-the-counter; e.g., iron, antibiotics, tranquilizers, antacids)
- Hiatal hernia is a common problem with adults over age 70. The diaphragmatic muscle weakens, and the lower portion of the esophagus slides from the abdominal cavity into the thoracic cavity. The gastroesophageal sphincter does not constrict efficiently, and gastric contents regurgitate into the lower esophagus. Epigastric pain and burning are common complaints, especially at night or during prolonged periods in a supine position.

- Major aging changes associated with the gastrointestinal system include the following:
  1. Decrease in total volume of acid secretion
  2. Decreased hunger contractions
  3. Delayed gastric emptying
  4. Diminished tone of bowel wall
  5. Decreased peristalsis
  6. Decreased abdominal muscle strength
  7. Decreased anal sphincter tone
- Other special problems related to aging are the following:
  1. Diminished esophageal swallow reflex, especially in the lower third of the esophagus; may result in difficulty swallowing (choking) or dilation of the lower esophagus with retention of food in this area.
  2. Increased swallowing of air, often associated with anxiety; may result in frequent eructation, abdominal distention, or flatus.
  3. Atrophic gastritis and diminished gastric acid content may be associated with diminished absorption of vitamin B_{12} (pernicious anemia). Malabsorption of iron can also occur in an alkaline gastric medium.
  4. Medications may decrease gastric secretions or gastrointestinal motility.
  5. Diverticulosis, an outpouching of a weakened area of the bowel wall, is a common condition with the elderly. It is frequently asymptomatic but may be associated with decreased intestinal contractions and resulting flatulence and heartburn.

In many instances the changes just listed do not produce any signs or symptoms that are significant to the client or the examiner. These changes take place at different rates with different individuals and are not predictable on a chronological basis. However, all symptoms should be explored carefully and not assumed to be "functional" disorders by the examiner. Elderly clients may manifest less pain and less abdominal rigidity in acute or chronic conditions. Details related to the major symptoms are covered in Chapter 17.

CLINICAL VARIATIONS: THE OLDER ADULT

CHARACTERISTIC OR AREA EXAMINED	NORMAL FINDINGS	DEVIATIONS FROM NORMAL
General behaviors of client	Appears relaxed Facial muscles relaxed Lying quietly Respirations even and slow	Marked restlessness Marked immobility or rigid posture Knees drawn up Facial grimacing Respirations rapid, uneven, or "grunting"
Abdomen		
1. Inspection of abdominal surface		
a. Skin color	May be paler than other parts because of lack of exposure	Jaundice Redness (inflammation) Lesions, bruises, discoloration, cyanosis (localized at umbilicus or generalized)
b. Surface characteristics	Smooth, soft Silver-white striae (usually lower abdomen)	Rashes, lesions Glistening, taut appearance
c. Scars (configuration, location, length)		
d. Venous network	Faint fine network may be visible	Prominent venous pattern Engorgement of veins around umbilicus
e. Umbilicus		
(1) Placement	Centrally located	Displaced upward or downward
(2) Contour	Usually sunken, may protrude slightly	Visible hernia around or slightly above umbilicus
(3) Surface	Smooth, noninflamed	Inflamed
f. Contour	Flat Rounded Scaphoid (concave profile) (*Note:* Elderly individuals may have increased fat deposits over abdominal area even though subcutaneous fat is decreased over extremities.)	Distention (common distress signal in elderly clients) Marked concavity associated with general wasting signs or associated with anteroposterior rib expansion
g. Symmetry	Evenly rounded with maximum height of convexity at umbilicus	Distention of upper or lower half Visible masses or bulges in any area of abdominal surface
h. Surface motion		
(1) Peristalsis	Usually not visible	Visible
(2) Pulsation	Upper midline pulsation may be visible in thin people	Marked pulsation
i. General movement with respirations	Smooth, even movements Women exhibit chiefly costal movement Men exhibit chiefly abdominal movement	Grunting, labored Respirations accompanied by restricted abdominal movement
2. Instruct client to take a deep breath and hold it	Contour remains smooth and symmetrical	Bulges or masses appear
3. Instruct client to raise head without using arms for support	Rectus abdominis muscles prominent Midline bulge may appear	Appearance of bulges through muscle layer

Continued.

CLINICAL VARIATIONS: THE OLDER ADULT—cont'd

CHARACTERISTIC OR AREA EXAMINED	NORMAL FINDINGS	DEVIATIONS FROM NORMAL
Abdomen—cont'd		
4. Auscultatory bowel sounds: quality	Usually 5 to 34/min Irregular in timing Gurgles, clicks Quality of sound varies greatly	Absence of sound established after 5 minutes of listening Note sounds that are infrequent High-pitched, tinkling noises
5. Vascular sounds a. Arterial: concentrate in epigastric area, in area surrounding umbilicus, over liver, and at posterior flank		Bruits (usually high-pitched, soft, swishing sound, and systolic in timing) (*Note:* Bruit will continue as client is moved into various positions.)
b. Venous		Venous hum (lower in pitch, softer, and continuous sound)
6. Friction rubs		Infrequently heard sound associated with respirations (soft, and may be confused with normal breath sounds)
7. Percussion tones over entire abdomen	General distribution of tympany (depending on amount of air and solid material in bowel) Suprapubic dullness heard over distended bladder	Marked dullness in local area
8. Liver a. Lower border percussion	Lower border of liver usually at costal margin or slightly below; however, if elderly client has distended lungs, liver border will descend 1 to 2 cm into abdominal cavity	Lower border of liver exceeds 2 to 3 cm below costal margin
b. Upper border percussion	Upper border of liver usually begins in fifth to seventh intercostal space Upper border may descend 1 to 2 cm if liver has lowered with diaphragm, associated with distended lungs	Upper border lowered Dullness extending above fifth intercostal space
c. Midclavicular liver span	6 to 12 cm (2½ to 4½ inches) Normal liver span usually greater in men than women and greater in taller individuals	Span exceeds 12 cm
d. Right midaxillary liver percussion	Liver dullness may be felt in fifth to seventh intercostal space	Dull percussion note exceeds limits of fifth to seventh intercostal space
e. Midsternal liver span	Ranges from 4 to 8 cm (1½ to 3 inches)	Span exceeds 8 cm
f. Liver descent with deep inspiration (*Note:* Deep inspiration may be difficult for elderly client.)	Lower border of liver should move inferiorly by 2 to 3 cm	Liver does not move with inspiration or movement less than 2 cm
9. Spleen percussion a. At left posterior midaxillary line	Small area of splenic dullness may be heard at sixth to tenth rib, or tone may be tympanic (colonic)	Dullness extends above sixth rib, or dullness covers large area between sixth rib and costal margin

CHARACTERISTIC OR AREA EXAMINED	NORMAL FINDINGS	DEVIATIONS FROM NORMAL
b. At lowest left intercostal space in anterior axillary line (performed after client takes deep breath)	Area usually tympanic	Tympany changes to dullness during inspiration (An enlarged spleen is brought forward during inspiration to produce a dull percussion note.)
10. Percussion of gastric "bubble" in left lower rib cage	Tympanic and varies in size	
11. Palpation		
a. Muscle tone	Elderly clients often manifest a more lax abdominal tone	Involuntary resistance Elderly clients may not manifest rigidity response to extent that younger client does; rigidity may be replaced by distention
b. Tenderness	Not present during light or moderate palpation Deep palpation may cause discomfort in midline near xiphoid process Over cecum Over sigmoid colon	Cutaneous (superficial areas of hypersensitivity) or deep pain response in local or generalized area
c. Surface characteristics	Smooth	Induration Nodules Rough texture
d. General tone and location of major structures	Abdomen surface feels smooth, and tension under palpating hand feels consistent throughout	Localized areas of rigidity, distention, or increased tension
e. Masses	Aorta often palpable at epigastrium and pulsates in forward direction Borders of rectus abdominis muscles Feces in ascending or descending colon Sacral promontory	Masses that descend during inspiration Pulsatile masses Laterally mobile masses Fixed masses Aortic pulsations directed laterally
f. Umbilicus	Umbilical ring round, with no irregularities or bulges Umbilicus may be inverted or slightly everted	Masses, bulges Umbilical ring may be incomplete or may feel soft in center
12. Specific organ identification		
a. Liver palpation		
(1) Border and contour	Liver often not palpable Liver often "bumps" against finger during inspiration (especially with thin clients) Liver commonly palpated 1 to 2 cm below costal margin in clients with distended lungs and lowered diaphragm	Greatly enlarged liver may lie under examiner's hand as it extends downward into abdominal cavity
(2) Border surface	Smooth	Irregular, nodular surface or edge
(3) Tenderness	None	Tenderness elicited (*Note:* Client's inspiration may be abruptly halted if pain exists.)
b. Spleen palpation	Spleen not normally palpable	

Continued.

CLINICAL VARIATIONS: THE OLDER ADULT—cont'd

CHARACTERISTIC OR AREA EXAMINED	NORMAL FINDINGS	DEVIATIONS FROM NORMAL
Abdomen—cont'd		
c. Kidney palpation	Kidneys rarely palpated in elderly clients Lower pole of right kidney may be felt in very thin clients; if palpated, contour smooth and no associated tenderness	
d. Inguinal nodes (horizontal and vertical)		
(1) Presence	Small, mobile Nontender nodes often present	Tender, enlarged
(2) Contour	Smooth or nonpalpable	
(3) Consistency (*Note:* Femoral pulses can also be palpated at this time. Techniques and palpable qualities are discussed in Chapter 9.) (*Note:* Special maneuvers for assessing fluid in abdominal cavity and abdominal pain are conducted in same manner as described on p. 358.)	Soft or nonpalpable	
Anal/rectal region		
1. Inspection of sacrococcygeal and perianal areas for skin and surface characteristics	Surface smooth and clear	Lumps Rash Inflammation Scars Pilonidal dimpling Tuft of hair at pilonidal area
2. Palpation of coccygeal area for tenderness	No tenderness	Tender
3. Inspection of anus for surface characteristics	Increased pigmentation Coarse skin	Inflammation Lesions Scars Skin tags Fissures Lumps Swelling Excoriation Hemorrhoids Mucosa (pinkish-red in color) bulges through anal ring
4. Ask client to strain down to assess sphincter tone	Sphincter tightens evenly around examiner's finger with minimal discomfort to client	Client unable to tighten sphincter around finger or experiences discomfort with tightening
5. Palpation of anal muscular ring for surface characteristics	Smooth, even pressure on finger	Nodules Irregularities
6. Palpation of all four rectal walls	Continuous smooth surface with minimal discomfort to client	Nodules Masses

CHARACTERISTIC OR AREA EXAMINED	NORMAL FINDINGS	DEVIATIONS FROM NORMAL
(*Note:* Prostate examination is discussed in Chapter 12.)		(*Note:* Cervix is sometimes palpable on anterior wall. Do not mistake for a mass. (*Note:* Elderly clients often have rectal polyps; however, they are soft and sometimes difficult to palpate.)
7. As finger is extracted, note characteristics of any stool		
a. Color	Brown	Presence of blood, pus Black, tarry stool Pale or yellow stool Mucus on stool surface
b. Consistency	Soft	

Study Questions

General

1. Complete the illustration on the right by drawing the following organs:
   a. Liver
   b. Stomach
   c. Spleen
   d. Ascending colon
   e. Transverse colon
   f. Descending colon
   g. Bladder (distended)
   h. Aorta

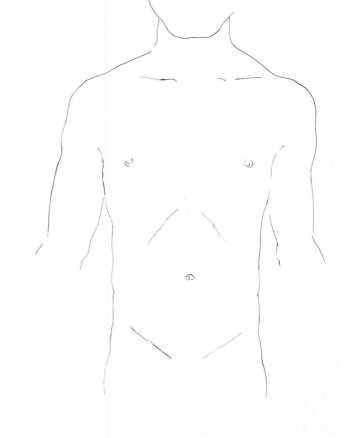

2. Describe five activities or conditions that contribute to client comfort and relaxation in preparation for an abdominal examination, beginning with:
   a. Recently emptied bladder
   b. _____
   c. _____
   d. _____
   e. _____
   f. _____

3. Which of the following statement(s) is/are true about findings associated with inspection of the abdomen:
   - ☐ a. Silvery, white striae are often considered to be a finding within normal limits.
   - ☐ b. A scaphoid abdominal contour may be a normal finding.
   - ☐ c. A fine venous network may normally be visualized on the abdominal surface.
   - ☐ d. A visible aortic pulsation may be a normal finding.
   - ☐ e. A diastasis recti may be a normal finding.
   - ☐ f. a, b, and d
   - ☐ g. All of the above
   - ☐ h. All except e
   - ☐ i. All except d
   - ☐ j. c and e

4. Which of the following statement(s) is/are true:
   - ☐ a. The normal liver span in the midclavicular line is 6 to 12 cm.
   - ☐ b. The normal liver span in the midsternal line is 4 to 8 cm.
   - ☐ c. The liver span is usually greater in tall people than in short people.
   - ☐ d. Gas in the colon can obscure the liver border.
   - ☐ e. During inspiration, the liver span will shift inferiorly 2 to 3 cm.
   - ☐ f. All except c
   - ☐ g. All of the above
   - ☐ h. All except e
   - ☐ i. b, c, and d
   - ☐ j. a, d, and e

5. Auscultation of the abdomen precedes percussion and palpation:
   - ☐ a. Only when one is examining an infant
   - ☐ b. When the examiner suspects that a pulsatile mass is present
   - ☐ c. Because the latter maneuvers may distort bowel sounds
   - ☐ d. Because palpation may displace organs and blood vessels

The Newborn

6. A gap felt between a newborn's rectus muscles and diastasis recti indicates that the infant:
   - ☐ a. May be crying
   - ☐ b. May have sepsis
   - ☐ c. Has a hernia
   - ☐ d. Has a diaphragmatic hernia

7. Kidneys in the newborn are normally palpable:
   - ☐ a. 1 to 2 cm above the xiphoid
   - ☐ b. 1 to 2 cm above the umbilicus
   - ☐ c. 3 to 4 cm above the symphysis pubis
   - ☐ d. 3 to 4 cm above the spleen

The Child

8. The rectal examination in the child is routinely done in which of the following situations:
   - ☐ a. At 1-year evaluation
   - ☐ b. At preschool evaluation
   - ☐ c. At time of puberty
   - ☐ d. None of the above

9. Which of the following children should be referred for further evaluation:
   - ☐ a. 2-month-old with 1 cm umbilical hernia
   - ☐ b. 5-year-old black boy with 2 cm umbilical hernia
   - ☐ c. 6-month-old whose liver is palpable 2 cm below the right costal margin
   - ☐ d. 3-year-old with 1 inch gap in rectus abdominis muscles
   - ☐ e. 18-month-old whose spleen is palpable 1 cm below the left costal margin
   - ☐ f. None of the above
   - ☐ g. a, b, and e
   - ☐ h. b, c, and d

The Childbearing Woman

10. Ballottement of the fetus usually occurs at:
    - ☐ a. 1 to 2 months gestation
    - ☐ b. 2 to 3 months gestation
    - ☐ c. 4 to 5 months gestation
    - ☐ d. 6 to 7 months gestation

11. Outline of the fetus is usually seen after the:
    - ☐ a. Fourth month of gestation
    - ☐ b. Fifth month of gestation
    - ☐ c. Sixth month of gestation
    - ☐ d. Seventh month of gestation

12. Fetal heart tones are usually heard through the Doppler around the:
    - ☐ a. Sixth to eighth week of gestation
    - ☐ b. Eighth to tenth week of gestation
    - ☐ c. Tenth to twelfth week of gestation
    - ☐ d. Twelfth to fourteenth week of gestation

13. Hemorrhoids usually resolve:
    - ☐ a. Immediately after delivery
    - ☐ b. 2 to 4 days postpartum
    - ☐ c. 1 week postpartum
    - ☐ d. 1 to 3 weeks after giving birth

The Older Adult

14. Elderly individuals often describe constipation as a concern. Which of the following might be a contributing factor:
    - ☐ a. Depression
    - ☐ b. Decreased abdominal muscle tone
    - ☐ c. Erratic eating habits
    - ☐ d. Inactivity
    - ☐ e. Insufficient bulk in diet
    - ☐ f. b and e
    - ☐ g. All of the above
    - ☐ h. All except a
    - ☐ i. c, d, and e

15. When examining the abdomen of a healthy older individual, the examiner is likely to find:
    - ☐ a. A liver span that is 1 to 2 cm longer than in a younger client
    - ☐ b. Moderate abdominal distention
    - ☐ c. Kidneys less readily palpable than in a younger client
    - ☐ d. A palpable gallbladder
    - ☐ e. Tenderness (during deep palpation) over the epigastrium at the xiphoid process

SUGGESTED READINGS
General

AH Robins GI series: Physical examination of the abdomen, Richmond, Va, 1974, AH Robins Co.

Bates B: *A guide to physical examination,* ed 4, Philadelphia, 1987, JB Lippincott.

Malasanos L, Barkauskas V, Stoltenberg-Allen K: *Health assessment,* ed 4, St Louis, 1990, Mosby–Year Book.

Pender NJ: *Health promotion in nursing practice,* ed 2, Norwalk, Conn, 1987, Appleton & Lange.

Prior JA, Silberstein JS, Stang JM: *Physical diagnosis: the history and examination of the patient,* ed 6, St Louis, 1981, Mosby–Year Book.

Smith C: Abdominal assessment: a blending of science and art, *Nurs '81* 11(2):42, 1981.

Thompson JM, McFarland GK, Hirsch JE, and others: *Mosby's manual of clinical nursing,* ed 2, St Louis, 1989, Mosby–Year Book.

The newborn

Auvenshine MA, Enriquez MG: *Maternity nursing: dimensions of change,* Belmont, Calif, 1985, Wadsworth.

Bobak IM, Jensen MD: *Essentials of maternity nursing,* ed 3, St Louis, 1991, Mosby–Year Book.

Judd JM: Assessing the newborn from head to toe, *Nurs '85* 15(12):34, 1985.

Kiernan BS, Scoloveno MA: Assessment of the neonate, *Top Clin Nurs* 8(1):1, 1986.

The Organization for Obstetrical, Gynecological and Neonatal Nurses (NAACOG): *Physical assessment of the neonate,* OGN nursing practice resource, Oct. 1986, The Association.

Pillitteri A: *Maternal-newborn nursing: care of the growing family,* ed 3, Boston, 1985, Little, Brown.

Scanlon JW, and others: *A system of newborn physical examination,* Baltimore, 1979, University Park Press.

Seidel HM, Ball JW, Dains JE, Benedict GW: *Mosby's guide to physical examination,* ed 2, St Louis, 1991, Mosby–Year Book.

Whaley LF, Wong DL: *Nursing care of infants and children,* ed 4, St Louis, 1991, Mosby–Year Book.

The child

Barness L: *Manual of pediatric physical diagnosis,* ed 5, Chicago, 1991, Mosby–Year Book.

Bates B: *A guide to physical examination,* ed 4, Philadelphia, 1987, JB Lippincott.

DeAngelis C: *Basic pediatrics for the primary health care provider,* ed 2, Boston, 1984, Little, Brown.

Prior JA, Silberstein JS, Stang JM: *Physical diagnosis: the history and examination of the patient,* ed 6, St Louis, 1981, Mosby–Year Book.

Whaley LF, Wong DL: *Essentials of pediatric nursing,* ed 3, St Louis, 1989, Mosby–Year Book.

The childbearing woman

Auvenshine MA, Enriquez MG: *Maternity nursing: dimensions of change,* Belmont, Calif, 1985, Wadsworth.

Bobak IM, Jensen MD: *Essentials of maternity nursing,* ed 3, St Louis, 1991, Mosby–Year Book.

Pillitteri A: *Maternal-newborn nursing: care of the growing family,* ed 3, Boston, 1985, Little, Brown.

Pritchard JA, MacDonald PC: *Williams' obstetrics,* ed 17, New York, 1985, Appleton-Century-Crofts.

Seidel HM, Ball JW, Dains JE, Benedict GW: *Mosby's guide to physical examination,* ed 2, St Louis, 1991, Mosby–Year Book.

Whitley N: *A manual of clinical obstetrics,* Philadelphia, 1985, JB Lippincott.

The older adult

Burnside IM, editor: *Nursing and the aged,* ed 3, New York, 1988, McGraw-Hill.

Carotenuto R, Bullock J: *Physical assessment of the gerontologic client,* Philadelphia, 1980, FA Davis.

Ebersole P, Hess P: *Toward healthy aging,* ed 3, St Louis, 1990, Mosby–Year Book.

Eliopoulos C: *Gerontological nursing,* ed 2, Philadelphia, 1987, JB Lippincott.

Shuran M, Nelson RA: Updated nutritional assessment and support of the elderly, *Geriatrics* 41(7):48, 1986.

Thompson JM, McFarland GK, Hirsch JE, and others: *Mosby's manual of clinical nursing,* ed 2, St Louis, 1989, Mosby–Year Book.

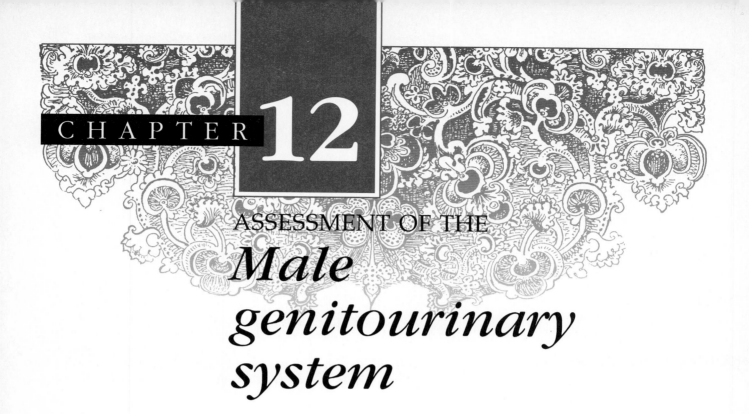

CHAPTER 12

ASSESSMENT OF THE
Male genitourinary system

VOCABULARY

anuria Absence of urine production or the inability to produce more than 250 ml of urine per day.

balano- Combining form denoting the glans penis.

> EXAMPLE: *Balanitis* means inflammation of the glans penis.

chordee Ventral curvature of the penis; congenital anomaly caused by a restrictive band of tissue between the meatus and the glans; usually associated with hypospadias.

cryptorchism (undescended testis) Failure of one or both of the testicles to descend into the scrotum.

dysuria Difficulty, pain, or burning sensation with urination.

enuresis Any involuntary urination, especially during sleep.

epididymitis Inflammation of the epididymis (tightly coiled, comma-shaped, structure overlying posterolateral surface of testis); infection can be acute or chronic; area is extremely tender, usually involving the scrotal wall and occasionally extending along the spermatic cord.

epispadias Congenital defect in which the urinary meatus opens on the dorsum of the penis; opening may be located on the glans or anywhere along the penile shaft, or extend into the pubic symphysis.

hematuria Presence of blood in the urine.

hernia Abnormal opening in a muscle wall or cavity that permits protrusion of its contents.

> *direct inguinal hernia* Protrusion of abdominal contents through external ring of inguinal canal, usually in region superior to the canal.
>
> *indirect inguinal hernia* Protrusion of abdominal contents into internal ring of inguinal canal; contents may remain in the canal, emerge through external ring, or extend downward into scrotal sac; occurs more commonly than direct inguinal herniation.
>
> *femoral hernia* Protrusion of abdominal contents through femoral canal (below inguinal ligament); occurs more often with women than men and is less common than inguinal hernias.

hydrocele Nontender, serous fluid mass located within the tunica vaginalis (layered, hollow membrane adjacent to testis); examiner's finger can get above the mass within the scrotum.

hypospadias Congenital defect in which the urinary meatus opens on the ventral aspect of the penis; opening may be located in the glans, penile shaft, scrotum, or perineum.

oliguria Inadequate production or secretion of urine (usually less than 400 ml in a 24-hour period).

orchi- Combining form denoting the testes.

> EXAMPLE: *Orchitis* means inflammation of one or both of the testes.

paraphimosis Condition characterized by the inability to pull the foreskin forward from a retracted position; glans is usually swollen and inflamed.

phimosis Tightness of the foreskin that results in an inability to retract it; usually caused by adhesions of the prepuce to the underlying glans.

pyuria Presence of white cells (pus) in the urine.

refractory period Rest interval following nerve excitation or muscle contraction.

> EXAMPLE: In sexual intercourse the refractory period is the phase that follows orgasm; it refers to the normal loss of erection after ejaculation and the time required before another ejaculation can occur.

smegma Accumulation of bacteria, urine, and cellular debris underneath the foreskin; sometimes associated with phimosis and resulting irritation and inflammation.

spermatocele (epididymal cyst) ainless, fluid-filled epididymal mass that contains spermatozoa.

tenesmus Rectal or anal spasm characterized by pain and a sensation of urgency; overly vigorous digital examination can cause anal sphincter spasms;

rectal tenesmus may be associated with prostatitis and resulting perirectal inflammation.

torsion (of spermatic cord) Twisting of the spermatic cord resulting in an infarction of the testis; severe pain, redness, and swelling are present; loss of the

testis can be prevented if the condition is diagnosed and treated quickly.

varicocele Abnormal tortuosity and dilation of spermatic veins; spermatic cord is described as feeling like a bag of worms; condition is not painful but involves a pulling or dragging sensation.

ANATOMY AND PHYSIOLOGY REVIEW

The male reproductive system includes the internal structures of two vas deferens, two seminal vesicles, the ejaculatory duct, the prostate gland, and two bulbourethral (Cowper) glands (Fig. 12-1). The urethra, the duct that conveys urine and ejaculated semen, extends from the urinary bladder to the urethral meatus at the tip of the penis. The external genitalia include the penis and the scrotum, which contains the testes and the epidid-

ymides where sperm are produced and transported through the vas deferens into the pelvis.

The scrotum is a pouch covered with thin, darkly pigmented, rugous (wrinkled) skin that is divided into two compartments by a septum. Each half contains a testis and an epididymis, which is suspended by the spermatic cord—a network of nerves, blood vessels, and the vas deferens (Fig. 12-2). The testes exist outside of the body because sperm production requires a temper-

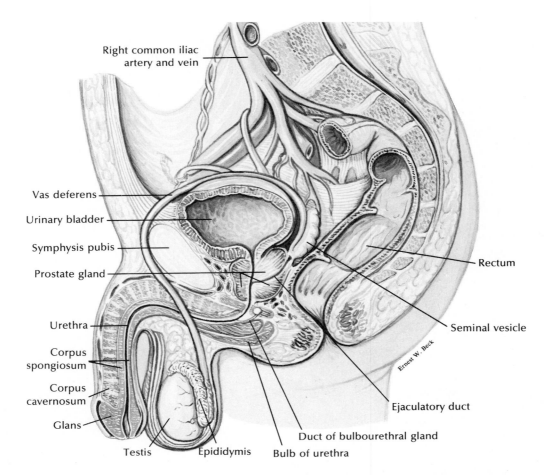

Fig. 12-1 Male pelvic organs. (From Anthony CP, Thibodeau GA: *Textbook of anatomy and physiology,* ed 12, St Louis, 1987, Mosby—Year Book.)

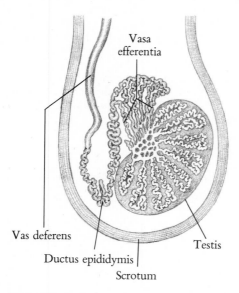

Fig. 12-2 Sagittal section of a mature testis. (From Seidel HM, Ball JW, Dains JE, Benedict GW: *Mosby's guide to physical examination,* ed 2, St Louis, 1991, Mosby–Year Book.)

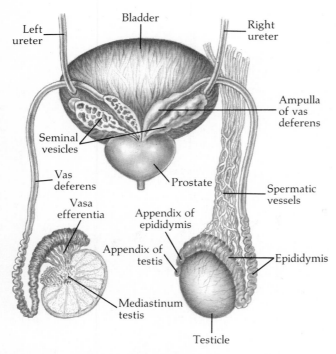

Fig. 12-3 Anatomical relation of vas deferens to bladder (posterior view). (From Thompson JM, McFarland GK, Hirsch JE, and others: *Mosby's manual of clinical nursing,* ed 2, St Louis, 1989, Mosby–Year Book.)

ature slightly below body temperature. A layer of muscle under the scrotal skin contracts when the outside temperature is cold and retracts the pouch and its contents upward toward the body. The wrinkled surface of the sac allows it to relax, expand, and drop downward in a warm environment when body heat is elevated. The left side of the scrotum usually lies slightly lower than the right side. Each testis is approximately 4.5 × 3 × 2 cm, ovoid, rubbery in texture, and smooth on the surface. The testis contains a series of coiled ducts (seminiferous tubules), where sperm production (spermatogenesis) occurs. The sperm move toward the center of the testis and into the efferent tubules adjacent to the epididymis. The comma-shaped epididymis is about 5 cm long and usually lies on the posterolateral surface of each testis. The sperm receive nutrients and mature in an elaborate, coiled duct within the epididymis. They are stored in the ductus epididymis and eventually travel through the vas deferens into the pelvis.

The vas deferens emerges from the tail of the epididymis and ascends from the scrotum through the external inguinal ring to the posterior aspect of the bladder, where it terminates in the ejaculatory duct at the prostate gland (Fig. 12-3). The seminal vesicles are pouches that lie between the rectum and the posterior bladder wall. They also join the ejaculatory duct at the base of the prostate (see Fig. 12-1). Secretions and nutrients are produced by the vas deferens, the seminal vesicles, the prostate, and the bulbourethral glands to provide semen that maximizes the health, life span, and motility of the sperm. The prostate gland is a trilobed, fibromuscular organ that is approximately 3.5 cm long, 4.5 cm wide, and 2.5 cm deep. It lies at the base of the bladder, and its posterior surface is adjacent to the anterior rectal wall, so it can be palpated during a rectal examination (see Fig. 12-12). The three lobes are not well defined, but the palpable portion manifests right and left vertical lobes divided by a sulcus (a slight groove). The prostate surrounds the urethra as it emerges from the bladder. This gland can obstruct urinary flow if it enlarges and constricts the urinary duct.

The body of the penis contains three cylindrical bodies of spongy tissue, the corpora cavernosa and the corpus spongiosum, which encircles the urethra (Fig. 12-4). The spongy tissue feels smooth and of a semifirm consistency on palpation of a flaccid penis, but the tissue becomes engorged with blood when the penis is erect. The skin covering the penis is thin, loosely adhered to the shaft, hairless, and usually darker in color. The glans penis, the end of the penis, is a lighter pink and is exposed when the prepuce (the foreskin) is pulled back or surgically removed (circumcision). The corona is the ridge that separates the glans from the shaft of the penis.

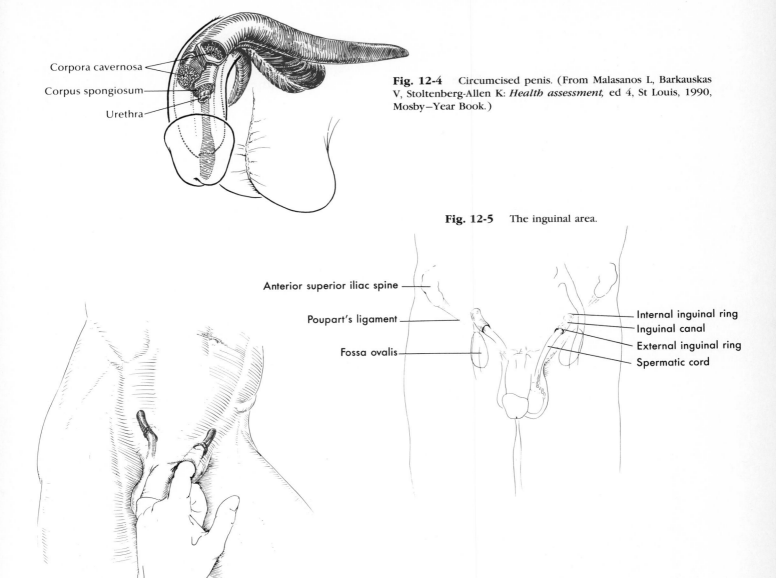

Fig. 12-4 Circumcised penis. (From Malasanos L, Barkauskas V, Stoltenberg-Allen K: *Health assessment,* ed 4, St Louis, 1990, Mosby—Year Book.)

Fig. 12-5 The inguinal area.

Fig. 12-6 Examination of a male client for indirect inguinal hernia. (From Malasanos L, Barkauskas V, Stoltenberg-Allen K: *Health assessment,* ed 4, St Louis, 1990, Mosby—Year Book.)

The Inguinal Area

The inguinal canal is a 4 to 6 cm tube that encases the vas deferens as it passes from the scrotum through the abdominal muscles into the pelvis (Fig. 12-5). The canal runs parallel to the inguinal ligament (Poupart's ligament), which connects the pubic tubercle and the superior iliac spine. The external inguinal ring is an area of weakness where a hernia may occur if abdominal contents bulge or protrude. The area of the external ring is palpable; the internal ring is not. A direct hernia emerges from behind the external ring and through the ring to the surface. An indirect hernia enters the internal ring and descends through the canal, sometimes down into the scrotal sac. The examiner can sometimes feel a bulge if a finger is inserted into the inguinal area at the point of the external ring as the client holds his breath and bears down (Fig. 12-6). (*Note:* Beginning examiners cannot usually differentiate between an indirect and a direct hernia through palpation.) Hernias can occur also at the fossa ovalis, an opening from the abdominal area that admits the femoral artery and vein to pass through to the leg. The site of a femoral hernia is just medial to the femoral artery.

The Urinary Tract

The urinary tract includes the kidneys, ureters, the urinary bladder, and the urethra. The kidneys interact with the cardiac, endocrine, and nervous systems to conserve body nutrients, remove waste materials, and regulate body substances, fluids, and blood pressure. This is accomplished in the kidneys through an elaborate microscopic filter and pressure system that eventually produces urine. The kidneys are paired organs located outside of the peritoneal cavity at spinal levels T12 through L3 (Fig. 12-7). The right kidney is slightly lower than the left because of displacement by the overlying liver. Each kidney is approximately 11 × 6 × 3 cm, is cushioned in a protective fatty mass, and is attached to the posterior abdominal wall with fascia.

The interior of the kidney is composed of the hilum, the outer cortex, the inner medulla, and the pelvis (Fig. 12-8). A renal artery branches from the aorta and enters the kidney through the hilum. The artery eventually branches into specialized arterioles, which enter thousands of microscopic units called *nephrons*, where fluid is filtered from the blood and nutrients are reabsorbed

back into the blood. Glomeruli, the central filtering units of each nephron, are located in the cortex. Glomeruli empty into tubules, where urine is concentrated and diluted, and nutrients are reabsorbed. The tubules empty into collecting ducts that form the renal pyramids in the medulla. The collecting ducts empty into a calyx, which leads to the flow of urine into the ureter. Renal veins exit the kidney at the hilum. The amount of urine produced is approximately 1 ml per minute, but this varies greatly with the needs and the activities of the individual moment by moment.

The ureters continue out of the renal pelvis and extend for approximately 24 to 30 cm to an insertion point at the base of the bladder. The ureters expedite the flow of urine by means of peristaltic waves that originate in the renal pelvis and are stimulated by renal output. The bladder is located anterior to the rectum and sits on top of the prostate gland (Fig. 12-9). The urethra extends out of the base of the bladder, through the prostate gland, into the pelvic floor, and through the penile shaft. The length of the urethra is approximately 18 to 20 cm from bladder to meatus. The size of the bladder varies

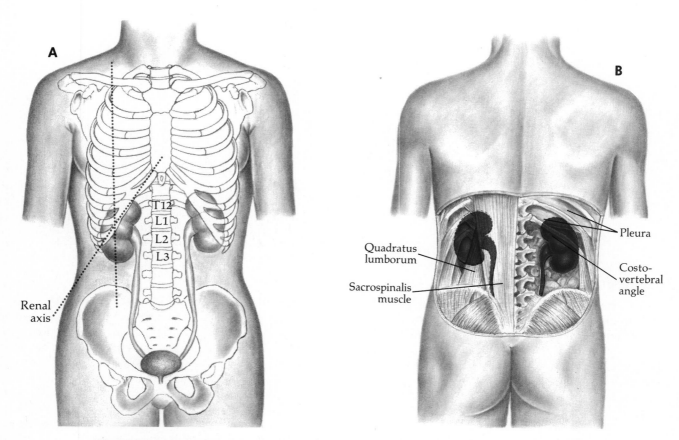

Fig. 12-7   Location of kidneys, ureters, and bladder. **A,** Anterior view. **B,** Posterior view. (From Thompson JM, McFarland GK, Hirsch JE, and others: *Mosby's manual of clinical nursing,* ed 2, St Louis, 1989, Mosby–Year Book.)

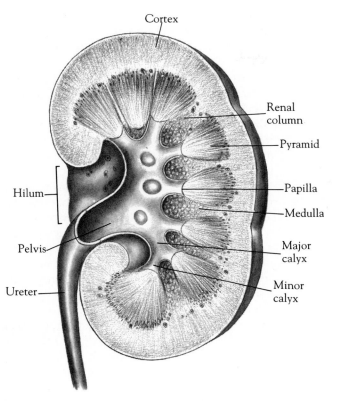

Fig. 12-8 Cross section of the kidney. (From Thompson JM, McFarland GK, Hirsch JE, and others: *Mosby's manual of clinical nursing,* ed 2, St Louis, 1989, Mosby–Year Book.)

according to the amount of urine it contains. About 300 ml of urine causes the internal sphincter to relax and alerts the individual with an urge to void.

COGNITIVE OBJECTIVES

At the end of this chapter the learner will demonstrate knowledge of assessment of the male genitourinary system by the ability to do the following:

- Apply the terms that are listed in the vocabulary section.
- Identify and locate the major internal and external structures of the male genitourinary system.
- Point out observable and palpable characteristics of normal penis and scrotal contents.
- Identify major inguinal and lower abdominal structures associated with assessment for hernias.
- Locate on a drawing the three common pelvic area hernia sites.
- Identify palpable characteristics of the normal prostate gland.
- Identify the major structures and functions of the urinary tract.
- Identify common selected variations for the newborn, the child, and the older adult.

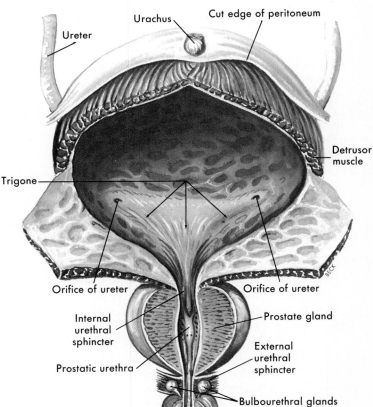

Fig. 12-9 The urinary bladder in relation to the prostate gland. (From McCance KL, Huether SE: *Pathophysiology: the biological basis for disease in adults and children,* St Louis, 1990, Mosby–Year Book.)

CLINICAL OUTLINE

At the end of this chapter the learner will perform a systematic assessment of the male genitourinary system, demonstrating the ability to do the following:

- Obtain a pertinent history from a client.
- Inspect and palpate the pubic region for the following:
  1. Hair distribution
  2. Parasites
  3. Surface characteristics
- Inspect and palpate the penis for the following:
  1. Surface characteristics
  2. Foreskin
  3. Meatus location
  4. Discharge
  5. Tenderness
- Inspect and palpate the scrotum and scrotal contents for the following:
  1. Size and contour
  2. Testes
     a. Size
     b. Contour
     c. Mobility
     d. Tenderness
  3. Epididymides
  4. Vas deferens
  5. Additional scrotal contents
- Transilluminate scrotal contents.
- Evaluate inguinal region for hernias: palpate external inguinal ring and femoral area.
- Inspect and palpate sacrococcygeal and perianal area for surface characteristics and tenderness.
- Inspect and palpate the anus for the following:
  1. Sphincter tone
  2. Tenderness
  3. Surface characteristics
- Palpate distal rectal walls for surface characteristics.
- Palpate the prostate gland for the following:
  1. Size
  2. Contour
  3. Consistency
  4. Tenderness
- Summarize results of the assessment with a written description of findings.

HISTORY

- Reproductive functions and sexuality. The examiner should screen all clients for sexual needs or problems by initially posing a broad, nondirective question. The question might be worded in this way: "Do you have any concerns regarding sexual practices or values that you would like to discuss?" This lets the client know that he can share his problems if he wishes to, and it does not direct him toward any specific area of concern. Anyone posing this question should be prepared

to follow through with intervention skills in this area.

A more specific detailed assessment will help to clarify general concerns and can supplement the original data base.

1. Present practices and values
   a. Are you comfortable with your intimate relationships (with or without sexual activity)? Do you have difficulty meeting your needs for intimacy (or affection)?
   b. Are you having a sexual relationship with anyone at present?
   c. Do you feel satisfied with this relationship? (For example, do you and your partner share similar feelings about the methods and variety of sexual acts you perform; about the frequency of sex; about the kind and amount of affection displayed; about initiating sex? Do you talk about sexual feelings with your partner? Is there anything you would change about this relationship?)
   d. If you do not have a sexual partner, are your sexual needs being met?
   e. Do you have more than one sexual partner? If so, is this a satisfactory arrangement?
   f. How many partners have you had in the past year?
   g. How do you feel about homosexuality (i.e., is it a personal issue with you)?
   h. How do you feel about masturbation?
   i. Have there been any recent changes in your sexual desire (arousal patterns), specific sexual acts or behaviors, frequency of sexual experiences, choice of sexual partners?
   j. Do you and/or your partner(s) use contraception? What method do you use? Do you have questions or difficulty with this?
   k. Do you have any questions about male sexuality, sexual function, female sexuality, sterility, venereal disease, other?
2. History
   a. Describe your personal experience with sex education. Was sexuality discussed with family members? Was it discussed openly? Were there others outside the family who informed or influenced you sexually? Explain.
   b. Were your parents affectionate with each other?
   c. What were your early experiences with masturbation; wet dreams; sex play with other children; adolescent relationships; dating (feeling comfortable with girls); petting?
   d. How old were you when you first had sexual intercourse? How did you feel about it?
   e. Have you ever had a homosexual experience? Describe.

f. How many sexual partners have you had?

3. Genital health
   a. Do you examine your penis and your scrotum (testicles)? How often? (*Note:* It is more helpful to allow the client to demonstrate how he examines himself during the physical assessment rather than to have him describe the procedure.)
   b. Do you have any general concerns about your genitalia (e.g., size, shape, surface characteristics, texture)?
   c. Are you able to pull back (and replace) the foreskin on your penis?
   d. Have you ever noticed any sores, rashes, swellings, lumps, or discharge?
   e. Have you felt any itching, burning, or stinging in your penis?
   f. Are you able to have an erection? Do you have difficulty attaining or maintaining an erection?
   g. Do you experience pain with an erection (either in your penis or scrotum)?
   h. Do you ever have prolonged painful erections? If so, are they associated with sexual arousal?
   i. When you have an erection, does your penis curve downward or to the side?
   j. Do you have any difficulty with ejaculation (e.g., premature, inadequate, painful)?
   k. Describe the fluid that discharges at the time of ejaculation (color, consistency, odor, amount).
   l. Do you ever feel any irregularities, lumps, soreness, or heaviness in your testicles?
   m. Have you ever been treated for (or ever been exposed to) any venereal diseases: gonorrhea, syphilis, herpes simplex, venereal warts? If so, describe symptoms, treatment, follow-up procedures.
   n. Do you take any precautions to prevent exposure to sexually transmitted diseases?
   o. Do you have specific questions or concerns about symptoms or disease transmission?

- AIDS (acquired immune deficiency syndrome).
  1. Screening for high-risk candidates. AIDS has become an urgent universal health concern. At present, the client's right to privacy (i.e., personal sexual life-style and health status) and anonymity (i.e., results of AIDS screening results) differs according to legal definitions in various states. Local policy (or law) may dictate (or confine) screening practices in local health agencies. (*Note:* A laboratory test for antibodies is the only way to confirm a positive exposure to the disease. Some authorities estimate that only 20% to 30% of those individuals exposed to the disease will manifest a positive antibody reaction.)

RISK FACTORS FOR AIDS

Because AIDS can be dormant (or asymptomatic), screening clients for high-risk status would involve identifying one (or more) of the following risk factors:
- Male homosexual practice (a higher risk exists with a history of multiple partners or having a partner with a history of multiple partners)
- Drug addicts who share contaminated needles
- A history of multiple heterosexual partners, especially without the use of a condom
- A history of contacts with prostitutes, especially without the use of a condom
- A history of frequent/multiple blood transfusions

---

2. At present, AIDS is usually diagnosed when the disease becomes active and symptomatic. The following symptoms are commonly reported:
   a. Chronic fatigue
   b. Chronic intermittent fever
   c. Night sweats
   d. Unexplained weight loss (10% to 15% of total body weight in 1 or 2 months)
   e. Oral candidiasis (white patches on the tongue or buccal membranes)
   f. Purple patches/discoloration of the skin (especially on the legs and ankles) or of the mucous membrane in the mouth
   g. Chronic dry cough
   h. Shortness of breath
   i. Bruising
   j. Unexplained bleeding under the skin or from any orifice

- Sexually transmitted diseases (STDs).
  1. Signs and symptoms of STD vary widely, and an individual can present with a combination of diseases or infections. Following is a categorization of signs and symptoms to be alert for:
     a. Localized
        (1) External: Lesions may appear as large ulcers or coalesced multiple ulcers. Vesicles, pustules, cysts, abscesses or condylomas (warts) may appear. The glans penis is a common site; however, the prepuce or the shaft of the penis may be involved. Lesions may appear also around the lips or in the perianal area. Pubic infestations may include scabies, nits, or pediculosis, accompanied by excoriation.
        (2) Internal: Urethritis or infection/inflammation/lesions within oral or anal mucosa can be accompanied by burning on urination

RISK FACTORS FOR MAJOR SEXUALLY TRANSMITTED DISEASES (STDs)

- Young, sexually active male or female (age range 15 to 30 years)
- Multiple sexual partners
- Urban dweller
- Low income
- Unmarried
- Early onset of sexual activity
- History of previous STD

and/or discharge that may be watery, mucopurulent, serosanguineous, or malodorous. Chronic inflammation may result in phimosis or urinary retention.

    b. Systemic: Lymphatic dissemination may result in inguinal node inflammation, fistulas, or a generalized adenitis. A generalized infection can produce fever, headache, malaise, joint pain, abdominal pain, focal neurological signs, or seizures. Endocarditis, meningitis, septicemia, and arthritis are some of the major manifestations of infection.

- Genitourinary symptoms.
  1. Urinary frequency. How many times do you void (urinate) in a 24-hour period? Does this frequency involve sleeping hours as well as waking hours? Can you estimate the volume voided each time? Has the volume increased or decreased?
  2. Nocturia. How many times do you have to urinate at night? Is this a *change* of habit for you? Has your daytime or nighttime fluid intake changed?
  3. Urgency. Does urgency occur with every urination, occasionally, or rarely? Does urgency occur without voiding? Is it associated with other symptoms, such as frequency, dysuria, or incontinence?
  4. Hesitancy. Do you have to wait a while for your stream to start? Once you have started, can you pass 80% to 90% of your urine in a continuous stream? Do you have to strain to start or to maintain your stream?
  5. Flow of urinary stream. Have you had any decrease in the size of your stream? Are you having to stand closer to the toilet to avoid urinating on the floor? (The examiner is concerned with the force as well as caliber of the stream.)
  6. Urethral discharge. What color is it? Has the amount of discharge increased or decreased since it started? Is the discharge associated with pain? With urination? Is an unusual odor associated with discharge? Describe.
  7. Hernia. If you feel a lump in your scrotum, are you able to push the lump back inside? Does the lump ever change size? How long has it been since you were able to push the lump back inside (a day, a week)? Do you have a heavy feeling or dragging sensation in your scrotum?

Text continues on p. 392.

CLINICAL GUIDELINES

ASSESSMENT PROCEDURE	NORMAL FINDINGS	EVALUATION
		DEVIATIONS FROM NORMAL

1. Assemble equipment
  a. Gloves
  b. Lubricant
  c. Penlight
  d. Rectal gloves
2. Put on gloves before beginning examination
3. Inspect and palpate the general pubic region (Palpation of inguinal lymphatics is described in Chapter 11.)
  a. Hair distribution
	Variable in adults
	Diamond-shaped pattern often extending to umbilicus
		Patchy growth or loss
		Absence of hair
		Female configuration: triangular, with base over pubis

b. Parasites	Absent	Nits, pubic lice

| | EVALUATION | |
ASSESSMENT PROCEDURE	NORMAL FINDINGS	DEVIATIONS FROM NORMAL
c. Skin surface characteristics	Smooth, clear	Scars Lower abdominal or inguinal lesions Rash (especially in folds) (*Note:* Tinea cruris ["jock itch"] is a common fungal infection found in the groin. Large, clearly margin-ated, reddened patches are pru-ritic and often associated with "athlete's foot." Monilial infections, which are red, eroded patches with scaling and pustules, also are often seen; they are associated with immobility and disability, systemic antibiotics, and immuno-logical deficits.)
4. Inspect the penis a. Skin color and surface character-istics	Usually dark Hairless Wrinkled; surface vascularity may be apparent	Reddened Lesions Swelling Nodules
b. Foreskin	Uncircumcised: prepuce present and folded over glans (Fig. 12-10) Circumcised: prepuce often absent, or small flaps remain at corona (Fig. 12-11)	

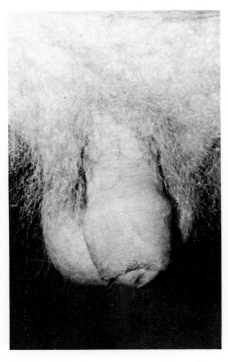

Fig. 12-10   Uncircumcised penis.

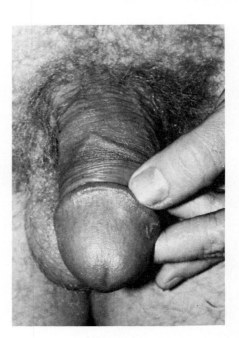

Fig. 12-11   Circumcised penis. *(Un-gloved hand is that of the client.)*

Continued.

CLINICAL GUIDELINES—cont'd

	EVALUATION	
ASSESSMENT PROCEDURE	**NORMAL FINDINGS**	**DEVIATIONS FROM NORMAL**
5. Ask client to retract foreskin if present (Fig. 12-12)	Foreskin retracts easily to expose glans and returns to original position with ease	Failure to retract; discomfort with retraction Difficulty returning prepuce to original position
6. Inspect glans and under prepuce fold	Glans smooth, pink, bulbous Prepuce fold wrinkled, loosely attached to underlying glans, darker in color than glans (*Note:* Circumcised penises have varying lengths of foreskin remaining; some have multiple folds and others have few or none.)	Lesions Crusting under fold or around tip of glans Redness, swelling
7. Inspect urethral meatus for: a. Location	Central, at distal tip of glans	Dorsal location Ventral location
b. Discharge	Usually not present	Yellow-green discharge Milky-white discharge Discharge with foul odor
8. Ask client to compress glans anteroposteriorly to open distal end of urethra (Fig. 12-13); inspect for surface characteristics	Pink, smooth No discharge	Reddened, swollen Discharge Crusting
9. Palpate entire penis between thumb and first two fingers for palpable characteristics	Nontender Smooth, semifirm consistency	Tenderness Swelling Nodules Induration
10. Ask client to hold penis out of the way; inspect scrotum for size and contour	Sac divided in half by septum Left scrotal sac may be longer than right Size varies: may appear pendulous Scrotal contents contracted when surface temperature cool	

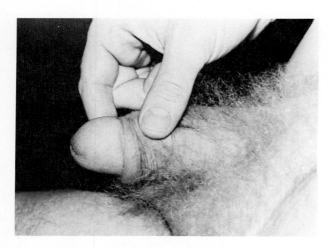

Fig. 12-12   Client retracting foreskin.

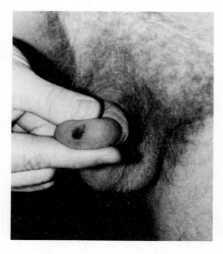

Fig. 12-13   Client compressing glans to open urethral meatus.

ASSESSMENT PROCEDURE	EVALUATION	
	NORMAL FINDINGS	DEVIATIONS FROM NORMAL
11. Lift scrotum to examine underside surface characteristics (spread rugated surface for better view) (*Note:* While viewing surface of scrotum, visualize scrotal contents: placement, proximity, size; tactile maneuvers will be more efficient [Fig. 12-14].)	Deeply pigmented Hairless Rugous surface	Reddened Edematous Rugae not present Rash Lesions
12. Palpate each half of scrotum for surface characteristics	Nontender Thin, loose skin over muscular layer	Marked tenderness Swelling, redness (*Note:* Scrotal inflammation can exacerbate quickly into cellulitis and gangrene. If scrotum is inflamed, examine rugated surface carefully for fissures or breaks in the skin. Refer immediately for treatment.)
	No pitting	Pitting
13. Palpate testes simultaneously between thumb and first two fingers (Fig. 12-15)		
a. Presence	Present in each sac	Not present
b. Size	Approximately $4 \times 3 \times 2$ cm ($1\frac{1}{2} \times 1 \times \frac{3}{4}$ inches) Equal in size	Enlarged (unilaterally/bilaterally) Atrophied
c. Tenderness	Mildly sensitive to moderate compression	Markedly tender
d. Contour	Smooth, ovoid	Nodular, irregular
e. Mobility	Movable	Fixed

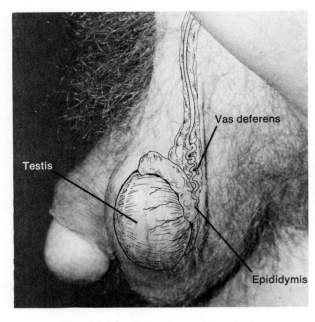

Fig. 12-14   Palpable scrotal contents.

Testis

Vas deferens

Epididymis

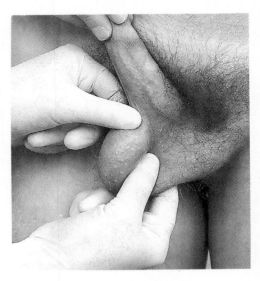

Fig. 12-15   Examiner palpating scrotum. (From Seidel HM, Ball JW, Dains JE, Benedict GW: *Mosby's guide to physical examination,* ed 2, 1991, Mosby—Year Book.)

Continued.

CLINICAL GUIDELINES—cont'd

ASSESSMENT PROCEDURE	EVALUATION	
	NORMAL FINDINGS	DEVIATIONS FROM NORMAL
14. Palpate epididymides for palpable characteristics	Nontender Usually located on posterolateral surface of each testis Discretely palpable Comma shaped Smooth	Tender Irregular Enlarged Indurated Nodular
15. Palpate vas deferens for palpable characteristics (use thumb and forefinger)	Nontender Discretely palpable from epididymis to external inguinal ring Smooth and cordlike Movable	Tender Tortuous Thickened; beaded Indurated
16. Palpate for additional scrotal contents; transilluminate each scrotal sac if mass or irregularity is suspected	None Testes and epididymides do not transilluminate	Mass distal or proximal to testis; either tender or nontender Hydrocele ⎱ Transilluminate Spermatocele ⎰ Tumors ⎱ Hernias ⎬ Do not transilluminate Epididymitis ⎰
17. Evaluate inguinal region for hernia; if possible, client should be standing and examiner sitting		
18. Inspect inguinal region for bulges; then ask client to strain, and continue to inspect area		Bulges at area of external ring, Hesselbach triangle, femoral area
19. Palpate both right and left inguinal rings: use index finger or little finger of hand on client's corresponding side; client should be standing if possible, and examiner seated (Fig. 12-16); ask client to strain	Finger follows spermatic cord upward to triangular, slitlike opening, which may or may not admit finger	Palpable mass touches examiner's fingertip or pushes against side of finger
20. Palpate each femoral area (fossa ovalis) for bulges; ask client to strain		Soft bulge emerges at fossa

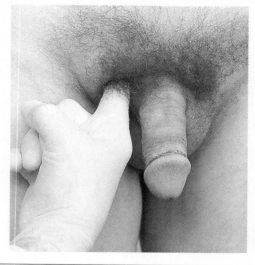

Fig. 12-16 Palpation for inguinal hernia. (From Seidel HM, Ball JW, Dains JE, Benedict GW: *Mosby's guide to physical examination,* ed 2, St Louis, 1991, Mosby–Year Book.)

| | EVALUATION | |
ASSESSMENT PROCEDURE	NORMAL FINDINGS	DEVIATIONS FROM NORMAL
21. Evaluate anal and rectal region (also described in Chapter 11)		
a. Inspect sacrococcygeal and perianal areas (client lying on left side with right hip and knee flexed) for skin and surface characteristics	Surface smooth and clear	Lumps Rash Inflammation Scars Pilonidal dimpling Tuft of hair at pilonidal area
b. Palpate coccygeal area for tenderness	No tenderness	Tenderness
c. Spread buttocks with both hands and inspect anus for surface characteristics (penlight can be used)	Increased pigmentation Coarse skin	Inflammation Lesions Scars Skin tags Fissures Lumps Swelling Excoriation
d. Ask client to strain down; place gloved and lubricated finger at anal opening; as sphincter relaxes, slowly insert finger pointing toward client's umbilicus; ask client to tighten sphincter around finger to assess tone	Sphincter tightens evenly around finger with minimal discomfort to client	Hemorrhoids Mucosal bulging Hypotonic sphincter Hypertonic sphincter with marked tenderness
e. Rotate finger to examine anal muscular ring for surface characteristics	Smooth, even pressure on finger	Nodules Irregularities
f. Insert finger further to palpate all four rectal walls	Continuous, smooth surface with minimal discomfort to client	Nodules Masses Tenderness
g. Palpate entire prostate gland (Fig. 12-17) at anterior surface for:		

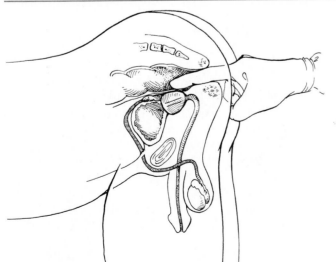

Fig. 12-17   Prostate palpation. (Modified from Malasanos L, Barkauskas V, Stoltenberg-Allen K: *Health assessment,* ed 4, St Louis, 1990, Mosby—Year Book.)

Continued.

CLINICAL GUIDELINES—cont'd

ASSESSMENT PROCEDURE	EVALUATION	
	NORMAL FINDINGS	DEVIATIONS FROM NORMAL
(1) Size	Approximately 4 cm (1½ inches) in diameter; projecting less than 1 cm into rectum	Projects more than 1 cm into rectal wall
(2) Contour	Symmetrical Bilobed with palpable sulcus	Asymmetrical Median sulcus obliterated
(3) Consistency	Firm, smooth	Boggy feeling Irregular Nodules
(4) Tenderness	Nontender	Tender
h. Ask client to strain; palpate area above prostate if possible		Masses or bulges touch finger
i. Slowly withdraw finger and examine any fecal material adhering to glove	Stool brown, soft	Presence of blood, pus Black, tarry stool Pale or yellow stool Light tan or gray stool

CLINICAL TIPS AND STRATEGIES

- **The female practitioner may have emotional discomfort with examination of male genitalia:** One way of avoiding discomfort is to be well prepared with the baseline cognitive data. Read carefully about surface, consistency, and contour characteristics of male genitalia. Have a clear mental picture of the size, location, contour, and palpable characteristics of scrotal contents before engaging in physical assessment. It is also helpful to observe an experienced examiner during the process of examination.
- **The male genital examination should be considered a routine part of any physical examination:** One author indicates that male genitalia examinations are often deferred for some of the following reasons: "...patient refused...will do later...too cold in room...no time...patient too nervous...VIP."*
- **Educating a client to examine his own genitalia regularly is important:** Self-examination on a weekly or a monthly basis is advisable. A regular time and place for self-assessment is helpful. Examination during the shower or bath might be convenient and simple. Many clients are not familiar with their scrotal contents and do not know what normal structures would feel like. The actual process of the examination is an excellent opportunity to explain the procedure and why it is being done. It is helpful to guide the client through the process of self-examination.
- **The examiner must have short fingernails!**

*Warren MM: Testicular tumors, *Continuing Ed,* March 1975, p 31.

SAMPLE RECORDING: NORMAL FINDINGS

Circumcised penis with no lesions, induration, or discharge. Scrotal contents palpated without tenderness or masses. External inguinal canals palpated without masses, bulges, or tenderness.

Sacrococcygeal, perianal, and anal surfaces present no lesions, rash, inflammation, masses, or hemorrhoids. Good anal sphincter tone. Anal and distal rectal mucosa are smooth with no masses. Bilobed prostate is firm, not enlarged, and nontender to palpation.

 The Newborn

HISTORY AND CLINICAL STRATEGIES

- Characteristics of male genitalia are used to help determine gestational age at birth. Premature infants may have undescended testes and few or no rugae. Full-term neonates have fully rugated and brownish-pigmented scrotums.
- Breech-delivered infants may have scrotal edema and ecchymoses. Observation for penile edema, inflammation, or bleeding should be done, especially after circumcision.
- Infants should not be circumcised if hypospadias is present, since foreskin may be used for corrective surgery.

CLINICAL VARIATIONS: THE NEWBORN

CHARACTERISTIC OR AREA EXAMINED	NORMAL FINDINGS	DEVIATIONS FROM NORMAL
	Full-term testes pendulous, deep rugae Scrotum may be edematous	Preterm infant may have undescended testes, no or little rugae Cryptorchism (testes not in scrotum in full-term infant) Priapism (constant erect penis)
	Urethra at tip of penis Penis about 3 to 4 cm long, 1 to 1.3 cm wide Uncircumcised foreskin (prepuce) covers glans	Epispadias (urethra at dorsal surface) Hypospadias (urethra at ventral surface) Torsion (twisting) of testes Hydrocele (fluid)
2. Excretion	Should void within 24 hours of birth Urine is dilute, clear; may have uric acid crystals	Cloudy, concentrated urine, hematuria Urine from perineum or abdomen (implies fistulous tract)
	Patent anus; passes meconium within 24 hours of birth	Imperforate anus, covered or closed anus; no meconium

The Child

HISTORY AND CLINICAL STRATEGIES

- The examiner must assess two types of clients in this area. One will be the infant or little boy and the second the maturing developing adolescent. Although the techniques of examination are similar, the observations and histories are unique.
- The examiner must ask the parents of the male infant or little boy the following questions:
  1. Does the child have difficulty voiding?
  2. Is the stream straight?
  3. Does the child's urination stream seem adequate? (That is, is there a very fine high pressure stream or a heavier easy flow?)
  4. Does the child cry and hold his genitalia as if something were hurting?
  5. Has the parent ever noticed any swelling, discoloration, or sores about the penis or scrotum?
  6. Has the child ever had a urinary tract infection?
  7. Does the child have difficulty because of bed-wetting or wetting himself? How much of a problem is this? What has the parent done about it? Any tests for the problem? How does the child feel about the problem? Is there a family history of bed-wetting?
  8. To the parent's knowledge, are the child's testes descended?
  9. Has the parent ever been told that the child has a hydrocele or hernia?
  10. Has the parent ever noticed that the child's scrotum appears to swell or change size with crying or coughing?
  11. Has the child ever caused trauma to his genitalia either through injury or during play?
- For older boys, the examiner will fluctuate between asking significant subjective questions appropriate for the smaller boys and asking those appropriate for the adult male. Much will depend on the actual maturation, development, and interest of the client. For example, it would be appropriate to ask a mature 16-year-old who is known to be dating, "Do you have any concerns regarding sexual practices or values that you would like to discuss?" Other specific interview questions regarding sexuality are thoroughly discussed on p. 384.
- It should be anticipated that as boys mature, they will have many educational needs regarding what is happening to their own bodies, as well as how to sexually explore with others. The examiner should be alert to these needs and be prepared to develop a beginning profile of the boy's current knowledge and understanding. Not every boy will feel comfortable sharing this information with the examiner, but the examiner should be prepared for and alert to an adolescent asking for clarification and assistance. Profile questions should include items such as the following:
  1. Has he ever had education classes regarding the changes that boys' bodies go through? If so, is he able to describe the type of material presented?

2. Were girls involved in the education classes? Did they also study about the changes girls' bodies are undergoing?

3. How does his family feel about discussing this information at home?

4. Within his family, who does he talk with about sexual changes and dating?

5. If he needs information clarified, who does he go to?

6. He he ever had any classes or organized discussions about dating, petting, birth control?

7. What does he know about venereal disease?

- Most adolescents are not intimidated by direct questioning, as long as it does not appear that someone is pointing an accusing finger toward them. Therefore the level of questioning may relate directly to *normal* activities that the young adolescent may be experiencing, may feel guilty about, or may have incorrect information about, such as homosexual desires, masturbation, sexual fantasies, nocturnal emissions, or erections. The examiner may ask questions such questions as: "Many fellas your age are experiencing new and normal sensations, such as wanting to touch other boys or having wet dreams at night. Do you have any concerns that I could perhaps provide more information about?"*

- The examination strategies will vary with age.

1. Infants through age 2 years should present no problem; the assessment is usually done following the abdominal examination. The examiner simply moves from the abdomen to the genitalia and inguinal area.

2. Boys 3 to 8 years of age should be examined in their undershorts. After the abdominal examination, matter-of-factly tell the child what is going to happen and then slip down his pants to examine the genitalia and inguinal area. During and after the examination, the examiner should reassure the child that everything is normal and healthy.

3. For boys over age 8, provide them with a drape, just as you would for an adult. A reassurance of normal findings is also recommended.

- Evaluation for undescended testes

1. History. If the parent reports that at one time the testes were found in the scrotum, the testes should not be considered undescended.

2. Rugae. If the scrotum shows well-formed rugae, it usually means that the testes have descended at some time.

3. Techniques to force testes into the scrotum (palpation of scrotum should confirm presence)

   a. Have the child stand; slightly milk the inguinal canal region to pull the testes into the scrotum.

   b. Have the child sit on a chair or the examination table, feet next to the buttocks, with the knees pulled tight to the chest.

   c. Have the child sit cross-legged; this will relax the cremasteric reflex.

   d. Child may be placed into very warm water.

4. Palpate the inguinal canal. If the testis is located in the inguinal canal but cannot be pushed down or if no testis is felt, an undescended testis is very likely.

5. Boys whose testes have not descended by age 4 years should be referred to a physician.

- If the testis is palpated momentarily in the scrotum but it quickly slips up into the inguinal canal before adequate assessment, the examiner may block the slippage by gently placing the index finger of the left hand over the inguinal canal and palpating the testis with the right hand.

- Inguinal hernias are fairly common in children. Generally, the parent will describe a bulge in the child's inguinal region. The inguinal region of a larger boy may be palpated in the same manner as for the adult. For the smaller boy it is better to try to produce the hernia or bulge by external techniques, such as the following:

1. Instruct the child to stand; give him a balloon to blow up.

2. Have the infant or toddler in a standing position on the examination table. The examiner should place one hand behind the child's back and with the other hand pump in and out on the child's abdomen. The external abdominal pressure may produce the inguinal bulge.

3. Instruct the child to sit on the examination table and pull his knees to his chest. The examiner then tries to straighten the leg on the questionable side. Again, intraabdominal pressure should fill the hernia sac and produce a bulge.

- Hydroceles are a common finding in children under 2 years of age. Any child with what appears to be a large scrotum should be evaluated for a hydrocele. To do this, the examiner must darken the examination room and transilluminate the scrotum. A fluid-enlarged scrotum shows a pink, light shadow. With scrotal palpation the examiner is not able to reduce the fluid.

*Daniel (1977) provides an excellent discussion of the normal experimentation of adolescent males.

CLINICAL VARIATIONS: THE CHILD

CHARACTERISTIC OR AREA EXAMINED	NORMAL FINDINGS	DEVIATIONS FROM NORMAL
1. Pubic region a. Skin surface b. Hair distribution	Smooth, clear Variable as male develops (Figs. 12-18 and 12-19)	Scars, rashes, lesions Patchy growth or loss Female configuration: triangle with base over pubis

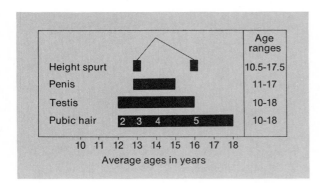

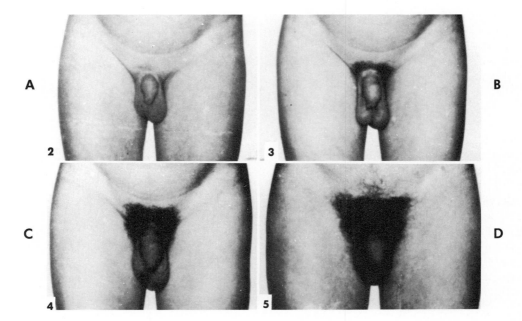

Fig. 12-18 Development of male genitalia and pubic hair. See Fig. 12-19 for description of stages of development of pubic hair. (From Tanner JM: *Growth at adolescence,* ed 2, Oxford, England, 1962, Blackwell Scientific Publications.)

Fig. 12-19 Pubic hair development in males. Preadolescent stage 1 (not shown): no pubic hair. **A,** Stage 2: scant, long, slightly pigmented. **B,** Stage 3: darker, starting to curl, small amount. **C,** Stage 4: resembles adult but less quantity, coarse, curly. **D,** Stage 5: adult distribution, spread to medial surface of thighs. (From Tanner JM: *Growth at adolescence,* ed 2, Oxford, England, 1962, Blackwell Scientific Publications.)

Continued.

CLINICAL VARIATIONS: THE CHILD—cont'd

CHARACTERISTIC OR AREA EXAMINED	NORMAL FINDINGS	DEVIATIONS FROM NORMAL
2. Penis a. Skin color and surface characteristics	Variable as male develops (Fig. 12-20)	Reddened Lesions Swelling Nodules

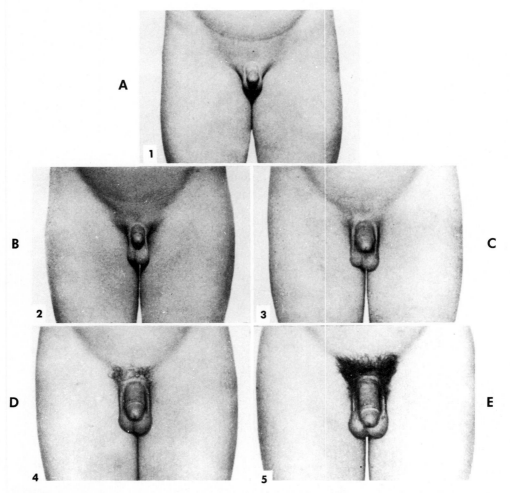

Fig. 12-20 Penis and testes/scrotum development in males. **A,** Stage 1: penis, testes, and scrotum (preadolescent). **B,** Stage 2: enlargement of scrotum and testes, texture alteration; scrotal sac reddens; penis usually does not enlarge. **C,** Stage 3: further growth of testes and scrotum; penis enlarges and becomes longer. **D,** Stage 4: continued growth of testes and scrotum; scrotum becomes darker; penis becomes longer; glans and breadth increase in size. **E,** Stage 5: adult in size and shape. (From Tanner JM: *Growth at adolescence,* ed 2, Oxford, England, 1962, Blackwell Scientific Publications.)

CHARACTERISTIC OR AREA EXAMINED	NORMAL FINDINGS	DEVIATIONS FROM NORMAL
b. Foreskin and foreskin retraction	Uncircumcised: prepuce present and folded over glans (Fig. 12-21)	Continually retracted foreskin in uncircumcised male
	Circumcised: prepuce often absent, or small flap remains at corona	
	For uncircumcised males after age 3, be gentle; if tissue resists, do not force	Unable to retract, or very tightly attached foreskin of child over 3 years of age
	Foreskin retracts easily to expose glans and returns to original position with ease	Failure to retract; discomfort with retraction
		Difficulty returning prepuce to original position
c. Glans and under prepuce fold		Lesions
		Crusting under fold or around tip of glans
		Redness, swelling
		Pinpoint opening
d. Urethral meatus		
(1) Location	Central, at distal tip of glans	Pinpoint opening
		Dorsal location
		Ventral location
(2) Discharge	Usually not present	Yellow-green discharge
		Milky white discharge
		Discharge with foul odor
e. Penile shaft palpation	Nontender	Tenderness
	Smooth, semifirm consistency	Swelling
		Nodules
		Induration

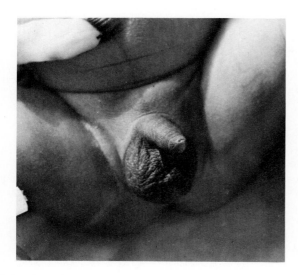

Fig. 12-21   Uncircumcised penis in newborn.

Continued.

CLINICAL VARIATIONS: THE CHILD—cont'd

CHARACTERISTIC OR AREA EXAMINED	NORMAL FINDINGS	DEVIATIONS FROM NORMAL
3. Scrotum		
a. Contour	Sac divided in half by septum Left scrotal sac may be longer than right Scrotal contents and scrotum may retract upward with cool temperature	
b. Size	Size varies; may appear pendulous	Fluctuates greatly in size with crying or coughing Hydrocele common in boys under 2 years of age; nontender mass
4. Scrotum and testes palpation	Testis present in each sac	Hydrocele, unable to reduce (see "Clinical Tips and Strategies," p. 392) Solid scrotal mass Testes not present in sac (see "Clinical Tips and Strategies," p. 392)
a. Size	11 to 18 years: 3.5 to 4.5 cm (1½ to 2 in) Equal in size	Unilateral or bilateral difference in testicle size
b. Tenderness	Mildly sensitive to slight compression	Markedly tender
c. Contour	Smooth, ovoid	Nodular Irregular
d. Mobility	Movable	Fixed
5. Epididymis	Nontender Usually located on posterolateral surface of each testis Discretely palpable Comma shaped Smooth	Tender Irregular shape Enlarged Indurated Nodular
6. Vas deferens	Nontender Discretely palpable from epididymides to external inguinal ring Smooth and cordlike Movable	Tender Tortuous Thickened; beaded Indurated
7. Inguinal hernia inspection (see "Clinical Tips and Strategies," p. 390); older boys may palpate right and left inguinal rings *if hernia is suspected;* child should stand and bear down after finger is in place	With little finger, follow spermatic cord upward to triangular, slitlike opening; opening may or may not admit finger	Bulges appearing at area of external ring, Hesselbach triangle, femoral area Palpable mass touches examiner's fingertip or pushes against side of finger

HISTORY RELATED TO POTENTIAL MALE PARENTS

- Adult males may wish to reproduce offspring. If an infertility problem is suspected, sperm tests may be performed.
- Signs of sexually transmitted diseases should be assessed. Pregnant female partners who are exposed to diseases may transfer them to their unborn infants.

 The Older Adult

HISTORY AND CLINICAL STRATEGIES

- Sexual functions. Physiological changes occurring in the aging male result in sexual function alterations.
  1. Erections develop more slowly in response to stimulation. Erection time may be longer or may be delayed until shortly before ejaculation.
  2. The erection may feel less full or firm.
  3. Ejaculation is less intense, invoking fewer contractions.
  4. The volume of seminal fluid expelled is lessened. The production of spermatozoa diminishes.
  5. The refractory phase is longer, lasting for about 12 hours to several days.

Note that the changes described occur gradually and at different rates according to the individual. Despite testosterone level decreases, an elderly man is capable of sexual function indefinitely if he is generally healthy and is within a sexually stimulating environment.

The questions posed to the adult male regarding his sexual and reproductive functions are generally appropriate for the elderly client (p. 384).

The questions about early childhood and adolescent experiences may not have as much bearing on present sexual concerns as they would with a younger client. An older man may be preoccupied with his present needs for intimacy and sexual activity. Some of the variables that could alter sexual function follow:
  1. Feelings of being too old or too frail to engage in sexual activity; election to withdraw from all sexual encounters or stimulation
  2. Loss of spouse, isolation, unavailability of a sexual partner, or a sexually restrictive environment
  3. Depression related to sexual or other concerns
  4. Physical illness resulting in fatigue, anxiety about health status, or pain (from arthritis, respiratory or cardiac problems, etc.)
  5. Effects of certain diseases (neurogenic or vascular impairment, diabetes mellitus)
  6. Side effects of drugs (e.g., some antihypertensive drugs, sedatives, tranquilizers, alcohol)
  7. Surgery for prostatism (may or may not affect erection status); retrograde ejaculation is a possible concern

8. Inadequate nutrition
9. Diminished strength of muscles associated with the act of intercourse

Several authors have stated that the majority of men requesting help for impotence offer no organic basis for the problem. It is imperative that the examiner be well informed about sexual needs and behaviors of the geriatric client and prepared to follow through with a thorough assessment in this area.

- Genitourinary symptoms. The symptoms of urinary frequency, nocturia, urgency, hesitancy, abnormal flow of urinary stream, urethral discharge, and scrotal masses are described on p. 386. Additional concerns or questions follow:
  1. Nocturnal frequency is a common concern. Ask the client what amount and type of fluids he drinks in the evening. Also, ask if he is taking diuretics.
  2. Incontinence. Was the onset sudden or slow? Does the client feel (or sense) any warning that he has to urinate?
- Prostatism. Early symptoms include the following:
  1. Hesitancy in initiating stream
  2. Diminished force of stream
  3. Urinary frequency
  4. Nocturia

These symptoms may be subtle, ignored, or tolerated by the client. The later symptoms of hematuria or urinary tract infection alarm the client. (*Note:* The size of the prostate gland [as estimated when palpated] may not be indicative of the degree of obstruction of the urethra. The number and intensity of symptoms offered by the client may not correlate with the estimated palpatory enlargement of the gland.)
- Cancer of the prostate gland. This condition is often asymptomatic.
- Pain associated with genitourinary illness. This symptom may be ill defined or vague, located in the groin, low back, perineum, abdomen, or flank.

CLINICAL VARIATIONS: THE OLDER ADULT

The assessment procedure and physical findings for the geriatric male are the same as for the younger client. The following alterations may be noted:

- The genital examination should be preceded by an abdominal assessment to palpate and percuss the bladder for fullness (after the client has been asked to urinate), discomfort, or dullness.
- The scrotal sac may appear elongated or pendulous. Elderly clients sometimes have the problem of sitting on the scrotum, resulting in trauma or excoriation of the surface.
- The testes may feel slightly softer than in a younger man and may be slightly smaller.
- The prostate gland may feel larger than in a younger client.

Study Questions

General

Match the lettered structures (in the illustration below) with the corresponding numbered label:

1. _____ Scrotum
2. _____ Shaft of penis
3. _____ Epididymis
4. _____ Anus
5. _____ Vas deferens
6. _____ Urethra
7. _____ Bladder
8. _____ Urethral meatus
9. _____ Prepuce
10. _____ Pubis
11. _____ Glans
12. _____ Corona
13. _____ Testis
14. _____ Rectum
15. _____ Prostate gland

16. Scrotal skin is:
    ☐ a. Pale
    ☐ b. Deeply pigmented
17. Scrotal skin is:
    ☐ a. Thick
    ☐ b. Thin
18. Normal testes are _____ sensitive to mild compression:
    ☐ a. Markedly
    ☐ b. Never
    ☐ c. Slightly
19. The epididymides are usually located _____ to the testes:
    ☐ a. Posterolateral
    ☐ b. Anteromedial

20. The vas deferens is usually:
    ☐ a. Taut or fixed to surrounding tissue
    ☐ b. Movable

The Newborn

21. Full-term testes are normally:
    ☐ a. Flat
    ☐ b. Edematous
    ☐ c. Pendulous
    ☐ d. Undescended
22. Newborns should pass urine and meconium within the first:
    ☐ a. 6 hours of life
    ☐ b. 12 hours of life
    ☐ c. 18 hours of life
    ☐ d. 24 hours of life

The Child

23. The *average* age for the beginning development of pubic hair in males is:
    ☐ a. 9 years
    ☐ b. 10 years
    ☐ c. 11 years
    ☐ d. 12 years
    ☐ e. 13 years
24. When examining the uncircumcised male, the examiner should attempt to retract the foreskin after which of the following ages:
    ☐ a. 6 weeks
    ☐ b. 2 months
    ☐ c. 4 months
    ☐ d. 6 months
    ☐ e. Never
25. Which of the following techniques should be used to attempt to force the testes back into the scrotum of a boy who is being evaluated for undescended testes:
    ☐ a. Child should stand; examiner attempts to milk testes into scrotum.
    ☐ b. Child is sitting on examination table, feet against buttocks, pulling knees tight to chest.
    ☐ c. Child sits cross-legged to relax cremasteric reflex.
    ☐ d. Child stands and examiner pushes on child's abdomen.
    ☐ e. Place child in tub of warm water.
    ☐ f. All of the above
    ☐ g. a, c, and d
    ☐ h. All except c
    ☐ i. All except d
    ☐ j. b, d, and e

The Older Adult

26. Physiological sexual function changes that normally occur with the aging male include:
    ☐ a. An extended erection period
    ☐ b. Slow detumescence
    ☐ c. Longer refractory phase
    ☐ d. Decrease in volume of seminal fluid at time of ejaculation
    ☐ e. Loss of ability to maintain erection
    ☐ f. a and b
    ☐ g. a and d
    ☐ h. c and e
    ☐ i. a, c, and d
    ☐ j. All except e

SUGGESTED READINGS
General

Bates B: *A guide to physical examination,* ed 4, Philadelphia, 1987, JB Lippincott.

Bennett JA: What we know about AIDS, *Am J Nurs* 86(9):1016, 1986.

Holmes KK, Karon JM, Kreiss J: The increasing frequency of heterosexually acquired AIDS in the United States: 1983-88, *Am J Public Health* 80(7):858, 1990.

Malasanos L, Barkauskas V, Stoltenberg-Allen K: *Health assessment,* ed 4, St Louis, 1990, Mosby—Year Book.

McCance KL, Huether SE: *Pathophysiology: the biological basis for disease in adults and children,* St Louis, 1990, Mosby—Year Book.

Prior JA, Silberstein JS, Stang JM: *Physical diagnosis: the history and examination of the patient,* ed 6, St Louis, 1981, Mosby—Year Book.

Seidel HM, Ball JW, Dains JE, Benedict GW: *Mosby's guide to physical examination,* ed 2, St Louis, 1991, Mosby—Year Book.

Thompson JM, McFarland GK, Hirsch JE, and others: *Mosby's manual of clinical nursing,* ed 2, St Louis, 1989, Mosby—Year Book.

Williams HA: Screening for testicular cancer, *Pediatr Nurs,* p 38, Sept-Oct, 1981.

The newborn

Auvenshine MA, Enriquez MG: *Maternity nursing: dimensions of change,* Belmont, Calif, 1985, Wadsworth.

Bobak IM, Jensen MD: *Essentials of maternity nursing,* ed 3, St Louis, 1990, Mosby—Year Book.

Judd JM: Assessing the newborn from head to toe, *Nurs '85* 15(12):34, 1985.

Kiernan BS, Scoloveno MA: Assessment of the neonate, *Top Clin Nurs* 8(1):1, 1986.

The Organization for Obstetrical, Gynecological and Neonatal Nurses (NAACOG): *Physical assessment of the neonate,* OGN nursing practice resource, Oct 1986, The Association.

Pillitteri A: *Maternal-newborn nursing: care of the growing family,* ed 3, Boston, 1985, Little, Brown.

Scanlon JW, and others: *A system of newborn physical examination,* Baltimore, 1979, University Park Press.

Seidel HM, Ball JW, Dains JE, Benedict GW: *Mosby's guide to physical examination,* ed 2, St Louis, 1991, Mosby—Year Book.

Whaley LF, Wong DL: *Nursing care of infants and children,* ed 4, St Louis, 1991, Mosby—Year Book.

The child

Alexander M, Brown MS: *Pediatric history taking and physical diagnosis for nurses,* ed 2, New York, 1979, McGraw-Hill.

Barness L: *Manual of pediatric physical diagnosis,* ed 6, Chicago, 1990, Mosby—Year Book.

Marshall WA, Tanner JM: Variations in the patterns of pubertal changes in boys, *Arch Dis Child* 45:13, 1970.

Seidel HM, Ball JW, Dains JE, Benedict GW: *Mosby's guide to physical examination,* ed 2, St Louis, 1991, Mosby—Year Book.

Whaley LF, Wong DL: *Nursing care of infants and children,* ed 4, St Louis, 1991, Mosby—Year Book.

The older adult

Carotenuto R, Bullock J: *Physical assessment of the gerontologic client,* Philadelphia, 1980, FA Davis.

Ebersole P, Hess P: *Toward healthy aging,* ed 3, St Louis, 1990, Mosby—Year Book.

Eliopoulos C: *Gerontological nursing,* ed 2, Philadelphia, 1987, JB Lippincott.

Steinberg FU, editor: *Care of the geriatric patient,* ed 6, St Louis, 1983, Mosby—Year Book.

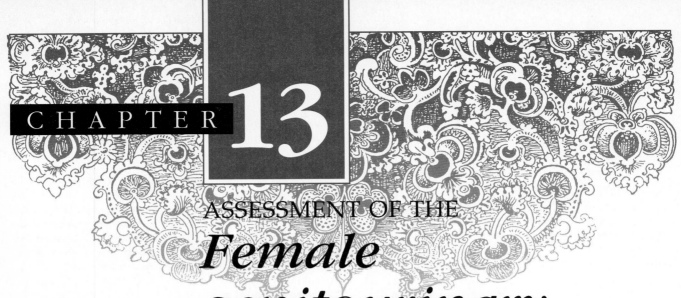

13

ASSESSMENT OF THE

Female genitourinary system

VOCABULARY

adnexa General term meaning adjacent or related structures.

> EXAMPLE: The ovaries and fallopian tubes are adnexa of the uterus.

amenorrhea The absence of menstruation.

Bartholin glands Two mucus-secreting glands located within the posterolateral vaginal vestibule.

condyloma acuminatum (wart) Soft, warty, papillomatous projection that appears on the labia and within the vaginal vestibule; viral in origin and sexually transmitted.

condyloma latum Slightly raised, moist, flattened papules that appear on the labia or within the vaginal vestibule; a sign of secondary syphilis; sexually transmitted.

cystocele Bulging of the anterior vaginal wall caused by protrusion of the urinary bladder through relaxed or weakened musculature.

dysmenorrhea Abnormal pain associated with the menstrual cycle. Mild, self-limiting premenstrual pain is considered normal. Pain becomes abnormal when it is severe, disabling, or accompanied by other severe symptoms, such as nausea, vomiting, fainting, or intestinal cramping.

dyspareunia Pain associated with sexual intercourse. The term is most often applied to female conditions, including vaginal spasms, lack of lubrication, or genital lesions.

escutcheon General term meaning a surface that is shield shaped. In female anatomy it denotes the visible surface of the lower abdomen, the mons pubis, and the inverted-triangle—shaped patch of hair covering the area.

fornix (plural: fornices) General term designating a fold or an archlike structure. The vaginal fornix is the ringed recess (pocket) that forms around the cervix as it projects into the vaginal vault; although continuous, this fornix is anatomically divided into the anterior, posterior, and lateral fornices.

fourchette Small fold of membrane connecting the labia minora in the posterior part of the vulva.

gravida Denotes number of pregnancies.

> EXAMPLE: *Multigravida* designates more than one pregnancy.

hymenal caruncles Small, irregular, fleshy projections that are remnants of a ruptured hymen; they are a normal phenomenon and may or may not be present at the vaginal introitus in varied sizes and shapes.

introitus General term denoting an opening or the orifice of a cavity or hollow structure.

> EXAMPLE: Vaginal introitus.

leukorrhea White, vaginal discharge; can be a normal phenomenon that occurs (or increases) with pregnancy, the use of birth control medication, or as a post-menstrual phase; can also be an abnormal sign indicating malignancy or infection.

menarche Onset of menstruation in adolescence or young adulthood.

menorrhagia Abnormally heavy or extended menstrual periods.

metrorrhagia Any uterine bleeding that is not related to menstruation.

> EXAMPLE: A bleeding lesion within the vagina, cervix, or uterus.

nabothian cyst (retention cyst) Small, white or purple, firm nodule that commonly appears on the cervix; forms within the mucus-secreting nabothian glands, which are present in large numbers on the uterine cervix.

oligomenorrhea Abnormally light or infrequent menstruation.

parity Denotes the number of viable births.

> EXAMPLES: *Nulliparous* means having experienced no viable births (also indicated as *para 0*; *multiparous* designates more than one viable birth.

pudendum Collective term denoting the external genitalia; for the female it includes the mons pubis, labia majora, labia minora, vaginal vestibule, and vestibular glands.

rectocele Bulging of the posterior vaginal wall caused by protrusion of the intestinal contents through relaxed or weakened musculature.

Skene glands (periurethral) Mucus-secreting glands that lie just inside the urethral orifice; not visible during examination.

vaginitis Inflammation of the vaginal vault; has various causes.

> **atrophic** Associated with aging and diminished vaginal lubrication; itching, redness, a thin, yellow discharge, and superficial erosions may be present; leukoplakia or petechiae may appear.

> **monilial** Related to a common yeastlike organism *(Candida albicans)*, normally present in mucous membranes, that may cause a superficial infection; presenting symptoms are itching, redness, swelling, a white, cheesy discharge, and white patches that bleed when scraped off.

> **trichomoniasis** Caused by a protozoan parasite that is sexually transmitted; itching, burning, and a malodorous, frothy, yellow-green discharge are commonly seen.

> **nonspecific** Presenting symptoms are redness and a thin, gray discharge.

NOTE: Diagnosis of vaginitis is confirmed with smears and cultures of vaginal secretions; its signs and symptoms may not be as concise or predictable as presented here.

ANATOMY AND PHYSIOLOGY REVIEW
External Genitalia

The external female genitalia, collectively called the *pudendum* or *vulva*, include the mons pubis, clitoris, labia majora, labia minora, vaginal vestibule, and the vestibular glands (Fig. 13-1). The mons pubis (or mons veneris) is a fatty cushion that covers the symphysis pubis. After puberty this surface is covered with coarse hair that extends down over the outer labia to the perineum. The labia majora are adipose folds that extend downward from the mons pubis, surround the vestibule, and meet at the perineum. The inner surfaces are hairless, smooth, and moist. The labia minora are darker, hairless inner folds that form the prepuce (overlying fold of skin) and the frenulum of the clitoris. They extend downward, encircle the vaginal vestibule, and join at the fourchette. They are usually flattened and folded together to cover the vestibule. The clitoris is a cylindrical, fibromuscular body that corresponds to the male penis. It is partially covered with a prepuce, sensitive to touch, and responds to stimulation with blood engorgement and erection. It is approximately 2 cm in length and 0.5 cm in diameter.

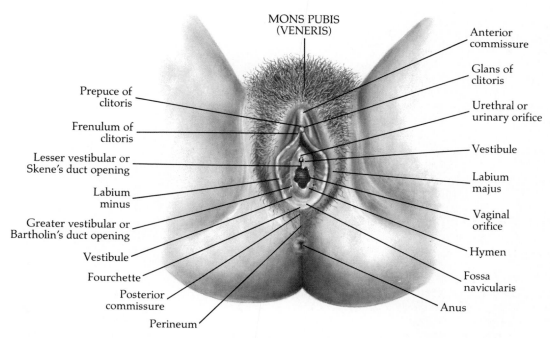

Fig. 13-1 External female genitalia. (From Bobak IM, Jensen MD: *Essentials of maternity nursing*, ed 3, St Louis, 1991, Mosby—Year Book.)

The vestibule, a surface enclosed by the labia minora, contains the urethral (urinary) orifice, the vaginal orifice (introitus), and hymenal tissue. The urethral opening is usually about 2 cm below the clitoris and appears as an irregularly shaped slit.

The hymen is a fold of mucous membrane that lies over the vaginal opening. In virgins it usually manifests a small opening or is, in rare instances, imperforate. The insertion of a tampon or the act of coitus enlarges the opening or tears the hymenal tissue, leaving small, irregular, fleshy projections around the introitus.

The vestibular glands include Skene glands, with ducts that lie on each side of the urethral meatus; and Bartholin glands, with ducts located on either side of the vaginal orifice. The ducts are usually not visible. Bartholin glands secrete a mucoid material during sexual excitement, and Skene glands lubricate the urinary meatus.

The perineal surface is the triangular-shaped area between the vaginal opening and the anus.

Internal Genitalia

The internal genitalia include the vagina, uterus, fallopian tubes, and ovaries (Fig. 13-2). The vagina is a distensible, rugated tube that extends posteriorly from the vestibule to the uterus. Its posterior length is approximately 9 to 10 cm, and its anterior length is 6 to 8 cm. It is lined with a moist mucous membrane. The uterine cervix juts into the anterior vaginal cavity so that a circular pocket (fornix) forms around the cervix (Fig. 13-3).

The uterus is a thick, muscular organ suspended and stabilized in the pelvic cavity by four sets of ligaments. It is usually loosely suspended in an anteverted position, but the positions of the organ may normally vary in individuals, from anteverted to midposition, anteflexed, retroflexed, or retroverted (see Figs. 13-16 through 13-20, pp. 419 and 420). The uterus is approximately 5.5 to 8 cm long and 3.5 to 4 cm wide. The body of the uterus is composed of three sections: the fundus, the bulbous top portion; the main body, the corpus, which extends to the lower section; and the isthmus, the narrow neck adjacent to the cervical os. The fundus, which is usually palpable at the level of the pubis, maintains its anterior position by the attached round ligaments, which are occasionally palpable on either side of the uterus (Fig. 13-4). The fundus is thick, rounded, and smooth. The inner lining of the uterus (endometrium) proliferates and sloughs in response to sex hormones on a monthly cycle to produce menstruation. The endometrial layer extends to the cervical os, which is lined with columnar epithelial cells. This layer may be visible to the examiner and appears as a symmetrical, circumscribed, reddened area surrounding the os. The colum-

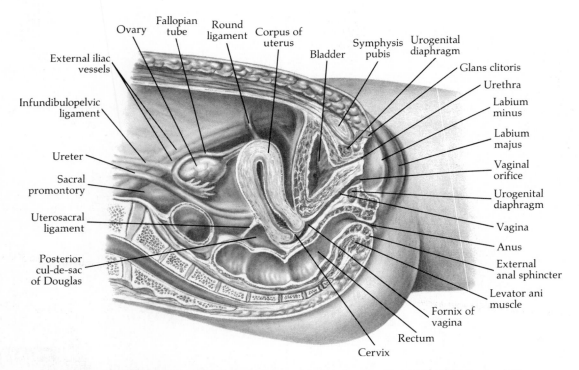

Fig. 13-2 Midsagittal view of internal genitalia—supine position. (From Bobak IM, Jensen MD: *Essentials of maternity nursing*, ed 3, St Louis, 1991, Mosby—Year Book.)

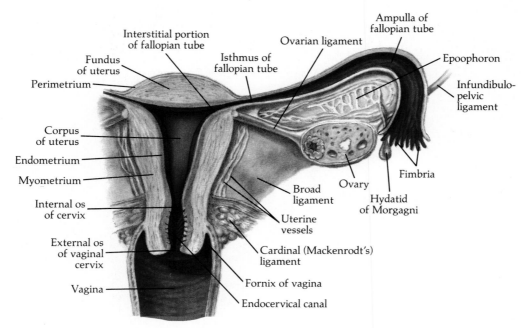

Fig. 13-3 Cross section of internal genitalia. (From Bobak IM, Jensen MD: *Essentials of maternity nursing*, ed 3, St Louis, 1991, Mosby–Year Book.)

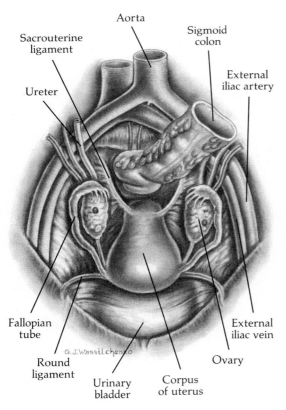

Fig. 13-4 Female pelvic contents viewed from above. (From Thompson JM, McFarland GK, Hirsch JE, and others: *Mosby's manual of clinical nursing*, ed 2, St Louis, 1989, Mosby–Year Book.)

nar mucosa joins the squamous epithelium, which lines the vagina at the endocervical canal (see Fig. 13-3). This is called the *squamocolumnar junction* and is a common site for cervical cancer. The cervix projects into the vaginal tube about 1 to 3 cm and creates a 1 to 3 cm fornix that surrounds the os.

The fallopian tubes are 10 cm long and extend from the uterine body to a space under the ovaries. The ends of the fallopian tubes are fringed (fimbriated) to draw ova into the tube for fertilization. The fallopian tubes are not palpable.

The ovaries are connected to the uterine body by the ovarian ligaments. The ovaries are approximately 4 cm in length and are often palpable in the lower, lateral abdominal quadrants.

The Urinary Tract

The urinary tract includes the kidneys, ureters, the urinary bladder, and the urethra. The kidneys interact with the cardiac, endocrine, and nervous systems to conserve body nutrients, remove waste materials, and regulate body substances, fluids, and blood pressure. This is accomplished in the kidneys through an elaborate microscopic filter and pressure system that eventually produces urine. The kidneys are paired organs located outside of the peritoneal cavity at spinal levels T12 through L3 (Fig. 13-5). The right kidney is slightly lower than the left because of displacement by the overlying liver. Each kidney is approximately 11 × 6 × 3 cm, is cushioned in a protective fatty mass, and is attached to

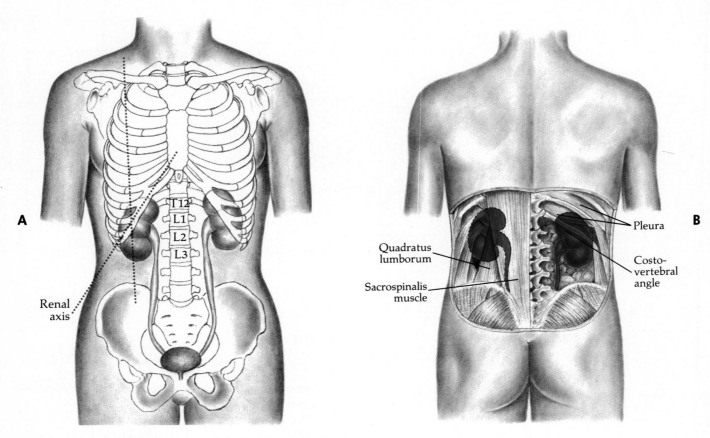

Fig. 13-5 Location of kidneys, ureters, and bladder. **A,** Anterior view. **B,** Posterior view. (From Thompson JM, McFarland GK, Hirsch JE, and others: *Mosby's manual of clinical nursing*, ed 2, St Louis, 1989, Mosby—Year Book.)

Fig. 13-6 Cross section of the kidney. (From Thompson JM, McFarland GK, Hirsch JE, and others: *Mosby's manual of clinical nursing*, ed 2, St Louis, 1989, Mosby—Year Book.)

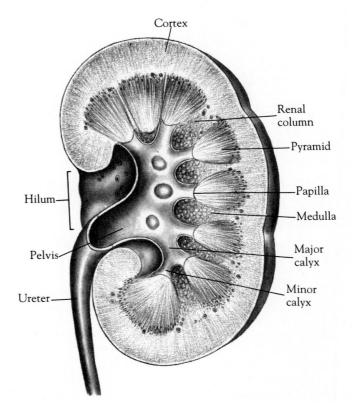

the posterior abdominal wall with fascia.

The interior of the kidney is composed of the hilum, the outer cortex, the inner medulla, and the pelvis (Fig. 13-6). A renal artery branches from the aorta and enters the kidney through the hilum. The artery eventually branches into specialized arterioles that enter thousands of microscopic units called *nephrons*, where fluid is filtered from the blood and nutrients are reabsorbed back into the blood. Glomeruli, the central filtering units of each nephron, are located in the cortex. Glomeruli empty into tubules, where urine is concentrated and diluted, and nutrients are reabsorbed. The tubules empty into collecting ducts that form the renal pyramids in the medulla. The collecting ducts empty into a calyx, which leads to the flow of urine into the ureter. Renal veins exit the kidney at the hilum. The amount of urine produced is approximately 1 ml per minute, but this varies greatly moment by moment with the needs and the activities of the individual.

The ureters continue out of the pelvis and extend for approximately 24 to 30 cm to insertion points at the base of the bladder. The ureters expedite the flow of urine by means of peristaltic waves that originate in the renal pelvis and are stimulated by renal output.

The bladder is located anterior to the rectum and in front of the uterus. The size of the bladder varies according to the amount of urine it contains. When it is full, the bladder can be felt as a central "mass" that obscures palpation of the uterine fundus. The bladder contains an internal sphincter, which relaxes in response to a full bladder (about 300 ml of urine) and alerts the individual with an urge to void. The urethra extends out of the base of the bladder to the external meatus and is approximately 3 to 4 cm long.

COGNITIVE OBJECTIVES

At the end of this chapter the learner will perform a systematic assessment of the female genitourinary system and rectal/anal region, demonstrating the ability to do the following:

- Apply the terms that are listed in the vocabulary section.
- Identify and locate the major internal and external structures of the female genitourinary system.
- Point out observable and palpable characteristics of normal external genitalia and perineum.
- Identify observable and palpable characteristics of the following normal internal structures:
  1. Vagina
  2. Cervix
  3. Fornices
- Describe the major characteristics of normal vaginal discharge.
- Identify the appropriate and effective procedures for using a vaginal speculum.
- Name specific examiner behaviors that will minimize

client discomfort and enhance effectiveness of the pelvic examination.
- Identify common normal palpable findings elicited during a bimanual examination.
- Describe common normal deviations of findings related to pelvic examination associated with the following:
  1. Nulliparous clients
  2. Multiparous clients
  3. Early pregnant clients
- Identify major palpable characteristics of the anteverted, retroverted, anteflexed, and retroflexed uterus.
- Give the reasons for performing a rectovaginal examination.
- Identify the major structures and functions of the urinary tract.
- Identify common newborn, child, childbearing, and older adult variations of the female genitourinary system.

CLINICAL OUTLINE

At the end of this chapter the learner will perform a systematic assessment of the female genitourinary system and rectal/anal region, demonstrating the ability to do the following:
- Obtain a pertinent history from a client.
- Inspect the pubic region and external genitalia for the following:
  1. Hair distribution
  2. Parasites
  3. Inguinal skin surface characteristics
  4. Labia majora surface
  5. Labia minora surface
     a. Vestibule surface
     b. Clitoris size and surface
     c. Urethral meatus contour and surface
  6. Vaginal introitus contour and surface
  7. Perineal surface
  8. Anal surface
- Palpate external genitalia for the following:
  1. Labia and vestibule consistency and tenderness
  2. Urethral duct tenderness and discharge
  3. Bartholin gland tenderness, discharge, and swelling
  4. Perineum consistency and tenderness
- Palpate vaginal introitus and test for bulging (or straining) and urinary incontinence.
- Perform a vaginal examination and inspect for the following:
  1. Cervix
     a. Color
     b. Position
     c. Size
     d. Surface characteristics
     e. Os configuration
     f. Discharge color, odor, and texture

2. Vagina
   a. Color
   b. Surface characteristics
   c. Consistency
   d. Secretions: color, odor, and texture
- Obtain specimens for cervical cytological evaluation.
- Perform a bimanual vaginal examination to identify the following:
  1. Vaginal wall surface characteristics and tenderness
  2. Cervix
     a. Size
     b. Contour
     c. Consistency
     d. Surface texture
     e. Mobility
     f. Location in vaginal tube
     g. Os patency
  3. Uterus
     a. Fundus location, contour, surface consistency, shape, size, mobility, and tenderness
     b. Isthmus consistency
  4. Adnexa
     a. Ovary location and surface characteristics
     b. Masses
     c. Pulsations
- Perform a rectovaginal examination to identify the following:
  1. Rectovaginal septum and pouch characteristics
  2. Tenderness in pouch
  3. Rectal wall surface characteristics
  4. Anal sphincter surface and tone
  5. Tenderness
- Summarize results of the assessment with a written description of findings.

HISTORY

- Reproductive functions and sexuality. The examiner should screen all patients for sexual needs or problems by initially posing a broad, nondirective question. The question might be worded in this way: "Do you have any concerns regarding sexual practices or values that you would like to discuss?" This lets the client know that she can share her problems if she wishes to, and it does not direct her toward any specific area of concern. Please note that anyone posing this question should be prepared to follow through with intervention skills in this area.

  A more specific detailed assessment will help to clarify general concerns and can supplement the original data base.
  1. Present practices and values
     a. Are you comfortable with your intimate relationships (with or without sexual activity)? Do you have difficulty meeting your needs for intimacy (or affection)?
     b. Are you having a sexual relationship with anyone at present?
     c. Do you feel satisfied with this relationship? (For example, do you and your partner share similar feelings about the methods and variety of sexual acts you perform; about the frequency of sex; about the kind and amount of affection displayed; about initiating sex? Do you talk about sexual feelings with your partner? Is there anything you would change about this relationship?)
     d. If you do not have a sexual partner, are your sexual needs being met?
     e. Do you have more than one sexual partner? If so, is this a satisfactory arrangement?
     f. How many partners have you had in the past year?
     g. How do you feel about homosexuality (i.e., is it a personal issue with you)?
     h. How do you feel about masturbation?
     i. Have there been any recent changes in your sexual desire (arousal patterns), specific sexual acts or behaviors, frequency of sexual experiences, choice of sexual partners?
     j Do you and/or your partner(s) use contraception? What method do you use? Do you have questions or difficulty with this?
     k. Do you have any questions about male sexuality, sexual function, female sexuality, sterility, venereal disease, other?
  2. History
     a. Describe your personal experience with sex education. Was sexuality discussed with family members? Was it discussed openly? Were there others outside the family who informed or influenced you sexually? Explain.
     b. Were your parents affectionate with each other?
     c. What were your early experiences with masturbation; sex play with other children; adolescent relationships; dating (feeling comfortable with boys); petting?
     d. How old were you when you first had sexual intercourse? How did you feel about it?
     e. Have you ever had a homosexual experience? Describe.
     f. How many sexual partners have you had?
- Abnormal bleeding.
  1. If associated with menses, it might fall into one of the following categories:
     a. Too many periods (menstrual interval is less than 19 to 21 days)
     b. Infrequent menses (menstrual interval is over 37 days)
     c. Amenorrhea
     d. Extended menses (duration is over 7 days)

e. Intermenstrual bleeding

f. Flow pattern increased during menses

2. Amount of flow (normal or abnormal) is difficult to determine. Inquire about the nature of the *change* in the amount of flow. Ask about the number of pads or tampons used during the heavy flow in a 24-hour period. Find out if the pad or tampon is soaked when it is changed. Do clots accompany the bleeding?

3. Is there bleeding associated with intercourse? With douching?

• Premenstrual tension. Should be defined by the client. Is it associated with headaches? Weight change? Edema? Breast tenderness? Marked (or difficult) mood swings? Does it occur before every period or just occasionally? Are premenstrual problems incapacitating (e.g., do they interfere with activities of daily living)?

• Vaginal discharge. Discharge is normal with many women and often occurs in cycles, with an increase at midcycle or just before menses. If vaginal discharge is a complaint, establish the *change* that has occurred in terms of estimated amount, color, odor, consistency, and times or intervals of increased discharge.

1. Are you taking any medications for other problems (especially broad-spectrum antibiotics, metronidazole, or steroids)? Do you take birth control pills?

2. Do you douche? If so, how often, what solution, and what amount? Were you douching before or after the discharge?

3. Is the discharge associated with itching? (If itching is present, is there a family or client history of diabetes mellitus?)

4. Do you wear cotton or ventilated underwear or pantyhose?

5. Was the onset of the discharge sudden or gradual?

6. Does your sexual partner have any problem with discharge, itching, rash or lesions, pain?

• Birth control. If any measure is used, establish the type, the length of time it has been used, and the client's assessment of its effectiveness, convenience, noninterference with sexual activity, and noninterference with the client's general physical and mental health. More specific questions include the following:

1. Birth control pills. Do you take them regularly? Do you have any symptoms or physical problems associated with taking the pill?

2. Diaphragm. Are you able to use it each time you have intercourse? Do you use cream (or jelly) every time you use the diaphragm? Do you have any problems inserting, removing, or retaining it? Do you examine your diaphragm periodically for thinning or weak spots, cracks, holes, or tears? How long before intercourse do you insert it? How long do you leave it in place after intercourse? How long ago were you fitted with your diaphragm?

3. IUD. Do you insert your finger into your vagina to feel for the string periodically? How often? Do you have any problem with bleeding or spotting between periods? Do you have any problem with menstrual cramps?

• AIDS (acquired immune deficiency syndrome).

1. Screening for high-risk candidates. AIDS has become an urgent universal health concern. At present the client's right to privacy (i.e., personal sexual life-style and health status) and anonymity (i.e., AIDS screening results) differs according to legal definitions in various states. Local policy (or law) may dictate (or confine) screening practices in local health agencies. Because AIDS can be dormant (or asymptomatic), screening clients for high-risk status would involve identifying one (or more) risk factors. (*Note:* A laboratory test for antibodies is the only way to confirm a positive exposure to the disease. Some authorities estimate that only 20% to 30% of those individuals exposed to the disease will manifest a positive antibody reaction.)

RISK FACTORS FOR AIDS

• Sexual involvement with male who has engaged in homosexual activity (a higher risk exists with a history of multiple partners or having a partner with a history of multiple partners)

• Drug addicts who share contaminated needles

• A history of multiple heterosexual partners, especially without the use of a condom

• A history of contacts with prostitutes, especially without the use of a condom

• A history of frequent/multiple blood transfusions

---

2. At present AIDS is usually diagnosed when the disease becomes active and symptomatic. The following symptoms are commonly reported:

a. Chronic fatigue

b. Chronic intermittent fever

c. Night sweats

d. Unexplained weight loss (10% to 15% of total body weight in 1 or 2 months)

e. Oral candidiasis (white patches on the tongue or buccal membranes)

f. Purple patches/discoloration of the skin (especially on the legs and ankles) or of the mucous membrane in the mouth

g. Chronic dry cough

h. Shortness of breath

i Bruising

j. Unexplained bleeding under the skin or from any orifice

- Sexually transmitted diseases (STDs).

1. Signs and symptoms of STD vary widely, and an individual can present with a combination of diseases or infections. Following is a categorization of signs and symptoms to be alert for:

   a. Localized

   (1) External: Lesions may appear as single, large ulcers or coalesced, multiple ulcers. Vesicles, pustules, cysts, abscesses, or condylomas (warts) may appear. Lesions may appear on the vulva, around the lips or mouth, or in the perianal area. Pubic infestations may include scabies, nits, or pediculosis, accompanied by excoriation.

   (2) Internal: Urethritis or infection/inflammation/lesions; accompanied by burning on urination and/or discharge that may be watery, mucopurulent, serosanguineous, or malodorous.

   b. Systemic

   Lymphatic dissemination may result in painful inguinal node inflammation, fistulas, or a generalized adenitis. A generalized infection can produce fever, headache, malaise, joint pain, abdominal pain, focal neurological signs, or seizures. Endocarditis, meningitis, septicemia, and arthritis are some of the major manifestations of infection.

- Menopause. If it has been established that the client is approaching, in the midst of, or completing the menopausal phase, a general question about any concerns should be posed. More specific questions include the following:

1. Do you recall your mother experiencing menopause? How old was she? Did she describe her experience to you?

2. Do you have any concerns or problems with menstrual irregularity, mood changes, tension, back pain, hot flashes, painful intercourse, changes in sexual desire or sexual behaviors, other physical changes?

3. What kind of birth control measures are you using? Describe.

4. What general feelings do you have about menopause?

- Pelvic discomfort associated with the menstrual cycle. This is normal with some women. If the client complains of pain, establish the *change* that has occurred in terms of timing (with menstrual cycle) and location (e.g., vulvar or vaginal, localized in lower abdomen, or general pain). Is the pain associated with intercourse? If so, does it occur at the time of insertion, deep penetration throughout intercourse, and/or is there a residual pain after intercourse?

Text continues on p. 422.

RISK FACTORS FOR MAJOR SEXUALLY TRANSMITTED DISEASES (STDs)

- Young, sexually active male or female (age range 15 to 30 years)
- Multiple sexual partners
- Urban dweller
- Low income
- Unmarried
- Early onset of sexual activity
- History of previous STD

CLINICAL GUIDELINES

ASSESSMENT PROCEDURE	EVALUATION	
	NORMAL FINDINGS	DEVIATIONS FROM NORMAL

1. Assemble equipment
  a. Gloves
  b. Speculum
  c. Sterile cotton swabs
  d. Glass slides
  e. Wooden spatula
  f. Lubricant
  g. Cytology fixative
  h. Examining lamp
  i. Culture plates for gonorrhea screening		

	EVALUATION	
ASSESSMENT PROCEDURE	NORMAL FINDINGS	DEVIATIONS FROM NORMAL
2. Check with client to be certain that bladder has been recently emptied 3. Position draped client in lithotomy position (Fig. 13-7) (*Note:* Examiner may assist client in positioning her buttocks at edge of examining table after checking to see that client's feet are secure in stirrups.) 4. See that equipment is within easy reach, and arrange light for good visualization of external genitalia 5. Wear gloves on both hands; warn client that examiner is going to touch her to begin procedure 6. Inspect external genitalia a. Hair distribution	Variable in adults Usually inverse triangle with base over pubis; some hair may extend up midline toward umbilicus No parasites	Male hair distribution (diamond-shaped pattern) Patchy loss of hair Absence of hair in client over 16 years Nits, pubic lice
b. Inguinal and mons pubis skin surface characteristics	Smooth, clear	Scars Inguinal swelling, excoriation, lesions, rash
c. Labia majora surface characteristics	Darker pigmentation Shriveled or full Gaping or closed Usually symmetrical Skin surface smooth May appear dry or moist	Inflammation, ulceration Lesions Nodules Marked asymmetry

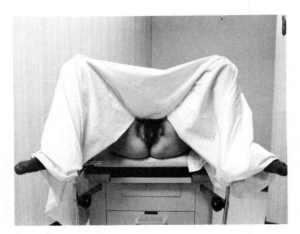

Fig. 13-7   Draped client in dorsal lithotomy position.

Continued.

CLINICAL GUIDELINES—cont'd

ASSESSMENT PROCEDURE	EVALUATION	
	NORMAL FINDINGS	DEVIATIONS FROM NORMAL
7. Spread labia to view:		
a. Inner surface of labia majora; labia minora and surface of vestibule (Fig. 13-8)	Dark pink pigmentation and moist Usually symmetrical	Inflammation Leukoplakia (white patches) Lesions Nodules Varicosities Marked asymmetry Swelling Excoriation
b. Clitoris (1) Size	2 cm (¾ inch) length visible 0.5 cm diameter	Enlargement Atrophy
(2) Surface	Medial aspect covered by prepuce	Inflamed
c. Urethral meatus and immediate surrounding tissue surface	Irregular opening or slit May be close to or slightly within vaginal introitus Usually located at midline	Discharge from surrounding glands (Skene) or urethral opening Polyp Inflammation Urethral caruncle Lateral position of meatus
d. Vaginal introitus and immediate surrounding tissue surface	Thin vertical slit or large orifice with irregular edges (hymenal caruncles) Moist tissue	Surrounding inflammation Profuse vaginal discharge Swelling Lesions
e. Perineal surface	Smooth or evidence of episiotomy Scar (midline or mediolateral) may be visible	Inflammation, fistula Lesions, mass
f. Anal surface	Increased pigmentation and coarse skin	Scars, skin tags Lesions, inflammation Fissures, lumps Excoriation

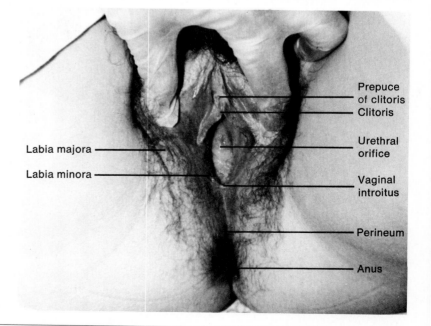

Fig. 13-8 Labia spread with thumb and fingers to view external genitalia.

| | EVALUATION | |
ASSESSMENT PROCEDURE	NORMAL FINDINGS	DEVIATIONS FROM NORMAL
8. Palpate external genitalia		
a. Labia and vestibule (Fig. 13-9)		
(1) Consistency	Soft, homogeneous	Irregular, nodular
(2) Tenderness	Nontender	Tender
b. Insert index finger in vagina, and milk urethral ducts (Fig. 13-10) to test for:		
(1) Tenderness	Nontender	Tender
(2) Discharge	No discharge	Discharge*

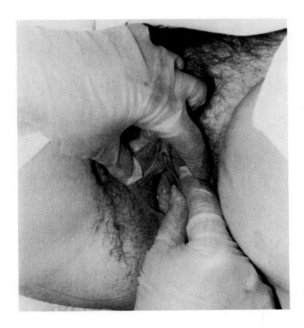

Fig. 13-9   Palpation of labia.

Fig. 13-10   Milking urethral duct.

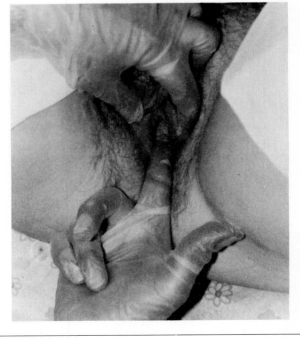

---

*Prepare a culture of any discharge.

Continued.

CLINICAL GUIDELINES—cont'd

ASSESSMENT PROCEDURE	EVALUATION	
	NORMAL FINDINGS	DEVIATIONS FROM NORMAL
c. Palpate lateral and posterior areas surrounding introitus (Fig. 13-11) to test for:		
(1) Tenderness	Nontender	Tender
(2) Discharge	No discharge	Discharge*
(3) Surface characteristics	Homogeneous	Swelling
d. Palpate perineum between index finger and thumb (Fig. 13-12) for:		
(1) Consistency	Nulliparous: thick, smooth Multiparous: thin, rigid Scarring	Paper thin
(2) Tenderness	Nontender	Tender
9. Ask client to squeeze vaginal orifice around examiner's finger; insert middle and index fingers into vagina; ask client to strain down or bear down to elicit:	Nulliparous client squeezes tightly Multiparous client demonstrates less tone	Client unable to constrict vaginal orifice around examiner's finger
a. Bulging	No bulging	Cystocele (anterior wall bulging) Enterocele Rectocele (posterior wall bulging) Uterine prolapse (cervix visible on straining, or uterus protrudes on straining)
b. Incontinence	No urinary incontinence	Urinary incontinence

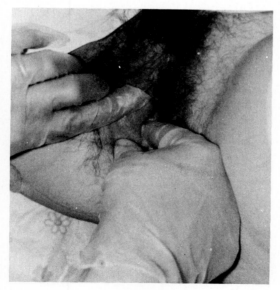

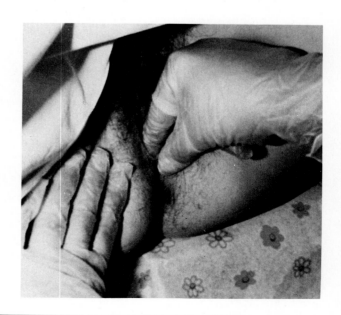

Fig. 13-11   Palpation of lateral and posterior areas surrounding vaginal introitus.

Fig. 13-12   Palpating perineum.

Prepare a culture of any discharge.

| | EVALUATION | |
ASSESSMENT PROCEDURE	NORMAL FINDINGS	DEVIATIONS FROM NORMAL
10. Select speculum of appropriate size, and warm and lubricate with water (if necessary)		
11. Place two fingers just inside vaginal introitus, and apply pressure over posterior wall (Fig. 13-13); wait for relaxation		
12. Insert closed speculum (held at oblique angle) over fingers and direct at 45° angle downward; remove fingers; lock speculum in place (Fig. 13-14, p. 416) to inspect cervix		
a. Color	Pink color evenly distributed Blue (in pregnancy) Symmetrical, circumscribed erythema surrounding os may indicate normal condition of exposed columnar epithelium; however, beginning examiners should consider any reddened appearance a problem for consultation	Inflamed Pale (associated with anemia) Cyanotic (other than pregnancy) Erythema, especially if patchy or if borders irregular or asymmetrical around os
b. Position	Midline Cervix and os may be pointed in anterior or posterior direction May project into vaginal tube 1 to 3 cm (resulting in 1 to 3 cm fornices surrounding cervix)	Cervix situated laterally Projection of over 3 cm (1 inch) into vaginal tube
c. Size	Usually 2.5 cm (1 inch) diameter	Over 4 cm (1½ inches) diameter

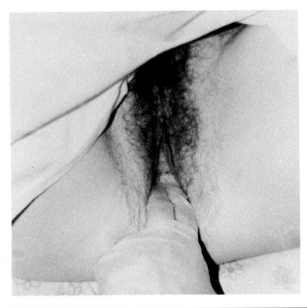

Fig. 13-13   Applying pressure with two fingers in posterior vaginal orifice.

Continued.

CLINICAL GUIDELINES—cont'd

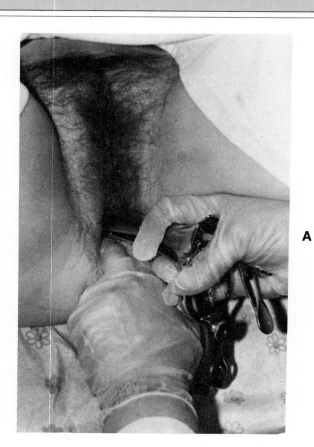

A

Fig. 13-14   A, Closed speculum is inserted over fingers. Insert speculum at oblique angle if vaginal opening is not relaxed. **B,** Fingers removed; closed speculum is inserted in downward (45° angle) direction. **C,** Speculum in place, locked, and stabilized. (Note cervix in full view.)

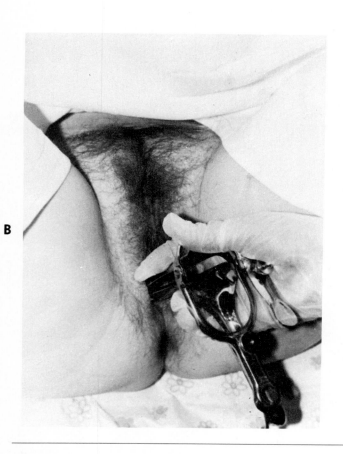

B

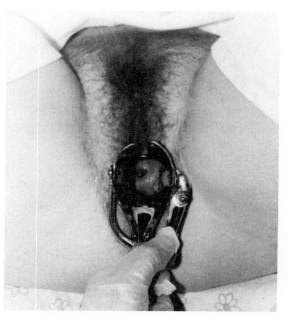

C

ASSESSMENT PROCEDURE	EVALUATION	
	NORMAL FINDINGS	DEVIATIONS FROM NORMAL
d. Surface	Smooth Occasional visible squamocolumnar junction (symmetrical reddened circle around os) Nabothian cysts (smooth, round, small, yellow raised areas)	Reddened granular area around os (especially asymmetrical) Friable tissue Red patches, lesions Strawberry spots White patches
e. Os	Nulliparous: small, evenly round Multiparous: slitlike, may be star shaped or irregular	
f. Cervical discharge	Mucous plug may be present at os Odorless Creamy or clear Thin, thick, or stringy Discharge often heavier at midcycle or immediately before menstruation	Odor Colored (yellow, green, gray)
13. Obtain specimens for: a. Papanicolaou smear b. Gonorrheal culture (See "Clinical Tips and Strategies," p. 422, if indicated.) 14. Inspect vagina: as unlocked, partially open speculum is rotated and slowly removed, it tends to close itself a. Color	Pink	Reddened Lesions Pallor (associated with anemia)
b. Surface	Transverse rugae (rugae diminish after vaginal deliveries) Moist, smooth	Leukoplakia Lesions, cracks Dried surface Bleeding
c. Consistency	Smooth, homogeneous	Nodular Swollen
d. Secretions	Thin Clear or cloudy Odorless	Thick, curdy, frothy Gray, green, yellow Foul odor
e. Amount of secretions	Minimal to moderate	Profuse
15. Perform bimanual vaginal examination a. Rise to standing position; remove glove from one hand, lubricate the other, and insert middle and index fingers into vaginal opening; compress posteriorly; wait for a moment and vaginal opening will relax; insert fingers gradually b. Palpate vaginal wall		
(1) Surface	Smooth, homogeneous	Nodules
(2) Tenderness	Nontender	Tender

Continued.

CLINICAL GUIDELINES—cont'd

ASSESSMENT PROCEDURE	EVALUATION	
	NORMAL FINDINGS	DEVIATIONS FROM NORMAL
16. Locate cervix with gloved hand; place palmar surface of other hand in abdominal midline, midway between umbilicus and pubis, and press lightly toward intravaginal hand		
17. Palpate cervix and fornices with palmar surface of both fingers (Fig. 13-15)		
a. Cervical size	2.5 to 4 cm	Enlarged
b. Contour	Evenly rounded Slightly ovoid	Irregular
c. Consistency and surface	Firm (like tip of nose), smooth	Soft, nodular Hard
d. Mobility	Cervix moves 1 to 2 cm in each direction without discomfort	Immobile (fixed), or discomfort associated with movement
e. Location	Anterior or posterior midline	Laterally displaced
18. Insert one finger gently into cervical os to evaluate:		
a. Patency	Os admits fingertip 0.5 cm	Os stenosed
b. Fornices (pockets surrounding cervical protrusion)	Pliable and smooth Nontender	Hardened, nodular, or irregular surface Tender on palpation
19. Palpate uterus: place intravaginal fingers in anterior fornix; slowly slide abdominal hand toward pubis with flattened fingers pressing downward to evaluate:		

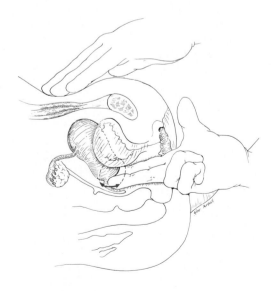

Fig. 13-15 Cervical palpation.

ASSESSMENT PROCEDURE	EVALUATION	
	NORMAL FINDINGS	DEVIATIONS FROM NORMAL
a. Location of fundus		
(1) Anteverted (Fig. 13-16)	Fundus at level of pubis palpated between abdominal and gloved hand; cervix aimed posteriorly (*Note:* Most women have an anteverted uterus. Fundus should be palpated at level of the pubis.)	
(2) Midposition (Fig. 13-17)	Fundus may not be palpable (depending on amount of abdominal adipose tissue and degree of abdominal muscle relaxation); cervix pointed along axis of vaginal canal	
(3) Anteflexed (Fig. 13-18)	Fundus palpable at pubis between abdominal and gloved hand; cervix pointed along axis of vaginal canal	

Fig. 13-16   Anteverted uterus.

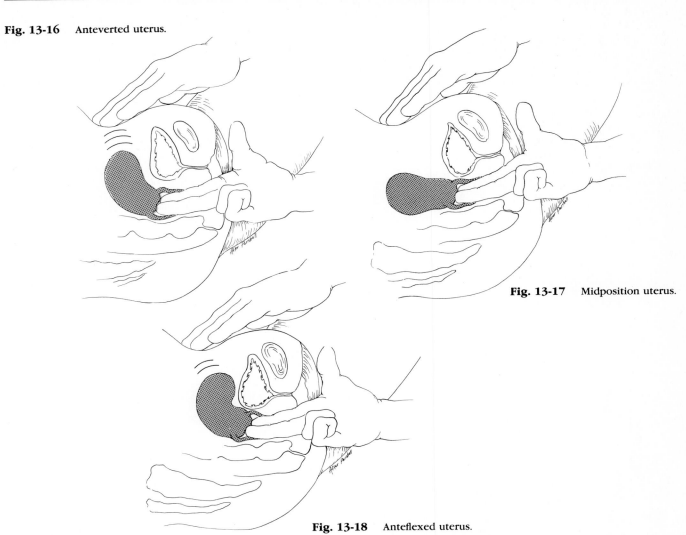

Fig. 13-17   Midposition uterus.

Fig. 13-18   Anteflexed uterus.

Continued.

CLINICAL GUIDELINES—cont'd

ASSESSMENT PROCEDURE	EVALUATION	
	NORMAL FINDINGS	DEVIATIONS FROM NORMAL
(4) Retroflexed (Fig. 13-19)	Fundus not palpable; cervix directed along axis of vaginal canal	
(5) Retroverted (Fig. 13-20)	Fundus not palpable; cervix aimed anteriorly	Enlarged; fundus above level of pubis
b. Contour of fundus	Rounded	Irregular
c. Consistency and surface of uterine wall	Firm, smooth	Soft, nodular Masses
20. After fundus is palpated, spread fingers within vagina, and press into and upward within posterior, anterior, and lateral fornices to palpate lateral uterine wall		
a. Shape and size of uterine wall	Pear shaped, 5.5 to 8 cm long Somewhat enlarged in multiparous client	Nodular Enlarged Tender on palpation
b. Consistency	Smooth	Nodular
21. Gently "bounce" uterus between intravaginal hand and abdominally placed hand for:		
a. Mobility	Freely movable	Fixed
b. Tenderness	Nontender	Tender

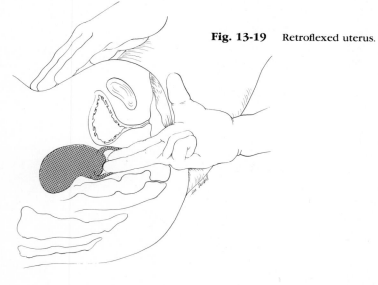

Fig. 13-19 Retroflexed uterus.

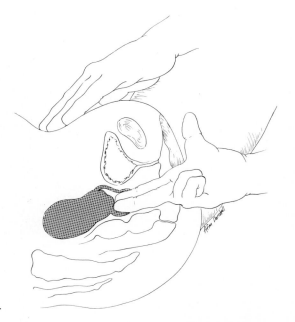

Fig. 13-20 Retroverted uterus.

	EVALUATION	
ASSESSMENT PROCEDURE	**NORMAL FINDINGS**	**DEVIATIONS FROM NORMAL**
22. Place outside hand in left lower abdominal quadrant and intravaginal hand in left fornix; slide flat portion of fingers toward intravaginal hand (Fig. 13-21) to evaluate:		
a. Left ovary	Slightly tender on palpation	Markedly tender
b. Palpable characteristics*	Not always palpable Firm, smooth, ovoid Walnut sized (approximately 4 cm) Mobile	Nodular Enlarged Immobile mass felt
c. Other organs, masses, pulsations	Usually no other structures palpable except occasional round ligaments	Masses Nodularity Pulsations Fallopian tubes usually not palpable; if palpated, may indicate problem
23. Repeat procedure for right side		
24. Withdraw fingers from vagina; examine secretions on fingers for:		
a. Odor	None	Foul odor
b. Color	Clear or creamy	Gray, yellow, frothy
c. Amount	Minimal to moderate	Profuse
25. Perform a rectovaginal examination: withdraw fingers; change glove; lubricate and reinsert index finger into vagina and middle finger into anus; place other hand on abdomen		

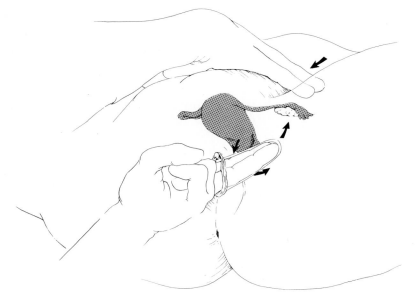

Fig. 13-21 Palpation of left adnexal area.

Remember, most palpation is done with the intravaginal *hand and the palmar surfaces of the fingers.*   *Continued.*

CLINICAL GUIDELINES—cont'd

	EVALUATION	
ASSESSMENT PROCEDURE	NORMAL FINDINGS	DEVIATIONS FROM NORMAL
26. Palpate anterior rectal wall for: a. Rectovaginal septum characteristics	Thin, smooth, pliable	Thickened, nodular
b. Rectovaginal pouch characteristics	Smooth Uterine body (occasionally the fundus) may be felt Nontender	Nodular Tenderness
27. Rotate finger in rectum to explore rectal wall for surface characteristics	Continuous smooth surface; minimal discomfort	Masses Nodules Induration Tenderness
28. Withdraw fingers slowly, noting: a. Anal sphincter tone	Sphincter evenly tight around finger	Sphincter markedly relaxed Nodules, induration, masses
b. Tenderness	Nontender	Tenderness
29. Examine gloved finger for stool	If present, brown	Black Blood present

CLINICAL TIPS AND STRATEGIES

- **Procedure for obtaining Papanicolaou smears**
  1. This procedure is performed after the cervix and surrounding tissue have been inspected and while the speculum is still in place in the vagina. The examiner should not apply lubricant to the speculum if the intent is to collect a Pap smear specimen.
  2. The bifid end of the wooden spatula is introduced into the vagina.
  3. The longer projection at the end of the spatula is inserted into the cervical os.
  4. The spatula is then rotated in a full circle, flush against the surrounding cervical tissue (light pressure is sufficient to keep the spatula in contact with the cervix).
  5. The spatula is then withdrawn, and the specimen is spread on a microscopic slide. A single light stroke with each side of the spatula enables the examiner to thin out the specimen over the slide surface. Avoid scraping the slide with back and forth motions.
  6. The slide is labeled and sprayed with a fixative solution or placed in a fixative solution container and labeled.
  7. The rounded end of the spatula is then introduced into the vagina and gently scraped over the posterior fornix area to collect a vaginal pool specimen.
  8. The spatula is withdrawn, and each side is lightly spread over another slide.
  9. This slide is labeled and sprayed or immersed in a fixative solution.

- **Procedure for obtaining a gonorrhea culture specimen**
  1. Endocervical culture
     a. The specimen for this culture can be collected immediately after the Papanicolaou smear procedure.
     b. A sterile cotton applicator is introduced into the vagina and inserted into the cervical os.
     c. The examiner holds the applicator in place for 10 to 30 seconds (there is no need to rotate the applicator).
     d. The applicator is withdrawn and spread (and rotated) in a large Z pattern over the medium of a Thayer-Martin plate, or the applicator is placed in a Thayer-Martin culture tube.
     e. The plate or tube is labeled.
     f. The examiner must be familiar with agency routines for keeping the specimen warm, cross-streaking, and immediate transport to the laboratory.

2. Anal culture
   a. The specimen for this culture is collected after the vaginal speculum has been removed.
   b. The sterile cotton-tipped applicator is inserted about 2.5 cm (1 inch) into the anal canal and rotated in a full circle. The applicator is also moved from side to side while inserted.
   c. The examiner holds the applicator in place for 10 to 30 seconds.
   d. The applicator is withdrawn and spread (and rotated) in a large Z pattern over the medium in a Thayer/Martin plate.
   e. The plate is labeled. (*Note:* If the swab contains feces, it must be discarded and another specimen taken.)
   f. The examiner must be familiar with agency routines for keeping the specimen warm, cross-streaking the medium, and transporting the specimen to the laboratory.

- **Mechanics of the pelvic examination**
   1. The examiner must decide which hand will insert and hold the speculum; then he or she must decide which will be the intravaginal hand during the bimanual examination. Once the decision is made, the examiner should maintain this routine. Often the dominant hand is more efficient with speculum insertion, as well as serving as the internal hand for the bimanual assessment.
   2. The beginning examiner should become familiar with the vaginal speculum before using it in a clinical setting. The metal speculum is very different from the disposable plastic speculum. The plastic

speculum base widens as a portion of it moves in an adjacent groove. When the base is stabilized, it goes into place with a resounding snap that often alarms both examiner and client! The metal speculum opens and stabilizes in position with the aid of twisting lever nuts and rods. It is most helpful to "play" with these instruments in advance until the examiner feels comfortable with them (Fig. 13-22).

- **Promoting client comfort**
   1. Inquire about whether the client has had a pelvic examination before, and ask if she has any concerns. Showing and explaining instruments, equipment, and the procedure will alleviate some anxiety.
   2. Assist the client in stabilizing her feet in the stirrups (she should wear her shoes). Help her to place her buttocks at the *edge* of the examining table.
   3. A client who is ill or weak may need assistance in maintaining her legs in position (an assistant may be necessary to support the client's legs).
   4. If the client is unable to assume the lithotomy position, as assessment can be accomplished while the client assumes the Sims' position.
   5. Be certain that the room is warm and privacy is ensured.
   6. When draping the client, be certain to cover her knees fully with the drape.
   7. Posing questions during the examination is difficult, particularly if you are unable to establish eye contact. However, we have found it helpful to

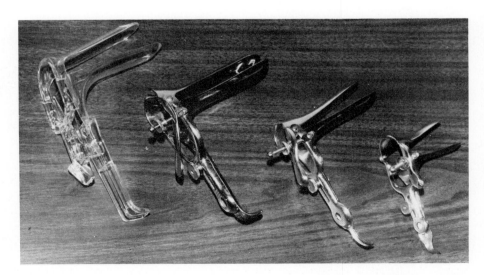

Fig. 13-22   Variety of metal specula in graduated sizes and plastic speculum *(left)*.

maintain a relaxed dialogue, describing our activities as we do them, so that the client feels included and informed.

8. Some practitioners carry small hand mirrors and offer the client the opportunity to view her own genitalia, with explanations and guidance from the examiner.

9. If the client becomes tense during the examination, stop the procedure but keep examining hands in place as you urge her to breathe slowly through her mouth and to concentrate on the breathing rhythm.

10. Be certain all equipment is close at hand before beginning the examination.

 The Newborn

HISTORY AND CLINICAL STRATEGIES

- Labia of neonates appear large. Characteristics of the genitalia are used to help determine gestational age. A full-term infant's labia minora cover the clitoris. When her legs are together, the labia majora cover the labia minora.

- Androgens and progestins may cause masculine characteristics in female infants. If genitalia are ambiguous, a history is obtained to determine maternal use of sex hormones during pregnancy and if any family history exists of adrenogenital syndrome. Chromosomal studies are used to determine sex if gender is not known.

SAMPLE RECORDING: NORMAL FINDINGS

External: Female hair distribution with no masses, lesions, scars, rash, or swelling in inguinal area. Labia, vestibule, urethral meatus are intact without inflammation, swelling, lesions, discharge, or tenderness. No bulging at vaginal orifice. Perineum intact with healed episiotomy scar.

Internal: Cervix multiparous, pink, firm, mobile, and midline without lesions. Vaginal surface rugous and moist without inflammation. No discharge visualized. Nonodorous. Uterine fundus anterior and firm under symphysis pubis, contour smooth, nontender. Ovaries and tubes not palpable. No masses or tenderness during palpation.

Rectovaginal: Septum smooth and firm. Cul-de-sac and rectum without nodules, tenderness, or masses. Good anal sphincter tone.

CLINICAL VARIATIONS: THE NEWBORN

CHARACTERISTIC OR AREA EXAMINED	NORMAL FINDINGS	DEVIATIONS FROM NORMAL
1. Characteristics	Full-term labia minora cover clitoris	Preterm infant has more prominent labia minora and uncovered clitoris
	Vulva may be edematous	Full-term infant with enlarged clitoris (may mean adrenogenital syndrome; hermaphroditism)
	One-fingertip space between vagina and anus	No space between anus and vagina (suggests ambiguous genitalia)
	Patent hymen; hymenal tag, bloody, mucoid, or milky discharge may be present (from maternal hormones)	Absence of vagina Labial fusion, lesions
2. Excretion	Should void within 24 hours of birth	Cloudy, concentrated urine, hematuria
	Urine is dilute, clear, may have uric acid crystals	
	Patent anus; should pass meconium within 24 hours of birth	Imperforate anus, covered or closed anus; no meconium

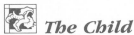
The Child

HISTORY AND CLINICAL STRATEGIES

- The extent of the gynecological examination of the child will depend on the child's age and presenting complaints. For the well child during a screening examination, the examination includes only inspection and palpation of the external genitalia. The vaginoscopy examination is done for a young child only when a problem is anticipated or for a teenager who is sexually active and requests birth control information or who is experiencing abdominal, gynecological, or urinary problems.

- Because of the complexity of the procedure, the vaginoscopy examination of the young child is beyond the scope of this text. Although it may at times become necessary to perform a speculum examination, it requires special equipment and a well-prepared and knowledgeable practitioner who frequently performs pediatric gynecological examinations.

- Examining the external genitalia of any child should be anticipated as a stressful event for both the client and her parent, if present. The examiner must explain to the child and the parent exactly what will be done before the examination, as well as continue to explain throughout inspection and palpation of the external genitalia. It may be necessary to explain to the parent that thorough inspection of the child's external genitalia is part of every complete examination.

  The young infant and child will usually participate cooperatively if the examination is completed in a matter-of-fact manner.

  By the time the child reaches 4 to 6 years of age, the examiner will need to spend even more time reassuring the child that the procedure involves only looking at her genitalia and touching her on the outside. If necessary, the examiner should enlist the help of the child by taking the child's hand and having her first touch herself; then the examiner can palpate the genitalia.

  A school-age or young teenage child will not like the examination but will allow it to occur uneventfully. The child's parent may or may not be present during the examination. If the child appears fearful or anxious, the parent may be able to provide comfort. If the child is older, the examiner should be alert to the child's embarrassment because her parent is present. The examiner should confer with the child before the examination and, if appropriate, ask the parent to wait outside.

  As the child begins to mature, she will become very interested in her own body and what she looks like. The examiner may use a mirror to allow the child to look at herself. Education could coincide with the examination.

  Older teenagers deserve to be examined without a parent present if they desire or if the examiner wants to talk with the adolescent alone. As for the younger adolescent, a mirror may be used as an educational tool and to involve the teenager in the actual assessment process.

- Positioning the child for the examination will depend on the child's age.

  1. Birth to 3 years of age. The child should be on the parent's lap with the child's back reclining at about a 45-degree angle against the parent's chest. The child should feel secure in this position, and the parent can help by holding the child's legs in a frog position up against her chest. This will allow the examiner full access to the external genitalia. The examiner should be opposite the parent and have an adequate light source.

  2. Three to 5 years. Because of the child's size, she will need to be moved to the examination table. If possible, the head of the table should be up about 30 degrees. The child should be resting back on the incline and her legs again help up by her parent in a frog position against her chest. The child does not need to be at the end of the examination table.

  3. Six to 15 years. The child should be on the examination table in a modified lithotomy position, lying flat or at an upward slight angle. Her legs must be flexed at the knee, and her heels should be close to her buttocks. The knees are then separated so that the genitalia may be viewed. If the parent is present, he or she should stand near the girl's head and assist in maintaining a spread-knee position. Depending on the child's age and the length of her legs, she may need to be toward the end of the table. If the examiner has difficulty visualizing the genitalia, a small pillow may be placed under the child's hips. Although the conventional gynecological stirrups are extremely convenient for the examiner, they are often frightening to the young adolescent and spaced too widely for comfort.

  4. Over age 15 years. The adolescent will require the same lithotomy positioning as the adult. The success and adequacy of this positioning will depend on the examiner's approach to the client.

- Frequently the examiner performs the first speculum examination for the teenage or young adult client. The first examination is perhaps the child's most important, since during that examination the client is developing perceptions that will remain with her for future examinations. Special preparations the examiner should make follow:

  1. Discuss the procedure with the client while she is still dressed.

  2. If possible, use illustrations or models to show ex-

actly what will happen and what the examiner will be observing.

3. Prepare all necessary equipment so that once the procedure is started, there will be no interruptions.

4. Use the appropriate size speculum.
   a. There are pediatric and virginal specula that are approximately 1 to 1.5 cm wide. They can be carefully inserted with minimal discomfort.
   b. A small adult speculum may be used if the client is sexually active.

• The history questions about the genitourinary system of the girls should focus on the following three areas:

1. Urinary functioning. Does the child have any difficulties with voiding, such as urinary incontinence, bed-wetting, inability to maintain a steady stream until the bladder is emptied, burning or urgency in urination? If any of these are present, explore in detail, including family history of similar problems, use of bubble bath, and frequency of urinary tract problems.

2. Vaginal itching or discharge. These are both frequent problems that require in-depth investigation. Common causes of them include inconsistent or inadequate cleansing of the area; foreign bodies, such as a toy, toilet tissue, crayons, or coins; sexual abuse or genital fondling. The parent and/or child must be questioned about these possibilities, and the examiner must be careful to consider them during the physical assessment.

3. Maturational changes. Girls over 9 years of age who are also showing breast and pubic hair development should be questioned about whether they have begun menstruation and whether they understand about the developmental changes their bodies are undergoing. Areas of specific investigation include the following:
   a. The girl's awareness and information about menstruation
   b. The girl's feelings about menstruation
   c. The girl's information regarding sexual activities and techniques to prevent pregnancy

CLINICAL VARIATIONS: THE CHILD

CHARACTERISTIC OR AREA EXAMINED	NORMAL FINDINGS	DEVIATIONS FROM NORMAL
1. Position child as discussed on p. 425		
2. Careful examination of external genitalia of the infant to make sure it is unambiguous		Inability to identify labia majora, labia minora, clitoris, urethra, vaginal introitus
3. Inguinal and mons pubis surface characteristics	Smooth, clear surface area Parasites absent	Poor perineal hygiene Scars, swellings, discolorations Excoriated surface Lesions, rash Lice
4. Hair distribution	See Figs. 13-23 (below) and 13-24 (p. 427) for maturational development	Absence of pubic hair by child's thirteenth birthday
5. Labia majora surface characteristics	Pink, smooth surface Symmetrical, dry appearance Becomes prominent and hair covered during puberty	Swelling, redness Discoloration, excoriated surface or rash

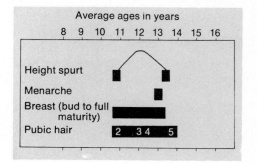

Fig. 13-23   Female maturational development. See Fig. 13-24 for description of stages of development of pubic hair. (From Tanner JM: *Growth at adolescence,* ed 2, Oxford, England, 1962, Blackwell Scientific Publications.)

CHARACTERISTIC OR AREA EXAMINED	NORMAL FINDINGS	DEVIATIONS FROM NORMAL
6. Labia minora	Very prominent in infants; general atrophy until puberty (may normally protrude from labia majora) By puberty labia minora recede to adult configuration Light pink color in infants and small children, changing to dark pink by puberty Symmetrical	Inflammation, swelling, nodules, varicosities Marked asymmetry Tissue appearing white and thin Labia fused by adhesions
7. Clitoris size	From 3 mm to 1 cm (¹⁄₂ inch) in length, depending on age and maturational development	Enlargement, atrophy Ambiguous appearance
8. Urethral meatus and surrounding tissue	Irregular opening or slit Usually located midline; may be close to or slightly within vaginal introitus	Redness, rashes, or lesions Lateral position of meatus Discharge from surrounding Skene glands or urethral opening
9. Vaginal introitus and immediate surrounding tissue	Moist tissue, even pink color Hymen may or may not be across or partially across vaginal opening; by menarche, opening should be at least 1 cm wide Vaginal opening present	If hymen intact (imperforate hymen), blue color or bulging behind hymen may mean presence of blood; most commonly found in (1) newborn: will generally reabsorb on own (2) adolescent: menstrual blood

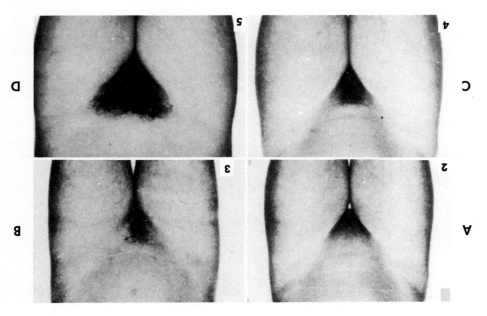

Fig. 13-24   Pubic hair development in females. Preadolescent stage 1 (not shown): none. A, Stage 2: sparse, lightly pigmented, straight along medial border of labia. B, Stage 3: darker, beginning to curl, increased amount. C, Stage 4: coarse, curly, abundant amount but less than adult. D, Stage 5: adult female triangle, spread to medial surface of thighs. (From Tanner JM: Growth at adolescence, ed 2, Oxford, England, 1962, Blackwell Scientific Publications.)

Continued

CHARACTERISTIC OR AREA EXAMINED	NORMAL FINDINGS	DEVIATIONS FROM NORMAL
10. Perineal surface	Smooth, pink	Lesions, redness, rashes, swelling
11. Anus	Deeper pigmentation and coarse skin	Lesions, rash, skin tags, inflammation, lumps, excoriation, unclean surface Presence of pinworms Inflammation, fistula, lesion, mass
12. External genitalia palpation a. Labia and vestibule	Soft, homogeneous, nontender	Nodular, tender
b. Skene glands	Not visible or palpable	Tender or swollen glands; presence of discharge
c. Bartholin glands	Not visible or palpable	Tender or swollen glands Unilateral swelling Presence of discharge
d. Vaginal discharge	Mucoid or sanguineous discharge in newborn Watery discharge present for 2 to 3 years before onset of menstruation Within 1 year after onset of menstruation, discharge as seen in adult	Thick or malodorous discharge; may be caused by a foreign body Any time imperforate hymen found, client should be referred

The Childbearing Woman

HISTORY AND CLINICAL STRATEGIES

• A pregnant woman should void for a random urine test at each prenatal and postpartum visit. Testing for ketones, protein, and sugar, and microscopic examinations of the urine should be performed. Ureter dilation and hypokinesis during pregnancy places women at risk for urinary tract infections. Catheterization should be avoided because it further increases the risk of infection.

• A thorough assessment of the reproductive system should be performed if pregnancy is suspected or confirmed. Data specific to pregnancy relate to the following:
1. Gravida and parity, including abortions
2. Exact date of last menstrual period (LMP)
3. Dates of sexual intercourse, if known
4. Any previous and current childbearing risks
5. Exact dates of quickening (when infant movement is felt) and lightening (setting of fetus into pelvis later in pregnancy)

• Assessment of fetal well-being relates to the following data:
1. Initial determination of pregnancy with cervical and uterine examination
2. Notation when fetal heartbeats or tones (FHB, FHT) can be heard; FHTs are taken at each visit
3. Fundal height and maternal weight measurements at each visit
4. Further gestational assessment if there are any risk factors

• Postpartum assessment concentrates on the following data:
1. Weight, vital signs, auscultation of heart and lungs, and condition of extremities (signs of fluid or edema require investigation)
2. Breast and nipple condition
3. Fundal position and abdominal condition
4. Lochia condition (signs of hemorrhage or infection require immediate investigation)
5. Perineum condition (e.g., lacerations, hemorrhoids, edema, episiotomy)
6. Voiding from bladder and bowels

CLINICAL VARIATIONS: THE CHILDBEARING WOMAN

CHARACTERISTIC OR AREA EXAMINED	NORMAL FINDINGS	DEVIATIONS FROM NORMAL
1. Renal	Urinary frequency: increased micturition subsides when uterus moves out of pelvis; occurs again with lightening Amount of urine increases during pregnancy Stress incontinence may occur Lactosuria (from mammary gland production)	Frequency, urgency, and burning (suggests infection; often caused by urinary stasis from dilated ureters) Dextrose, ketones, protein in urine, hematuria (suggests pregnancy-induced hypertension, diabetes, or other problem)
2. Renal (postdelivery)	Lessened urge to void (from decreased pressure, anesthesia) Lactosuria increases during early lactation Increased urination for a few days after delivery (from excess fluid)	Bladder distention: no voiding 12 to 24 hours after delivery (may result from edema, bruising, perineal injuries)
3. Vagina and cervix	Amenorrhea (missed period) Goodell's sign: softening of cervical os about second missed period (from edema and increased vascularity) Cervix darkens Vulva and perianal area darken Vaginal mucosa discolors Chadwick's sign: purplish-blue congestion (from vascularity) Anterior wall and vaginal opening thicken Leukorrhea; vaginal secretions increased	Increased discharge, odor, itching, burning (may be from infection, such as *Candida albicans,* resulting from lowered vaginal pH)

4. Uterus	Uterus becomes more anteflexed, soft, spongy; Hegar's sign: lower uterus softer than cervix, occurring around sixth week
	Braun von Fernwald's sign: irregular-shaped uterus at 5 weeks
	Piskacek's sign: asymmetric, softened, enlarged uterus (from placental growth)
	Increased size and weight:
	  About one fingerbreadth above pubis at 12 weeks
	  Between umbilicus and pubis at 16 weeks
	  At umbilical level at 20 to 22 weeks
	  Between umbilicus and xiphoid process at 28 weeks
	  At xiphoid process at 36 weeks
	(Breathing more difficult until lightening [fetus into pelvis]; see Gastrointestinal section)
		Early contractions; labor (may be confused with Braxton Hicks contractions)
		
		Decreased uterine growth (may be fetal growth retardation, oligohydramnios)
		Increased uterine size (may be multiple pregnancy, large fetus, polyhydramnios)

Continued.

CLINICAL VARIATIONS: THE CHILDBEARING WOMAN—cont'd

CHARACTERISTIC OR AREA EXAMINED	NORMAL FINDINGS	DEVIATIONS FROM NORMAL
5. Vagina, cervix, and uterus (post-delivery)	Pigmented changes may fade, but areas remain more darkened than before pregnancy	
	Postpartum lochia	
	Rubra is red, bloody for 1 to 3 days	Severe pooling of blood and clots (hemorrhage may be from retained placenta or clotting disorder)
	Serosa is pink-brown, no clots, lasting 5 to 7 days	
	Alba is yellow-brown, no odor, lasting 1 to 3 weeks	Lacerations may cause severe bleeding
	Breast-feeding mothers may progress through lochial changes faster than women who bottle feed; after cesarean section, women will have less lochia (from suctioning at surgery)	Hematomas (may require treatment)
	Uterine contractions: afterbirth pains may occur after delivery, especially when breast-feeding	Boggy fundus (may be from full bladder pressure)
		If fundus remains soft, intervention is needed
	Uterus 12 cm above symphysis pubis after delivery; it moves to umbilicus and descends 1 cm per day	
	Cervical os closes by 2 to 3 weeks	

 The Older Adult

HISTORY AND CLINICAL STRATEGIES

• Sexual history. The elderly woman is capable of sexual functioning during her entire lifetime. Changes associated with aging do occur in the external and internal genitalia, but they happen slowly and at different rates according to the individual. A summary of the aging changes follows:

1. The vaginal tube becomes shorter and narrower
2. Vaginal fluids lessen and may secrete at a slower rate in response to direct stimulation.
3. The vaginal walls are thinner and more friable.
4. Excitement phase: the time and extent of the expansion phase of the vagina is diminished.
5. Plateau phase: uterine elevation is reduced; vasocongestion of the labia is diminished.
6. Orgasmic phase: duration of orgasm is lessened, and the number of uterine contractures are fewer. Occasionally the uterine muscles will lapse into spasm, which can be painful.
7. Resolution phase: this phase is more rapid than in younger women.

Some of these changes mentioned accelerate if the woman experiences no sexual stimulation for an extended period of time (either with a sexual partner or through masturbation). Lack of a sexual partner can be a problem. Some older women, even though they have sexual needs and a desire for intimacy, are not comfortable with extramarital relationships, masturbation, or other life-style alterations if they have no sexual partner.

All the intimacy and sex-related questions listed on p. 408, are appropriate for the elderly woman. Additional questions might be considered if the client indicates that she is interested in pursuing the topic of sexuality.

1. If you have a male sexual partner, do you feel that he is comfortable with his sexual behaviors, responses, and capabilities?
2. Do you ever experience pain in response to direct stimulation of the vagina? During orgasm?
3. Do you have difficulty with urinary frequency or urgency during sexual stimulation?
4. Do you have other physical problems that interfere with sexual behavior (e.g., painful joints, fatigue, dyspnea, fear of injuring yourself or causing illness)?
5. Does your partner have any other physical problems that interfere with sexual behaviors?

6. Are adequate privacy and time available for you to meet your sexual needs?
7. Do you have any problems with family members objecting to your friendships or sexual habits? (*Note:* Some elderly women have consciously made the decision to discontinue sexual activity. An overly enthusiastic practitioner might create conflict and cause embarrassment. Other older females are quite creative and zealous in pursuing needs for sexual fulfillment. Homosexual encounters, masturbation, extramarital experiences, and creative sexual methods with a partner may be part of their life-style. The practitioner should be well informed about elderly individuals' needs and capabilities before pursuing a detailed sexual history.)

• Symptoms associated with the genitourinary system.
1. Vaginitis and/or vulvitis occur often with immobilization. Poor hygiene practices, urinary incontinence, poor nutrition, and obesity contribute to this problem. Medications (especially antibiotics), systemic diseases (e.g., diabetes or atherosclerosis), and atrophic changes also aggravate a potential inflammation. Any individuals who are immobilized should be examined *regularly* for itching and scratching (with resultant lichenification), redness, yellow or white discharge, leukoplakia, petechiae, and vaginal odors.
2. Vaginitis may occur because of limited vaginal secretions, increased alkaline condition (associated with diminished estrogen output), or pessary irritation. Symptoms are itching, pain during intercourse, general localized soreness, and perhaps a resulting increase in vaginal discharge that may be yellow or brown and malodorous.
3. Uterine cancer is first suspected with postmenopausal bleeding. *Any bleeding episode* is cause for immediate referral to a physician.

4. Genital prolapse may feel like pressure or heaviness in the genital area. Back pain, attacks of cystitis (urgency, frequency, burning during urination), urinary retention, urinary incontinence, and constipation may accompany this problem. (*Note:* The severity and number of complaints may not correlate with the severity of prolapse that the examiner observes.)
5. Stress incontinence is common. Involuntary urination may occur with coughing, sneezing, laughing, moving from sitting to standing position, or general movement.
6. The questions regarding vaginal discharge and pelvic pain, p. 410, are appropriate for the aging woman.
7. The client should be asked to share any concerns or information about her menopausal phase.
8. If the client is undergoing estrogen therapy, inquire specifically about bleeding episodes, fluid retention, breast enlargement, or pain. Ask the client to evaluate the effects and side effects of the therapy.

• Clinical strategies.
1. Many clients may assume the lithotomy position with help and support from the examiner. Another individual might be needed to support the client's legs, since they may tire easily when the hip joints remain in abduction for extended periods.
2. Clients with orthopnea will need their head elevated during the examination.
3. Disabled clients may assume the Sims' position for a pelvic examination if they are unable to maintain the dorsolithotomy pose.
4. Papanicolaou smears should be obtained for aging women with the same frequency as with younger women.
5. Read the "Clinical Tips and Strategies," p. 423, for further suggestions regarding client comfort and examination procedures.

CLINICAL VARIATIONS: THE OLDER ADULT

CHARACTERISTIC OR AREA EXAMINED	NORMAL FINDINGS	DEVIATIONS FROM NORMAL
1. External genitalia inspection		
a. Hair distribution	Pubic hair thinned, perhaps sparse, often gray Parasites absent	Patchy loss of hair Total absence of hair Nits, pubic lice
b. Inguinal mons pubis, skin surface characteristics	Smooth, clear	Scars Inguinal swelling, excoriation, lesions, rash
c. Labia majora surface characteristics	Labial folds flattened or may disappear into surrounding skin	Shrinkage accompanied by inflammation

Continued.

CLINICAL VARIATIONS: THE OLDER ADULT—cont'd

CHARACTERISTIC OR AREA EXAMINED	NORMAL FINDINGS	DEVIATIONS FROM NORMAL
	Decrease in subcutaneous fat in folds; usually corresponds to degree of loss of subcutaneous fat elsewhere on client's body	Thickening or induration of small areas
		Maceration, ulceration, lesions, nodules
	Symmetrical	Marked asymmetry
	Skin appears smooth, often shiny, and paler than in younger adult	
d. Inner surface of labia majora and labia minora	Shiny, usually dry, paler than in young adult	Inflammation
		Maceration
	Fewer folds	Lesions, nodules
	Usually symmetrical	Varicosities
		Swelling, thickening
		Induration
		Marked asymmetry
e. Clitoris size	Slightly smaller than in younger adult	Enlargement
		Marked atrophy
f. Clitoris surface	Medial aspect covered by prepuce	Inflammation
	Pink	
g. Urethral meatus and immediate surrounding tissue	Irregular opening or slit (relaxed perineal musculature may result in meatus being situated more posteriorly; very near or within vaginal introitus)	Discharge from surrounding glands or urethral opening
		Polyp
		Inflammation
	Midline location	Urethral caruncles fairly common, appearing as a bright red nodule near urethral meatus
		Lateral position of meatus
h. Vaginal introitus and immediate surrounding tissue	May be smaller (admit only one finger) than younger adult, or multiparous client may manifest gaping introitus with vaginal walls rolling toward opening	Surrounding inflammation
		Profuse vaginal discharge
		Swelling
		Lesions
		Large rectocele, cystocele, enterocele, or marked uterine prolapse will show mucosal tissue bulging through vaginal orifice
i. Perineal surface	Smooth, or episiotomy scar (midline or mediolateral) may be visible	Inflammation, fistula
		Lesions, mass
j. Anal surface	Increased pigmentation and coarse skin	Scars, skin tags
		Lesions, inflammation
		Fissures, lumps
		Excoriation
		Hemorrhoids
k. External genitalia palpation	Soft, homogeneous	Irregular, nodular
	Nontender	Tender
(1) Urethral duct	No discharge from urethral duct	Discharge*
	Nontender	Tenderness
(2) Bartholin gland area	No tenderness, no swelling, homogeneous tissue	Tender, swelling, nodules
	No discharge	Discharge*
(3) Perineum	Thin, rigid	Paper thin
	Lateral episiotomy scar may be visible	
	Nontender	Tender

*Prepare a culture of any discharge.

CHARACTERISTIC OR AREA EXAMINED	NORMAL FINDINGS	DEVIATIONS FROM NORMAL
(*Note:* At time of insertion of finger into vaginal orifice, estimate opening and vaginal orifice tone.)	Opening may be very narrow and admit one finger only Opening may be very relaxed; client has difficulty squeezing examiner's finger with voluntary vaginal constriction	
2. Insert middle finger and index finger (if possible) into vagina; press posteriorly with firm, gradual motion; ask client to strain down or bear down to elicit: a. Bulging	Vaginal wall may roll slighly outward	Bulge appears from anterior wall Bulge appears from posterior wall Uterus emerges at opening (cervix may be visible at opening or may protrude beyond opening) (*Note:* The cervix is often eroded and hypertrophied with marked uterine prolapse.)
b. Urinary incontinence	No incontinence	Incontinent
3. Internal inspection (*Note:* A speculum with narrow blades may need to be used if client has small introitus.) a. Cervix (1) Color	Paler than in younger woman; color evenly distributed Symmetrical, circumscribed erythema surrounding os may indicate normal condition of exposed columnar epithelium; however, beginning examiners should consider any reddened appearance a problem for consultation	Inflamed (red) in local areas or generally Markedly pale Cyanotic Erythema, especially if patchy or if borders irregular around os
(2) Position	Midline Cervix and os may be pointed in anterior or posterior direction Cervix protrudes less into vaginal tube; may be flush against back of vaginal wall Surrounding fornices diminish or may disappear	Situated laterally Projection of over 3 cm (1¼ inches) into vaginal tube
(3) Size	Cervix decreases in size with aging	Over 4 cm (1½ inches) in diameter
(4) Surface	Smooth; may appear paler than in younger woman Occasional visible squamocolumnar junction (symmetrical reddened circle around os) Nabothian cysts common (smooth, round, yellow, raised areas)	Reddened granular area around os (especially asymmetrical), friable tissue Red patches, lesions Strawberry spots White patches

Continued.

CLINICAL VARIATIONS: THE OLDER ADULT—cont'd

CHARACTERISTIC OR AREA EXAMINED	NORMAL FINDINGS	DEVIATIONS FROM NORMAL
(5) Os	Often very narrow or stenosed; in some instances may be obliterated	Absence of os should be reported as problem (*Note:* If secretions from uterus are trapped by nonfunctional os, the uterus may be enlarged and tender during palpation.)
(6) Cervical discharge	Often scanty; if present, should be clear or slightly opaque and odorless	Foul odor Colored (yellow, green, gray) Also note odor of stale urine Bloody discharge
b. Vagina	Length of tube shortens with aging	
(1) Color	Appears paler than in younger women	Reddened Lesions Pallor (associated with anemia)
(2) Surface	Less moisture Smooth (rugae diminish with aging) Shiny	Leukoplakia Dried surface Lesions, cracks, petechiae Bleeding
(3) Consistency	Smooth, homogeneous	Nodular Swollen
(4) Secretions	If present, should be clear or slightly opaque Odorless	Thick, curdy, frothy Gray, green, yellow Foul odor
(5) Amount of secretion	May be absent or sparse	Profuse
4. Bimanual examination		
a. Vaginal wall surface (*Note:* Examiner may be able to insert only one finger.)	Smooth, homogeneous Nontender	Nodular Tender
b. Cervix	Cervical protrusion into vaginal vault diminishes Cervix may be flush against back of vault In some instances examiner may not be able to palpate cervix	
(1) Size	Diminished	Enlarged
(2) Contour	Evenly rounded, may be slightly ovoid	Irregular in shape

CHARACTERISTIC OR AREA EXAMINED	NORMAL FINDINGS	DEVIATIONS FROM NORMAL
(3) Consistency and surface	Firm (like tip of nose) Smooth	Soft, nodular, or hard
(4) Mobility	Cervix remains mobile, but mobility may be less noticeable if protrusion into vaginal vault greatly diminished Movement should not cause discomfort	Immobile, fixed, or discomfort associated with movement
(5) Location	Midline	Laterally displaced
(6) Patency of os	Os may be smaller but should be palpable	Stenosis of os may be normal finding; however, beginning examiners should report this as problem
(7) Fornices surrounding cervix	Diminish (may disappear) with aging; if palpable, should be pliable, smooth, and nontender	Irregular or nodular surface, tender during palpation
c. Uterus	Greatly diminishes in size; most often not palpable at all If body of uterus palpated with internal hand, should be smooth, firm, freely movable, and nontender	Enlarged Nodular, irregular, hardened, or indurated areas; tender during palpation Fixed
d. Ovaries	Atrophy with age and rarely palpable in aging women Fallopian tubes not palpable	Marked tenderness in adnexal area Nodulation or mass palpated Pulsations Ascites and pleural fluid accumulation sometimes associated with adnexal masses
5. Rectovaginal examination: palpable characteristics	Rectal wall should feel smooth and homogeneous Nontender Rectovaginal septum should feel thin, smooth, and pliable Uterine body rarely palpated, and posterior fornix difficult to locate Anal sphincter tone may be somewhat diminished but should be nontender	Nodular, thickened Tender Pouching on anterior rectal wall Any palpated mass abnormal Uterus bulging into rectal wall Anal sphincter manifesting no tone

Study Questions

General

Match the lettered structures with the corresponding
numbered label.

1. _____ Anus
2. _____ Clitoris
3. _____ Labia minora
4. _____ Perineum
5. _____ Urethral meatus
6. _____ Prepuce
7. _____ Mons pubis
8. _____ Vaginal introitus
9. _____ Opening of the Skene gland
10. _____ Labia majora
11. _____ Vestibule
12. _____ Bartholin gland

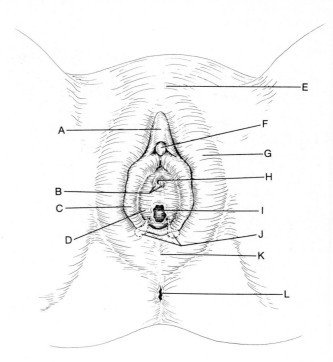

Match the lettered structures with the corresponding
numbered label.

13. _____ Uterus (isthmus)
14. _____ Introitus
15. _____ Ovary
16. _____ Rectum
17. _____ Cervix
18. _____ Uterus (fundus)
19. _____ Perineum
20. _____ Urethra
21. _____ Fallopian tube
22. _____ Vagina
23. _____ Rectouterine pouch
24. _____ Bladder
25. _____ Fornix

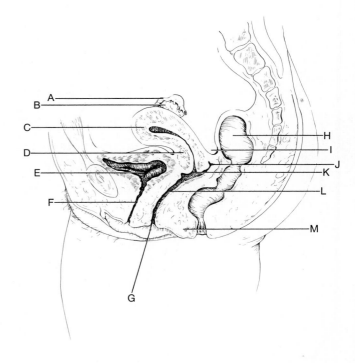

26. Which of the following statement(s) is/are true:
    - ☐ a. The vagina inclines posteriorly at about a 45-degree angle with the vertical plane of the body.
    - ☐ b. The anterior vaginal wall is more sensitive to pressure than the posterior wall.
    - ☐ c. Vaginal discharge is normally odorless.
    - ☐ d. A white, creamy vaginal discharge should be considered abnormal.
    - ☐ e. The vaginal surface often appears thinner and paler in an elderly client.
    - ☐ f. a, b, and c
    - ☐ g. c, d, and e
    - ☐ h. All except c
    - ☐ i. All of the above
    - ☐ j. All except d

27. Retroversion of the uterus:
    - ☐ a. Rarely occurs
    - ☐ b. Is a tilting backward of the entire uterus
    - ☐ c. Occurs with aging
    - ☐ d. When marked, may permit palpation of the fundus through the rectum
    - ☐ e. Results in the cervix facing more anteriorly in the vagina
    - ☐ f. b, d, and e
    - ☐ g. All except c
    - ☐ h. All except a
    - ☐ i. b, c, and d

28. Anteflexion of the uterus:
    - ☐ a. Results in the cervix facing more posteriorly in the vagina.
    - ☐ b. Results in easy palpation of the fundus
    - ☐ c. Is a tilting forward of the entire uterus
    - ☐ d. Occurs with aging
    - ☐ e. May permit palpation of the fundus through the rectum
    - ☐ f. All except e
    - ☐ g. a, b, and c
    - ☐ h. c and d
    - ☐ i. b and c

29. A normal cervix:
    - ☐ a. Is covered by a smooth, pink epithelium
    - ☐ b. Is a granular, vascular membrane
    - ☐ c. Has an os with a slitlike appearance after childbirth
    - ☐ d. Is immobile
    - ☐ e. Feels firm, like the tip of the nose
    - ☐ f. All except a
    - ☐ g. a, c, and e
    - ☐ h. b, d, and e
    - ☐ i All except b
    - ☐ j. a and d

30. Which of the following statement(s) is/are true about normal palpable findings during a bimanual examination:
    - ☐ a. The cervix is freely movable (1 to 2 cm in each direction) when manipulated by the examiner's fingers.
    - ☐ b. The normal cervical os is closed and will not admit a fingertip.
    - ☐ c. Approximately 85% of uteri are in an anteposition and can be palpated anteriorly.
    - ☐ d. Normal ovaries are 4 to 6 cm, firm to touch, and movable.
    - ☐ e. Round ligaments are sometimes palpated as cordlike structures.
    - ☐ f. a, d, and e
    - ☐ g. b and c
    - ☐ h. All except b
    - ☐ i. b, c, and d

31. The rectovaginal examination is performed:
    - ☐ a. To confirm the uterine position
    - ☐ b. To reassess adnexal areas
    - ☐ c. To palpate the rectovaginal cul-de-sac and septum
    - ☐ d. To palpate the rectal wall
    - ☐ e. To assess anal sphincter tone
    - ☐ f. All except c
    - ☐ g. All of the above
    - ☐ h. d and e
    - ☐ i. a, c, and d
    - ☐ j. All except b

The Newborn

32. Between the vagina and the anus of a neonate, there is usually:
    - ☐ a. No space
    - ☐ b. A one-fingertip space
    - ☐ c. A 2 cm space
    - ☐ d. A 3 mm space

33. Masculinization of a female neonate may be caused by maternal ingestion of:
    - ☐ a. Estrogen
    - ☐ b. Calcium
    - ☐ c. Iron
    - ☐ d. Progestin

The Child

Mark each statement as either "T" for true or "F" for false.

34. _____ By age 13 years all girls should start to develop pubic hair.

35. _____ All teens should have a speculum examination by age 16.

36. _____ The hymen must be perforated for the adolescent to menstruate.

37. _____ The best method to examine the external genitalia of a 2-year-old is to have the child on the parent's lap.

38. _____ The labia majora in the infant are more prominent than the labia minora.

The Childbearing Woman

39. The amount of urine during pregnancy and immediately postpartum usually:
    - ☐ a. Varies
    - ☐ b. Decreases
    - ☐ c. Increases
    - ☐ d. Remains unchanged

Match the terms in Column A with their signs in Column B.

	Column A	Column B
40. _____	Softening of the cervical os	a. Chadwick's sign
		b. Goodell's sign
41. _____	Blue vaginal mucosa	c. Hegar's sign
42. _____	Softening of the lower uterus	

Match the terms in Column A with their signs in Column B.

	Column A	Column B
43. _____	Red lochia, 1 to 3 days postpartum	a. Alba
		b. Rubra
44. _____	Pink-brown lochia, 5 to 7 days postpartum	c. Serosa
45. _____	Yellow lochia, 1 to 3 weeks postpartum	

The Older Adult

46. Common genital findings in the aging female are:
    - ☐ a. A flaccid, boggy uterus that can usually be palpated in the anterior rectal wall
    - ☐ b. Diminished vaginal secretions
    - ☐ c. Increased protrusion of the cervix into the vaginal vault, resulting in deep fornices surrounding the cervix
    - ☐ d. Paler appearing vaginal walls
    - ☐ e. Flatter labia majora and diminished skinfolds
    - ☐ f. All of the above
    - ☐ g. b, d, and e
    - ☐ h. a, c, and e
    - ☐ i. All except b
    - ☐ j. None of the above

47. Sexual functioning of the elderly female:
    - ☐ a. Usually ceases after age 65 years
    - ☐ b. Is not usually advisable if the client has osteoarthritis or cardiac disease
    - ☐ c. May be consciously relinquished by the individual
    - ☐ d. Should be rigorously promoted by the practitioner
    - ☐ e. None of the above

48. Vulvitis may occur because of:
    - ☐ a. Poor nutrition
    - ☐ b. Poor hygiene practices
    - ☐ c. Urinary incontinence
    - ☐ d. Excess vaginal secretions
    - ☐ e. Obesity
    - ☐ f. All of the above
    - ☐ g. None of the above
    - ☐ h. All except d
    - ☐ i. b and c

SUGGESTED READINGS
General

Bates B: *A guide to physical examination*, ed 4, Philadelphia, 1987, JB Lippincott.

Malasanos L, Barkauskas V, Stoltenberg-Allen K: *Health Assessment*, ed 4, St Louis, 1990, Mosby—Year Book.

McCance KL, Huether SE: *Pathophysiology: the biological basis for disease in adults and children*, St Louis, 1990, Mosby—Year Book.

Prior JA, Silberstein JS, Stang JM: *Physical diagnosis: the history and examination of the patient*, ed 6, St Louis, 1981, Mosby—Year Book.

Seidel HM, Ball JW, Dains JE, Benedict GW: *Mosby's guide to physical examination*, ed 2, St Louis, 1991, Mosby—Year Book.

Thompson JM, McFarland GK, Hirsch JE, and others: *Mosby's manual of clinical nursing*, ed 2, St Louis, 1989, Mosby—Year Book.

The newborn

Auvenshine MA, Enriquez MG: *Maternity nursing: dimensions of change*, Belmont, Calif, 1985, Wadsworth.

Bobak IM, Jensen MD: *Essentials of maternity nursing*, ed 3, St Louis, 1990, Mosby—Year Book.

Judd JM: Assessing the newborn from head to toe, *Nurs '85* 15(12):34, 1985.

Kiernan BS, Scoloveno MA: Assessment of the neonate, *Top Clin Nurs* 8(1):1, 1986.

The Organization for Obstetrical, Gynecological and Neonatal Nurses (NAACOG): *Physical assessment of the neonate*, OGN nursing practice resource, Oct. 1986, The Association.

Pillitteri A: *Maternal-newborn nursing: care of the growing family*, ed 3, Boston, 1985, Little, Brown.

Seidel HM, Ball JW, Dains JE, Benedict GW: *Mosby's guide to physical examination*, ed 2, St Louis, 1991, Mosby—Year Book.

Whaley LF, Wong DL: *Nursing care of infants and children*, ed 4, St Louis, 1991, Mosby—Year Book.

The child

Alexander M, Brown MS: *Pediatric history taking and physical diagnosis for nurses*, ed 2, New York, 1979, McGraw-Hill.

Barness I: *Manual of pediatric physical diagnosis*, ed 6, Chicago, 1990, Mosby—Year Book.

Daniel WA Jr: *Adolescents in health and disease*, St Louis, 1977, Mosby—Year Book.

Marshall WA, Tanner JM: Variations in patterns of pubertal changes in girls, *Arch Dis Child* 44:291, 1969.

Rauh J, Brookman RR: Adolescent development stages. In Johnson TR, Moore WM, Jefferies JE, editors: *Children are different: developmental physiology*, Columbus, Ohio, 1978, Ross Laboratories.

Seidel HM, Ball JW, Dains JE, Benedict GW: *Mosby's guide to physical examination*, ed 2, St Louis, 1991, Mosby—Year Book.

Whaley LF, Wong DL: *Essentials of pediatric nursing*, ed 3, St Louis, 1989, Mosby—Year Book.

The childbearing woman

Auvenshine MA, Enriquez MG: *Maternity nursing: dimensions of change*, Belmont, Calif, 1985, Wadsworth.

Beischer NA, MacKay EV: *Obstetrics and the newborn: an illustrated textbook*, ed 2, Philadelphia, 1986, WB Saunders.

Blair CL, and others: *Nursing assessment: interview principles, procedures, and tools*, Series 2: *Prenatal care, module 9; a staff development program in perinatal nursing care*, White Plains, NY, 1984, March of Dimes Birth Defects Foundation.

Bobak IM, Jensen MD: *Essentials of maternity nursing*, ed 3, St Louis, 1990, Mosby—Year Book.

Pillitteri A: *Maternal-newborn nursing: care of the growing family*, ed 3, Boston, 1985, Little, Brown.

Pritchard JA, MacDonald PC: *Williams' obstetrics*, ed 17, New York, 1985, Appleton-Century-Crofts.

Seidel HM, Ball JW, Dains JE, Benedict GW: *Mosby's guide to physical examination*, ed 2, St Louis, 1991, Mosby—Year Book.

Whitley N: *A manual of clinical obstetrics*, Philadelphia, 1985, JB Lippincott.

The older adult

Burnside IM, editor: *Nursing and the aged*, ed 3, New York, 1988, McGraw-Hill.

Carotenuto R, Bullock J: *Physical assessment of the gerontologic client*, Philadelphia, 1980, FA Davis.

Ebersole P, Hess P: *Toward healthy aging*, ed 3, St Louis, 1990, Mosby—Year Book.

Jain H, Shamoian CA, Mobarek A: Sexual disorders in the elderly, *Med Aspects Hum Sexuality* 21(3):14, 1987.

Steinberg FU, editor: *Care of the geriatric patient*, ed 6, St Louis, 1983, Mosby—Year Book.

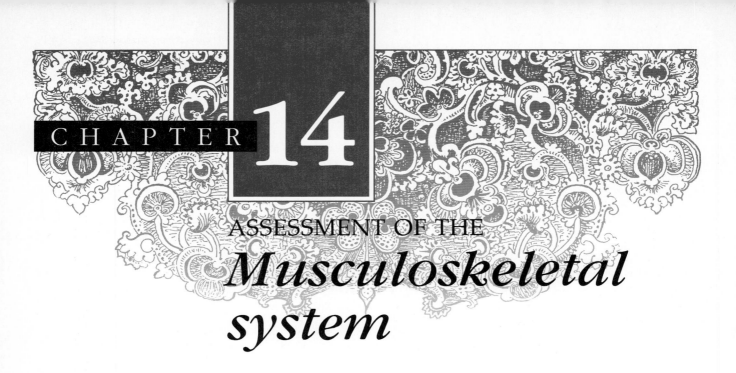

CHAPTER 14

ASSESSMENT OF THE
*Musculoskeletal
system*

VOCABULARY

abduction Movement of the limbs or the trunk and head away from the median plane of the body.

adduction Movement of the limbs or the trunk and head toward the median plane of the body.

ankylosis Fixation of a joint, often in an abnormal position, usually resulting from destruction of articular cartilage, as in rheumatoid arthritis.

bunion Abnormal prominence on the inner aspect of the first metatarsal head, with bursal formation; results in lateral or valgus displacement of the great toe.

bursa Fibrous, fluid-filled sac found between certain tendons and the bones beneath them.

bursitis Inflammation of a bursa.

carpal tunnel syndrome Painful disorder of the wrist and hand induced by compression of the median nerve between the inelastic carpal ligament and other structures within the carpal tunnel.

circumduction Circular movement of a limb.

clonus Spasmodic alternation of muscular contraction and relaxation.

cogwheel rigidity Abnormal motion in the muscle tissues characterized by jerky movements when the muscle is passively stretched.

crepitus Dry, crackling sound or sensation heard or felt as a joint is moved through its range of motion.

dorsiflexion Backward bending or flexion of a joint.

epicondyle Round protuberance above the condyle (at the end of a bone).

epiphysis End of a long bone that is cartilaginous during early childhood and becomes ossified during late childhood.

extension Movement that brings a limb into or toward a straight condition.

external rotation Outward turning of a limb.

fasciculation Localized, uncoordinated, uncontrollable twitching of a single muscle group innervated by a single motor nerve fiber.

flexion Movement that brings a limb into or toward a bent condition.

gait: stance During walking, the resting phase in which the feet, legs, and body are still.

gait: swing During walking, the process of lifting the foot in back, swinging it through, and placing it in front of the other foot.

gout Metabolic disease that is a form of acute arthritis; marked by inflammation of the joints.

internal rotation Inward turning of a limb.

kyphosis Abnormal convexity of the posterior curve of the spine.

lordosis Abnormal anterior concavity of the spine.

myalgia Tenderness or pain in the muscle.

osteoarthritis Form of arthritis in which one or many of the joints undergo degenerative changes.

plantar flexion Extension of the foot so that the forepart is depressed with respect to the position of the ankle.

pronate To turn the forearm so that the palm faces downward, or to rotate the leg or foot inward.

rheumatoid arthritis Chronic, destructive collagen disease characterized by inflammation, thickening, and swelling of the joints.

scoliosis Lateral curvature of the spine.

spondylitis Inflammation of one or more of the spinal vertebrae, usually characterized by stiffness and pain.

sprain Traumatic injury to the tendons, muscles, or ligaments around a joint; characteristics are pain, swelling, and discoloration of the skin over the joint.

strain Temporary damage to the muscles, usually caused by excessive physical effort.

subluxation Partial or incomplete dislocation.

supinate To turn the forearm so that the palm faces upward, or to rotate the foot and leg outward.

tendinitis Inflammation of a tendon.

tennis elbow Inflammation of the tissue at the lower end of the humerus at the elbow joint; caused by repetitive flexing of the wrist against resistance; also called *external humeral epicondylitis.*

valgus Bending outward.

varus Turning inward.

ANATOMY AND PHYSIOLOGY REVIEW

Bones give form to the body. The skeleton is composed of 206 bones, which are shaped to facilitate their functioning. They are held together by muscles, tendons, and ligaments. Many of the bones function as movable components to move the body. Other bones protect many of the body's vital organs (e.g., the rib cage, the skull, and the pelvis).

The skull, facial bones, auditory ossicles, vertebrae, ribs, sternum, and hyoid bone make up the *axial* skeleton; the *appendicular* skeleton consists of the bones in the upper and lower extremities (Fig. 14-1). Bones of the upper and lower extremities are shown in Fig. 14-2. Major muscle groups are seen in Fig. 14-3.

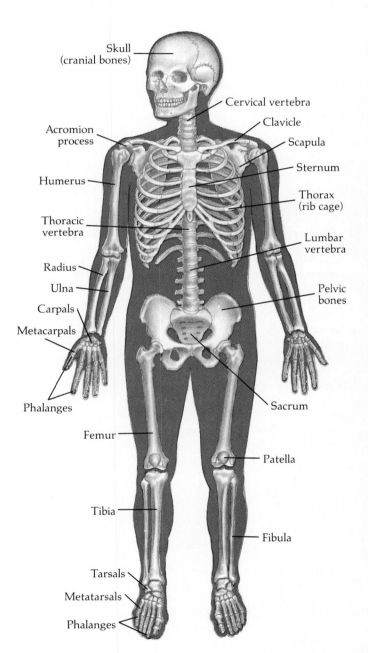

Fig. 14-1 Bones that make up axial and appendicular skeletons. (From Thompson JM, McFarland GK, Hirsch JE, and others: *Mosby's manual of clinical nursing,* ed 2, St Louis, 1989, Mosby–Year Book.)

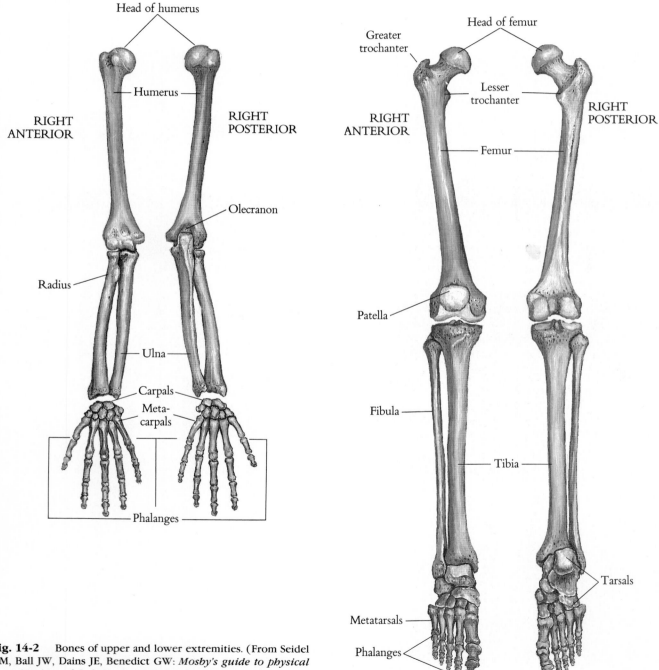

Fig. 14-2 Bones of upper and lower extremities. (From Seidel HM, Ball JW, Dains JE, Benedict GW: *Mosby's guide to physical examination,* ed 2, St Louis, 1991, Mosby–Year Book.)

A

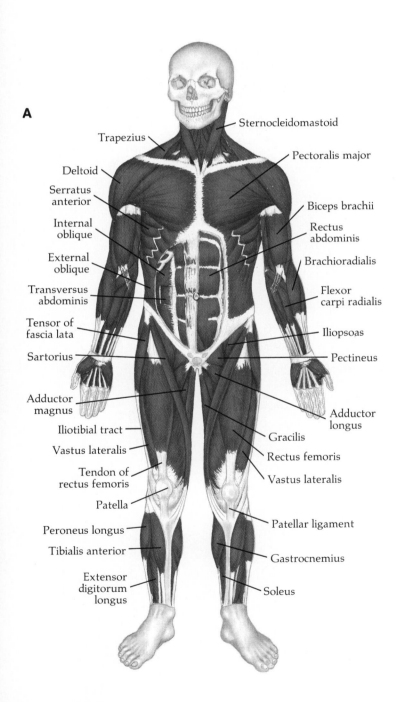

Trapezius

Sternocleidomastoid

Deltoid

Pectoralis major

Serratus
anterior

Biceps brachii

Internal
oblique

Rectus
abdominis

External
oblique

Brachioradialis

Transversus
abdominis

Flexor
carpi radialis

Tensor of
fascia lata

Iliopsoas

Sartorius

Pectineus

Adductor
magnus

Adductor
longus

Iliotibial tract

Gracilis

Vastus lateralis

Rectus femoris

Tendon of
rectus femoris

Vastus lateralis

Patella

Peroneus longus

Patellar ligament

Tibialis anterior

Gastrocnemius

Extensor
digitorum
longus

Soleus

Fig. 14-3 Muscles of body. **A,** Anterior view. (From Thompson JM, McFarland GK, Hirsch JE, and others: *Mosby's manual of clinical nursing,* ed 2, St Louis, 1989, Mosby–Year Book.) *Continued.*

B

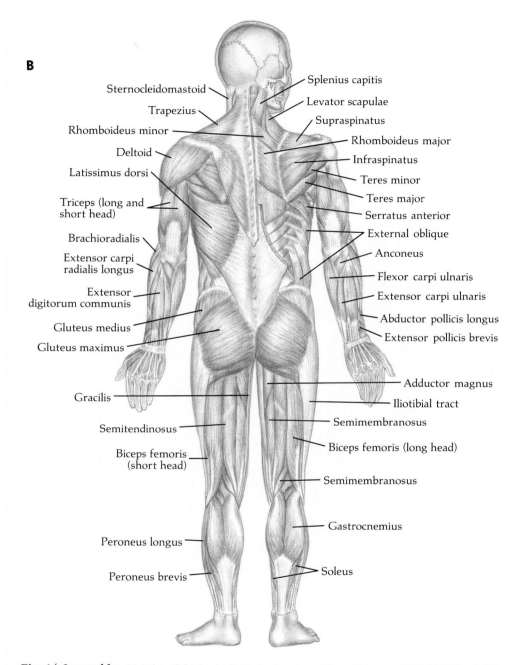

Sternocleidomastoid

Trapezius

Rhomboideus minor

Deltoid

Latissimus dorsi

Triceps (long and short head)

Brachioradialis

Extensor carpi radialis longus

Extensor digitorum communis

Gluteus medius

Gluteus maximus

Gracilis

Semitendinosus

Biceps femoris (short head)

Peroneus longus

Peroneus brevis

Splenius capitis

Levator scapulae

Supraspinatus

Rhomboideus major

Infraspinatus

Teres minor

Teres major

Serratus anterior

External oblique

Anconeus

Flexor carpi ulnaris

Extensor carpi ulnaris

Abductor pollicis longus

Extensor pollicis brevis

Adductor magnus

Iliotibial tract

Semimembranosus

Biceps femoris (long head)

Semimembranosus

Gastrocnemius

Soleus

Fig. 14-3, cont'd   Muscles of the body. **B,** Posterior view. (From Thompson JM, McFarland GK, Hirsch JE, and others: *Mosby's manual of clinical nursing,* ed 2, St Louis, 1989, Mosby—Year Book.)

Several joint formations facilitate joint movement. For example, the glenohumeral joint (shoulder) forms the articulation of the humerus and the glenoid fossa of the scapula; Fig. 14-4 shows the details of this joint. Note the bursae that cushion the ligaments of the joint capsule.

Joints are formed where two surfaces of bones come together and articulate. Joints are classified by degree of movement and are either immovable (synarthrotic), slightly movable (amphiarthrotic), or freely movable (diarthrotic). Examples of the three types of joints follow:

- synarthrotic: skull
- amphiarthrotic: symphysis pubis
- diarthrotic: most other joints of the body

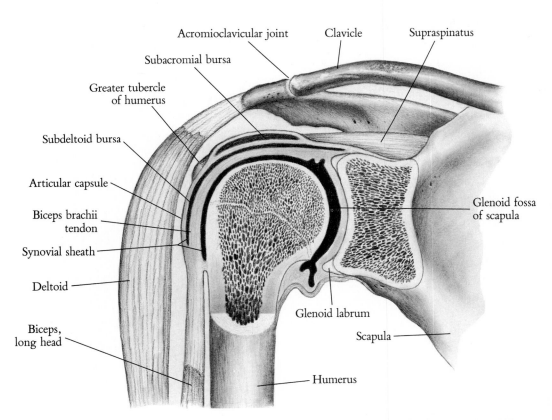

Fig. 14-4   Structures of glenohumeral and acromioclavicular joints. (From Seidel HM, Ball JW, Dains JE, Benedict GW: *Mosby's guide to physical examination,* ed 2, St Louis, 1991, Mosby-Year Book.)

Ligaments hold bones to bones (Fig. 14-5). The ligaments encircle the joint to add strength and stability around the joint.

Tendons hold muscles to bones (Fig. 14-6). They form at the ends of muscles and are strong, nonelastic cords of collagen.

Cartilage is a smooth, resilient supporting tissue made up of elastic fibers containing the protein *chondrin*. Cartilage serves as a smooth surface for articulating bones. Cartilage absorbs weight and stress. It contains no blood vessels and receives its nutrition from the synovial fluids.

A bursa is a small sac or cavity in the connective tissues (usually the tendons) surrounding or near a joint. The bursa is lined with synovial membrane and contains synovial fluid. Normally the bursa is part of the musculoskeletal tissues, but a bursa can also form as a result of pressure or friction over a prominent part.

• • •

Assessment of the musculoskeletal system can be performed on many levels, from gross observations of function to the electrical evaluation of selected muscle fiber groups. For the purpose of this chapter, musculoskeletal evaluation is directed toward functional assessment and detection of the presence, location, and extent of dysfunction. Emphasis is placed on observation of gait; symmetry and function of joints, bones, and muscles; and range of motion as it relates to activities of daily living.

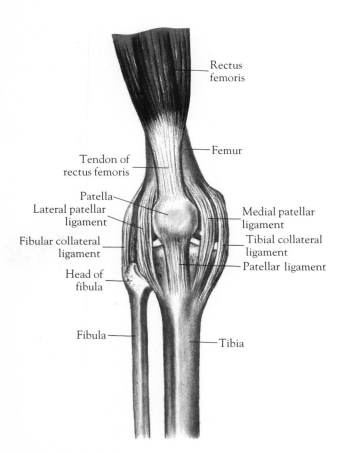

Fig. 14-5 Ligaments of knee joint. (From Thompson JM, McFarland GK, Hirsch JE, and others: *Mosby's manual of clinical nursing,* ed 2, St Louis, 1989, Mosby–Year Book.)

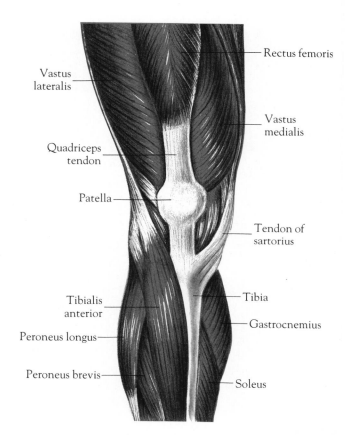

Fig. 14-6 Tendons and muscles around knee joint (anterior view). (From Thompson JM, McFarland GK, Hirsch JE, and others: *Mosby's manual of clinical nursing,* ed 2, St Louis, 1989, Mosby–Year Book.)

COGNITIVE OBJECTIVES

At the end of this chapter the learner will demonstrate knowledge of assessment of the musculoskeletal system by the ability to do the following:

- Apply the terms that are listed in the vocabulary section.
- State the anatomy and function of a joint.
- Describe assessment criteria for evaluating joint function.
- Describe selected methods of evaluating a symptomatic joint, including the drawer test, the McMurray test, and the Thomas test.
- List the normal range-of-motion position of the joints to be assessed during a screening examination.
- Describe a systematic method for evaluating the skeletal system.
- Explain a systematic method of evaluating muscle function during a screening evaluation using the make/break technique.
- Describe the normal gait sequence and assessment criteria for evaluating gait functioning.
- Identify selected characteristics of the newborn, the child, the childbearing woman, and the older adult.

CLINICAL OUTLINE

At the end of this chapter the learner will perform a systematic assessment of the musculoskeletal system, demonstrating the ability to do the following:

- Obtain a health history appropriate to the screening evaluation of the musculoskeletal system. This history should include demonstration of knowledge of the client's ability to perform the activities of daily living, as well as in-depth investigation of such symptoms as musculoskeletal pain and skeletal, muscle, or joint problems.
- Demonstrate inspection of the client's musculoskeletal system, including body build, bone structure and contour, symmetry, posture, gait, strength, and coordination.
- Demonstrate inspection of the client's range of motion of all joints. Communicate an interpretation of findings as related to normal.
- Demonstrate palpation of the client's musculoskeletal system, noting the following:
  1. Bone structure and contour
  2. Joint stability and characteristics and any deviations from normal
  3. Muscle mass, including hypertrophy or atrophy
- Demonstrate screening techniques to evaluate muscle strength of the fingers, hands, wrists, triceps, biceps, deltoids, feet, ankles, hips, hamstrings, gluteals, abductors, adductors, quadriceps, and trunk muscle groups.

- Demonstrate ability to perform special evaluation techniques for the knee, hip, and lower back, including:
  1. Knee fluid evaluation
  2. Drawer test
  3. McMurray test
  4. Thomas test
  5. Back pain evaluation techniques
- Summarize results of the assessment with a written description of findings.

HISTORY

- What is the client's employment situation, both past and present? What are the working conditions and risks (regarding lifting or accident likelihood) for the musculoskeletal system?
- To what extent does the client walk or exercise each day?
- Are there recent weight changes that could have stressed the musculoskeletal system?
- How well can the client perform activities of daily living? (The following activities are arranged according to function. If the interviewer receives a response indicating difficulty, that area should be evaluated further during the physical assessment.) Also refer to functional assessment in Chapter 17.
  1. Eating
     a. Opening containers
     b. Cutting meat
     c. Chewing and swallowing
     d. Preparing food
     e. Getting food to mouth
     f. Measuring and taking medications
  2. Bathing
     a. Running water and testing temperature
     b. Undressing self
     c. Getting into and out of tub or shower
  3. Dressing
     a. Getting clothes
     b. Putting on prosthesis
     c. Putting on clothes
     d. Using zippers
     e. Buckling
     f. Tying
     g. Buttoning
     h. Putting on shoes (shoelaces)
  4. Grooming
     a. Washing hair
     b. Brushing hair
     c. Brushing teeth
     d. Shaving
     e. Grooming nails
     f. Applying makeup
     g. Washing clothes

5. Elimination
   a. Bowel routine
   b. Bladder routine
6. Activity (consider safety factor)
   a. Walking
   b. Getting into and out of chair
   c. Getting into and out of bed
   d. Transferring
   e. Turning
7. Communication
   a. Speech
   b. Telephone

- Often clients complain of musculoskeletal problems. The following outline details the symptoms analysis profile for the complaint of *pain*. This profile may be slightly adapted to collect information about any client with a musculoskeletal complaint. Following the detailed pain analysis profile are numerous other musculoskeletal complaints. Accompanying each of the items listed are important evaluative components. These components may be added to or may replace certain components of the pain analysis profile.

1. Pain
   a. When was the client last well?
      (1) When did *this type* of pain start occurring?
      (2) How long has the client been bothered with musculoskeletal pain in general?
   b. Date of current problem onset
   c. Character of specific complaint
      (1) Pressure sensation
      (2) Stiffness
      (3) Numb, tingling sensation
      (4) Single area, multiple areas
      (5) Sharp versus dull or shooting pain
      (6) If radiation of pain occurs, note to where (hips, buttocks, or legs; unilateral versus bilateral)
   d. Nature of onset
      (1) Slow (over several weeks, days, hours)
      (2) Abrupt (over several minutes)
   e. Client's hunch of precipitating factors
      (1) Recent injury
      (2) Recent strenuous activity, exercise, lifting
      (3) Sudden movement
      (4) Stress
   f. Course of problem
      (1) Comes and goes
      (2) Becoming progressively worse or better
      (3) Relieved by medication, rest, exercise, etc.
   g. Location of problem
      (1) Anatomical location
      (2) Unilateral versus bilateral
   h. Relation to other entities
      (1) Clumsiness
      (2) Weakness
      (3) Paralysis
      (4) Anesthesia (hypoesthesia, hyperesthesia)
      (5) Gastroenterological complaints (ulcer disease, pancreatitis, bowel problems, biliary colic)
      (6) Gynecological complaints (e.g., endometriosis)
      (7) Urological complaints (calculi, prostatic disease)
      (8) Chills
      (9) Fever
      (10) General malaise
      (11) Stiffness
   i. Patterns
      (1) Worse with movement or better with activity
      (2) Worse after coughing or defecation
      (3) Worse in morning or evening (gets better or worse as day progresses)
      (4) Worse after exercise or specific movements
      (5) Worse when riding in car
      (6) Episodes of problem getting closer together and increasing in severity
      (7) Episodes of problem getting closer together but not increasing in severity
   j. Efforts to treat
      (1) Exercise program
      (2) Weight-reduction program
      (3) Rest
      (4) Medications
      (5) Physician evaluation
   k. How does pain interfere with client's activities of daily living?
2. Gait difficulty
   a. Clumsiness

b. Weakness

c. Client unaware of position in space

d. Pain

e. Stiffness

f. Systemic difficulty, such as dizziness or vision problem

3. Voluntary muscle complaints

   a. Muscle weakness or fatigue

   b. Stiffness

   c. Pain

   d. Wasting (atrophy)

   e. Paralysis

   f. Tremor

   g. Tic

   h. Cogwheel movement

   i. Spasms

   j. Aching muscles

   k. Muscle hypertrophy

4. Skeletal complaints

   a. Recent fractures

   b. Abnormalities in skeletal contour

   c. Absence of or change of movements in a part

   d. Crepitus

   e. Pain with movement

   f. Ecchymosis or hematoma of injured part

5. Joint complaints

   a. Recent injury (explore event in detail, including direction joint was stressed)

   b. Change in contour or size of joint

   c. Limitations of joint motion

   d. Swelling or redness of skin around joint

   e. Local pain or ache that increases with muscle contraction

- Any client complaining of vague or generalized musculoskeletal complaints should be questioned in detail regarding history of both self and family, social history, personal psychological history; a detailed review of systems should be performed.
- Any client with a musculoskeletal complaint should be questioned regarding activities of daily living and occupational history. Both areas should include questions about the type of work or activity (present and past), working conditions, injury proneness, and safety precautions.
- As well as evaluating clients with complaints or injuries, the examiner must develop a profile to identify clients at risk and intervene with preventive education techniques. Although the following is not an inclusive list, it represents the type of risk profile data that should be collected regarding the musculoskeletal system.

1. Client who exercises, jogs, plays tennis, etc., only sporadically or less than twice a week

2. Athlete playing contact sports without a structured conditioning program

3. Participation in athletics without proper supportive or protective equipment

4. Occupation requiring lifting of awkward or heavy items

5. Occupation requiring operation of press machines or equipment, such as farm machinery that could catch clothing or limbs, causing crushing or mutilating injury

6. Client overweight for height and body build

7. Family history of arthritis or musculoskeletal diseases

8. Pregnancy

9. Client with poor eyesight or unsafe environment (e.g., throw rugs or darkened stairway)

10. Client with systemic complaint, such as dizziness, light-headedness, or difficulty determining body position in space

11. Any client unable to perform activities of daily living

• • •

Before assessment of the musculoskeletal system, the practitioner must study and memorize several things: (1) the anatomy of the skeletal system and the names of the bones to be assessed, (2) the anatomy and normal range and degree of motion of the joints to be assessed, and (3) the major muscle groups to be evaluated and the anticipated normal response to each group. The student must be knowledgeable in these areas.

Because of the vast complexity of assessment of the musculoskeletal system, an integrated body-region approach will be used. During examination of each region, the bones, joints, and muscles will be evaluated. This approach should save the examiner time, as well as provide a more integrated assessment of each region.

Text continues on p. 473.

CLINICAL GUIDELINES

ASSESSMENT PROCEDURE	EVALUATION	
	NORMAL FINDINGS	DEVIATIONS FROM NORMAL
1. Have goniometer and tape measure at hand (if ranges of motion are to be measured) (*Note:* For musculoskeletal assessment, client should be undressed to underpants only or underpants and bra and gown.)		
2. Observe client walking into room (Fig. 14-7)	Gait smooth, coordinated, rhythmic Walks with ease, arms extended to sides, standing erect; gaze straight forward	Walks with difficulty or with assistance Fasciculations, tremors
3. Measure client's height and weight	(See Tables 2-1 and 2-2 on p. 40.)	
Trunk		
1. Observe client standing erect (front, back, and side) (Fig. 14-8)	Stands erect Symmetry of body parts Straight spine Normal spine curvature: cervical spine concave; thoracic spine convex; lumbar spine concave Knees in direct straight line between hips and ankles Feet flat on floor pointing directly forward	Unable to maintain straight posture Asymmetry Lateral spine curvature Asymmetry in height of shoulders or iliac crest Lordosis or kyphosis, varus or valgus deformity Medial or lateral rotation of feet

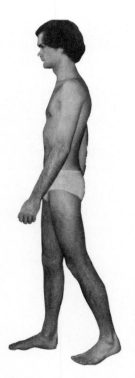

Fig. 14-7   Inspect client's gait.

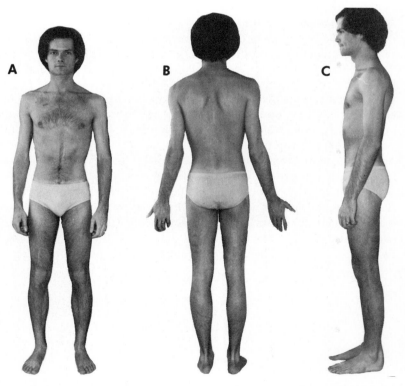

Fig. 14-8   **A,** Anterior inspection. **B,** Posterior inspection. **C,** Lateral inspection.

	EVALUATION	
ASSESSMENT PROCEDURE	**NORMAL FINDINGS**	**DEVIATIONS FROM NORMAL**
2. With client standing, observe spine from posterior as client bends from waist to touch toes; note range of motion and symmetry (Fig. 14-9)	Straight spine Iliac crests to equal height Shoulders of equal height Convexity of thoracic spine	Lateral deviation of spine Asymmetry of shoulder height ("razor back" deformity) (Fig. 14-10)

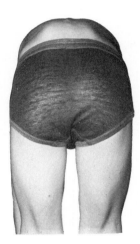

Fig. 14-9   Inspect shoulder and hip symmetry and spine straightness during forward bending.

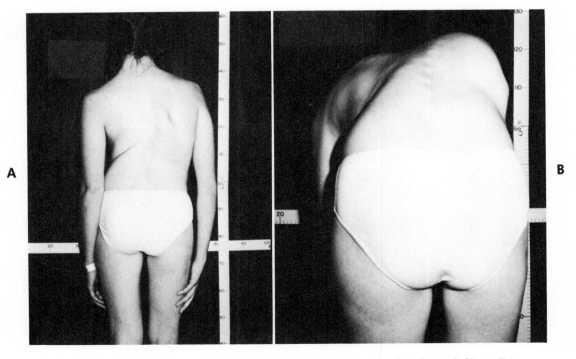

Fig. 14-10   **A,** Asymmetry of shoulder height. **B,** Same patient, bending forward. (From Prior JA, Silberstein JS: *Physical diagnosis: the history and examination of the patient,* ed 5, St Louis, 1977, Mosby–Year Book.)

Continued.

CLINICAL GUIDELINES—cont'd

ASSESSMENT PROCEDURE	EVALUATION	
	NORMAL FINDINGS	DEVIATIONS FROM NORMAL
Trunk—cont'd		
3. Observe client hyperextending spine (Fig. 14-11)	30° hyperextension from neutral position	Unable to hyperextend without losing balance; pain with hyperextension
4. Observe as client does right and left lateral bending; may be necessary to stabilize client's pelvis (Fig. 14-12)	35° flexion both ways from midline position	Decreased flexion degree or pain with bending

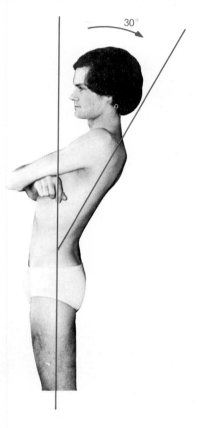

Fig. 14-11   Hyperextension of spine.

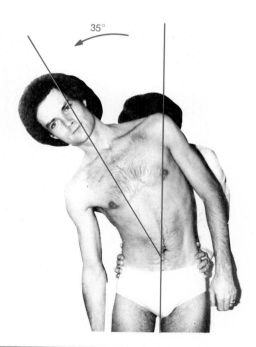

Fig. 14-12   Lateral bending of spine.

| | EVALUATION | |
ASSESSMENT PROCEDURE	NORMAL FINDINGS	DEVIATIONS FROM NORMAL
5. Observe as client rotates upper trunk (stabilize pelvis) to right and left (Fig. 14-13)	30° rotation in both directions from direct forward position	Decreased rotation capability Rotation with discomfort
6. Palpate along spinal processes and paravertebral muscles; may be helpful to have client hunch shoulders forward and slightly flex (Fig. 14-14)	Straight spine Nontender	Curvature of spine Tenderness Spasm of paravertebral muscles
Gait		
1. Have client walk across room and back; observe for rhythm and smoothness		
a. Gait phase	Conformity; ability to follow gait sequencing of both stance and swing	Pain or discomfort with gait
b. Cadence	Symmetry of gait Regular smooth rhythm	Unsteady Jerky
c. Stride length	Symmetry in length of leg swing	Asymmetry or irregularity
d. Trunk posture	Smooth swaying related to gait phase	Irregular or jerky
e. Arm swing	Smooth, symmetrical	Jerky, asymmetrical, or unrelated to gait

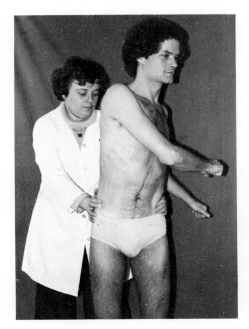

Fig. 14-14 Palpation of vertebral column.

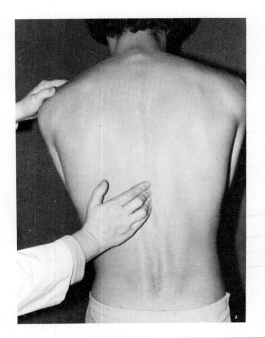

Fig. 14-13 Functional testing of trunk rotation; examiner stabilizes client's hips.

Continued.

CLINICAL GUIDELINES—cont'd

| | EVALUATION | |
ASSESSMENT PROCEDURE	NORMAL FINDINGS	DEVIATIONS FROM NORMAL
Head and neck		
1. With client sitting on examination table, observe musculature of face and neck	Symmetrical appearance	Asymmetry Atrophy or hypertrophy of muscles
2. Palpate each temporomandibular joint just anterior to tragus of ear while client opens and closes mouth (Fig. 14-15)	Smooth movement of mandible	Pain, limited range of motion, or crepitus of temporomandibular joint
3. Move behind client; inspect and palpate posterior neck, cervical spine, paravertebral and trapezius muscles; locate landmarks C7 and T1	Nontender cervical spine	Tenderness Nodules Muscular spasm
4. Evaluate range of motion of neck by asking client to:		
a. Flex chin to chest	45° from midline	Limited or painful range of motion
b. Extend head	55° from midline	Crepitus of cervical spine
c. Laterally bend neck to right and left	40° each way from midline	
d. Rotate chin to shoulders right and left	70° from midline	
5. Evaluate neck muscle strength		
a. Have client flex chin to chest; instruct client to maintain position while examiner tries to manually force head upright (Fig. 14-16)	With reasonable strength, unable to force head upright	Able to break muscular flexion before anticipated point
b. Have client hyperextend head; instruct client to maintain position while examiner tries to manually force head upright (Fig. 14-17)	With reasonable strength, unable to force head upright	Able to break muscular flexion before anticipated point

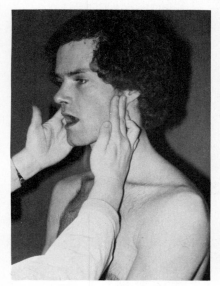

Fig. 14-15 Palpation of temporomandibular joint.

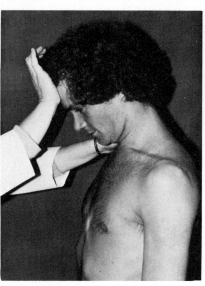

Fig. 14-16 Maintaining flexion of neck against resistance.

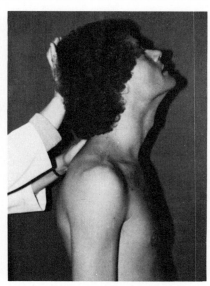

Fig. 14-17 Maintaining hyperextension of neck against resistance.

ASSESSMENT PROCEDURE	EVALUATION	
	NORMAL FINDINGS	DEVIATIONS FROM NORMAL
Hands and wrists 1. Observe and palpate hands and wrists, including joints	Smoothness; no swelling or deformities noted Fingers able to maintain full extension	Irregular finger contour Swelling Deformities (Fig. 14-18, *A*) Tenderness (Fig. 14-18, *B*) Muscular atrophy Heberden nodes (Fig. 14-18, *C*)

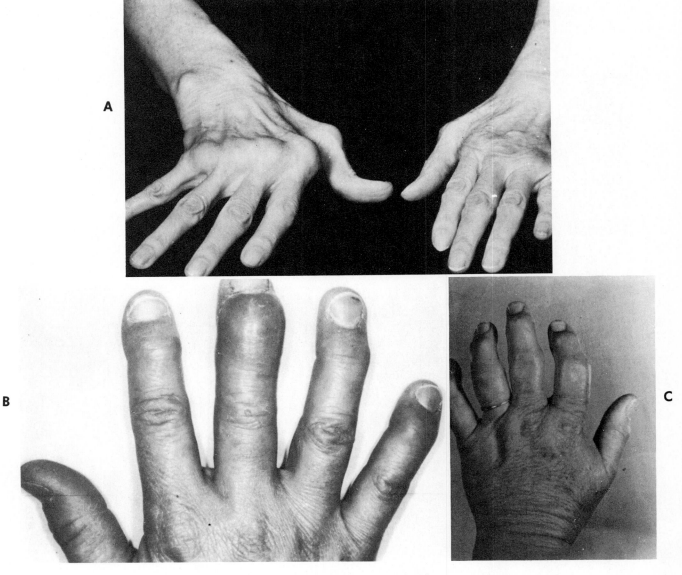

Fig. 14-18   **A,** Unilateral ulnar deviation of metacarpophalangeal joints of right hand secondary to rheumatoid arthritis. **B,** Inflammatory synovitis of distal joint of middle finger. **C,** Heberden nodules in osteoarthritis of the hand. (From Prior JA, Silberstein JS, Stang JM: *Physical diagnosis: the history and examination of the patient,* ed 6, St Louis, 1981, Mosby–Year Book.)

Continued.

CLINICAL GUIDELINES—cont'd

ASSESSMENT PROCEDURE	EVALUATION	
	NORMAL FINDINGS	DEVIATIONS FROM NORMAL
Hands and wrists—cont'd		
2. Observe muscular function and range of motion of fingers and hands; instruct client to:		
a. Extend and spread fingers of both hands (Fig. 14-19, *A*)	Symmetrical response Smooth movement without complaints of discomfort Full flexion and extension	Asymmetrical response Pain during movement
b. Make fist with thumb across fingers (Fig. 14-19, *B*)		
c. Grip examiner's first two fingers (Fig. 14-19, *C*) (see clinical strategy for muscle strength grading)	Bilaterally equal response Tight grip	Unequal response Decreased response

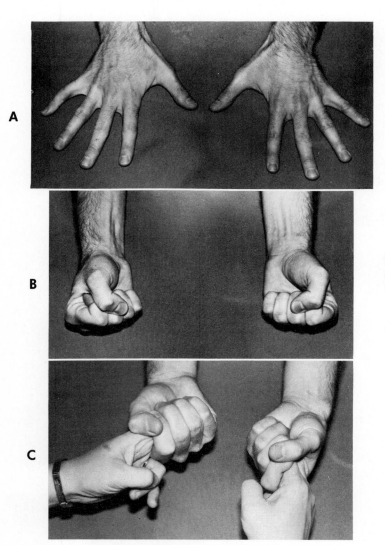

Fig. 14-19 Functional assessment of hands. **A,** Fingers extended and spread. **B,** Fist formation. **C,** Hand grip.

ASSESSMENT PROCEDURE	EVALUATION	
	NORMAL FINDINGS	DEVIATIONS FROM NORMAL
3. Observe range of motion of wrist a. Radial deviation (Fig. 14-20, *A*)	20° movement from central position	Pain with movement Decreased movement
b. Ulnar deviation (Fig. 14-20, *B*)	55° movement from central position	
c. Extension (Fig. 14-20, *C*)	70° movement from central position	
d. Flexion (Fig. 14-20, *D*)	90° movement from central position	

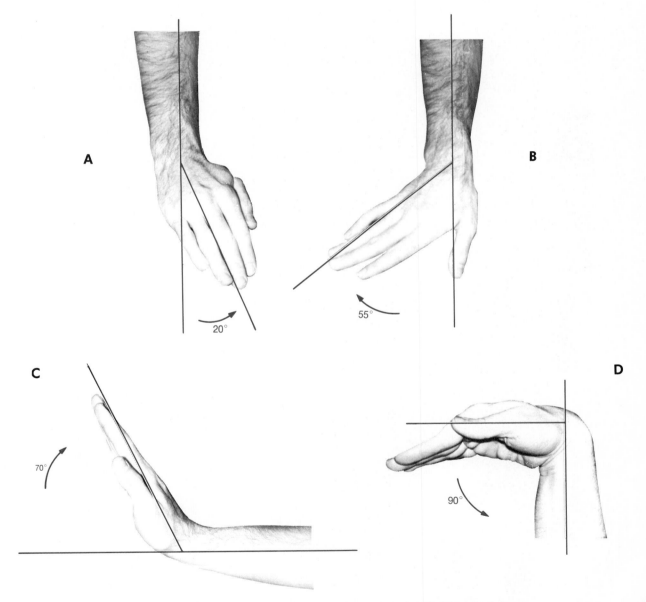

Fig. 14-20   Functional assessment of wrist. **A,** Radial deviation. **B,** Ulnar deviation.
C, Extension. **D,** Flexion.

Continued.

CLINICAL GUIDELINES—cont'd

ASSESSMENT PROCEDURE	EVALUATION	
	NORMAL FINDINGS	DEVIATIONS FROM NORMAL
Hands and wrists—cont'd		
4. Evaluate wrist strength; instruct client to maintain position against examiner's force by using make/break technique (see "Clinical Tips and Strategies," p. 473, for full explanation)		
a. Client flexes wrist; examiner attempts to straighten wrist by grasping client's hand and extending hand to position on a straight plane from client's forearm (Fig. 14-21, *A*)	Bilaterally strong Unable to break position	Asymmetrical response Able to break position easily
b. Client extends wrist; examiner grasps client's hand and attempts to flex hand to a position on a straight plane from client's forearm (Fig. 14-21, *B*)	Bilaterally strong Unable to break position	Asymmetrical response Able to break position easily
Elbows		
1. Flex client's arm and support; inspect and palpate elbow, including:		
a. Extensor surface of ulna	Skin intact	Swelling
b. Olecranon process	Smooth	Inflammation
c. Groove on either side of olecranon	Surface nontender without nodules or discomfort	General tenderness Subcutaneous nodules Point tenderness
d. Lateral epicondyle	Not tender or swollen	
e. Epitrochlear nodes (palpate lateral groove between biceps and triceps muscles)	Lymph nodes not palpable	Lymph nodes palpated

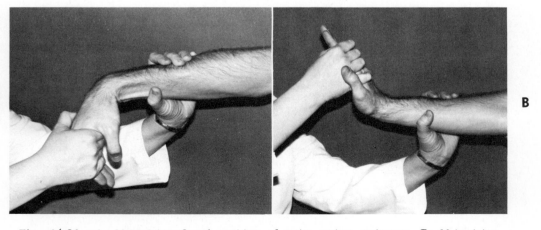

Fig. 14-21   **A,** Maintaining flexed position of wrist against resistance. **B,** Maintaining hyperextended position of wrist against resistance.

ASSESSMENT PROCEDURE	EVALUATION	
	NORMAL FINDINGS	DEVIATIONS FROM NORMAL
2. Evaluate range of motion		
a. Ask client to bend and extend elbow (Fig. 14-22)	160° full movement Bilaterally equal No discomfort	Limited range of motion Asymmetrical movement Pain at elbow
b. Bend client's elbow to 90° angle from shoulder; have client pronate and supinate forearm (Fig. 14-23)	90° each direction Bilaterally equal No discomfort	Limited range of motion Asymmetrical movement Pain at elbow

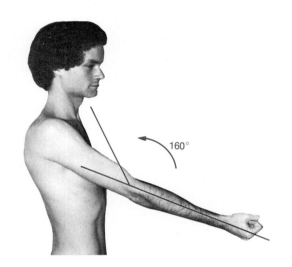

Fig. 14-22   Functional assessment of elbow extension.

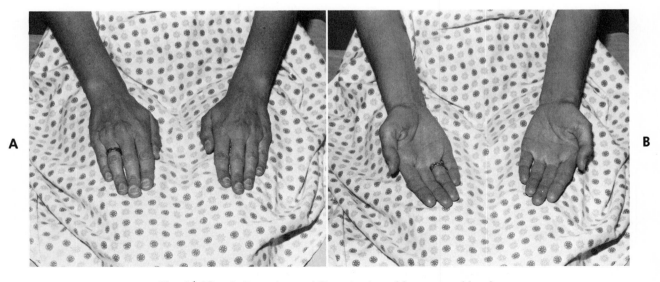

Fig. 14-23   **A,** Pronation, and **B,** supination of forearms and hands.

Continued.

CLINICAL GUIDELINES—cont'd

ASSESSMENT PROCEDURE	EVALUATION	
	NORMAL FINDINGS	DEVIATIONS FROM NORMAL
Shoulders		
1. Inspect shoulders, including shoulder girdle and acromioclavicular junction	Intact Smooth and regular Bilaterally symmetrical	Redness Swelling Nodules
2. Palpate shoulders, including sternoclavicular joint, acromioclavicular joint, shoulder in general, humerus, and biceps groove	Nontender Smooth and regular Bilaterally symmetrical	Tender, painful Swelling
3. Evaluate range of motion of shoulders		
a. Client extends arms straight up beside head (Fig. 14-24, *A*)	180° from resting neutral position Bilaterally equal No discomfort	Limited range of motion Pain with movement Crepitations with movement Asymmetry
b. Client hyperextends arms backward (Fig. 14-24, *B*)	50° Bilaterally equal No discomfort	Limited range of motion Pain with movement Crepitations with movement Asymmetry

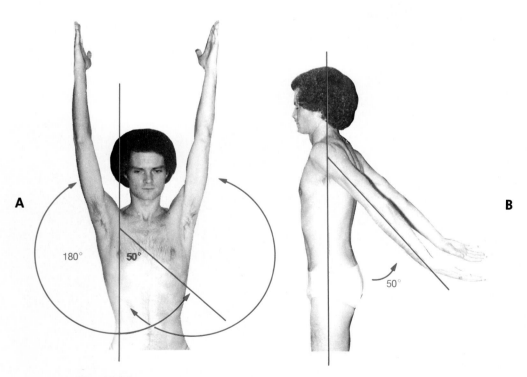

Fig. 14-24 **A,** Abduction and adduction. **B,** Hyperextension of shoulders.

| | EVALUATION | |
ASSESSMENT PROCEDURE	NORMAL FINDINGS	DEVIATIONS FROM NORMAL
c. External (outward or lateral) rotation: client starts in abducted location with arms extended directly forward from shoulder, then places hands behind head with elbows out (Fig. 14-24, *C*)	90° Bilaterally equal No discomfort	Limited range of motion Pain with movement Crepitations with movement Asymmetry
d. Internal (inward or medial) rotation: client starts with forearms extended in abducted location, then places hands behind small of back (Fig. 14-24, *D*)	90° Bilaterally equal No discomfort	Limited range of motion Pain with movement Crepitations with movement Asymmetry
Arm muscles (Using make/break technique) 1. Deltoids: client holds arms up while examiner attempts to push them down (Fig. 14-25)	Bilaterally strong Unable to break position	Symmetrically unequal Weak response Pain during technique Muscular spasm

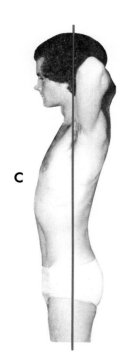
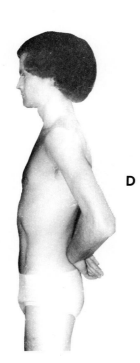

Fig. 14-24, cont'd   C, External rotation. **D**, Internal rotation.

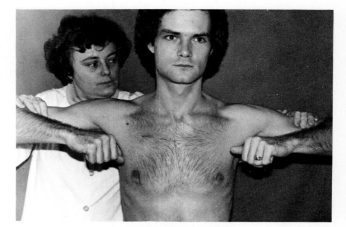

Fig. 14-25   Testing deltoid strength against resistance.

Continued.

CLINICAL GUIDELINES—cont'd

ASSESSMENT PROCEDURE	EVALUATION	
	NORMAL FINDINGS	DEVIATIONS FROM NORMAL
Arm muscles—cont'd		
2. Biceps: client tries to flex arm into fighting position while examiner tries to extend forearm (Fig. 14-26)	Bilaterally strong Unable to break position	Symmetrically unequal Weak response Pain during technique Muscular spasm
3. Triceps: client tries to straighten forearm while examiner attempts to flex forearm (Fig. 14-27)	Bilaterally strong Unable to break position	Symmetrically unequal Weak response Pain during technique Muscular spasm

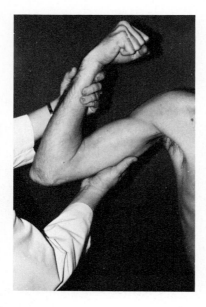

Fig. 14-26 Testing bicep strength against resistance.

Fig. 14-27 Maintaining extended position of forearm against resistance.

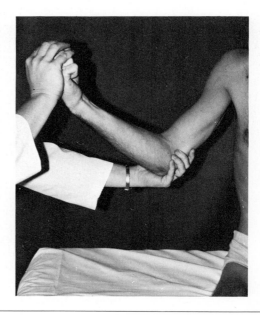

| | EVALUATION | |
ASSESSMENT PROCEDURE	NORMAL FINDINGS	DEVIATIONS FROM NORMAL
Feet and ankles		
1. Inspect feet and ankles with client lying down	Smoothness; no swelling or deformities noted Toes maintain extended and straight position Toenails intact and neatly trimmed Feet maintain straight position	Inflammation Swelling over any joint Gout (Fig. 14-28, *A*) Medial deviation of toes (Fig. 14-28, *B*) Hallux valgus (Fig. 14-28, *C*) Clawtoes (Fig. 14-28, *D*) Hammer toes Calluses
2. Palpate feet and ankles	Smooth Nontender	Tenderness (diffuse vs. pinpoint) Swelling Inflammation Ulcerations Nodules

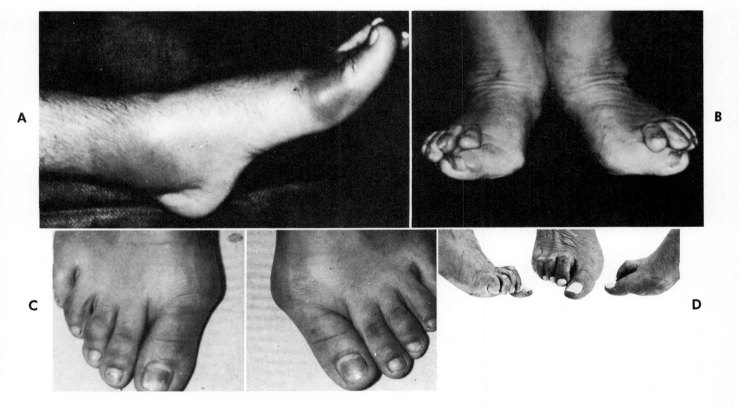

Fig. 14-28   **A,** Inflammatory response of acute gout of the great toe. **B,** Medial deviation of the great toes. **C,** Hallux valgus. **D,** Clawtoes. (**A** and **B** from Prior JA, Silberstein JS, Stang JM: *Physical diagnosis: the history and examination of the patient,* ed 6, St Louis, 1981, Mosby—Year Book; **C** from American Academy of Orthopaedic Surgeons: *Instructional course lectures,* vol 22, St Louis, 1973, Mosby—Year Book; **D** from Mann RA, editor: *Surgery of the foot,* ed 5, St Louis, 1986, Mosby—Year Book.)

Continued.

CLINICAL GUIDELINES—cont'd

ASSESSMENT PROCEDURE	EVALUATION	
	NORMAL FINDINGS	DEVIATIONS FROM NORMAL
Feet and ankles—cont'd 3. Evaluate range of motion of feet and ankles a. Client dorsiflexes and plantar flexes foot (Fig. 14-29)	Dorsiflexion 20° from midline position Plantar flexion 45° from midline position Bilaterally equal No discomfort	Limited range of motion Pain with movement Crepitations Asymmetry

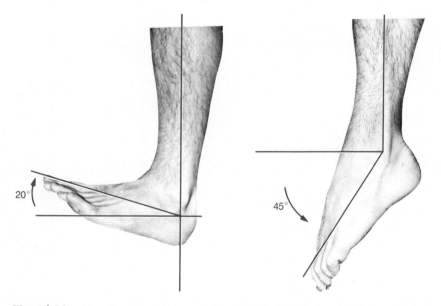

Fig. 14-29   Functional assessment of the ankle. **A,** Dorsiflexion. **B,** Plantar flexion.

ASSESSMENT PROCEDURE	EVALUATION	
	NORMAL FINDINGS	DEVIATIONS FROM NORMAL
b. Inversion and eversion of foot (stabilize heel) (Fig. 14-30)	Inversion 30° from midline position Eversion 20° from midline position Bilaterally equal No discomfort	Limited range of motion Pain with movement Crepitations Asymmetry
c. Flexion and extension of toes	Active movement without discomfort	Painful movement
4. Evaluate muscles of foot and ankle by make/break technique: client is instructed to flex foot upward and maintain position; examiner presses down on big toe (Fig. 14-31)	Bilaterally strong Unable to break position	Unequal Weak response Pain during technique

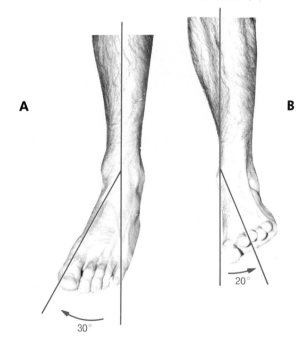

A **B**

Fig. 14-30   Functional assessment of the ankle. **A,** Inversion. **B,** Eversion.

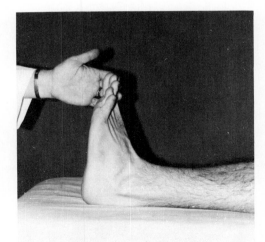

Fig. 14-31   Dorsiflexion of the foot against resistance.

Continued.

CLINICAL GUIDELINES—cont'd

ASSESSMENT PROCEDURE	EVALUATION	
	NORMAL FINDINGS	DEVIATIONS FROM NORMAL
Knee		
1. Inspect knees; note alignment and characteristics	Symmetrical Smooth Hollowness present adjacent to and above patella	Swelling Bowlegged Knock-kneed Thickness Bogginess Inflammation
2. Palpate knees a. Palpate suprapatellar pouch on each side of quadriceps (Fig. 14-32, *A* and *B*)	Smooth, nontender	Bogginess Thickening Tenderness Pain
b. Compress suprapatellar pouch with one hand; palpate each side of patella and over tibiofemoral joint space (Fig. 14-32, *C*)	Smooth, nontender	Bogginess Thickening Tenderness Pain
c. Palpate popliteal space	Smooth, nontender	Tenderness, redness Nodules and swelling

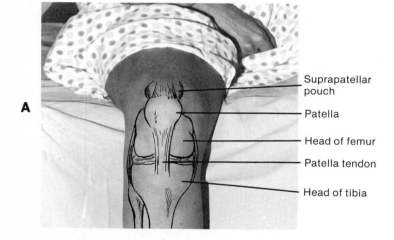

A

- Suprapatellar pouch
- Patella
- Head of femur
- Patella tendon
- Head of tibia

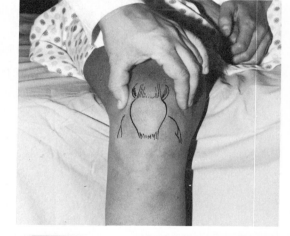

B

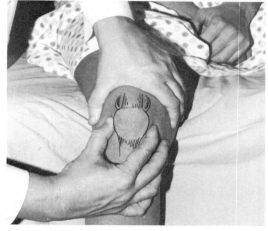

C

Fig. 14-32 **A,** Anatomical structures of the knee. **B,** Palpation of suprapatellar pouch. **C,** Stabilize suprapatellar pouch and palpate each side of patella and over tibiofemoral joint space.

| | EVALUATION | |
ASSESSMENT PROCEDURE	NORMAL FINDINGS	DEVIATIONS FROM NORMAL
3. Evaluate range of motion of knees by asking client to flex knees (Fig. 14-33) (*Note:* May postpone until hip range of motion is evaluated.)	130° from straight extended position No discomfort or difficulty	Decreased range of motion Pain with movement Crepitations
Hips and pelvis		
1. With patient lying down, inspect and palpate hips for position and stability (Fig. 14-34)	Bilaterally symmetrical Stable and painless with palpation	Painful hip area (diffuse vs. pinpoint tenderness) Crepitations

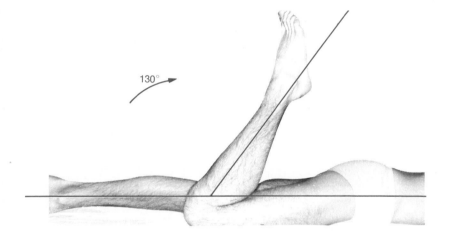

Fig. 14-33   Evaluating knee flexion.

Fig. 14-34   Evaluating pelvic stability.

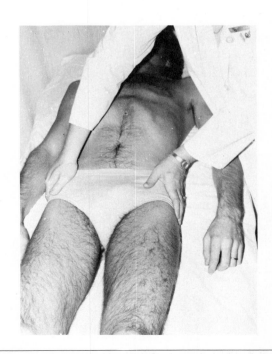

CLINICAL GUIDELINES—cont'd

ASSESSMENT PROCEDURE	EVALUATION	
	NORMAL FINDINGS	DEVIATIONS FROM NORMAL
Hips and pelvis—cont'd		
2. Evaluate range of motion of hip		
a. Instruct client to alternately pull each knee up to chest (Fig. 14-35)	120° from straight extended position	Limited range of motion Pain or discomfort with movement Flexion of opposite thigh Crepitations
b. Instruct client to flex hip as far as possible without bending knee (Fig. 14-36)	90° from straight extended position	Limited range of motion Pain or discomfort with movement Crepitations

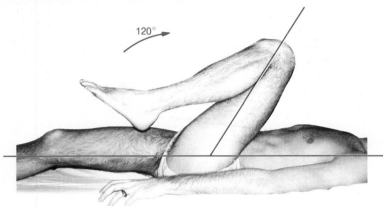

Fig. 14-35   Evaluating hip flexion.

Fig. 14-36   Evaluating hip flexion with leg extended.

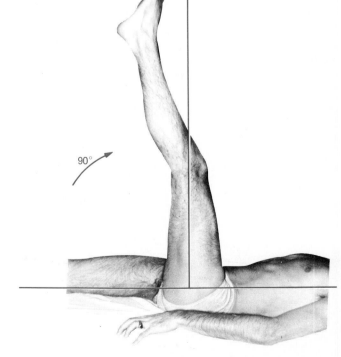

	EVALUATION	
ASSESSMENT PROCEDURE	**NORMAL FINDINGS**	**DEVIATIONS FROM NORMAL**
c. Instruct client to place foot on opposite patella; press knee down laterally (external hip rotation) (Patrick test) (Fig. 14-37)	40° from straight midline position	Limited range of motion Pain or discomfort with movement Crepitations
d. Instruct client to flex knee and turn medially (or inward); examiner pulls heel laterally (or outward) (internal hip rotation) (Fig. 14-38)	40° from straight midline position	Limited range of motion Pain or discomfort with movement Crepitations

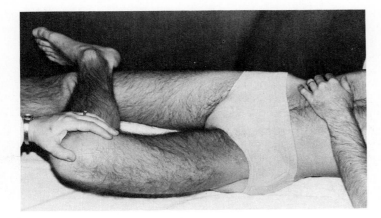

Fig. 14-37   Evaluating external rotation of hip.

Fig. 14-38   Internal hip rotation.

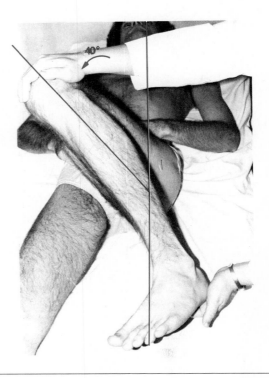

Continued.

CLINICAL GUIDELINES—cont'd

	EVALUATION	
ASSESSMENT PROCEDURE	**NORMAL FINDINGS**	**DEVIATIONS FROM NORMAL**
Leg, hip, and pelvis muscles (Using make/break technique)		
1. Hip strength: client in supine position attempts to raise legs while examiner tries to hold them down; evaluate one leg at a time	Bilaterally strong Unable to break position	Symmetrically unequal Weak response Pain during technique
2. Hamstrings, gluteals, abductors, and adductors: instruct client to sit and alternately cross legs (Fig. 14-39)	Able to perform Bilaterally equal and without difficulty	Unable to perform Performs with pain or great difficulty
3. Quadriceps: client extends leg at knee; examiner attempts to flex knee (Fig. 14-40)	Bilaterally strong Unable to flex knee	Symmetrically unequal Weak response Pain during technique
4. Hamstrings: client tries to bend knee while examiner attempts to straighten knee (Fig. 14-41)	Bilaterally strong Unable to flex knee	Symmetrically unequal Weak response Pain during technique

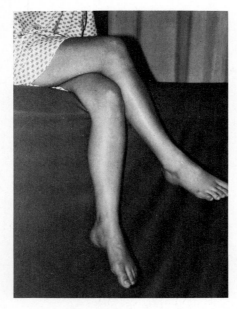

Fig. 14-39 Assessment of adductors and hamstring.

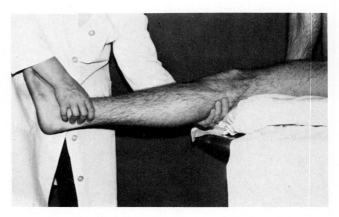

Fig. 14-40 Maintaining extended position of anterior thigh muscles against resistance.

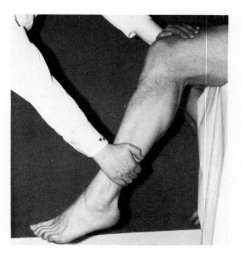

Fig. 14-41 Maintaining flexed position of hamstring against resistance.

| | EVALUATION | |
ASSESSMENT PROCEDURE	NORMAL FINDINGS	DEVIATIONS FROM NORMAL
Special techniques		
1. Knee evaluation		
a. Fluid within knee joint: extend knee; milk medial aspect of knee upward two or three times; then tap on lateral side of patella	No fluid waves or bulging on opposite side of joint	Fluid waves palpable on opposite side of joint
b. Drawer test (to evaluate intactness of cruciate ligaments): client in supine position, knee flexed at right angle; examiner sits on client's foot, thus fixing it on examining table		
(1) Instruct client to relax muscle in flexed leg		
(2) Press head of tibia forward or backward with both hands (Fig. 14-42)	Unable to displace its position	Tibia can be pulled anteriorly from under femur (indicates injury to anterior cruciate ligament) Tibia can be pushed posteriorly from under femur (indicates injury to posterior cruciate ligament)
c. McMurray test (to evaluate presence of damaged or torn meniscus): client is supine with knees and hips strongly flexed toward chest; stabilize one hand on client's knee with thumb and index finger on either side of joint space; with other hand, grasp client's heel; with both hands, externally rotate knee and abduct leg at same time (Fig. 14-43)	Stable knee No discomfort	Positive findings: pain, clicking feeling, or inability to extend lower leg

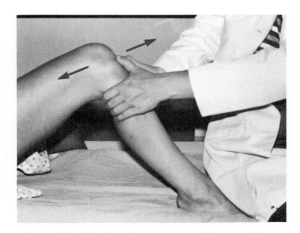

Fig. 14-42   Performing drawer test.

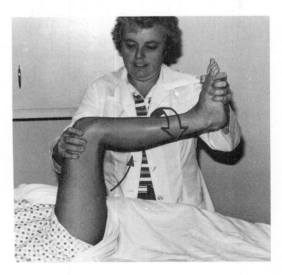

Fig. 14-43   Performing McMurray test.

Continued.

CLINICAL GUIDELINES—cont'd

ASSESSMENT PROCEDURE	EVALUATION	
	NORMAL FINDINGS	DEVIATIONS FROM NORMAL
Special techniques—cont'd		
2. Hip evaluation: Thomas test (to evaluate for flexion contractures of hip); client supine and pulls one knee up toward chest as far as possible	Easy flexion Opposite leg remains flat on table (Fig. 14-44, *A*)	Opposite leg and hip flex in response to flexing leg Note degree of flexion (Fig. 14-44, *B*)
3. Low back pain evaluation		
a. Four specific areas of assessment		
(1) Observe curvature of lumbar region	Lumbar lordosis: concavity of lumbar region	Reversal or flattening of lumbar curvature
(2) Observe trunk positioning	Upright trunk position	Slightly flexed back Slight lateral bending of trunk
(3) Palpate erector muscles of spine	Muscle not in spasm Nontender muscles	Muscle spasms of erector group Tender
(4) Evaluate range of motion of lumbar spine		Limited, difficult, or painful range of motion
b. Lasègue sign, or sciatic stretch test (to evaluate low back pain arising from nerve root irritation): client supine and performs single and alternating straight leg raising	Tightness may be felt, but there should be no pain	Pain felt with elevation of leg; then flex knee: pain should be gone as leg raised further
c. Evaluation of lumbar disk injury: client supine and performs alternating straight leg raising	Tightness may be felt, but there should be no pain	Pain felt with elevation of leg Dorsiflexion of foot causes feeling of pressure in lumbosacral area

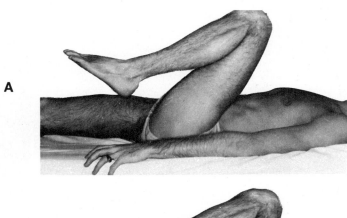

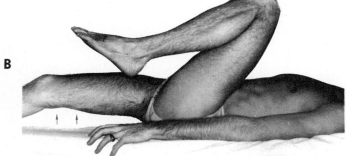

Fig. 14-44 Thomas test. **A**, Negative. **B**, Positive.

CLINICAL TIPS AND STRATEGIES

- **Assessment of the musculoskeletal system should begin as the client enters the examination room:** Use that time to observe ambulatory capabilities and body posturing.
- **Assessment of the musculoskeletal system involves an individual evaluation of bone stability, joint function, and muscle strength and function:** The clinical guidelines describe in detail what the examiner must do, as well as the anticipated response. It is essential that the examiner *continuously* keep in mind *what* bones, muscles, or joints are being evaluated, as well as the *normal* anticipated response.
- **Many clients complain of vague aches or muscular weakness:** The examiner must thoroughly explore the complaint, as well as perform a systematic evaluation. In addition, the examiner should watch how the client moves, postures, rises from a sitting position, takes off a coat, and so on.
- **A key consideration when evaluating the musculoskeletal system is symmetry.**
- **The client must be undressed:** This includes removal of shoes and socks.
- **A method of client assessment must be developed and maintained every time a client is evaluated:** It does not matter whether examination sequence is from the top down or vice versa.
- **How much and what type of musculoskeletal assessment each client requires will be individually determined:** A young athlete who comes to see the examiner for a college physical will require a basic screening evaluation, whereas a 67-year-old chronically ill woman will require a more thorough assessment. Many times the data collection and early inspection of the client's ability to ambulate, sit, and undress are keys for determining the necessary extent of the assessment.
- **The practitioner's purpose in collecting data about the musculoskeletal system is to assess the client's functional capabilities,** including activities of daily living: If the examiner isolates areas of distress or injury, the client should be referred to the physician for differential diagnosis.
- **While performing extremity evaluation, the examiner should incorporate the assessment of the skin, peripheral vascular system, and neurological system.**
- **If the examiner notes a difference in muscle size or in arm or leg diameter or length, a measurement should be recorded:** A circumference or length difference of more than 1 cm should be considered abnormal. The examiner *must* be careful to measure from the same spot bilaterally.
- **The technique for using a goniometer to mea-** sure the range of motion of a joint (Fig. 14-45) follows:
1. Start with joint in fully extended position.
2. When the joint is flexed as much as possible, the angle is measured. This is recorded as the angle of greatest flexion (AGF).
- **Although normal flexion angles of joints have been identified in this text, the examiner should realize that many deviations from these angles are considered normal for various individuals of different ages:** It is most important that the examiner compare one side of the client's body with the other when measuring angles and considering abnormal findings.
- **Many techniques can be used to measure muscle strength, from actual number scoring to evaluation of minimal or severe weakness:** We have used the make/break screening technique to grossly

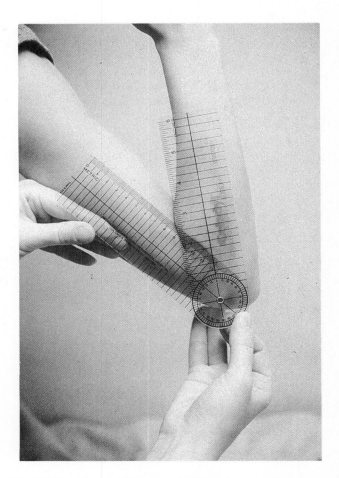

Fig. 14-45 Use of goniometer to measure joint range of motion. (From Seidel HM, Ball JW, Dains JE, Benedict GW: *Mosby's guide to physical examination,* ed 2, St Louis, 1991, Mosby—Year Book.)

evaluate the client's ability to make and maintain a flexed position while the examiner attempts to break the position. When using this technique, the examiner instructs the client to flex the limb or muscle group being tested and to maintain that position. Then the examiner exerts a steady, gentle retraction against the client's flexed position. The retraction should last 2 to 3 seconds for each position tested. The examiner should apply the same degree of retraction strength against each position being tested.

Although the results will be interpreted subjectively, the examiner will, with practice, determine what an abnormal response is for his or her own strength.

The following guidelines may be used to measure and grade muscle strength:

Grade	Normal (%)	Description
5	100	Full range of motion against gravity with extreme resistance
4	75	Full range of motion against gravity with some resistance
3	50	Full range of motion against gravity with no resistance
2	25	Full range of motion with gravity eliminated
1	10	Slight contraction visible
0	0	No contraction

An absolute baseline of muscle testing involves the client's ability to move the limbs or trunk against gravity (e.g., lifting the arm up in the air). Any client who has difficulty moving the trunk or limbs against gravity should be referred for further evaluation.

SAMPLE RECORDING: NORMAL FINDINGS

Muscular development and skeletal structure bilaterally equal, normal for age. No joint deformities, tenderness, or crepitations. Full active range of motion without pain. Normal spine curve without deformity. No spinal tenderness on palpation. Adequate muscle tone and strength bilaterally. McMurray, drawer, and Thomas tests negative.

 ## The Newborn

HISTORY AND CLINICAL STRATEGIES

- Neonates should be observed for general symmetry between their body sides (Fig. 14-46). Newborns assume their intrauterine positions (Fig. 14-47). Scoliosis, lordosis, or kyphosis is not normal and requires further investigation.

- Fractures may occur if the delivery is traumatic. Humeral, clavicular, and scapular areas should be examined carefully. Range of motion and spontaneous movement should be equal and symmetric. A lagging or flaccid extremity is abnormal (Fig. 14-48).

- Hips should be assessed for full range of motion (Fig. 14-49). Ankles and feet should be observed for signs of malformation. Preterm infants have limited ankle dorsiflexion.

- Neuromuscular factors help to assess gestational age. Posture, wrist motion, arm recoil, popliteal angle, scarf sign (arm movement in relation to head), and heel-to-ear motion provide half of the signs for determining maturity scores.

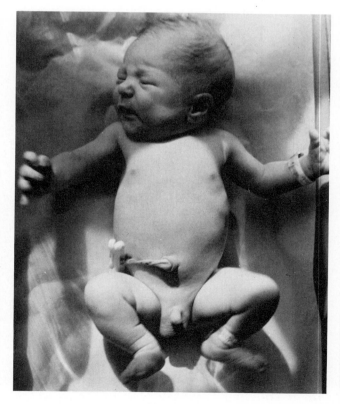

Fig. 14-46 Make a general observation of the musculoskeletal system of the neonate.

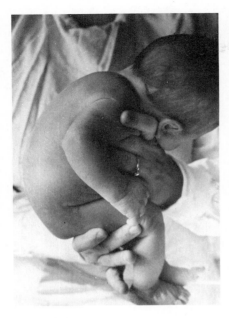

Fig. 14-47 Normal convex curvature of newborn's spine.

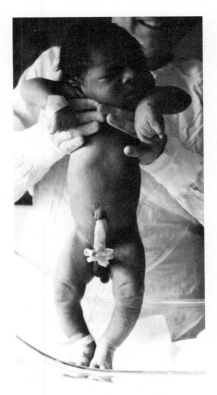

Fig. 14-48 Newborn shoulder muscle assessment.

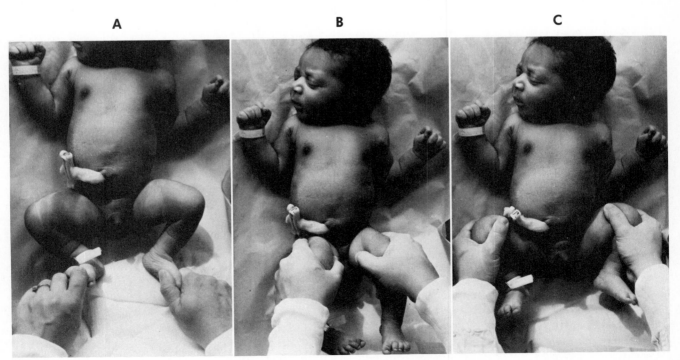

Fig. 14-49 Ortolani's test. **A,** Initial observation of symmetry.
B, Hips flexed at 90-degree angle. **C,** Hips externally rotated.

CLINICAL VARIATIONS: THE NEWBORN

CHARACTERISTIC OR AREA EXAMINED	NORMAL FINDINGS	DEVIATIONS FROM NORMAL
1. Spine	Spine is flexible; dorsal and sacral curves are convex No masses Easily moved in and out of fetal position	Asymmetric back curve (may mean absent vertebrae, ribs) Masses; hair tufts, dimples (may mean spinal bifida, pilonidal cyst, sinus) Posture: wrists, arms, heels, and popliteal angles vary with age of gestation
2. Extremities	Symmetric, equal Arms and legs kept flexed Full range of motion Five digits on each foot and hand No longitudinal foot arches Positional foot curves straighten with gentle pressure Hip and buttock creases even Arm and leg lengths even Abducts without difficulty	Preterm infant has no or few heel creases Asymmetry, limited movement Syndactyly (fused digits) Polydactyly (extra digits) Metatarsus varus (forefoot inversion) Talipes equinovarus (clubfoot) Erb's palsy (suggests birth trauma, shoulder dystocia) Uneven gluteal folds, hip clicks with abduction (hip dysplasia, dislocation)

The Child

HISTORY AND CLINICAL STRATEGIES

- Assessment of the child's musculoskeletal system can range from a basic functional screening examination to an extensive joint-by-joint evaluation. The extent of the actual evaluation should be determined for each individual child, based on subjective data as well as gross objective assessment. An active and coordinated toddler who demonstrates basic gross and fine motor functioning appropriate for age will require a less extensive musculoskeletal assessment than a 7-year-old complaining of joint pains and generalized weakness.
- To subjectively evaluate motor functioning appropriate for age, the examiner must be aware of normal values. Table 14-1 details the sequencing of motor development and approximate age of achievement. The practitioner should consider this sequence when collecting data base information. Any child who lags behind in two or more areas at any given age should be carefully evaluated. Although it is unrealistic to believe that all children develop at the normal rate, nonmastery of these criteria should serve as red flags indicating necessity of a thorough physical evaluation. Conversely, an active, playful, and maturing child who is on or ahead of schedule will need a less detailed evaluation. Some of the values in Table 14-1 have been extracted from the Denver Developmental Screening Test (DDST). Children who appear to be lagging behind in musculoskeletal development may be screened more closely through tests such as the DDST.

- The approach used to examine the musculoskeletal system in the child will vary greatly, depending on the child's age.
  1. Up to 6 months (see Fig. 14-46). Assessment should be done with the child undressed to the diaper and supine on the examining table or the parent's lap. Although the examiner should observe the symmetry and overall kicking and wiggling movement of the child, the actual palpation and joint and muscle evaluation is done with the child's passive participation. As the child becomes older, the examiner must position the child in a way that facilitates the evaluation. For example, place a 4-month-old in a prone position to evaluate his ability to push up on hands and roll from a prone to a supine position; place in a standing position to evaluate muscle strength of the legs.
  2. Six months to 1 year (see Fig. 14-71). Approach the child slowly. Start the evaluation by playing with his fingers and toes. As the child becomes accustomed to your touching, slowly move from distal limb evaluation to neck, hip, and spine evaluation. Much can be observed about the child's musculoskeletal and neurological systems by watching the child sitting and playing with hands and feet. If the examiner charges toward the child and frightens him, the child may stiffen up, cry, or decide not to cooperate. An inaccurate musculoskeletal evaluation will follow.

Text continues on p. 494

TABLE 14-1   Normal age and sequence of motor development in children

AGE	FINE MOTOR	GROSS MOTOR
4 weeks (1 month)	Following with eyes to midline	Turns head to side Keeps knees tucked under abdomen (Fig. 14-50) When pulled to sitting position, has gross head lag and rounded swayed back (Fig. 14-51)
8 weeks (2 months)	Follows objects well; may not follow past midline (major developmental milestone)	Holds head in same plane as rest of body (Fig. 14-52) Can raise head and maintain position; looks downward

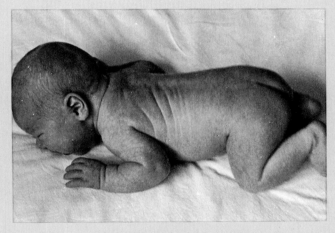

Fig. 14-50   From Whaley LF, Wong DL: *Nursing care of infants and children,* ed 4, St Louis, 1991, Mosby—Year Book.

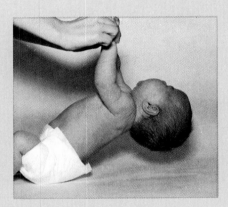

Fig. 14-51   From Whaley LF, Wong DL: *Nursing care of infants and children,* ed 4, St Louis, 1991, Mosby—Year Book.

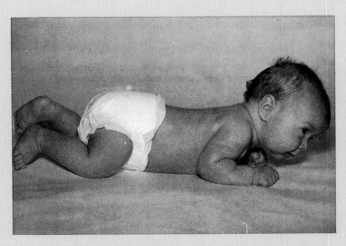

Fig. 14-52   From Whaley LF, Wong DL: *Nursing care of infants and children,* ed 4, St Louis, 1991, Mosby—Year Book.

Data from Frankenburg WK, Dodds JB: Denver Developmental Screening Test, *Denver, 1969, University of Colorado Medical Center.*

Continued.

TABLE 14-1   Normal age and sequence of motor development in children—cont'd

AGE	FINE MOTOR	GROSS MOTOR
12 weeks (3 months)	Follows past midline (Fig. 14-53) When in supine position, puts hands together; will hold hands in front of face	Raises head to 45° angle Maintains posture; looks around with head May turn from prone to side position When pulled into sitting position, shows only slight head lag (Fig. 14-54)
16 weeks (4 months)	Grasps rattle (Fig. 14-55) Plays with hands together	Actively lifts head up and looks around (Fig. 14-56) Will roll from prone to supine position When pulled to sitting position, no longer has head lag (Fig. 14-57) When held in standing position, attempts to maintain some weight support

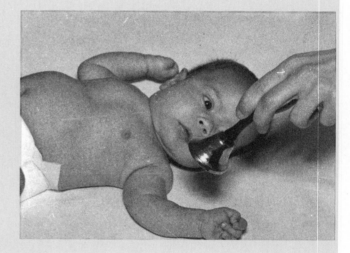

Fig. 14-53   From Whaley LF, Wong DL: *Nursing care of infants and children*, ed 4, St Louis, 1991, Mosby—Year Book.

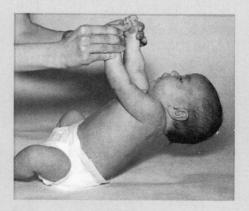

Fig. 14-54   From Whaley LF, Wong DL: *Nursing care of infants and children*, ed 4, St Louis, 1991, Mosby—Year Book.

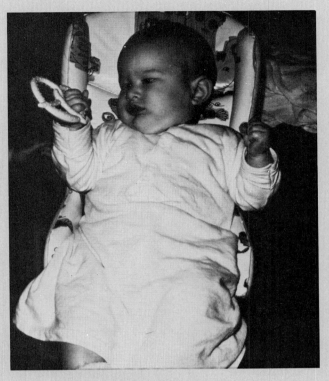

Fig. 14-55 From Bailey RA, Burton EC: *The dynamic self: activities to enhance infant development,* St Louis, 1982, Mosby—Year Book.

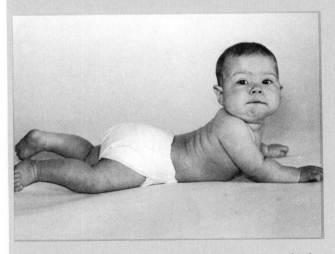

Fig. 14-56 From Whaley LF, Wong DL: *Nursing care of infants and children,* ed 4, St Louis, 1991, Mosby—Year Book.

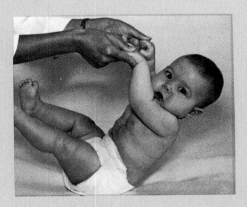

Fig. 14-57 From Whaley LF, Wong DL: *Nursing care of infants and children,* ed 4, St Louis, 1991, Mosby—Year Book.

Continued.

TABLE 14-1   Normal age and sequence of motor development in children—cont'd

AGE	FINE MOTOR	GROSS MOTOR
20 weeks (5 months)	Can reach and pick up object May play with toes (Fig. 14-58)	Able to push up from prone position and maintain weight on forearms (Fig. 14-59) Rolls from prone to supine and back to prone Maintains straight back when in sitting position (Fig. 14-60)

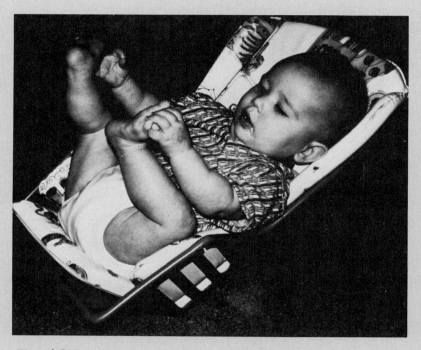

Fig. 14-58   From Bailey RA, Burton EC: *The dynamic self: activities to enhance infant development,* St Louis, 1982, Mosby–Year Book.

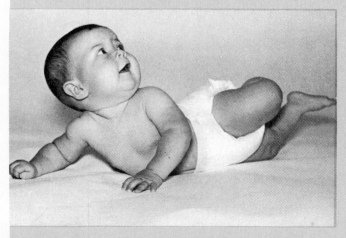

Fig. 14-59   From Whaley LF, Wong DL: *Nursing care of infants and children,* ed 4, St Louis, 1991, Mosby–Year Book.

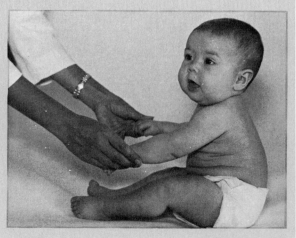

Fig. 14-60   From Whaley LF, Wong DL: *Nursing care of infants and children,* ed 4, St Louis, 1991, Mosby–Year Book.

AGE	FINE MOTOR	GROSS MOTOR
24 weeks (6 months)	Will hold spoon or rattle Will drop object and reach for second offered object	Begins to raise abdomen off table Sits, but posture still shaky May sit with legs apart and hands (arms straight) as prop between legs (Fig. 14-61) Supports almost full weight when pulled to standing position
28 weeks (7 months)	Can transfer object from one hand to another Grasps objects in each hand	Sits alone; still uses hand for support When held in standing position, bounces (Fig. 14-62) Pulls feet to mouth
32 weeks (8 months)	Beginning thumb-finger grasping (Fig. 14-63)	Sits securely without support (major developmental milestone) (Fig. 14-64)

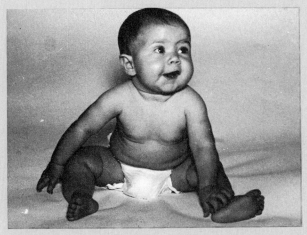

Fig. 14-61 From Whaley LF, Wong DL: *Nursing care of infants and children,* ed 4, St Louis, 1991, Mosby—Year Book.

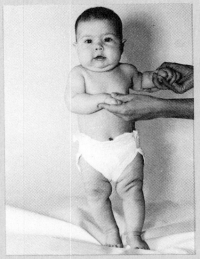

Fig. 14-62 From Whaley LF, Wong DL: *Nursing care of infants and children,* ed 4, St Louis, 1991, Mosby—Year Book.

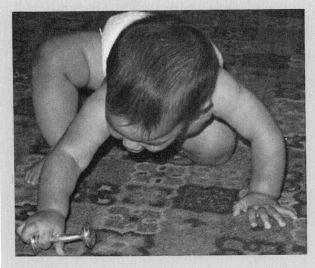

Fig. 14-63 From Whaley LF, Wong DL: *Nursing care of infants and children,* ed 4, St Louis, 1991, Mosby—Year Book.

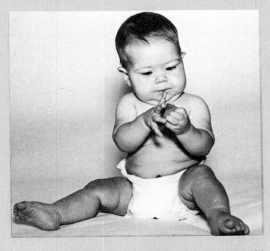

Fig. 14-64 From Whaley LF, Wong DL: *Nursing care of infants and children,* ed 4, St Louis, 1991, Mosby—Year Book.

Continued.

TABLE 14-1   Normal age and sequence of motor development in children—cont'd

AGE	FINE MOTOR	GROSS MOTOR
36 weeks (9 months)	Continued development of thumb-finger grasp May bang objects together	Steady sitting; can lean forward and still maintain position Begins creeping (Fig. 14-65); abdomen off floor (Fig. 14-66) Can stand holding onto stabilizing object when placed in that position; still may not be able to pull self into standing position
40 weeks (10 months)	Practices picking up small objects (Fig. 14-67) Points with one finger Will offer toys to people but unable to let go of object	Can pull self into standing position; unable to let self down again (Fig. 14-68)

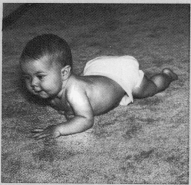

Fig. 14-65   From Whaley LF, Wong DL: *Nursing care of infants and children,* ed 4, St Louis, 1991, Mosby—Year Book.

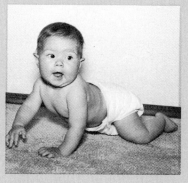

Fig. 14-66   From Whaley LF, Wong DL: *Nursing care of infants and children,* ed 4, St Louis, 1991, Mosby—Year Book.

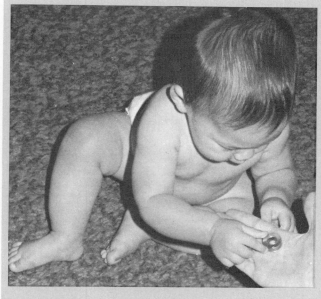

Fig. 14-67   From Whaley LF, Wong DL: *Nursing care of infants and children,* ed 4, St Louis, 1991, Mosby—Year Book.

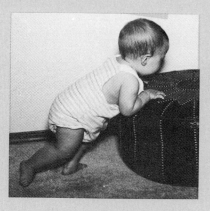

Fig. 14-68   From Whaley LF, Wong DL: *Nursing care of infants and children,* ed 4, St Louis, 1991, Mosby—Year Book.

AGE	FINE MOTOR	GROSS MOTOR
44 weeks (11 months)		Moves about room holding onto objects Preparing to walk independently, wide-base stance (Fig. 14-69) Stands securely, holding on with one hand

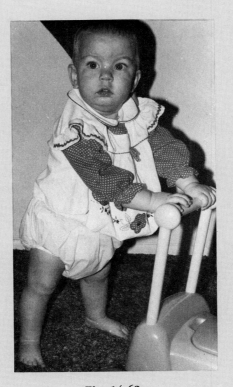

Fig. 14-69

Continued.

TABLE 14-1   Normal age and sequence of motor development in children—cont'd

AGE	FINE MOTOR	GROSS MOTOR
48 weeks (12 months)	May hold cup and spoon and feed self fairly well with practice (Fig. 14-70) Can offer toys and release them (Fig. 14-71)	Able to twist and turn and maintain posture Able to sit from standing position May stand alone at least momentarily

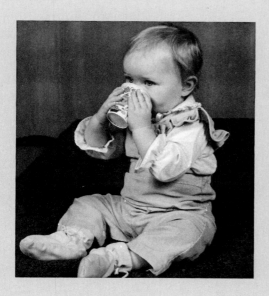

Fig. 14-70   From *The baby checkup book* by Sheila Hillman. Copyright © 1982 by Hillman Press. By permission of Bantam Books. All rights reserved.

Fig. 14-71

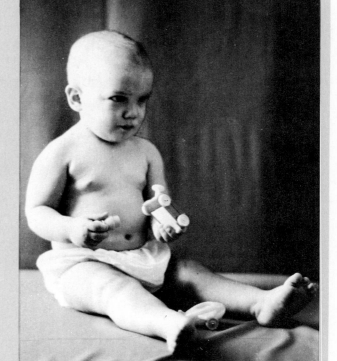

AGE	FINE MOTOR	GROSS MOTOR
15 months	Can put raisins into bottle Will take off shoes and pull toys (Fig. 14-72)	Walks alone well (Fig. 14-73) Able to seat self in chair (Fig. 14-74)

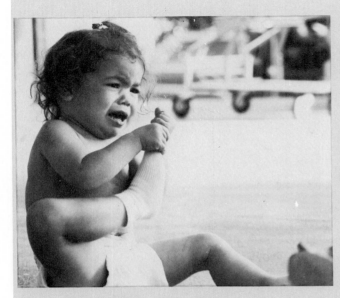

Fig. 14-72 From Powell ML: *Assessment and management of developmental changes and problems in children,* ed 2, St Louis, 1981, Mosby—Year Book.

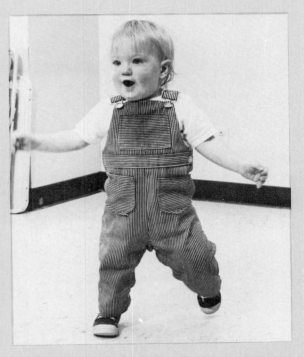

Fig. 14-73 From Powell ML: *Assessment and management of developmental changes and problems in children,* ed 2, St Louis, 1981, Mosby—Year Book.

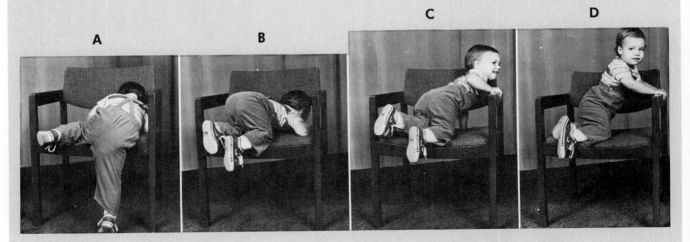

Fig. 14-74 From *The baby checkup book* by Sheila Hillman. Copyright © 1982 by Hillman Press. By permission of Bantam Books. All rights reserved.

Continued.

TABLE 14-1 Normal age and sequence of motor development in children—cont'd

AGE	FINE MOTOR	GROSS MOTOR
18 months	Holds crayon Scribbles spontaneously (major developmental milestone) (Fig. 14-75)	May walk up and down stairs holding a hand May show running ability (Fig. 14-76)

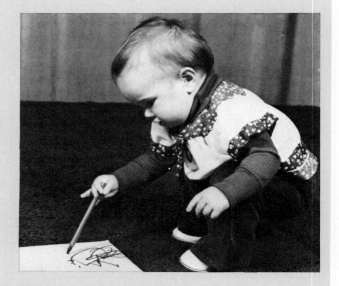

Fig. 14-75 From *The baby checkup book* by Sheila Hillman. Copyright © 1982 by Hillman Press. By permission of Bantam Books. All rights reserved.

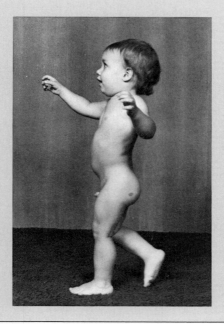

Fig. 14-76 From *The baby checkup book* by Sheila Hillman. Copyright © 1982 by Hillman Press. By permission of Bantam Books. All rights reserved.

AGE	FINE MOTOR	GROSS MOTOR
2 years	Able to turn doorknob Able to take off shoes and socks (Fig. 14-77) Able to build two-block tower (Fig. 14-78) Dumps raisin from bottle after demonstration	May walk up stairs by self, two feet on each step Able to walk backward Able to kick ball (Fig. 14-79)

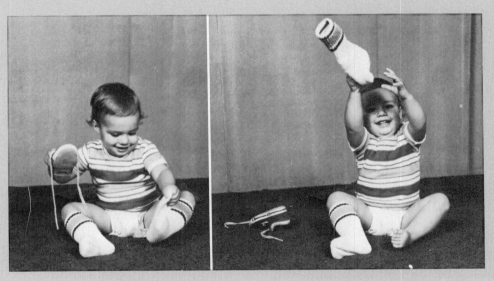

Fig. 14-77   From *The baby checkup book* by Sheila Hillman. Copyright © 1982 by Hillman Press. By permission of Bantam Books. All rights reserved.

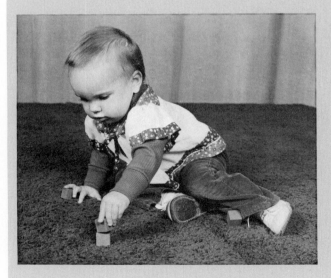

Fig. 14-78   From *The baby checkup book* by Sheila Hillman. Copyright © 1982 by Hillman Press. By permission of Bantam Books. All rights reserved.

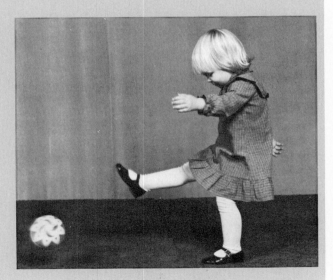

Fig. 14-79   From *The baby checkup book* by Sheila Hillman. Copyright © 1982 by Hillman Press. By permission of Bantam Books. All rights reserved.

Continued.

TABLE 14-1   Normal age and sequence of motor development in children—cont'd

AGE	FINE MOTOR	GROSS MOTOR
2½ years	Able to build four-block tower Scribbling techniques continue (Fig. 14-80) Feeding self with increased neatness (Fig. 14-81) Dumps raisins from bottle spontaneously	Able to jump from object Walking becomes more stable; wide-base gait decreases (Fig. 14-82) Throws ball overhanded

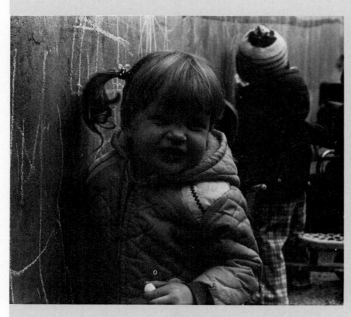

Fig. 14-80   From Weiser MG: *Group care and education of infants and toddlers,* St Louis, 1982, Mosby—Year Book.

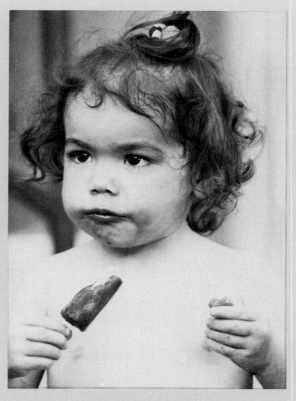

Fig. 14-81   From Powell ML: *Assessment and management of developmental changes and problems in children,* ed 2, St Louis, 1981, Mosby—Year Book.

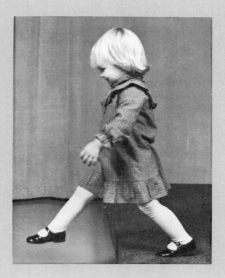

Fig. 14-82   From *The baby checkup book* by Sheila Hillman. Copyright © 1982 by Hillman Press. By permission of Bantam Books. All rights reserved.

AGE	FINE MOTOR	GROSS MOTOR
3 years	Can unbutton front buttons Copies vertical line within 30° Copies "O" Able to build eight-cube tower (Fig. 14-83)	Walks upstairs, alternating feet on steps Walks downstairs, two feet on each step Pedals tricycle Jumps in place Able to perform broad jump

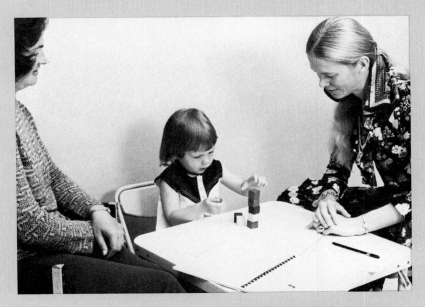

Fig. 14-83   From Powell ML: *Assessment and management of developmental changes and problems in children,* ed 2, St Louis, 1981, Mosby—Year Book.

Continued.

TABLE 14-1   Normal age and sequence of motor development in children—cont'd

AGE	FINE MOTOR	GROSS MOTOR
4 years	Able to copy " + " Picks longer line three out of three times Draws a stick man (Fig. 14-84)	Walks downstairs, alternating feet on steps (Fig. 14-85) Able to button large front buttons Able to balance on one foot for approximately 5 seconds (Fig. 14-86)

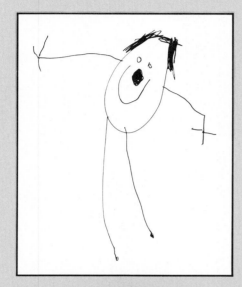

Fig. 14-84

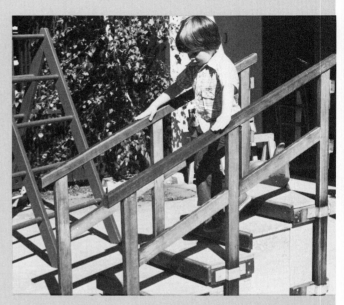

Fig. 14-85   From Powell ML: *Assessment and management of developmental changes and problems in children,* ed 2, St Louis, 1981, Mosby—Year Book.

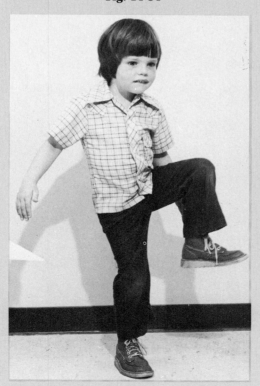

Fig. 14-86   From Powell ML: *Assessment and management of developmental changes and problems in children,* ed 2, St Louis, 1981, Mosby—Year Book.

AGE	FINE MOTOR	GROSS MOTOR
5 years	Able to dress self with minimal assistance (Fig. 14-87) Able to draw three-part human figure Draws ☐ following demonstration Colors within lines	Hops on one foot Catches ball bounced to child two out of three times Able to demonstrate heel-toe walking
6 years	Copies ☐ Draws six-part human figure (Fig. 14-88) Printing skills improve	Jumps, tumbles, skips, hops Able to walk straight line Able to skip rope with practice Able to ride two-wheel bicycle Able to demonstrate heel-toe backward walking
7 years	Able to read small print Able to print well (Fig. 14-89) Able to write in script with practice (Fig. 14-90)	Able to play hopscotch and to skip well Running, climbing abilities improve; becoming more coordinated

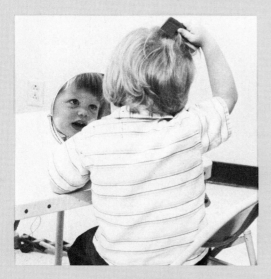

Fig. 14-87   From Powell ML: *Assessment and management of developmental changes and problems in children*, ed 2, St Louis, 1981, Mosby–Year Book.

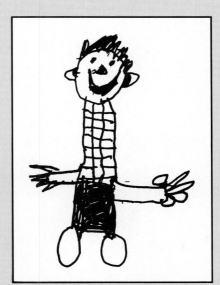

Fig. 14-88

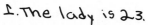

Fig. 14-89

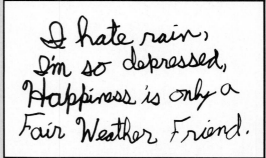

Fig. 14-90

Continued.

TABLE 14-1   Normal age and sequence of motor development in children—cont'd

AGE	FINE MOTOR	GROSS MOTOR
8 years	Handwriting skills show maturity	Movements become more graceful
9 years	Writing and drawing skills continue to show maturity and less awkwardness (Fig. 14-91)	Development of hand-eye coordination; assists with playing baseball, basketball, soccer (Fig. 14-92)

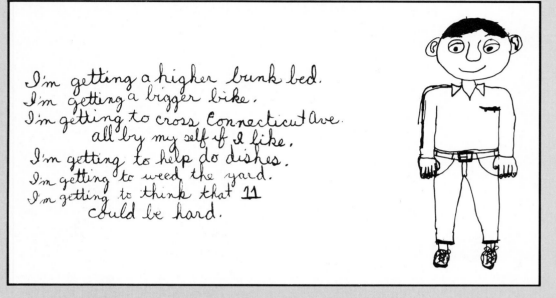

Fig. 14-91

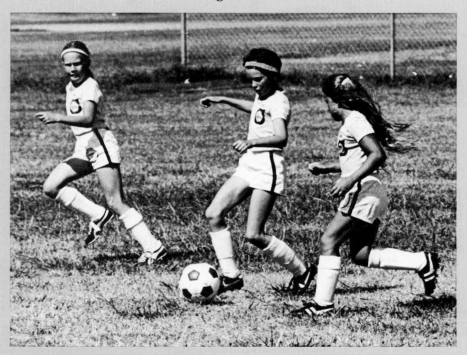

Fig. 14-92   From Klafs CE, Lyon MJ: *The female athlete: a coach's guide to conditioning and training,* ed 2, St Louis, 1978, Mosby—Year Book.

AGE	FINE MOTOR	GROSS MOTOR
10 years		Girls taller than boys
		Continued sports and coordinated activities (Fig. 14-93)
		Physically more active
11 years		May appear awkward because of preadolescent growth spurt
		May do less well in sports
12 years		Growth spurt begins
		Coordination decreases (Fig. 14-94)
13 years		Continues to have coordination difficulty
		Poor posture may become problem

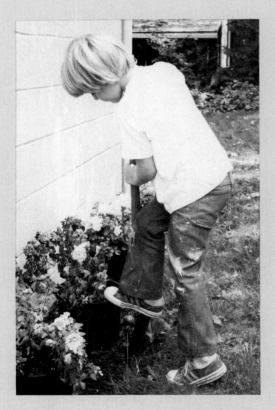

Fig. 14-93 From Powell ML: *Assessment and management of developmental changes and problems in children,* ed 2, St Louis, 1981, Mosby—Year Book.

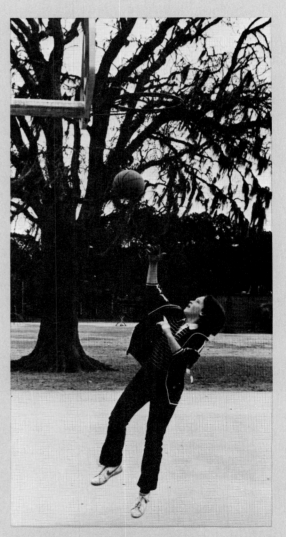

Fig. 14-94 From Godow AG: *Human sexuality,* St Louis, 1982, Mosby—Year Book.

3. One to 3 years (Fig. 14-95). The examiner should let the toddler show off a little: watch him walk, play with blocks, and climb onto the examining table. Much can be learned about the development and functioning of the musculoskeletal system through observation.

   Once the child is situated for the examination, the examiner should again start with the hands and feet. To evaluate the child's range of motion and ability to follow directions, a game of limitation might follow: instruct the child to "Do as I do;" if that does not work, games, such as catching and kicking a ball, building a tower of blocks, and playing peek-a-boo, may facilitate the examination.

4. Three to 6 years (Fig. 14-96). A slow, "let's play" approach is still helpful for the unsure preschooler. The examiner should watch the child undress and climb onto the examination table. The child should be ready to play hopping games and jumping, squatting, and bending exercises that will facilitate the physical evaluation. The challenge for the examiner with this age child is to invent techniques that will evoke cooperation from the child. Sometimes a game of "Simon Says" works. For example, say "Simon says keep your arm as stiff as a tree and don't let me push it down."

5. Over age 6 years. These children should be ready to cooperate fully with the examiner. The degree of cooperation will usually depend on how the examiner approaches the child. The brisk examiner may get less cooperation and fewer data than will the examiner who takes a few minutes to play with the child, watch him write his name, and demonstrate how strong he is by allowing him to show off his muscles and squeeze the examiner's hand.

• Many parents may express concern that their children

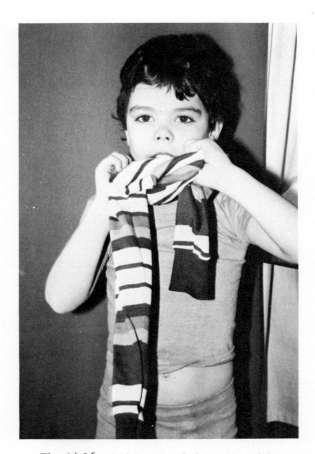

Fig. 14-96 Make a general observation of the musculoskeletal system of the preschooler.

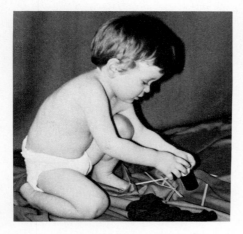

Fig. 14-95 Make a general observation of the musculoskeletal system of the toddler.

have foot problems. Following are some principles of foot evaluation:

1. Examine the foot for complete range of motion.
2. Do not limit the evaluation to the foot only; also evaluate for stability, deformity, and range of motion of the knee, hip, and spine.
3. Palpate the underside of the foot to evaluate for deformities of the forefoot or the hindfoot.
4. Observe for tibial torsion or bowing.
5. Observe the older infant or child walking without shoes. (*Note:* a cold floor on bare feet may distort the child's gait.)
6. Observe for muscular weakness or asymmetry.
7. Inspect the child's shoes for evidence of abnormal wear. Normal heel-toe gait wears the shoes more on the outer border of the heel and the inner border of the toe. Toddlers will normally wear down the medial edge of the shoe first.
8. Inspect the child's shoes for size and general fit.
   a. High shoes that cover the ankle are necessary only if the child walks out of low-cut shoes. The ankles are not supported by high shoes, nor is the support necessary.
   b. Shoes should be long enough to allow the thumb to be pressed between the end of the big toe and the end of the shoe while the child maintains a weight-bearing position.
9. Evaluate for flat feet.
   a. Before a child begins to walk, the foot does not actually have any arch.
   b. When a child first begins to stand, the feet normally pronate slightly inward (Fig. 14-97). The child assumes a wide-base stance, and the weight line normally falls toward the inner side of the foot.
   c. Between 12 and 30 months, the arch strengthens and the weight bearing falls more directly with the middle of the foot (Fig. 14-98).

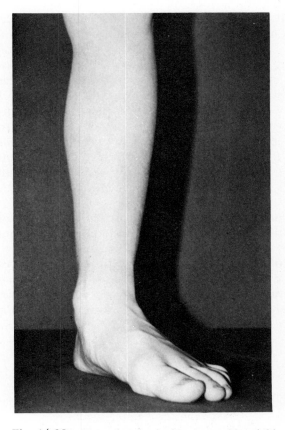

Fig. 14-98   Normal arch of a foot in an older child.

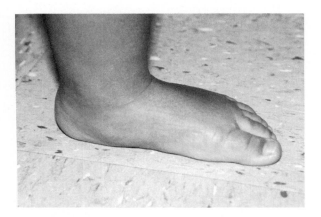

Fig. 14-97   Normal pronation of a toddler's foot.

d. Any child older than 30 months whose feet maintain a pronated medial position in which the medial border of the foot becomes prominent should be referred for further evaluation.

10. Evaluate for pigeon toes.
    a. Many children may demonstrate inward bending of the foot (either of the ankle or toes), the tibia (tibial torsion), or the femur (femoral torsion).
    b. If the examiner notes any inward bending of any of these areas, the child should be referred for further evaluation.

11. Evaluate toe walking. Babies and older children may demonstrate toeing downward or toe walking techniques. Toe walking may be normal, or it may be found in children with spastic diseases, congenital shortening of the Achilles tendon, early muscular dystrophy, or infantile autism. The examiner should manually dorsiflex the child's foot to evaluate the stretchability of the Achilles tendon. Any child with a tight or shortened Achilles tendon (dorsiflexion less than 20 degrees) should be referred. Likewise, any child demonstrating other musculoskeletal or neurological problems should be referred.

- Children may complain of muscular aches and pains. Although a thorough history and physical evaluation are mandatory, the examiner must also be aware of normal "growing pains." Boys between 11 and 18 years and girls between 9 and 16 years experience rapid growth spurts. At times the skeletal system grows faster than the muscular system; therefore the children may feel discomfort in their limbs.

- Curvature of the spine is a common finding in children, particularly during puberty. There are two types of scoliosis:
  1. Functional: this is the most common type found in young children. The spine is curved when the child stands, but if the child bends over to touch his toes, the curvature disappears.
  2. Idiopathic: the spine remains curved when the child is sitting, as well as when bending forward. There is pelvic tilt, and there may be a shortened leg.

     Even though all children must be evaluated for lateral spinal bending, teenagers are at high risk. Teenage girls (12 to 13 years old) are at highest risk to show development of scoliosis. Any child with noted spinal curvature should be referred for further evaluation. Most studies have shown that the approximate time of spinal curvature development is the same time that pubic hair develops. Each child deserves a careful inspection and palpation of the spine.

- Hip evaluation for possible congenital hip dislocation (Ortolani's test).
  1. Problem is found more in girls than boys.
  2. Parent may report difficulty diapering the child.
  3. Infant should be checked at every visit from newborn stage until about 2½ years of age.
  4. Technique (see Fig. 14-49).
     a. Baby supine, knees brought to 90-degree angle with back
     b. Examiner's hands on knees, index finger along

lateral thigh to feel click vibration if present
  c. Knees brought up, then flexed laterally; a newborn's knees should lie almost flat on bed (160 degrees to 175 degrees)
5. Abnormal findings:
  a. Pop, click, or snap during manipulation technique
  b. Bilaterally unequal response
  c. Sudden cry of pain during procedure
• Hip and knee evaluation for teenage boys, who are at risk for two specific types of skeletal problems:
1. Slipped capital femoral epiphysis. Even though this is a hip injury, the boy will usually have pain in the knee or lateral distal thigh. Many times this injury is precipitated by an activity, such as jumping off an object. Any boy with these complaints should be referred. Objective assessment data include the following:
  a. Deep palpation to the hip causes pain and tenderness.
  b. There is increased pain with abduction, internal or external rotation, or flexion of the hip.
  c. In severe cases the examiner may see a shortening of the affected leg caused by muscle spasm and upward displacement of the femoral head.
2. Osgood-Schlatter disease. This condition affects young athletic teenagers. The child will usually complain of knee pain at a point inferior to the knee on the head of the tibia. The pain may not be associated with a specific injury, but is usually aggravated with running or jumping.

  a. Inspection of the area will reveal a slight elevation.
  b. Tapping the area with the knuckles will cause pain.

• • •

The clinical guidelines for the musculoskeletal system of children vary greatly, depending on age and motor development. The examiner will spend a great deal of time developing routines for examining different ages. The guidelines and motor development sequence presented here represent normal findings for children of various ages.

Special techniques for evaluation of feet and shoes, muscle aches and pains, scoliosis, and hips have been discussed under "Clinical Tips and Strategies," p. 473. They must be incorporated into the following guidelines.

To use the guidelines, the examiner must know the developmental norms for the age of the child being examined and have the cleverness to collect these data during the examination. If the examiner does not have the cooperation of the child, an inaccurate evaluation will result.

By age 6 years a child should be able to cooperate fully with the examiner. Evaluation of a child less than 6 years of age will require flexibility in performing evaluation guidelines. The examiner must watch the child walk, climb, play patty-cake, jump, and skip to gather the necessary data. Other more specific suggestions, such as "kiss your knee" or "touch the toes," will aid specific joint and muscle evaluation.

Text continues on p. 508

CLINICAL VARIATIONS: THE CHILD

CHARACTERISTIC OR AREA EXAMINED	NORMAL FINDINGS	DEVIATIONS FROM NORMAL
1. Weighing and measuring child	(See Figs. 14-99 and 14-100.)	

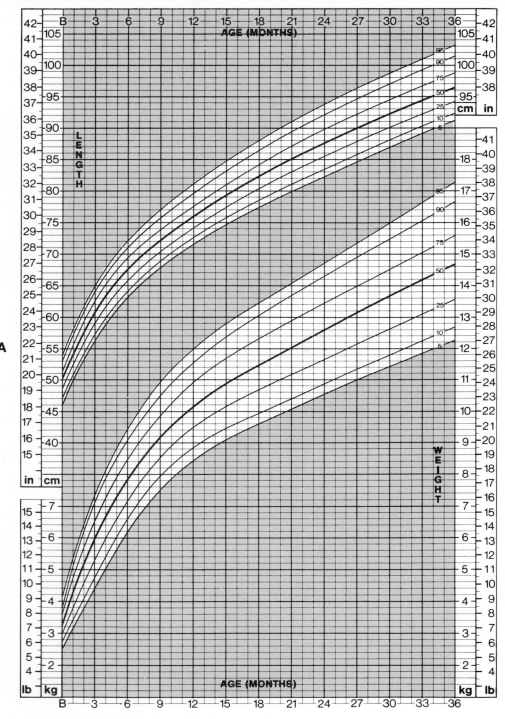

Fig. 14-99   A, Boys: birth to age 36 months—physical growth (length, weight), National Center for Health Statistics percentiles. (Modified from Hamill PVV and others: *Am J Clin Nutr* 32:607, 1979. Data from the Fels Research Institute, Wright State University School of Medicine, Yellow Springs, Ohio. Provided as a service of Ross Laboratories, 1980.)

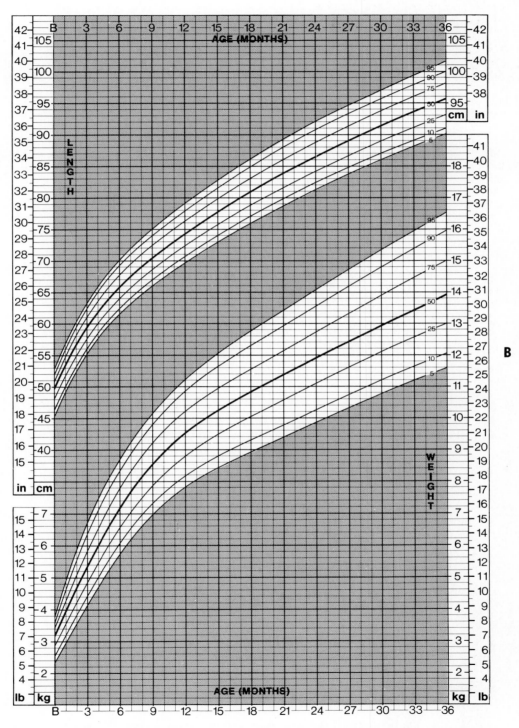

Fig. 14-99, cont'd **B,** Girls: birth to age 36 months—physical growth (length, weight), National Center for Health Statistics percentiles. (Modified from Hamill PVV and others: *Am J Clin Nutr* 32:607, 1979. Data from the Fels Research Institute, Wright State University School of Medicine, Yellow Springs, Ohio. Provided as a service of Ross Laboratories, 1980.)

Continued.

CLINICAL VARIATIONS: THE CHILD—cont'd

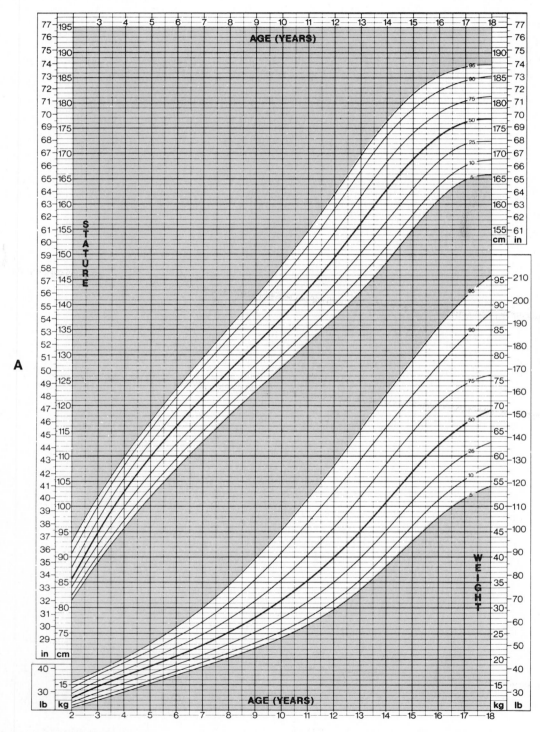

Fig. 14-100 A, Boys: ages 2 to 18—physical growth (stature, weight), National Center for Health Statistics percentiles. (Modified from Hamill PVV and others: *Am J Clin Nutr* 32:607, 1979. Data from the Fels Research Institute, Wright State University School of Medicine, Yellow Springs, Ohio. Provided as a service of Ross Laboratories, 1980.)

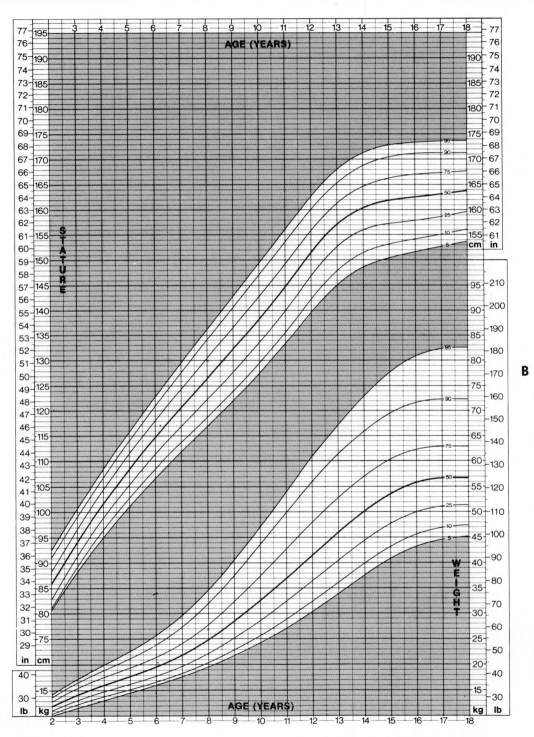

Fig. 14-100, cont'd **B,** Girls: ages 2 to 18—physical growth (stature, weight), National Center for Health Statistics percentiles. (Modified from Hamill PVV and others: *Am J Clin Nutr* 32:607, 1979. Data from the Fels Research Institute, Wright State University School of Medicine, Yellow Springs, Ohio. Provided as a service of Ross Laboratories, 1980.)

CLINICAL VARIATIONS: THE CHILD—cont'd

CHARACTERISTIC OR AREA EXAMINED	NORMAL FINDINGS	DEVIATIONS FROM NORMAL
2. Trunk (child lying or standing): spine	Spine straight 3 to 4 months: cervical curve develops as child holds head up 12 to 18 months: lumbar curve develops as child learns to walk (Fig. 14-101) Lumbar lordosis in toddlers Beyond 18 months: cervical spine concave; thoracic spine convex, but less than that of adult; lumbar spine concave, like that of adult (Fig. 14-102) No dimpling or bulges along spine Black children may more frequently show lordosis	Dimpling or bulges along spine, or thickening Lumbar lordosis in children over 6 years Curved spine either in standing or bent-over position
a. Bending to touch toes	Straight spine, both in upright and bending position Iliac crests of equal height Shoulders equal height Convexity of thoracic spine	Functional vs. idiopathic scoliosis (see "Clinical Tips and Strategies," p. 473) Unequal iliac crests in either standing or bent-over position

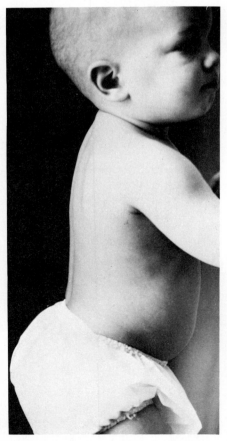

Fig. 14-101   Normal lumbar curvature of toddler's spine.

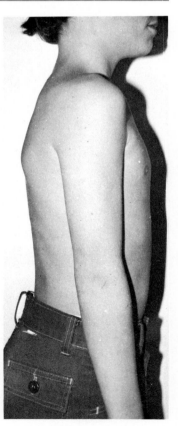

Fig. 14-102   Adult curvature in school-age child.

CHARACTERISTIC OR AREA EXAMINED	NORMAL FINDINGS	DEVIATIONS FROM NORMAL
b. Hyperextension	30° hyperextension from neutral position	Unable to hyperextend without losing balance or experiencing pain with hyperextension
c. Lateral bending	35° flexion both ways from midline position	Decreased flexion degree or experiencing pain with bending
d. Lateral rotation	30° rotation in both directions from forward position	Decreased rotation capability Rotation with discomfort
e. Spinal process palpation	Straight spine Nontender	Curvature of spine Tenderness Spasm of paravertebral muscles
3. Gait	Newly walking babies and toddlers have wide stance and wide-waddle gait pattern, which tends to disappear by approximately 2 to 2½ years (see Fig. 14-69) Gait should become progressively stronger, steadier, and smoother as child matures; any deviation from this or history of increasing falls or balance problems should be considered abnormal (also evaulate shoes; see "Clinical Tips and Strategies," p. 473) Smooth, regular gait with symmetrical arm swing	Unsteady or jerky Pain or discomfort Irregular or jerky trunk posturing Asymmetrical or jerky arm swing unrelated to gait
4. Head and neck a. Musculature	Symmetrical appearance	Asymmetry Atrophy or hypertrophy of muscles
b. Temporomandibular joint	Smooth movement of mandible	Pain, limited range of motion, or crepitus of temporomandibular joint
c. Posterior neck	Locating landmarks may be difficult in small child because of short neck and excess baby fat Locate C7, T1; nontender cervical spine	Tenderness, spasms Nodules
d. Range of motion of neck (1) Chin flexion	45° from midline	Limited or painful range of motion
(2) Head extension	55° from midline	Crepitus of cervical spine
(3) Lateral bending	40° each way from midline	
(4) Rotation of chin to shoulders	70° from midline	
e. Muscle strength of back (1) Chin flexion, position maintenance	With reasonable strength, unable to force head upright	Able to break muscular flexion before anticipated point
(2) Head hyperextension, position maintenance	With reasonable strength, unable to force head upright	Able to break muscular flexion before anticipated point
5. Hands and wrists	Smoothness; no swelling or deformities noted Fingers able to maintain full extension position	Irregular finger contour Swelling Deformities Tenderness

Continued.

CLINICAL VARIATIONS: THE CHILD—cont'd

CHARACTERISTIC OR AREA EXAMINED	NORMAL FINDINGS	DEVIATIONS FROM NORMAL
		Muscular atrophy
		Heberden nodes
		Long, spider or short, clubbed fingers
a. Range of motion of fingers and wrists		
(1) Finger extension	Symmetrical response	Asymmetrical response
	Smooth movements without complaints of discomfort	Pain during movement
	Full flexion and extension	
(2) Fist	Bilaterally equal response	Unequal response
		Decreased response
(3) Grip	Tight grip	Pain with movement
(4) Radial deviation	20°	Decreased movement
(5) Ulnar deviation	55°	
(6) Extension	70°	
(7) Flexion	90°	
b. Wrist strength		
(1) Wrist flexion, position maintenance	Bilaterally strong	Asymmetrical response
	Unable to break position*	Able to break position easily
(2) Wrist extension, position maintenance	Bilaterally strong	Asymmetrical response
	Unable to break position	Able to break position easily
6. Elbows		
a. Palpation	Skin intact	Swelling
	Smooth	Inflammation
	Surface nontender, without nodules or discomfort	General tenderness
		Subcutaneous nodules
	Lymph nodes not palpable	Point tenderness
		Lymph nodes palpated
b. Range of motion		
(1) Extension and flexion	160° full movement	Limited range of motion
	Bilaterally equal	Asymmetrical movement
	No discomfort	Pain at elbow
(2) Pronation and supination	90° each direction	Limited range of motion
	Bilaterally equal	Asymmetrical movement
	No discomfort	Pain at elbow
7. Shoulders		
a. Inspection	Skin intact	Redness
	Skin smooth and regular	Swelling
	Bilaterally symmetrical	Nodules
b. Palpation	Nontender	Tender, painful
	Smooth and regular	Swelling
	Bilaterally symmetrical	
c. Range of motion		
(1) Extension	180° from resting neutral position	Limited range of motion
	Bilaterally equal	Pain with movement
	No discomfort	Crepitations with movement
		Asymmetry
(2) Hyperextension	50°	Limited range of motion
	Bilaterally equal	Pain with movement
	No discomfort	Crepitations with movement
		Asymmetry

Throughout pediatric guidelines, according to resistance appropriate for age.

CHARACTERISTIC OR AREA EXAMINED	NORMAL FINDINGS	DEVIATIONS FROM NORMAL
(3) External rotation	90° Bilaterally equal No discomfort	Limited range of motion Pain with movement Crepitations with movement Asymmetry
(4) Internal rotation	90° Bilaterally equal No discomfort	Limited range of motion Pain with movement Crepitations with movement Asymmetry
8. Arm muscles: use make/break technique a. Deltoids	Bilaterally strong Unable to break position	Symmetrically unequal Weak response Pain during technique Muscular spasm
b. Biceps	Bilaterally strong Unable to break position	Symmetrically unequal Weak response Pain during technique Muscular spasm
c. Triceps	Bilaterally strong Unable to break position	Symmetrically unequal Weak response Pain during technique Muscular spasm
9. Shoulder muscles: lift infant under arms	Infant able to maintain position on examiner's hands	If muscles weak, child will slip through examiner's hands
10. Feet and ankles a. Inspection	Smoothness; no swelling or deformities noted Toes maintain extended and straight position Toenails intact and neatly trimmed Feet maintain straight position (See "Clinical Tips and Strategies," p. 473, for additional observation criteria)	Inward or lateral deviation of feet or toes; tight Achilles tendons Flat feet
b. Palpation	Smooth Nontender	Tenderness: diffuse vs. point Swelling Inflammation Nodules
c. Range of motion (1) Dorsiflexion and plantar flexion	Dorsiflexion 20° from midline position Plantar flexion 45° from midline position Bilaterally equal No discomfort	Dorsiflexion less than 20° because of tight tendon Limited range of motion Pain with movement Crepitations Asymmetry
(Instruct child to stand on toes) (2) Inversion	Inversion 30° from midline position	Inversion or eversion when foot at rest
(3) Eversion	Eversion 20° from midline position Bilaterally equal No discomfort	Limited range of motion Pain with movement Asymmetry

Continued.

CLINICAL VARIATIONS: THE CHILD—cont'd

CHARACTERISTIC OR AREA EXAMINED	NORMAL FINDINGS	DEVIATIONS FROM NORMAL
d. Muscular evaluation: maintain dorsiflexed position against opposite pull	Bilaterally strong Unable to break position	Unequal Weak response Pain during technique
11. Knee	Knees in direct straight line between hip, ankle, great toe	Deviation of line so that it maintains position of hip, knee, ankle, fourth or fifth toe Rotation of feet or lower legs (see "Clinical Tips and Strategies," p. 473) May be seen with systemic diseases such as polio, rickets, syphilis
	Valgus: medial malleolus >2.5 cm (1 inch) apart with knees touching; normal for children 2 to 3½ years old (may be present and normal in some children up to 12 years) (Fig. 14-103) Varus: medial malleolus touching, knees >2.5 cm (1 inch) apart; needs further evaluation for tibial torsion (may be normal until 18 months to 2 years of age)	

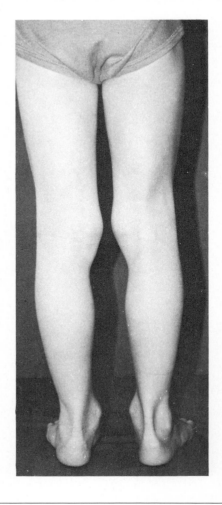

Fig. 14-103   School-age child: normal valgus position.

CHARACTERISTIC OR AREA EXAMINED	NORMAL FINDINGS	DEVIATIONS FROM NORMAL
	Smooth, symmetrical	Swelling, thickness
		Inflammation
		Inflamed, painful joints in black children may be sign of sickle cell anemia
		Enlargement of tibial tubercles in teenage boys may be sign of Osgood-Schlatter disease
a. Palpation of knees and popliteal space	Smooth, nontender	Bogginess
		Thickening
		Tenderness, redness
		Painful
		Nodules and swelling
b. Range-of-motion evaluation	130° from straight extended position	Decreased range of motion
	No discomfort or difficulty	Pain with movement
		Crepitations
12. Hips and pelvis		
a. Inspection and palpation		
(1) Babies to 3 years	Gluteal folds bilaterally equal	Difference in height of gluteal folds
	No click, snap, or dislocation felt	Click, snap felt
	Hip rotation of 160° to 175° bilaterally equal	Unequal range of motion
		Sudden cry during procedure
(2) Children over 3 years: use adult technique to evaluate		
(a) Knee to chest	120° from straight extended position	Limited range of motion
		Pain or discomfort with movement
		Flexion of opposite thigh
		Crepitations
(b) Hip flexion without bending knee	90° from straight extended position	Limited range of motion
		Pain or discomfort with movement
		Crepitations
(c) External rotation	40° from straight midline position	Limited range of motion
		Pain or discomfort with movement
		Flexion of opposite thigh
		Crepitations
		In teenage boys with slipped femoral epiphysis: much pain with external rotation or abduction of hip
(d) Internal rotation	40° from straight midline position	Limited range of motion
		Pain or discomfort with movement
		Crepitations
b. Muscular evaluation		
(1) Hips: flexion against examiner's pushing	Bilaterally strong	Symmetrically unequal
	Unable to break position	Weak response
		Pain during technique
(2) Hamstring		
(a) Leg crossing	Able to perform	Unable to perform
	Bilaterally equal and without difficulty	Performs with pain or great difficulty
(b) Bending of knee against examiner's pushing	Bilaterally strong	Symmetrically unequal
	Unable to flex knee	Weak response
		Pain during technique
(3) Quadriceps: extension of lower leg against examiner's pushing	Bilaterally strong	Symmetrically unequal
	Unable to flex knee	Weak response
		Pain during technique

The Childbearing Woman

HISTORY AND CLINICAL STRATEGIES

- Pregnant women should be assessed for musculoskeletal conditions that may complicate childbearing. A limp or unequal gait may indicate a pelvic deformity and a contracted pelvis, making vaginal delivery difficult.
- Often during pregnancy there is decreased thoracic cage expansion with thoracic kyphosis. Heart and lungs may be compressed, decreasing vital capacity.

CLINICAL VARIATIONS: THE CHILDBEARING WOMAN

CHARACTERISTIC OR AREA EXAMINED	NORMAL FINDINGS	DEVIATIONS FROM NORMAL
1. Predelivery	Lordosis, curvature of spine, is caused by weight of uterus Full-term uterus weighs about 12 pounds Backache; posture may cause musculoskeletal discomfort Ligaments and joints of spinal column and pelvis soften (from hormonal influence) causing strain and pelvic instability May feel aching, numbness, weakness in extremities Pulling of ulnar and median nerves from neck flexion and shoulder girdle slumping Muscle cramps, especially at night (may be from temporary blood shunting, hypocalcemia)	Strain (may be caused from exaggerated posture or activity) Preexisting conditions may become worse or exaggerated
2. Postdelivery	Neck, arms, and legs may ache from delivery posture and activity Posture and comfort soon return to state before pregancy	

 The Older Adult

HISTORY AND CLINICAL STRATEGIES

- The normal aging process is accompanied by numerous musculoskeletal changes:
  1. Decrease in bone mass, which results in increased vulnerability to stress in weight-bearing areas and predisposes to fractures
  2. Thinning (possible collapse) of intervertebral disks
  3. Calcification within cartilage and ligaments
  4. Less elastic tendons
  5. Decrease in muscle mass, tone, and strength (however, at age 60 the decrease usually does not exceed a 10% to 20% loss)
     a. Less ability to perform intense, sudden exercise
     b. Decreased endurance with exercise (less ability to hold isometric contractions)
     c. Decreased agility
- Risk factors. As with all other aging changes, these alterations occur at different rates in different individuals. The changes are gradual and not often presented as a complaint. The rate of change is greatly affected by a number of variables or risk factors.
  1. General physical health of client
     a. Decreased respiratory capacity and reserve
     b. Diminished circulatory supply
     c. Arthritic changes accompanied by symptoms

   d. Neurogenic disorders affecting voluntary muscle response or sensory alterations

   e. Other physical changes that are accompanied by symptoms that interfere with body function or fitness; pain, diminished vision, fatigue, and weakness

2. Obesity

3. Immobility, either short-term (2 to 3 weeks), related to injury or episodic illness, or long-term

4. Sedentary life-style (a hypokinetic state can perpetuate itself)

5. Depression

6. Inadequate nutrition and/or fluid intake

7. Mind-altering drugs (e.g., tranquilizers, sedatives, alcohol)

8. Fear of falling

9. Confusion or altered mental state (inattentiveness)

All the variables mentioned contribute to reduced physical activity, which in turn promotes and hastens the changes associated with the aging musculoskeletal system.

• Presenting symptoms related to musculoskeletal problems:

1. The major symptoms to inquire about are listed in the geriatric data base in Chapter 2, p. 47. These complaints relate to the following:
   a. General feeling of well-being
   b. Muscle function
   c. Joint and bone function and appearance
   d. Extremity function
   e. Back and spine function
   f. Gait
   g. Sleeping patterns

2. Further details about the following symptoms are offered on p. 448:
   a. Pain
   b. Gait difficulty
   c. Voluntary muscle function complaints
   d. Skeletal complaints
   e. Joint complaints

3. Additional symptoms that should be explored in detail follow:
   a. Weakness
     (1) Onset sudden or slow?
     (2) Isolated to a specific body part or generalized (e.g., difficulty swallowing, lid drooping, unilateral weakness, or weakness in feet, ankles, hands)?
     (3) Associated with any particular activity (e.g., stair climbing [how many], rising from a chair, walking on level ground)?
     (4) Occur at onset of activity or after activity has been sustained (how long or how much)?

  (5) Associated symptoms (e.g., dizziness, "black-outs," numbness or tingling, pain, tics or fasciculations, tremors, shortness of breath)

  (6) Associated stiffness of joints, spasms, or muscle tension (do these symptoms occur at night?)

  (7) Associated weight gain or loss

  (8) Associated mood or mental changes

  (9) Medications being taken

  b. "Restless" legs (usually at night)
    (1) Associated symptoms of back pain, muscle cramps in legs, numbness or coldness of extremities?
    (2) How is this condition relieved?

  c. History of injuries, falls (inquire specifically about all accidents, minor "spills," or injuries that are recent; client may not be aware that a pattern of increased stumbling, falls, or limited agility is emerging if injuries are not obvious or incapacitating)

  d. Decrease in height (ask client to estimate number of inches over last few years; last year)

• Osteoarthritis is described as a universal aging process that is usually noninflammatory and involves deterioration and abrasions of the articular cartilage and possibly formation of new bone at the joint surfaces. The examiner must determine whether joint and bone changes are creating symptoms or signs that alter the physical functioning of the client. It is estimated that 50% of individuals over age 60 years and 78% of those over age 78 years manifest signs or symptoms related to arthritis.

1. Risk factors:
   a. Advancing age
   b. History of excessive use of a given joint (or group of joints)
   c. Obesity
   d. Family history of arthritis (especially with involvement of hands and fingers)
   e. History of injuries to a given joint (or group of joints)
   f. History of joint abnormalities (e.g., laxness of ligaments)

2. Joints most frequently involved with symptomatic arthritic changes are weight-bearing areas:
   a. Knees
     (1) Client frequently notices crepitation. (*Note:* Crepitation can also be heard or palpated in normal joints.)
     (2) Pain, stiffness, and/or joint enlargement may be evident.
     (3) Quadriceps may atrophy because of disuse resulting from pain.

b. Hips
   (1) Pain may be local or referred to buttock or inner aspect of thigh.
   (2) Hip may be held in partially flexed and adducted position.
   (3) Hip extension and rotation are diminished.
c. Spine (cervical and lumbar areas most frequently affected)
   (1) Cervical crepitation during movement is noticed by client. Weakness, numbness, or sensory changes may be noticed in upper arm, forearm, and thumb and fingers. "Black-out" spells occasionally occur with neck rotation.
   (2) Spinal changes may result in stiffness, loss of lordotic curve, or exaggerated kyphosis.
d. Fingers
   (1) Fingers may manifest outward changes, especially distal joint enlargement or node formation (Fig. 14-104).
   (2) Range of motion may be limited because of pain.
   (3) Interosseous spaces may be atrophied as a result of decrease in use of fingers and hands.
e. Shoulders: pain experienced during movement, especially abduction
f. Ribs: arthritic changes in the costovertebral joint may produce localized pain during palpation or referred pain to chest wall
3. Symptoms are often increased by weather changes or prolonged immobility.
4. Temporary relief is often completely or partially provided by rest, heat application, or analgesics. (*Note:* Heat application can be a risk if the client does not check temperature of water or heating device; the client's sensitivity to heat may be impaired. Also, gastrointestinal complaints may result from frequent use of some analgesics.)

- Osteoporosis is described as a decrease in mass and density of the skeleton, affecting approximately 29% of the aging female population and 18% of aging males.* Involvement is more intense in the long bones and vertebral column.
1. Risk factors:
   a. Postmenopausal state (especially early menopause)
   b. Positive family history
   c. Smoking
   d. Alcohol consumption
   e. Small, thin stature
   f. Immobility

g. Cushing syndrome
h. Advanced diverticulitis (interferes with calcium absorption)
i. Hyperthyroidism (increased bone resorption)
j. History of limited calcium dietary intake
k. Heparin
l. Diabetes mellitus
2. Symptoms are often absent or mild; vague discomfort in back is experienced.
3. Vulnerability to fractures (of spine, femur, and pelvis) is greatly increased.
4. Loss of height occurs as a result of kyphotic changes and vertebral fractures.
5. Point tenderness of the spine is a signal of acute vertebral problems.

- If the examiner is confronted with a client who is disabled or incapacitated with discomfort or reduced function, the need for safety and performance of activities of daily living should be assessed. Detailed questions regarding activities of daily living are offered on p. 9 in Chapter 1, and inquiries and concerns for safety are described on p. 10 of Chapter 1.
- Physical assessment. The aging client who is not afflicted with illness or arthritic changes should be able to participate in the musculoskeletal assessment as it is described on p. 448. Normal range of motion of joints and muscular strength and tone should be the same as with the younger adult. Even if muscular strength is reduced by 10% to 20%, the client should be able to sustain the opposition of the examiner in the testing for muscular strength. The following general patterns may be noted:
1. Response to examiner commands may be slower.
2. General muscle bulk may be reduced. The arms and legs may appear thinner and flabby. (*Note:* Many "normal" clients [including young adults] cannot

*Smith RW Jr, Eyler WR, Melinger RC: *Ann Intern Med 52:773,* 1960.

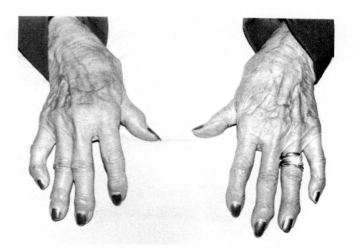

Fig. 14-104 Distal joint deformities associated with osteoarthritis.

touch their toes as they bend forward from the waist.)

- Early signs of musculoskeletal deviations. As physical disability and/or advanced aging changes encroach on the elderly client, the response to musculoskeletal physical assessment manifests an increasing number of deviations from normal findings. Some of the early (or more subtle) signs are the following:

1. Posture (stance) (Fig. 14-105). The appearance is one of general flexion (any or all of these signs may be evident).
   a. Head and neck thrust forward
   b. Dorsal kyphosis or kyphoscoliosis
   c. Flexion at the elbow and wrist
   d. Hips slightly flexed
   e. Knees flexed
   f. Broad stance (feet spread farther apart)
2. Gait should be carefully evaluated in *all* clients; they should be permitted to wear shoes.
   a. Gait phases
      (1) Heel strike (Fig. 14-106). Dorsiflexors that normally decelerate the foot before striking may be weakened. The flat of the foot strikes the floor. The client may lift the leg farther off the floor with each step.
      (2) Foot at midstance; other foot is pushing off (Fig. 14-107). Weakened quadriceps may not be able to stabilize the knee while the foot is bearing weight. Lateral and antero-posterior hip stability may not be maintained if gluteus muscles are weakened.

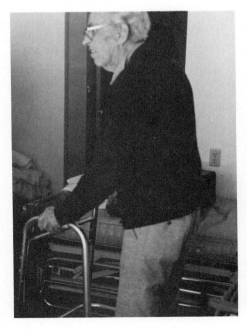

Fig. 14-105 Posture (stance) featuring head and neck thrust forward, dorsal kyphosis, hip flexion, and knees slightly flexed.

   (3) Foot is pushing off (Fig. 14-108). Weakened gastrocnemius and soleus unable to elevate the body to permit the other foot to swing freely.
      (4) Swing phase (Fig. 14-109). Swing may be shortened, foot may be lifted farther off the ground (marching style), or foot may just fall or slide forward (shuffling pattern).
   b. Arms may be held out to assist with balance or move in a rowing motion.
   c. Arm movement may be limited or absent.
   d. Normal vertical body motions that accompany push-off and stance phases tend to diminish.
   e. Upper torso may sway from side to side to assist with maintaining balance.
   f. Feet may be farther apart (broadened base to maintain balance).
   g. Steps may be uneven or tottering.
   h. Shortened step and shuffling propulsive gait with limited arm movement are associated with parkinsonism.
   i. Individuals who are weak or unsteady watch their feet as they walk.
3. Range of motion
   a. Most often limited because of pain (client stops movement abruptly).
   b. Weight-bearing joints (knees, hips, and lumbar spine) are frequently affected. Joints that are frequently used (cervical spine, shoulder, elbow, and fingers) may have limited range or pain associated with movement.
   c. Loss of full spinal range of motion, particularly in the lumbar area.
4. Muscle appearance and function
   a. Muscle wasting may be evident near immobile joints or in extremities that have limited motion (e.g., deep interosseous spaces often appear in severely arthritic hands).
   b. Mild bilateral muscle weakness (particularly of lower extremities) may not be noticed by the examiner during the opposition testing. Careful evaluation of gait and stair climbing may reveal more subtle weaknesses.

- Functional testing for activities of daily living. The examiner will be assessing many elderly clients who have permanent muscle or joint function loss or other altered health states that contribute to diminished physical ability. Beyond the assessment of body parts for functional capacity, the examiner needs to assess the client's ability to move about and to perform essential functions at home. The client often compensates for weakened muscle groups by altering posture or assisting movement with other body parts or special devices (e.g., cane, walker). The following assessment tests the ability and combination of major muscle groups to perform vital activities of daily living.

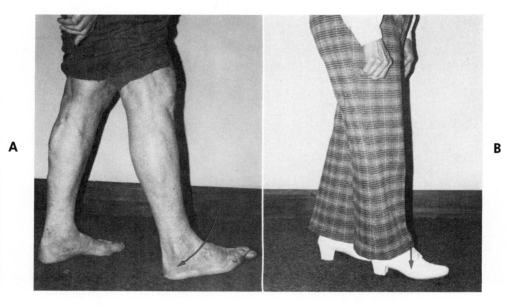

Fig. 14-106   **A,** Right foot demonstrating normal heel strike; left foot is bearing weight. **B,** Weakened dorsiflexors allow flat of right foot rather than heel to strike the floor.

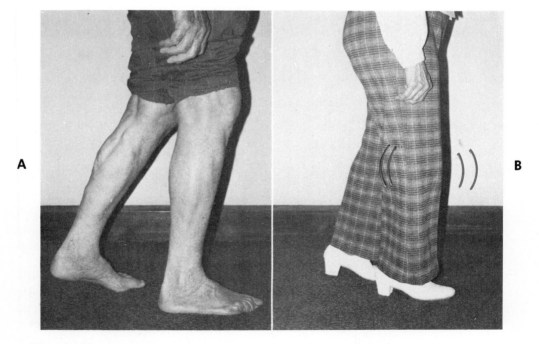

Fig. 14-107   **A,** Weight is shifted to the right foot, which is in midstance. **B,** Weakened right leg is wobbly while bearing weight (midstance phase). A weakened or painful leg or foot results in a shortened stride, since that weight can be shifted quickly back to the other foot.

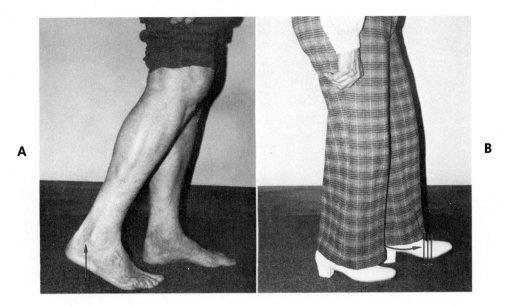

Fig. 14-108 **A,** Right foot demonstrates normal body lift at the end of push phase; left leg has swung free to a new step position. **B,** Weakened right leg is unable to lift the body sufficiently to permit left foot to swing freely.

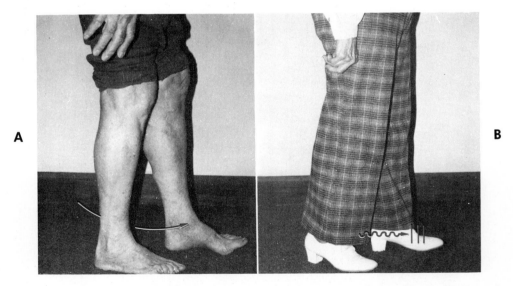

Fig. 14-109 **A,** Left leg demonstrates normal free swing. **B,** Left leg demonstrates shuffle-forward rather than free swing. Stride is shortened.

CLINICAL VARIATIONS: THE OLDER ADULT

CHARACTERISTIC OR AREA EXAMINED	COMMENTS
1. Client rising from lying to sitting position (Fig. 14-110)	Often rolls to one side and pushes with arms to raise elbow position Grabbing siderail or adjacent table may help client to pull up to full sitting position
2. Client rising from chair to standing position (Fig. 14-111)	May supplement weakened leg muscles by pushing with arms (*Note:* Chairs without arms provide no support for clients who need to push away to rise to a standing position.) Upper torso thrusts forward before body rises; feet spread far apart to provide broad support base

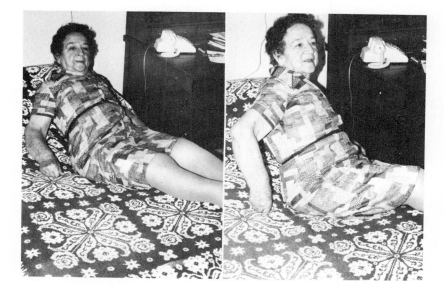

Fig. 14-110

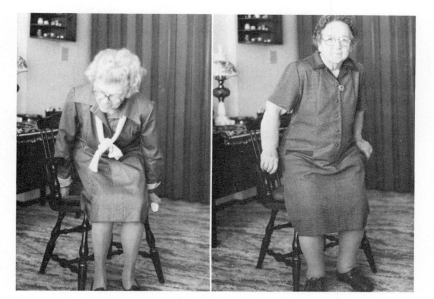

Fig. 14-111

CHARACTERISTIC OR AREA EXAMINED	COMMENTS
3. Client walking (Fig. 14-112)	Note heel midstance, push-off, swing phase, arm motion, and upper trunk motion (See comments about gait phases on p. 453)
4. Client climbing step (Fig. 14-113)	May use favorite leg (stronger one) to climb stair Will usually hold handrail for balance and may pull body up and forward with that arm
5. Client descending step (Fig. 14-114)	Often descends steps sideways, lowering weaker leg first and holding rail with both hands If unsteady or insecure, client often watches feet while lowering and standing on them

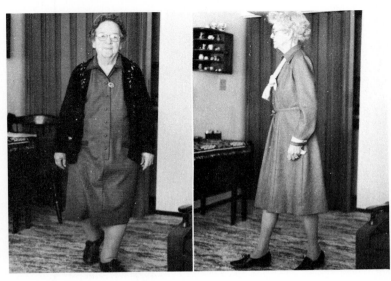

Fig. 14-112

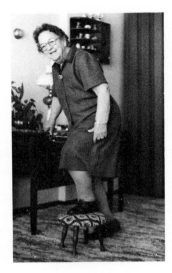

Fig. 14-113

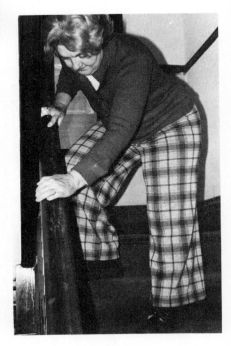

Fig. 14-114

Continued.

CLINICAL VARIATIONS: THE OLDER ADULT—cont'd

CHARACTERISTIC OR AREA EXAMINED	COMMENTS
6. Client picking up item from floor (Fig. 14-115)	Grasps or leans on table or handrail for support while lowering body; one hand may be firmly supported on thigh to assist in lowering and in elevating upper torso to standing position; client may avoid bending knees and stoop from waist
7. Client tying shoes while seated (Fig. 14-116)	Tests for manual dexterity and flexibility of spine Client may use footstool to reduce need for spinal flexion (*Note:* Velcro-fastened shoes are effectively used as substitutes for laces.)
8. Client putting on and pulling up trousers (or stockings) (Fig. 14-117)	Clothing often pulled over feet while client seated; final act of pulling up clothing demonstrates shoulder and upper arm strength

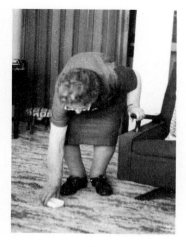

Fig. 14-115

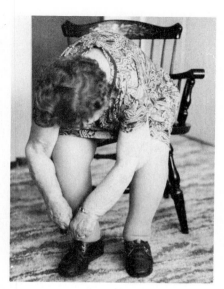

Fig. 14-116

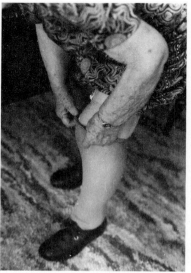

Fig. 14-117

CHARACTERISTIC OR AREA EXAMINED	COMMENTS
9. Client putting on sweater or jacket (Fig. 14-118)	Often applies first sleeve to weaker arm or shoulder; may use internal or external shoulder rotation to reach remaining sleeve and to thrust arm into it
10. Client zipping dress in back (Fig. 14-119) (or fastening brassiere)	Some individuals discard all garments that fasten in back; others find someone else to zip them up This maneuver tests ability to rotate shoulders

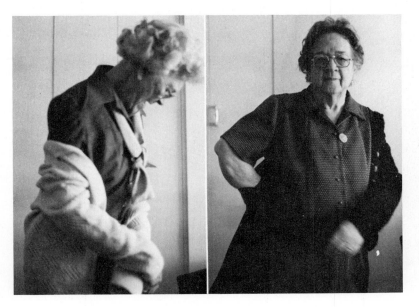

Fig. 14-118

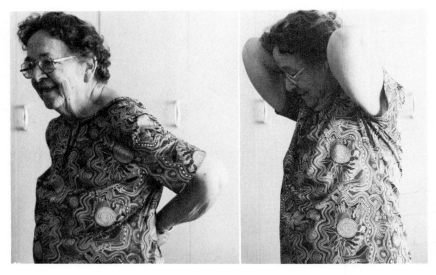

Fig. 14-119

Continued.

CLINICAL VARIATIONS: THE OLDER ADULT—cont'd

CHARACTERISTIC OR AREA EXAMINED	COMMENTS
11. Client combing hair in back and at sides (Fig. 14-120)	Shows ability to grasp and maneuver brush or comb, wrist flexion, pronation/supination of forearm, and shoulder rotation Some clients will turn back of head toward comb to accommodate diminished external shoulder rotation
12. Client pushing chair away from table (while seated in chair) (Fig. 14-121)	Demonstrates upper arm, shoulder, and lower arm strength and wrist motion; some clients will rise to standing position and ease chair out with torso

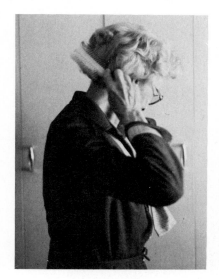

Fig. 14-120

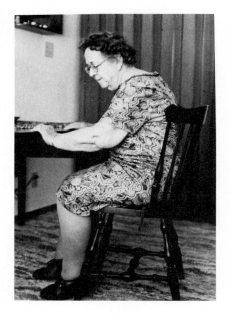

Fig. 14-121

CHARACTERISTIC OR AREA EXAMINED	COMMENTS
13. Client buttoning button, writing name, picking up paper from table (Fig. 14-122) (*Note:* Tooth brushing can be used to show a combination of manual dexterity, grip strength, wrist range of motion, and strength of forearm.)	Shows manual dexterity and finger-thumb opposition (*Note:* Velcro fasteners and pull-on styles are sometimes substituted for buttons.)

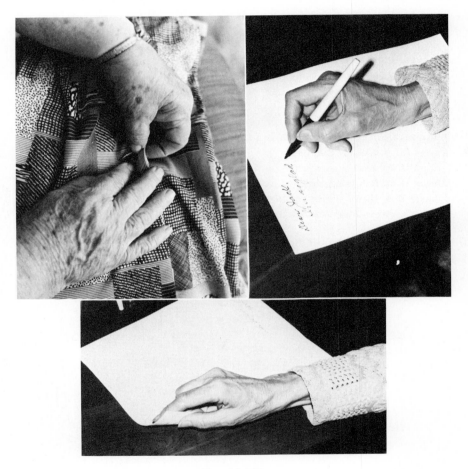

Fig. 14-122

Study Questions

General

Mark each statement as either "T" for true or "F" for false.

1. _____ The two articulating surfaces of a joint are cartilage.
2. _____ It is important to examine muscles both during relaxation and during contraction.
3. _____ *Varus* is a term used to describe an angular deviation of an extremity.
4. _____ Another name for kyphosis is *swayback.*
5. _____ Where there is muscle disease, the tendon stretch reflex is greatly altered.
6. _____ As the client ages, decreased muscle strength is caused by an increased amount of collagen in the muscle tissue, followed by fibrosis of the connective tissue.
7. _____ The kind of arthritis that occurs many times with the aging process is called *rheumatoid arthritis.*
8. _____ The normal lumbar curve is convex.
9. _____ The straight leg raise test is generally a good test to use in evaluation of a disk problem.
10. _____ The curvature seen in scoliosis is considered to be a varus deformity.
11. Painless nodules commonly found around the tendon sheaths of the wrist are:
    - ☐ a. Ganglia
    - ☐ b. Fovea
    - ☐ c. Tophi
    - ☐ d. Tenalgia
    - ☐ e. Rheumatoid nodules
12. The best instruction you can offer to a client who wants to know what to do in a case of a muscle cramp is:
    - ☐ a. Tell him to stretch the muscle fibers of the cramping muscle by placing the limb in a position that will stretch the affected muscle
    - ☐ b. Rub the area vigorously until the cramp goes away
    - ☐ c. Apply ice to the cramping muscle
    - ☐ d. Apply heat to the cramping muscle
    - ☐ e. None of the above

13. Basic evaluation of the musculoskeletal system of an asymptomatic adult should at minimum include:
    - ☐ a. Assessment of activities of daily living
    - ☐ b. Gait
    - ☐ c. Spinal curvature
    - ☐ d. Joint evaluation
    - ☐ e. Tissue evaluation around joints
    - ☐ f. Muscle mass evaluation
    - ☐ g. Muscle strength evaluation (make/break technique)
    - ☐ h. All of the above
    - ☐ i. All except e
    - ☐ j. All except f
    - ☐ k. All except g
    - ☐ l. All except c

The Newborn

14. Hip and buttock creases in a newborn should be:
    - ☐ a. Asymmetric
    - ☐ b. Uneven
    - ☐ c. Even
    - ☐ d. Unequal
15. A newborn's spine is normally:
    - ☐ a. Convex
    - ☐ b. Asymmetric
    - ☐ c. Dimpled
    - ☐ d. Inflexible

The Child

16. Which of the following children should be referred because of a lag in motor development:
    - ☐ a. Four-month-old Kara, who is unable to sit by herself
    - ☐ b. Eight-month-old William, who is unable to roll from prone to supine position and back to prone position
    - ☐ c. Nine-month-old Ryan, who is unable to pull himself into a standing position
    - ☐ d. Two-year-old Lynn, who is unable to build a four-block tower
    - ☐ e. Jason, age 3½ years, who is unable to skip

17. Behaviors for evaluating the gross motor development of 3-year-old Stephen are:
    - ☐ a. Able to jump in place
    - ☐ b. Able to walk up stairs, alternating feet on steps
    - ☐ c. Able to walk down stairs, two feet on each step
    - ☐ d. Able to pedal a tricycle
    - ☐ e. Able to walk a straight line, one foot in front of other
    - ☐ f. All of the above
    - ☐ g. All except c
    - ☐ h. All except e
    - ☐ i. a, b, and e
    - ☐ j. c, d, and e

The Childbearing Woman

18. Weight of a pregnant uterus may cause temporary:
    - ☐ a. Lordosis
    - ☐ b. Crepitus
    - ☐ c. Kyphosis
    - ☐ d. Arthritis

19. During pregnancy, ligaments and joints of the spinal column and pelvis:
    - ☐ a. Harden
    - ☐ b. Soften
    - ☐ c. Shorten
    - ☐ d. Shrink

20. Susan Mulligan, a 24-year-old pregnant client, comes to you because of a repeated "charley horse" in her right leg. Which of the following techniques would you recommend to her for stopping the muscle cramp: (Select the *best* answer.)
    - ☐ a. Massage the leg
    - ☐ b. Plantar flex the right foot
    - ☐ c. Dorsiflex the right foot
    - ☐ d. Elevate the leg from the hip

The Older Adult

21. By the time an individual is 70 years old:
    - ☐ a. He usually manifests a 50% loss of muscle strength
    - ☐ b. Arthritis of the hip and knee joints are symptomatic
    - ☐ c. He often manifests a longer endurance rate with isometric contractions
    - ☐ d. None of the above

22. Some of the risk factors associated with diminished physical functioning in elderly individuals are:
    - ☐ a. Sedentary life-style
    - ☐ b. Altered mental state
    - ☐ c. Obesity
    - ☐ d. Pain
    - ☐ e. Diminished circulatory supply to body parts
    - ☐ f. a, d, and e
    - ☐ g. a, b, and c
    - ☐ h. All of the above
    - ☐ i. a, c, and d

23. Early or mild weakness of lower extremities:
    - ☐ a. Is usually easily validated with make/break assessment procedures
    - ☐ b. Is always unilateral
    - ☐ c. May be identified by asking the client to climb a step
    - ☐ d. None of the above

24. The joints most commonly involved with symptomatic arthritis are:
    - ☐ a. Wrists
    - ☐ b. Knees
    - ☐ c. Hips
    - ☐ d. Ankles
    - ☐ e. Lumbar spine
    - ☐ f. b, c, and e
    - ☐ g. b, c, and d
    - ☐ h. a, d, and e
    - ☐ i. All of the above

25. In a normally functioning gait:
    - ☐ a. The gluteus maximus helps to stabilize the hip while one foot is in stance position
    - ☐ b. The tibial dorsiflexors decelerate the foot as it approaches heel strike
    - ☐ c. The upper torso often sways from side to side to maintain balance
    - ☐ d. None of the above
    - ☐ e. a and b

SUGGESTED READINGS
General

Bates B: *A guide to physical examination,* ed 4, Philadelphia, 1987, JB Lippincott.

Debrunner HU: *Orthopaedic diagnosis,* Chicago, 1982, Mosby–Year Book.

DeGowin E, DeGowin R: *Bedside diagnostic examination,* ed 4, New York, 1981, Macmillan Publishing.

Ebersole P, Hess P: *Toward healthy aging: human needs and nursing response,* ed 3, St Louis, 1990, Mosby–Year Book.

Freidmann LW, Cassvan A: Diagnosis: low back pain, *Hosp Med* 144, Nov. 1984.

Judge RD, Zuidema G, editors: *Methods of clinical examination: a physiologic approach,* ed 3, Boston, 1989, Little, Brown, p 285.

Kelley WN, and others: *Textbook of rheumatology,* ed 2, Philadelphia, 1985, WB Saunders.

Malasanos L, Barkauskas V, Stoltenberg-Allen K: *Health assessment,* ed 4, St Louis, 1990, Mosby–Year Book.

Norkin C, Levangie P: *Joint structure and function,* Philadelphia, 1983, FA Davis.

Prior JA, Silberstein JS, Stang JM: *Physical diagnosis: the history and examination of the patient,* ed 6, St Louis, 1981, Mosby–Year Book.

Rodts MF: An orthopedic assessment you can do in fifteen minutes, *Nurs '83* 13(5):65, 1983.

Strickland A: Examination of the knee joint, *Physiotherapy* 70(4):144, 1984.

Tanner JM, Davies PSW: Clinical longitudinal standards for height and weight velocity for North American children, *J Pediatr* 107(3):317, 1985.

The newborn

Auvenshine MA, Enriquez MG: *Maternity nursing: dimensions of change,* Belmont, Calif, 1985, Wadsworth.

Ballard JL: A simplified score for assessment of fetal maturation of newly born infants, *J Pediatr* 95:769, 1979.

Bobak IM, Jensen MD: *Essentials of maternity nursing,* ed 3, St Louis, 1991, Mosby–Year Book.

Judd JM: Assessing the newborn from head to toe, *Nurs '85* 15(12):34, 1985.

Kiernan BS, Scoloveno MA: Assessment of the neonate, *Top Clin Nurs* 8(1):1, 1986.

The Organization for Obstetrical, Gynecological and Neonatal Nurses (NAACOG): *Physical assessment of the neonate,* OGN Nursing Practice Resource, Oct. 1986, The Association.

Pillitteri A: *Maternal-newborn nursing: Care of the growing family,* ed 3, Boston, 1985, Little, Brown.

Scanlon JW, and others: *A system of newborn physical examination,* Baltimore, 1979, University Park Press.

Seidel HM, Ball JW, Dains JE, Benedict GW: *Mosby's guide to physical examination,* ed 2, St Louis, 1991, Mosby–Year Book.

Whaley LF, Wong DL: *Nursing care of infants and children,* ed 4, St Louis, 1991, Mosby–Year Book.

The child

Barnes L: *Manual of pediatric physical diagnosis,* ed 6, Chicago, 1990, Mosby–Year Book.

DeAngelis C: *Pediatric primary care,* ed 3, Boston, 1984, Little, Brown.

Frankenburg WK, and others: The newly abbreviated and revised Denver Developmental Screening Test, *J Pediatr* 99(6):995, 1981.

Nickel RA, and others: The infant motor screening, *Dev Med Child Neurol* 31:35, 1979.

Pillitteri A: *Nursing care of the growing family: a child health text,* Boston, 1977, Little, Brown.

Powell ML: *Assessment and management of developmental changes and problems in children,* ed 2, St Louis, 1981, Mosby–Year Book.

Whaley LF, Wong DL: *Essentials of pediatric nursing,* ed 3, St Louis, 1989, Mosby–Year Book.

The childbearing woman

Auvenshine MA, Enriquez MG: *Maternity nursing: dimensions of change,* Belmont, Calif, 1985, Wadsworth.

Bobak IM, Jensen MD: *Essentials of maternity nursing,* ed 3, St Louis, 1991, Mosby–Year Book.

Pillitteri A: *Maternal-newborn nursing: care of the growing family,* ed 3, Boston, 1985, Little, Brown.

Pritchard JA, MacDonald PC: *Williams' obstetrics,* ed 17, New York, 1985, Appleton-Century-Crofts.

Seidel HM, Ball JW, Dains JE, Benedict GW: *Mosby's guide to physical examination,* ed 2, St Louis, 1991, Mosby–Year Book.

The older adult

Burnside, IM: *Nursing and the aged,* ed 3, New York, 1988, McGraw-Hill.

Cohen SB: Arthritis—but what sort? *Geriatrics* 37(12):49, 1982.

Ebersole P, Hess P: *Toward healthy aging: human needs and nursing response,* ed 3, St Louis, 1990, Mosby–Year Book.

Eliopoulos C: *Gerontological nursing,* ed 3, Philadelphia, 1987, JB Lippincott.

Gilmore RL: Recognizing problems of the aging spine, *Geriatrics* 35(11):83, 1980.

Reich ML: Arthritis: avoiding diagnostic pitfalls, *Geriatrics* 37(6):46, 1982.

Reich N, Otten P: What to wear: a challenge for disabled elders, *Am J Nurs* 87(2):207, 1987.

Steinberg FU, editor: *Care of the geriatric patient,* ed 6, St Louis, 1983, Mosby–Year Book.

Tideiksaar R, Kay AD: What causes falls? a logical diagnostic procedure, *Geriatrics* 41(12):32, 1986.

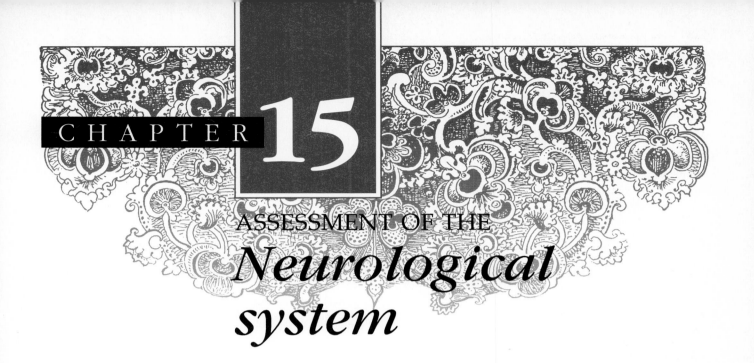

15

ASSESSMENT OF THE

Neurological system

VOCABULARY

ageusia Absence or impairment of the sense of taste.

anesthesia Partial or complete loss of sensation.

anosmia Absence or impairment of the sense of smell.

aphasia Absence or impairment of the ability to communicate through speech.

ataxia Inability to coordinate muscular movement.

athetosis Condition in which there are slow, irregular, involuntary movements in the upper extremities, especially the hands and fingers.

cerebellar system Receives sensory and motor input and coordinates muscular activity; also helps to maintain posture and equilibrium.

clonus Abnormal pattern of neuromuscular functioning characterized by rapidly alternating involuntary contraction and relaxation of skeletal muscles.

dura mater Tough, fibrous connective tissue that lies directly beneath the periosteum of the cranium.

dysesthesia Sensation of something crawling on the skin or of pricks of pins and needles.

dysmetria Inability to fix the range of movement in a muscular activity.

dyssynergia Failure of muscular coordination; also known as *ataxia*

extrapyramidal system Motor pathways lying outside the pyramidal tract that help to maintain muscle tone and to control body movements such as walking; includes nerve pathways between the cerebral cortex, basal ganglia, brain stem, and spinal cord.

fasciculation Localized, uncontrollable twitching of one muscle group that is innervated by a single motor nerve.

graphesthesia Ability to recognize symbols, numbers, or letters traced on the skin.

hyperesthesia Abnormally increased sensitivity to sensory stimuli, such as touch or pain.

hyperkinesis Hyperactivity or excessive muscular activity.

hypoesthesia Decreased or dulled sensitivity to stimulation.

hyposmia Defective sense of smell.

kinesthetic sensation Ability to detect the position of a body part when it is moved through space.

lower motor neurons Nerve cells that originate in the anterior horn cells of the spinal column and travel to innervate the skeletal muscle fibers. Injury or disease of this area will result in decreased muscle tone, reflexes, or strength.

myoclonus Twitching or clonic spasm of a muscle group.

paresthesia Abnormal sensation, such as numbness or a tingling feeling.

proprioception Awareness of posture, movement, and changes in equilibrium.

pyramidal tract Bundle of upper motor neurons that coordinate voluntary movements originating in the motor cortex of the brain; nerve fibers travel through the brain stem and the spinal cord, where they synapse with anterior horn cells, responsible for the coordinated response of voluntary movements; also called *corticospinal tract.*

Romberg test Evaluates an individual's ability to maintain a given position when standing erect with feet together and eyes closed.

spasticity Increased tone or contractions of muscles causing stiff and awkward movements; seen with upper motor neuron lesions.

stereognosis Ability to recognize objects by the sense of touch.

tic Spasmodic muscular contraction most commonly involving the face, head, neck, or shoulder muscles.

tremor Continuous involuntary trembling movement of a part or parts of the body.

two-point discrimination Ability to identify being touched by two sharp objects simultaneously.

upper motor neurons Nerve cells that originate in the cerebral cortex and project downward; make up the corticobulbar and pyramidal tracts and end in the anterior horn of the spinal cord; responsible for the fine and discrete conscious movements.

vertigo Sensation of moving around in space (subjective vertigo) or of objects moving about oneself (objective vertigo); results in disturbance of the individual's equilibrium.

ANATOMY AND PHYSIOLOGY REVIEW

The nervous system is divided into two fairly distinct structural categories: the central nervous system, which consists of the brain and the spinal cord; and the peripheral nervous system, which is made up of 12 pairs of cranial nerves, 31 pairs of spinal nerves, and the sympathetic and parasympathetic subdivision of the autonomic nervous system. The examination actually evaluates six major areas, as follows:

- Cranial nerves
- Proprioception
- Cerebellar function
- Motor function
- Sensory pathways
- Spinal cord and arc reflexes

Cranial Nerves

The twelve pairs of cranial nerves form the peripheral nerves of the brain (Fig. 15-1 and Table 15-1). Five pairs of the cranial nerves have only motor fibers, three pairs have only sensory fibers, and four pairs have both sensory and motor fibers.

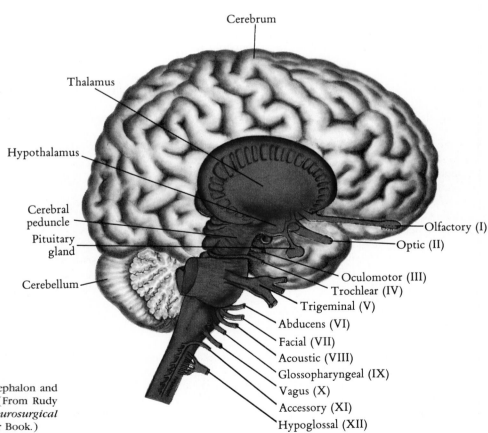

Fig. 15-1 Structures of the diencephalon and location of the cranial nerve roots. (From Rudy EB: *Advanced neurological and neurosurgical nursing,* St Louis, 1984, Mosby–Year Book.)

TABLE 15-1   The cranial nerves

NUMBER	NERVE	FUNCTION
CN I	Olfactory	Sense of smell
CN II	Optic	Vision
CN III	Oculo-motor	Pupillary constriction; extra-ocular movements
CN IV	Trochlear	Downward, inward movements of the eyes
CN V	Trigeminal	Motor—temporal and masseter muscles and lateral movement of the jaw Sensory—facial (ophthalmic, mandibular, and maxillary)
CN VI	Abducens	Lateral deviation of the eye
CN VII	Facial	Motor—muscles of the face except jaw; close eyes Sensory—taste: anterior two thirds of tongue
CN VIII	Acoustic	Hearing
CN IX	Glosso-pharyn-geal	Motor—voluntary muscles of swallowing and phonation Sensory—sensation of nasopharynx gag reflex; taste: posterior one third of tongue Parasympathetic—secretion of salivary glands; carotid reflex
CN X	Vagus	Motor—voluntary muscles of phonation and swallowing Sensory—sensation behind ear and part of external ear canal Parasympathetic—secretion of digestive enzymes; peristalsis; carotid reflex; involuntary action of the heart, lungs, and digestive tract
CN XI	Spinal accessory	Motor—turn head; shrug shoulders; some actions for phonation and swallowing
CN XII	Hypoglossal	Motor—tongue movement for speech sound articulation and swallowing

Adapted from Rudy EB: Advanced neurological and neurosurgical nursing, *St Louis, 1984, Mosby–Year Book.*

Proprioception, Cerebellar Function, and Motor Function

Proprioception, cerebellar function, and motor function affect three areas of coordination and motor function:
• General function
• Upper extremity function
• Lower extremity function

Motor function depends on the intactness of three areas:
• Muscles
• Functioning of the neuromuscular junction
• Cranial and spinal nerves

More specifically, proprioception and cerebellar function depend on the intactness of the upper and lower neurons and the cerebellar system.

The *upper motor neurons* originate in the cerebral cortex and project downward. These neurons make up the corticobulbar tract, which ends in the brain stem, and the corticospinal tract (or pyramidal tract), which ends in the anterior horn of the spinal cord. This tract is responsible for particularly fine and discrete conscious movement.

Malfunctioning within the corticospinal tract will cause a paralysis or spasticity response. Deep tendon reflexes will increase, voluntary functioning of fine motor ability will decrease.

The *lower motor neurons* originate in the anterior horn cells of the spinal cord, leave the spinal cord, and travel to and innervate the muscle fibers. Injury or disease affecting the lower motor neurons will result in decreased or absent muscle tone, reflexes, or strength. Local or general muscle wasting and atrophy, as well as fasciculations of affected areas, will be observed.

The *extrapyramidal motor neurons* originate in the cerebral cortex but lie outside the pyramidal or corticospinal tracts. Their function is to help maintain muscle tone and gross body movements, such as walking. Gross body functioning may still be maintained in the presence of a disease of the pyramidal tract because of the intactness of the extrapyramidal and lower motor neurons.

If the extrapyramidal system is being used to function, slow or sluggish voluntary movement, slowed coordination, and decrease in fine motor functioning will usually be observed. The reflexes will be normal.

The *proprioception* and *cerebellar systems* function to maintain posture and balance. Any malfunctioning of this area would impair muscle coordination or the ability to perform movements smoothly. Muscle tone may be decreased, and after the deep tendon reflex examination the limb tends to "swing."

Sensory Pathways

Intactness of the dermatomes and major peripheral nerves affects sensory function. Knowledge of the normal dermatome areas and the spinal nerves represented, as well as the major peripheral nerves and areas of sensation (Fig. 15-2), is essential for the evaluation of sensory function.

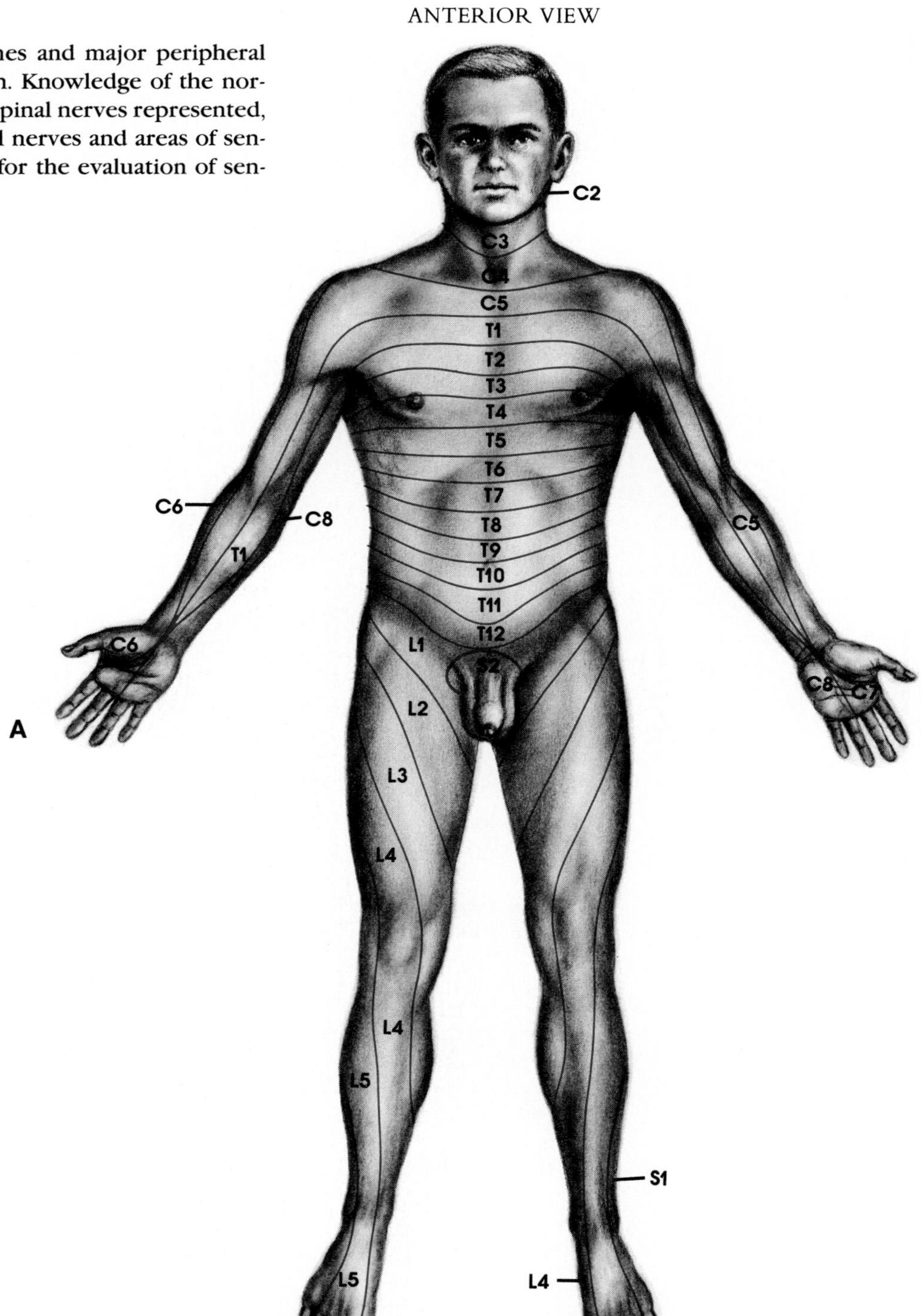

ANTERIOR VIEW

Fig. 15-2   Dermatomes of the body—the area of body surface innervated by particular spinal nerves; C1 usually has no cutaneous distribution. **A,** Anterior view. **B,** Posterior view. It appears that there is a distinct separation of surface area controlled by each dermatome, but there is almost always overlap between spinal nerves. (From Rudy EB: *Advanced neurological and neurosurgical nursing,* St Louis, 1984, Mosby—Year Book.)

POSTERIOR VIEW

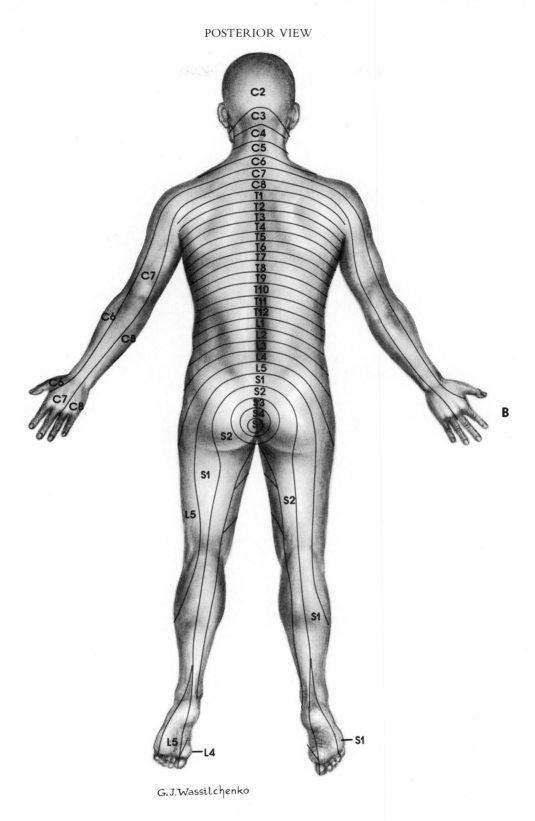

G.J.Wassilchenko

The sensory pathways start with the receptor sensors in the skin. This sensation is stimulated by the sensory receptors located in the skin, mucous membranes, muscles, tendons, and viscera.

The sensory fibers of the dorsal root carry impulses from sensory receptors of the body to the spinal cord. From here the impulses travel to the brain for interpretation by the cerebral sensory cortex. The impulses may alternatively initiate a reflex action when it synapses immediately with the motor fiber after a stimulus such as a tap on a stretched muscle tendon. In this case, the impulse is transmitted outward by the motor neuron in the anterior horn of the spinal cord via the spinal nerve and peripheral nerve of the skeletal muscle, stimulating a brisk contraction. Such a reflex is dependent on intact afferent nerve fibers, functional synapses in the spinal cord, intact motor nerve fibers, functional neuromuscular junctions, and competent muscle fibers.*

Spinal Cord and Reflex Arc

Assessment of the deep tendon reflexes allows the examiner to obtain information about the function of the reflex arcs and spinal cord segments without implicating other cord segments of higher neural structures. The reflex arc consists of five steps:

1. The receptor cells of the tendon are stimulated.
2. The nerve impulse travels along an afferent (sensory) neuron from the receptor cells by means of the dorsal root until it synapses with an anterior horn cell.
3. After the synapse the impulse is transmitted directly or indirectly to an efferent neuron.
4. The impulse travels along the efferent (motor) neuron by means of the ventral root until it innervates a skeletal muscle.
5. The skeletal muscle contracts.

*From Seidel HM, Ball JW, Dains JE, Benedict GW: *Mosby's guide to physical examination,* ed 2, St Louis, 1991, Mosby–Year Book.

Neural circuits in the spinal cord, when activated, display specific sets of motor responses. Reflex arcs form basic units that respond to stimuli and provide protective circuitry for motor output. Structures mandatory for a reflex arc are a receptor, an afferent (sensory) neuron, an efferent (motor) neuron, and an effector muscle or gland (Fig. 15-3).

The examiner should know the segmental levels of the following deep tendon reflexes:

Biceps reflex	C5, C6
Brachioradialis	C5, C6
Triceps	C6, C7, C8
Abdominal reflex	T8, T9, T10, T11, T12
Patellar reflex	L2, L3, L4
Achilles tendon reflex	L5, S1, S2
Plantar reflex	L4, L5, S1, S2

• • •

Although the techniques of the neurological examination are fairly easy to implement, the interpretation of findings is complex. The examiner is challenged to understand the physiological interpretations of the elicited responses during neurological testing. References for response interpretations are listed under the suggested readings for this chapter.

Assessment of the neurological system may range from a basic screening of function to a highly detailed and lengthy process. This chapter details the process for performing a *screening* neurological examination for asymptomatic clients. The examination evaluates six major areas:

• Mental assessment and speech patterns
• Cranial nerves
• Proprioception and cerebellar function
• Muscular function
• Sensory function
• Reflex function

If the examiner identifies abnormalities in any of the findings, a more detailed evaluation and referral are warranted.

Fig. 15-3   Cross section of the spinal cord showing a simple reflex arc. (From Rudy EB: *Advanced neurological and neurosurgical nursing,* St Louis, 1984, Mosby–Year Book.)

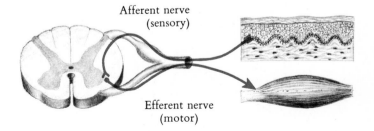

Afferent nerve (sensory)

Efferent nerve (motor)

COGNITIVE OBJECTIVES

At the end of this chapter the learner will demonstrate knowledge of assessment of the neurological system by the ability to do the following:

- Apply the terms that are listed in the vocabulary section.
- List each of the 12 cranial nerves and define the tests used to assess their integrity and the normal and abnormal responses.
- List the functions of the cerebellum and define the tests used to assess its integrity and the normal and abnormal responses.
- Describe the differences between the upper and lower motor neurons.
- Describe the differences between the pyramidal and extrapyramidal tracts and define the tests used to assess their integrity and the normal and abnormal responses.
- List the sensory modalities usually tested during a screening neurological examination and discuss the normal and abnormal responses.

CLINICAL OUTLINE

At the end of this chapter the learner will perform a systematic assessment of the neurological system, demonstrating the ability to do the following:

- Obtain a health history appropriate to the screening evaluation of the neurological system.
- Demonstrate testing of the cranial nerves.
- Demonstrate testing methods to evaluate the intactness of the proprioception and cerebellar systems.
  1. Use two techniques to evaluate general intactness
  2. Use two techniques to evaluate upper extremity intactness.
  3. Use one method to evaluate lower extremity intactness.
- Demonstrate testing methods to evaluate the intactness of sensation, including:
  1. Light-touch sensation
  2. Painful sensation
  3. Vibratory sensation
- Demonstrate one method for evaluating cortical and discriminatory forms of sensation.
- Demonstrate testing of the deep tendon reflexes, including biceps, triceps, brachioradialis, patellar, and Achilles reflexes.
- Demonstrate testing of pathological reflexes, including Babinski response and the test for ankle clonus.
- Summarize results of the assessment with a written description of findings.

HISTORY

- Any positive finding collected during the screening history should be further explored to describe its characteristics, as well as its relation to the client's ability to function. For example, if a client complains of shooting pains in the right leg, the examiner should describe (1) the characteristics of the leg pain (symptom analysis) and (2) how that leg pain interferes with activities of daily living.
- Complaints such as weakness, nervousness, tremors, or tics should be fully investigated regarding symptoms analysis, as well as how they interfere with the client's ability to maintain activities of daily living.
- Clients with complaints of balance problems need further questioning to determine how that problem is precipitated (i.e., position, time of day, related activity).
- The term *convulsions* has many meanings. If the client gives this complaint, in-depth data must be collected to document what this term means to the client. Note the following:
  1. What happens to the client's eyes during a convulsion?
  2. Parts of the body involved?
  3. Muscles flaccid versus stiff; tense versus twitching?
  4. How long does it last?
  5. How many times during the past day, week, month, year, years?
  6. Current medications?
  7. Cause?
  8. Interference with activities of daily living, driving, occupation?
- Head injury and headache history profiles are discussed under "History" in Chapter 4, p. 93.
- For the client complaining of pain associated with the neurological system, symptom analysis should be performed. The following may be helpful in evaluating the characteristics of that pain:
  1. Quality of pain: dull ache, throbbing, sharp or stabbing, burning, pressing, stinging, cramping, gnawing, pricking, shooting
  2. Associated manifestation: crying, decreased activities, sweating, muscle rigidity or tremor, impaired mental processes or concentration
- Objective data can be collected during the history session by noting evidence of such factors as abnormalities in speech, language function, memory, emotional status, and judgment.

Text continues on p. 548.

CLINICAL GUIDELINES

ASSESSMENT PROCEDURE	EVALUATION	
	NORMAL FINDINGS	DEVIATIONS FROM NORMAL

1. Gather equipment necessary to perform the screening neurological examination
  a. Penlight
  b. Tongue blade
  c. Safety pin
  d. Tuning fork (200 to 400 cps)
  e. Cotton wisp
  f. Percussion hammer
  g. Aromatic materials		

Mental and speech pattern (Mental health status was discussed in Chapter 2) 1. Speech pattern: assess during data base collection	Client gives information requested Speech smooth and flowing Logical thought process Able to relate past events Voice tone has inflections Strong voice; able to increase volume Clear voice	Error in choice of words or syllables Difficulty in articulation: may involve thought process, tongue, or lips Slurred speech (tone sounds slurred) Poorly coordinated or irregular speech Monotone voice Weak voice Nasal tone, rasping or hoarse, whisper voice Stuttering
Cranial nerves 1. CN I: olfactory nerve—obtain information through history or instruct client to close eyes and properly identify aromatic substance (coffee, toothpaste, orange, oil of clove) held under the nose (Fig. 15-4); test one nostril at a time	Client correctly identifies item and odor	Unable to smell anything Incorrect identification of odor being tested

2. CN II: optic nerve (Fig. 15-5) (described in Chapter 7)
  a. Test visual acuity
  b. Funduscopy examination
  c. Visual fields by confrontation
	As discussed in Chapter 7	As discussed in Chapter 7

3. CN III: oculomotor nerve (Fig. 15-6) (described in Chapter 7)	As discussed in Chapter 7	As discussed in Chapter 7
4. CN IV: trochlear nerve (Fig. 15-7) (described in Chapter 7)	As discussed in Chapter 7	As discussed in Chapter 7

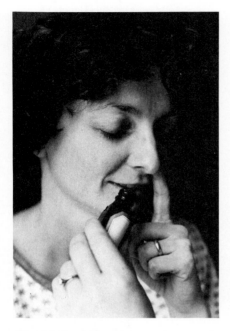

Fig. 15-4 Evaluating CN I (olfactory).

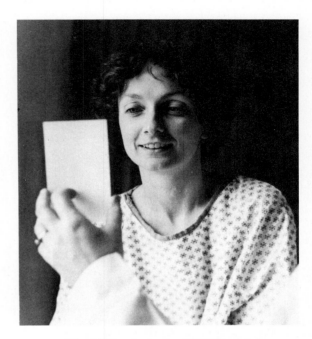

Fig. 15-5 Evaluating CN II (optic).

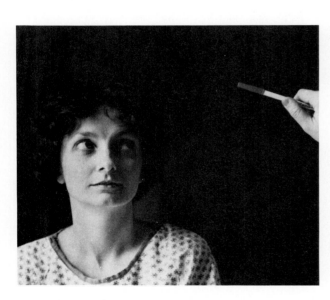

Fig. 15-6 Evaluating CN III (oculomotor).

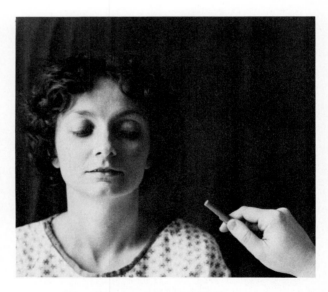

Fig. 15-7 Evaluating CN IV (trochlear).

Continued.

CLINICAL GUIDELINES—cont'd

ASSESSMENT PROCEDURE	EVALUATION	
	NORMAL FINDINGS	DEVIATIONS FROM NORMAL
Cranial nerves—cont'd		
5. CN V: trigeminal nerve		
a. Test *motor* function, instructing client to clench the teeth; then palpate temporal and masseter muscles (Fig. 15-8)	Bilaterally strong muscle contractions	Inequality in muscle contractions Pain with muscle contractions Twitching Asymmetry in movement of jaw
b. Test *sensory* function with client's eyes closed		
(1) Light sensation: wipe cotton wisp lightly over client's anterior scalp and paranasal sinuses (Fig. 15-9)	Tickle sensation equally present over palpated areas	Decreased or unequal sensation

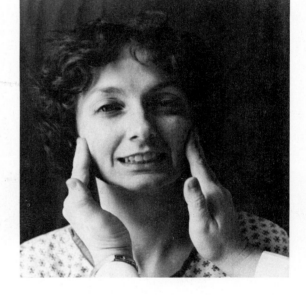

Fig. 15-8   Evaluating CN V (trigeminal—motor).

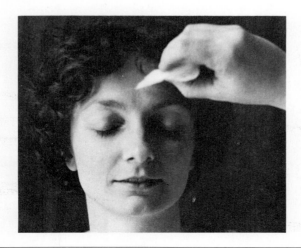

Fig. 15-9   Evaluating CN V (trigeminal—light sensory).

	EVALUATION	
ASSESSMENT PROCEDURE	**NORMAL FINDINGS**	**DEVIATIONS FROM NORMAL**
(2) Deep sensation: use alternating blunt and sharp ends of safety pin over client's forehead and paranasal sinus areas (Fig. 15-10)	Able to feel pressure and pain equally throughout Able to differentiate between sharp and dull	Decreased or unequal sensation
(3) Corneal reflex: use cotton wisp on cornea; instruct client to look up (approach from side) (Fig. 15-11)	Bilateral blink to corneal touch	No blink (make sure abnormal response not caused by contact lenses)
6. CN VI: abducens nerve (described in Chapter 7) (Fig. 15-12)	As described in Chapter 7	As described in Chapter 7
7. CN VII: facial nerve		
a. Inspect face both at rest and during conversation	Symmetry of face	Asymmetry, unequal movements, facial weakness Drooping on one side of face or mouth Unable to maintain position until instructed to relax

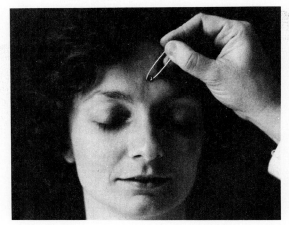

Fig. 15-10   Evaluating CN V (trigeminal—deep sensory).

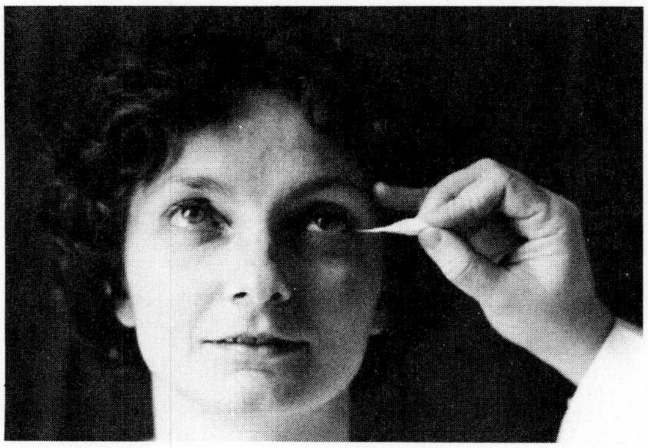

Fig. 15-11   Evaluating CN V (trigeminal—corneal reflex).

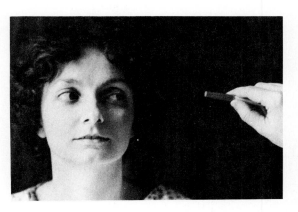

Fig. 15-12   Evaluating CN VI (abducens).

Continued

CLINICAL GUIDELINES—cont'd

| | EVALUATION | |
ASSESSMENT PROCEDURE	NORMAL FINDINGS	DEVIATIONS FROM NORMAL

Cranial nerves—cont'd
b. Instruct client to: (Fig. 15-13)
    (1) Raise eyebrows
    (2) Frown
    (3) Close eyes tightly
    (4) Show teeth
    (5) Smile
    (6) Puff out cheeks
	Able to correctly follow command
	Symmetry of face
		Asymmetry, unequal movements

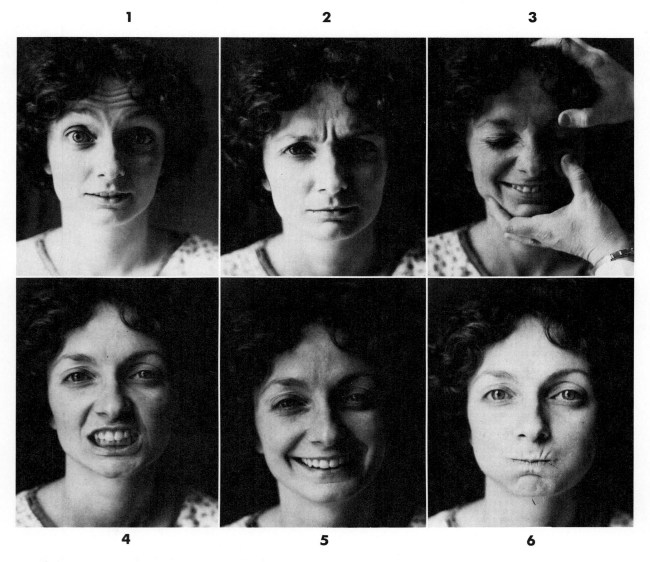

Fig. 15-13 Evaluating CN VII (facial).

ASSESSMENT PROCEDURE	EVALUATION	
	NORMAL FINDINGS	DEVIATIONS FROM NORMAL
c. Evaluate taste over anterior half of tongue (sensory branch of facial nerve) with sugar, salt, lemon juice; instruct client to stick tongue out and leave it out during testing process; use cotton applicator to place small quantity of substance on client's tongue	Able to correctly identify taste	Unable to identify substance Consistently identifies substance incorrectly
8. CN VIII: acoustic nerve (Fig. 15-14); hearing assessment described in Chapter 6	As discussed in Chapter 6	As discussed in Chapter 6
9. CN IX: glossopharyngeal nerve CN X: vagus nerve (CN IX and CN X tested together)		
a. Instruct client to say "ah" (Fig. 15-15)	Bilaterally equal upward movement of soft palate and uvula Speech smooth Gag will occur	Asymmetry of soft palate movement or tonsillar pillar movement; lateral deviation of uvula Gag reflex absent
b. If posterior portion of tongue or pharynx is stimulated: taste—posterior third of tongue (by history)	Able to taste sweet, salt, sour	Unable to differentiate tastes

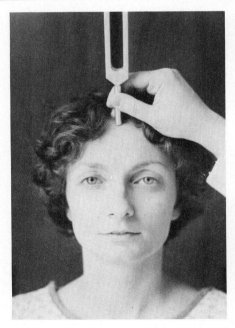

Fig. 15-14   Evaluating CN VIII (acoustic).

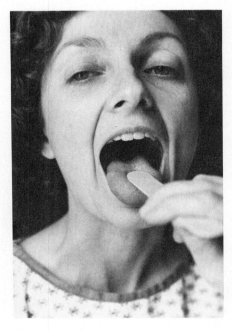

Fig. 15-15   Evaluating CN IX (glossopharyngeal) and CN X (vagus).

Continued.

CLINICAL GUIDELINES—cont'd

	EVALUATION	
ASSESSMENT PROCEDURE	**NORMAL FINDINGS**	**DEVIATIONS FROM NORMAL**
Cranial nerves—cont'd		
10. CN XI: spinal accessory nerve		
a. Instruct client to shrug shoulders upward against examiner's hand (Fig. 15-16, *A*)	Strength and symmetry of contraction of trapezius muscles	Muscle weakness: unilateral, bilateral Pain or discomfort
b. Have client turn head to side against examiner's hand; repeat with other side (Fig. 15-16, *B*)	Observe contraction of opposite sternocleidomastoid muscle; note force of movement against examiner's hand	Unable to maintain contracted muscle position Asymmetry, difficulty of movement
11. CN XII: hypoglossal nerve: motor development of tongue—instruct client to stick tongue out and move from side to side (Fig. 15-17)	As discussed in Chapter 5	As discussed in Chapter 5

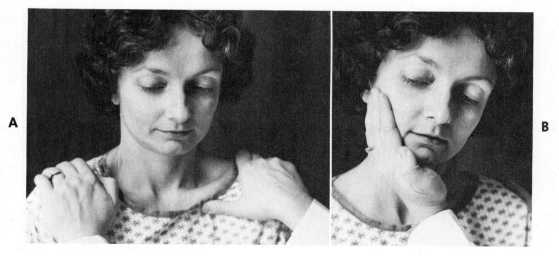

Fig. 15-16 Evaluating CN XI (spinal accessory).

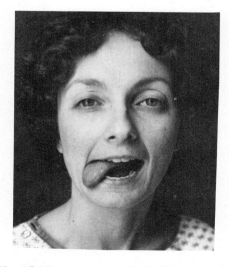

Fig. 15-17 Evaluating CN XII (hypoglossal).

	EVALUATION	
ASSESSMENT PROCEDURE	**NORMAL FINDINGS**	**DEVIATIONS FROM NORMAL**
Proprioception, cerebellar function, and motor function 1. For the asymptomatic client, at least *two* techniques should be used for each area to be assessed. The choice of which two to use may depend on the age and overall physical ability of the client. For example, it is not necessary for every client to perform deep knee bends. 2. General (use two tests for screening of gross motor and balance testing) a. Assess client's gait function by asking client to walk across room, turn, and walk back	Maintains upright posture; walks unaided, maintaining balance, opposing arm swing	Poor posturing, ataxia, unsteady gait, rigid or no arm movements, wide-base gait, trunk and head held tight, legs bend from hips only, lurches or reels, scissors gait, steppage gait, staggering gait, parkinsonian gait (stooped posture, flexion at hips, elbows, knees)
b. Perform Romberg test: ask client to stand with feet together, arms resting at sides, first with eyes open, then with eyes closed (Fig. 15-18)	Slight swaying, but upright posture and foot stance maintained	Unable to maintain foot stance; moves to wider foot base to maintain posture
c. Instruct client to walk a straight line, placing heel of one foot directly against toes of other foot (Fig. 15-19)	Able to maintain heel-toe walking pattern along straight line	Unable to maintain heel-toe walking pattern Steps to wider-base gait to maintain upright posture

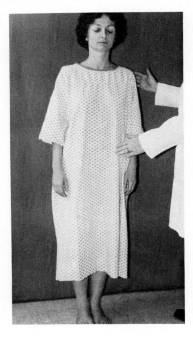

Fig. 15-18 Balance testing using Romberg test.

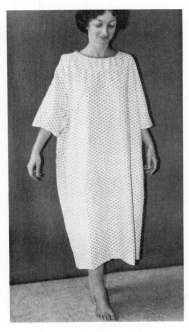

Fig. 15-19 Evaluating balance by having client walk a straight line.

Continued.

CLINICAL GUIDELINES—cont'd

| | EVALUATION | |
ASSESSMENT PROCEDURE	NORMAL FINDINGS	DEVIATIONS FROM NORMAL
Proprioception, cerebellar function, and motor function—cont'd		
d. Instruct client to close eyes and stand on one foot and then other (Fig. 15-20)	Able to maintain position for at least 5 seconds	Unable to maintain single-foot balancing for 5 seconds
e. Hopping in place: instruct client to hop first on one foot and then other (Fig. 15-21)	Able to follow directions successfully Muscle strength adequate to follow through	Unable to hop or to maintain single-leg balance
f. Knee bends: instruct client to hold hands outward and perform several shallow or deep knee bends (Fig. 15-22)	Able to follow directions successfully Muscle strength adequate to follow through	Unable to perform activity because of balance difficulty or decreased muscle strength
g. Walk on toes, then heels	Able to follow directions by walking several steps on toes and then heels May need to use hands to maintain balance	Unable to maintain balance Poor muscle strength Unable to complete activity

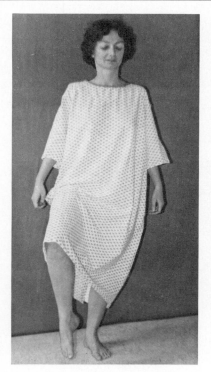

Fig. 15-20 One-foot balance testing with eyes closed.

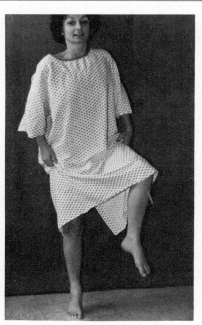

Fig. 15-21 Evaluating balance by having client hop in place.

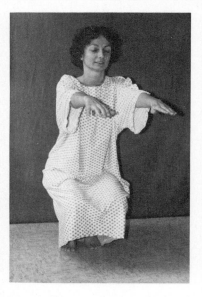

Fig. 15-22 Balance testing by having client perform deep knee bends.

ASSESSMENT PROCEDURE	EVALUATION	
	NORMAL FINDINGS	DEVIATIONS FROM NORMAL
3. Upper extremity testing (use two tests for screening of upper extremity and fine motor testing)		
a. Using pronation and supination of hands, instruct client to alternately tap knees (do both hands together); use rapid movement (see Fig. 14-23)	Bilaterally equal timing Purposeful movement Able to maintain rapid pace	Unequal movement Uncoordinated or increasingly uncoordinated movement Unable to maintain rapid pace
b. Instruct client to stretch arm outward and to use index fingers to alternately touch nose (eyes closed) rapidly (Fig. 15-23)	Able to repeatedly touch nose Rhythmic response	Uncoordinated response Misses nose many times Arms unable to maintain testing position, drift downward
c. Evaluate client's ability to perform rapid rhythmic alternating movement of fingers (test each hand separately); ask client to touch each finger to thumb, in rapid sequence (Fig. 15-24)	Can rapidly and purposefully touch each finger to thumb	Unable to coordinate fine, discrete, rapid movement

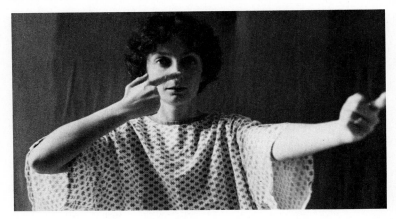

Fig. 15-23 Evaluating fine-motor function by having client touch nose with alternating hands.

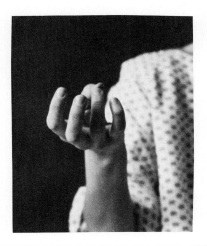

Fig. 15-24 Evaluating fine-motor function by rapid, rhythmic alternating movement of fingers.

Continued.

CLINICAL GUIDELINES—cont'd

ASSESSMENT PROCEDURE	EVALUATION	
	NORMAL FINDINGS	DEVIATIONS FROM NORMAL
Proprioception, cerebellar function, and motor function—cont'd		
d. Instruct client to rapidly move index finger back and forth between client's nose and examiner's finger (approximately 46 cm [18 inches] apart); test one hand at a time (Fig. 15-25)	Able to maintain activity with conscious coordinated effort	Unable to maintain continuous touch with both own nose and examiner's finger Unable to maintain rapid movement Coordination difficulty obvious
4. Lower extremity testing for fine motor function: instruct seated client to place heel of one foot just below opposite knee on tibia; then instruct client to run heel down shin to foot; repeat with other foot (Fig. 15-26)	Able to run heel down opposite shin purposefully Bilaterally equal coordination	Unable to coordinate activity Heel keeps moving off shin Unequal responses Tremors or awkwardness
Muscular function		
Muscle function and strength testing described in Chapter 14	As discussed in Chapter 14	As discussed in Chapter 14

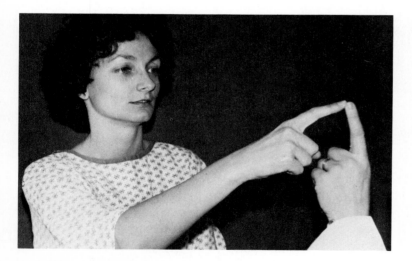

Fig. 15-25 Evaluating fine-motor function by rapid movement of client's finger between own nose and examiner's finger.

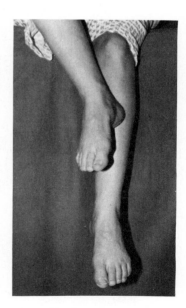

Fig. 15-26 Evaluating fine-motor function by having client run heel of one foot down tibia of other leg.

	EVALUATION	
ASSESSMENT PROCEDURE	**NORMAL FINDINGS**	**DEVIATIONS FROM NORMAL**

Sensory function
1. Test the peripheral extremities in several areas for sensation; if sensation is intact, no further extremity evaluation is necessary; if the peripheral sensation is impaired, move up the extremities, testing periodically until a level or area of sensation is identified; beyond the extremities, also evaluate the forehead, cheeks, and abdomen; if a deviation is identified, try to map out the area involved
2. Compare bilateral responses in each of the following sensation testing categories:
  a. Primary sensory screening
    (1) Light touch sensation: use cotton wisp to lightly touch each designated area (client's eyes closed) (Fig. 15-27)
    (2) Painful sensation: using pointed tip of a pin, lightly prick each designated area (client's eyes closed) (Fig. 15-28); it may be helpful to alternate light and pain sensations to more accurately evaluate client's response
	Client perceives light sensation
	Client able to correctly point to spot where touched
	
	Client perceives pain
	Client able to correctly point to spot where touched
		Unable to perceive touch
		Incorrectly identifies touched location
		Asymmetrical response
		Unable to perceive pain sensation
		Incorrectly identifies touch location
		Asymmetrical response

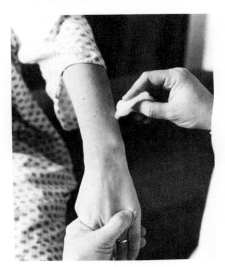

Fig. 15-27 Evaluating light sensory function of forearm (eyes closed).

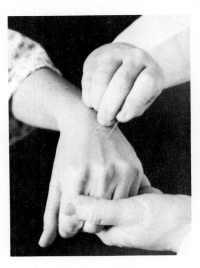

Fig. 15-28 Evaluating pain sensation (eyes closed).

Continued.

CLINICAL GUIDELINES—cont'd

| | EVALUATION | |
ASSESSMENT PROCEDURE	NORMAL FINDINGS	DEVIATIONS FROM NORMAL
Sensory function—cont'd		
(3) Vibration sensation: have client verbalize what is felt when a vibrating tuning fork is placed on a bony area of wrist, ankle, and sternum (Fig. 15-29)	Client feels sense of vibration (decreased sensation may be normal response in older adults)	Unequal or decreased vibratory sensations
b. Cortical and discriminatory forms of sensation (use one for screening)		
(1) Stereognosis: place small, familiar object in client's hand and ask client to identify it (Fig. 15-30)	Appropriate identification	Unable to correctly identify object
(2) Two-point discrimination: with two sharp objects (client's eyes closed) touch selected parts of the body simultaneously; ask client if one or two objects are used (Fig. 15-31)	Can distinguish two-point discrimination Fingertips: 2.8 mm Palms: 8 to 12 mm Chest/forearm: 40 mm Back: 40 to 70 mm Upper arm/thigh: 75 mm	Unable to tell two-point discrimination within normal limits

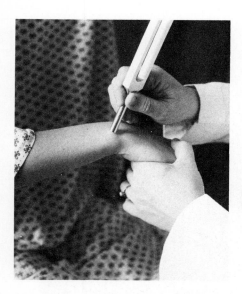

Fig. 15-29 Evaluating vibratory sensation over bony prominence.

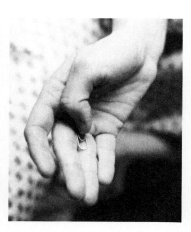

Fig. 15-30 Evaluating stereognosis by client's ability to properly identify a familiar object placed in the hand (eyes closed).

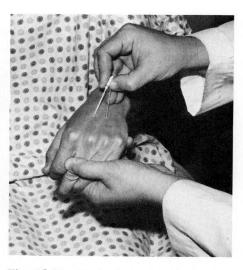

Fig. 15-31 Evaluating two-point discrimination of dorsal surface of hand (eyes closed).

	EVALUATION	
ASSESSMENT PROCEDURE	**NORMAL FINDINGS**	**DEVIATIONS FROM NORMAL**
(3) Graphesthesia: use blunt instrument to draw number or letter on client's hand, back, or other area (client's eyes closed) (Fig. 15-32)	Client able to recognize drawn number or letter	Client unable to distinguish number or letter
(4) Kinesthetic sensation: with client's eyes closed, grasp client's finger and move its position (Fig. 15-33)	Client able to describe how finger position has changed	Unable to distinguish position change

Reflex status

1. Irritation or disruption to any portion of the reflex arc will result in disruption of the reflex response; this includes the areas discussed regarding corticospinal, sensory, or lower motor neuron disturbances. (See "Clinical Tips and Strategies", p. 548, for a description of percussion technique and the use of reinforcement.)

   Deep tendon reflex responses are commonly scored as follows:
   a. 4+ or + + + +: brisk, hyperactive, clonus
   b. 3+ or + + +: more brisk than normal but not necessarily indicating disease
   c. 2+ or + +: normal
   d. 1+ or +: low normal; sluggish response
   e. 0: no response

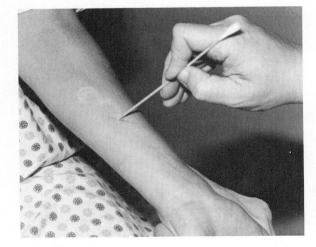

Fig. 15-32 Evaluating discriminatory sensation by using graphesthesia (eyes closed).

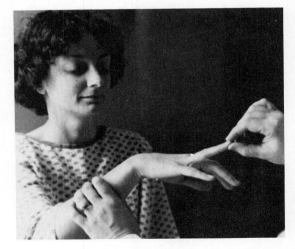

Fig. 15-33 Evaluating discriminatory sensation by using kinesthesia (eyes closed).

Continued.

CLINICAL GUIDELINES—cont'd

| | EVALUATION | |
ASSESSMENT PROCEDURE	NORMAL FINDINGS	DEVIATIONS FROM NORMAL
Reflex status—cont'd		
It will take a beginning examiner much practice and working with a preceptor to determine the actual clinical criteria for this scoring; in attempting to elicit an accurate response, the examiner must be confident that the technique being used is correct		
2. Deep tendon reflexes (all are to be tested; client to be seated)		
a. Biceps reflex (tests C5 and C6): client's arm should be partially flexed at elbow, with palms down; examiner places thumb on biceps tendon and strikes reflex hammer on thumb toward tendon (Fig. 15-34)	Bilaterally equal response; responds rapidly Contraction of biceps	Hyperactive or diminished response Unequal response bilaterally
b. Triceps tendon (tests C6, C7, and C8): flex client's arm at elbow, palm relaxed at side of body; abduct elbow; strike triceps tendon above elbow (Fig. 15-35)	Extension of elbow and contraction of triceps muscle Bilaterally equal response	Hyperactive or diminished response Unequal response bilaterally

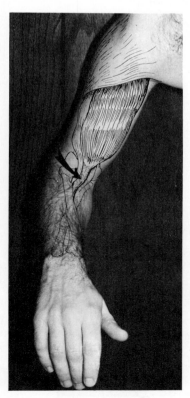

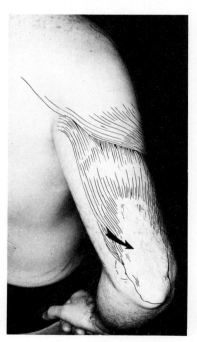

Fig. 15-34 Tendon of biceps brachialis muscle. (Percuss at arrow.)

Fig. 15-35 Tendon of triceps muscle. (Percuss at arrow.)

| | EVALUATION | |
ASSESSMENT PROCEDURE	NORMAL FINDINGS	DEVIATIONS FROM NORMAL
c. Brachioradialis tendon (tests C5 and C6): with client's forearm resting on abdomen or lap (palm down), strike radius 2.5 to 5 cm (1 to 2 inches) above wrist over tendon (Fig. 15-36)	Flexion of elbow and pronation of forearm Bilaterally equal response	Hyperactive or diminished response Unequal response bilaterally
d. Abdominal reflexes (tests T8, T9, T10, T11, and T12): with client lying, lightly stroke with sharp instrument both above and below umbilicus in directions as indicated (Fig. 15-37)	Abdominal muscles contract slightly Umbilicus moves slightly toward area of stimulus Bilaterally equal response	Absent or unilateral response

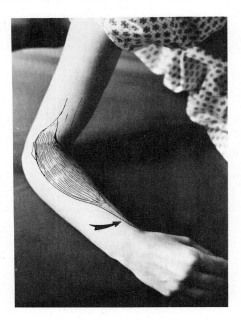

Fig. 15-36 Tendon of brachioradialis muscle. (Percuss at arrow.)

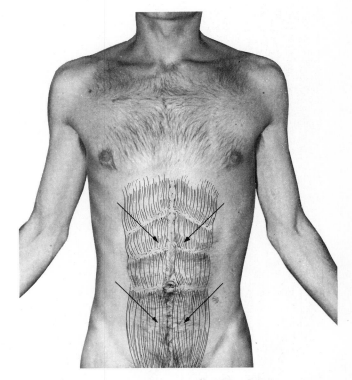

Fig. 15-37 Assessment of abdominal reflexes.

Continued.

CLINICAL GUIDELINES—cont'd

ASSESSMENT PROCEDURE	EVALUATION	
	NORMAL FINDINGS	DEVIATIONS FROM NORMAL
Reflex status—cont'd		
e. Knee (patellar) reflex (tests L2, L3, and L4): with client sitting or lying and knee flexed and relaxed, tap patellar tendon just below patella (Fig. 15-38)	Contraction of quadriceps with extension of lower leg from knee Bilaterally equal response	Hyperactive or diminished response Unequal response bilaterally
f. Ankle (Achilles) reflex (tests S1 and S2): with leg somewhat flexed at knee, dorsiflex ankle; strike Achilles tendon (Fig. 15-39)	Plantar flexion of foot at ankle Bilaterally equal response	Hyperactive or diminished response Unequal response bilaterally

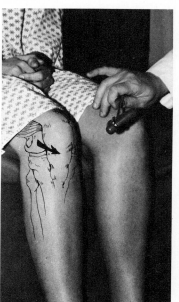

Fig. 15-38 Assessment of patellar tendon. (Percuss at arrow.)

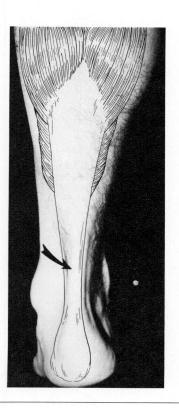

Fig. 15-39 Achilles tendon. (Percuss at arrow.)

	EVALUATION	
ASSESSMENT PROCEDURE	**NORMAL FINDINGS**	**DEVIATIONS FROM NORMAL**
3. Pathological reflexes		
a. Plantar (Babinski) response: using moderately sharp object, stroke lateral aspect of sole from heel to ball of foot, curving medially across ball (Fig. 15-40)	Flexion of great toe, with fanning of other toes	Extension of great toe, with fanning of other toes Indicates pyramidal tract disease
b. Test for ankle clonus (if reflexes are hyperactive): support knee in partly flexed position; with other hand, sharply dorsiflex foot and maintain in flexion (Fig. 15-41)	No movement of foot	Rhythmic oscillations between dorsiflexion and plantar flexion

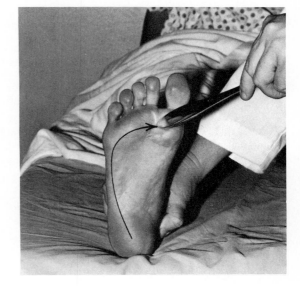

Fig. 15-40 Evaluating for plantar (Babinski) reflex.

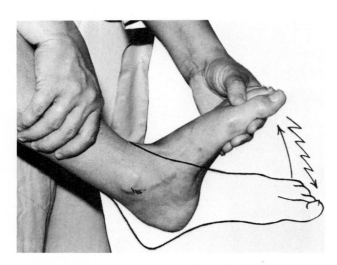

Fig. 15-41 Evaluating for ankle clonus.

CLINICAL TIPS AND STRATEGIES

- **Symmetry is the key!**
- **Numerous tests can be done to screen the various neurological systems:** Which specific set the examiner chooses is up to the individual. The client's functional ability should be considered to understand and follow through. For example, deep knee bends or rapid alternating hand movements would not be appropriate for an older adult with osteoarthritis.
- **It is important to provide selected screening exercises in each of the designated areas:** To skip a total area of assessment is inappropriate.
- **Develop a *method* to examine the neurological system and follow that general method every time:** This will prevent missing any aspect.
- **The percussion hammer, like all other assessment tools, must be correctly used to obtain the desired response:** Following are several strategies:
  1. The client must be relaxed and the extremities loose.
  2. The limb should be positioned to cause slight tension on the tendon to be evaluated. For example, flex the knee to approximately 90 degrees before testing the patellar tendon.
  3. The examiner should hold the percussion hammer loosely between the thumb and index finger so that, as the examiner taps the desired tendon, the hammer can move in a smooth and rapid, yet controlled, direction.
  4. The action of percussion with a hammer should be just like the percussion used on the thorax or abdomen. The examiner should use a rapid wrist-flick motion to percuss the desired tendon. The tap should be quick, firm, and well directed. As soon as the tendon is tapped, the examiner should flick the wrist back so that the hammer doesn't remain on the tendon.
  5. Before the actual percussion, the examiner should palpate the desired tendon so that the precise location will be percussed (Fig. 15-42).
- **If the client is heavy, deep tendon reflexes (DTRs) may be very difficult to elicit:** The examiner should spend time trying to locate the tendon specifically before striking it with the hammer.
- **If the examiner has difficulty eliciting the deep tendon reflex in a client who shows no signs of neurological dysfunction, several techniques may be tried.**
  1. Change the client's position. If the client was sitting, try the technique with the client lying down.

Any position may be used, as long as there is slight tension of the muscle or tendon being tested.

2. If the examiner has difficulty eliciting the deep tendon reflex response of the lower extremity, it may be helpful to use the Jendrassik maneuver of reinforcement. The client locks the fingers together and pulls one hand against the other while the examiner attempts to elicit the lower leg reflexes.
3. Reinforcement for the upper extremities may include instructing the client to tightly clench the teeth or tighten the muscles in the legs.
4. If the examiner continues to have difficulty, the percussion technique should be reexamined.

- **Because of the vast complexity of the neurological examination, it must be reemphasized that the clinical guidelines presented in this chapter are meant to be used for well-adult screening:** If the examiner is expected to examine a client with neurological dysfunction, additional skills are required.

SAMPLE RECORDING: NORMAL FINDINGS

Alert, oriented × 3, CN intact I to XII, coordinated movements and gait, negative Romberg. Cerebellar, sensory, and motor testing intact and bilaterally equal for both upper and lower extremities.

DTRs intact, bilaterally equal, neither diminished nor hyperactive.

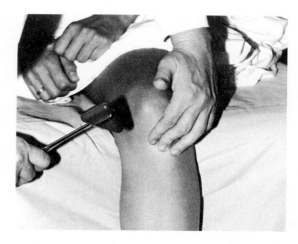

Fig. 15-42   Percussing tendon.

The Newborn

HISTORY AND CLINICAL STRATEGIES

- Neuromuscular assessment is an important part of a newborn's examination. Apart from muscle tone and gestational age assessment, a newborn's state of alertness and reflexes should be carefully observed. Cranial nerves I through XII should be intact.
- A full-term, healthy neonate is capable of the following:
  1. Yawning
  2. Stretching
  3. Sneezing
  4. Burping
  5. Hiccupping
  6. Rooting (movement toward stroked cheek)
  7. Sucking and swallowing
  8. Moro reflex (sudden movement response of symmetric retroflexion)
  9. Tonic neck (arm extension toward turned head; not always noticeable in newborn)
  10. Traction (infant pulled up by wrist grasp)
  11. Trunk incurvature (infant turns pelvis toward stroked side)
  12. Palmar grasp
  13. Plantar response (flexion of toes with pressure on ball of foot)
  14. Placing (touch leg to table; knee flexes to allow foot on table)
  15. Stepping (infant upright with feet touching surface; looks like infant is trying to walk)
- All senses (vision, hearing, touch, taste, smell) and kinesthetic abilities should be present at birth.

CLINICAL VARIATIONS: THE NEWBORN

CHARACTERISTIC OR AREA EXAMINED	NORMAL FINDINGS	DEVIATIONS FROM NORMAL
1. Responses	Responds to touch, pressure, and temperature Will yawn, blink, sneeze, hiccup	Inappropriate or no response (may be neurological problem or related to disease or other disorder)
2. Reflexes	Symmetric posture and movement Adductor spread of knee jerk, rooting, sucking, palmar and plantar grasp, Moro, placing, and stepping (clonus) reflexes intact (see Table 15-1)	Asymmetric, weak, inappropriate, or absent reflexes (may be neurologic problem or related to disease or other disorder)
3. Muscle tone	Will hold head at 45° angle or less until at upright sitting position; then head will flop forward Ventral suspension: infants will dorsiflex back and elevate head with feet and legs flexed Arm and leg recoil, square window, popliteal angle, ankle dorsiflexion, and heel-to-ear maneuver	Infants have less tone if younger than 40 weeks gestational age Muscle tone varies with gestational age; preterm infant has scarf sign Neurological problem is suspected if reflexes or muscle tone is abnormal for gestational age

TABLE 15-1 Infantile reflexes

REFLEX	TECHNIQUE FOR EVALUATION	APPEARANCE AGE	DISAPPEARANCE AGE	NORMAL RESPONSE
Reflexes to evaluate position and movement				
Moro (Fig. 15-43)	Startle infant by making loud noise, jarring examination surface, or slightly raising infant off examination surface and letting him fall quickly back onto examining table	Birth	1 to 4 months	Infant abducts and extends arms and legs; index finger and thumb assume C position; then infant pulls both arms and legs up against trunk as if trying to protect self
Tonic neck (Fig. 15-44)	Infant supine; rotate head to side so that chin is over shoulder	Birth to 6 weeks	4 to 6 months	Arm and leg on side to which head turns extend; opposite arm and leg flex; infant assumes fencing position (some normal infants may never show this reflex)

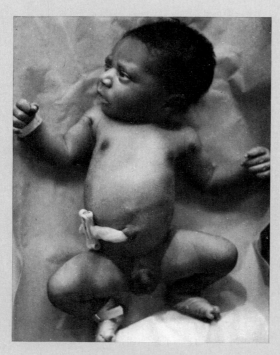

Fig. 15-43

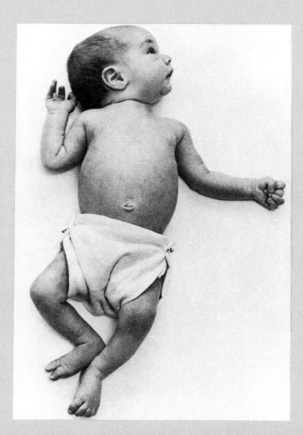

Fig. 15-44   Courtesy Mead Johnson & Co., Evansville, Ind.

REFLEX	TECHNIQUE FOR EVALUATION	APPEARANCE AGE	DISAPPEARANCE AGE	NORMAL RESPONSE
Plantar grasp (Fig. 15-45)	Touch object to sole of infant's foot	Birth	8 to 10 months	Toes will flex tightly downward in attempt to grasp
Palmar grasp (Fig. 15-46)	Touch object against ulnar side of infant's hand; then place finger in palm of hand	Birth	3 to 4 months	Infant will grasp finger with his finger; grasp should be tight, and examiner may be able to pull infant into sitting position by infant's grasp
Babinski (Fig. 15-47)	Stroke lateral surface of infant's sole, using inverted J curve from sole to great toe	Birth	18 months	Infant response: positive response showing fanning of toes
		Starting 18 months		Adult response: occurs after child has been walking for some time; flexion of great toe with slight fanning of other toes

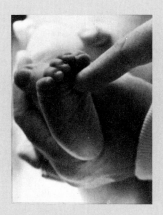

Fig. 15-45

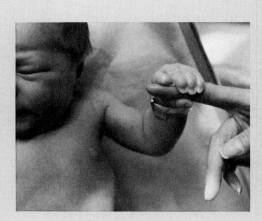

Fig. 15-46

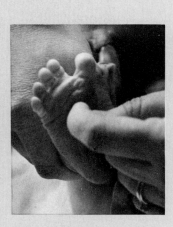

Fig. 15-47

Continued.

TABLE 15-1 Infantile reflexes—cont'd

REFLEX	TECHNIQUE FOR EVALUATION	APPEARANCE AGE	DISAPPEARANCE AGE	NORMAL RESPONSE
Reflexes to evaluate position and movement—cont'd				
Step in place (Fig. 15-48)	Infant in upright position, feet flat on surface	Birth	3 months	Will pace forward using alternating steps
Clonus	Dorsiflex foot; pinch sole of foot just under toes	Birth	4 months	May get clonus movement of foot (not always present)
Feeding reflexes				
Rooting response (awake)	Brush infant's cheek near corner of mouth	Birth	3 to 4 months	Infant will turn head in direction of stimulus and will open mouth slightly
Rooting response (asleep) (Fig. 15-49)		Birth	7 to 8 months	
Sucking	Touch infant's lips	Birth	10 to 12 months	Sucking motion follows with lips and tongue

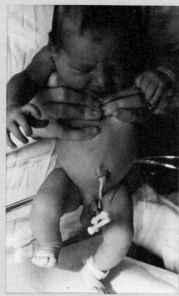

Fig. 15-48

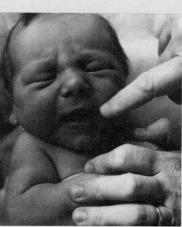

Fig. 15-49

 The Child

HISTORY AND CLINICAL STRATEGIES

- The neurological assessment of the child is unlike that of the adult because the central nervous system of babies and very young children is incompletely developed and in fact operates at a subcortical level. The newborn neurological examination reflects brain stem and spinal cord activity. As the child develops, and with increased myelinization and maturation of the neurological system, the examination becomes more like that for the adult client. The clinical guidelines for assessment of the pediatric client have four components: (1) assessment of infants under 1 year of age, (2) assessment of children 1 to 3 years of age, (3) assessment of children over age 3 years, and (4) screening assessment of neurological "soft" signs.

- The data base history provides evaluative characteristics to assess accurately the maturational and neurological status of the child. In addition, the examiner should inquire about the mother's pregnancy when assessing a newborn or infant. Specifically, the mother should be queried regarding history of drug usage, infections, trauma, intoxication, and metabolic disturbances. A careful family history should be gathered regarding seizure disorders or systemic diseases, such as muscular dystrophy or cerebral palsy.
- Ask the parents if the child has continued to grow and mature normally and ask how this child's development compares with that of siblings.
- Has the parent noted any clumsiness, unsteady gait, progressive muscular weakness, or unexplained falling? Describe.
- Has the child experienced learning or school difficulties associated with attention, interest, activity level, or ability to concentrate?
- Has the child had a head injury or neurological problems, such as seizure, tremor, or weakness, in the past? Describe in detail.
- Has the parent noticed or has the child complained of any problems when going up and down stairs? Is there muscular weakness or weakness when getting up from a lying position on the floor? These are screening questions for muscular dystrophy and should be asked during an examination.
- The neurological examination, like the musculoskeletal examination, begins as the examiner first meets the child. The examiner should note overall alertness, coordination, and body muscle tone. Observe the child undressing or the parent undressing the child. The examiner should observe for gross floppiness, incoordination, or weakness.
- In older children, the examiner should evaluate language, as well as adaptive and motor behavior.
- In younger children the examiner should watch the child at play. Observe the infant lying on the examination table or sitting in the parent's lap. Observe the toddler moving around the room, taking off shoes, and using a pincer grip. Observations should include purposefulness of movements, symmetry, and motor tone.
- The examiner must get a general impression of the child's abilities and responsiveness.
- Even for young children there must be some structure to neurological assessment. Although the examiner must be alert to neurological function and maturational development throughout the examination, a time should be designated for actual reflex testing, motor tone evaluation, and cerebellar functioning. When

the examiner incorporates these techniques does not matter. We recommend placing them in the middle of the examination. Although they are not considered intrusive procedures, such as the ear and throat examination, their accuracy depends on the full cooperation and enthusiasm of the child.

- The Denver Developmental Screening Test (DDST) (Fig. 15-50) or the Denver Developmental Screening Test Revised (short form; DDST-R) (Fig. 15-51) should be used to evaluate the personal/social, fine motor/adaptive, language, and gross motor functioning of all children from 1 month through 6 years. An abbreviated form called the *Denver Prescreening Developmental Questionnaire (PDQ)* may be used to determine which children require the DDST or the DDST-R. These evaluations are meant to uncover "red flags" that indicate lags in the child's development. The DDST-R was released in 1981. The purpose of this new, shortened version is to collect screening data without the lengthy procedure required by the DDST. The examiner is encouraged to use the DDST-R first and then progress to the full DDST for those children who require a more extensive evaluation. The directions and equipment for using either of the DDST forms are extremely important in attaining valid and reliable results. The material on pp. 556-557 provides an overview of the procedures. Every examiner should become familiar with them and other similar screening tests, such as the Goodenough Draw-a-Person test (see box on p. 558), and incorporate them into practice on a regular basis.
- Table 15-2 lists the milestones associated with normal neurological development. Note that the fine and gross motor criteria are the same as listed in Chapter 14 in Table 14-1, on assessment of the musculoskeletal system. These criteria reflect items tested by the Denver Developmental Screening Test.
- Table 15-3 lists "red flags," or warning signs, to determine whether the child's neurological development is lagging. Although every expert would agree that children mature at different rates, norms for lag limits must be developed. If the examiner encounters a child who seems to have difficulty, special attention should be given to a thorough neurological examination, implementation of the Denver Developmental Screening Test or similar tool, and, finally, referral to a physician.
- As with the adult examination, the following clinical guidelines reflect screening procedures for the healthy child. If the child shows significant signs of neurological difficulty, referral and in-depth evaluation are warranted.

Text continues on p. 563.

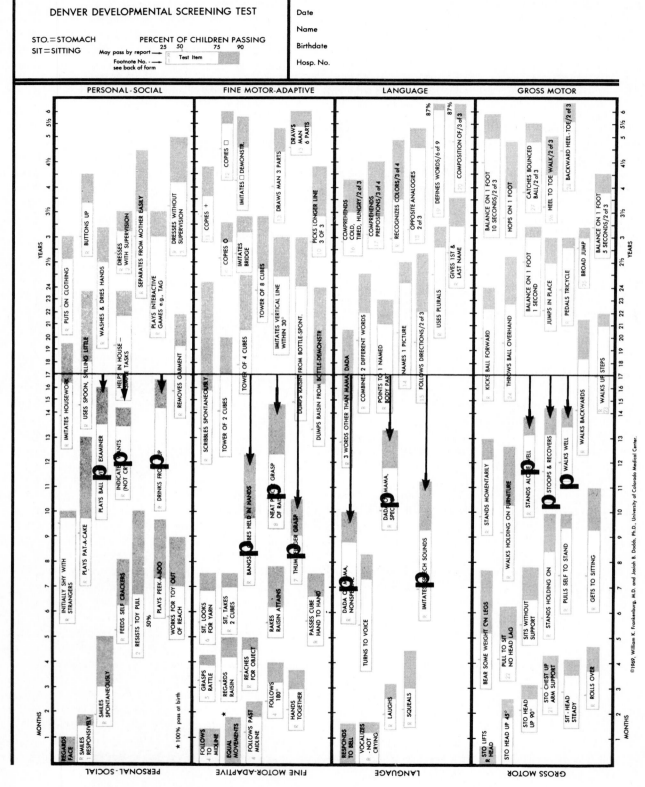

Fig. 15-50   A, Denver Developmental Screening Test (DDST). (From Frankenburg WK, Sciarillo W, Burgess D: *J Pediatr* 99[6]:995, 1981.)

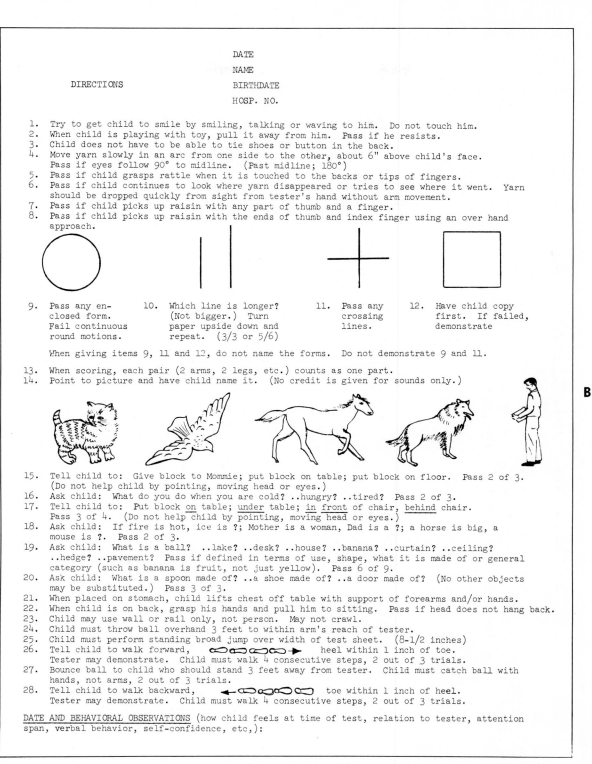

DIRECTIONS

DATE

NAME

BIRTHDATE

HOSP. NO.

1. Try to get child to smile by smiling, talking or waving to him. Do not touch him.
2. When child is playing with toy, pull it away from him. Pass if he resists.
3. Child does not have to be able to tie shoes or button in the back.
4. Move yarn slowly in an arc from one side to the other, about 6" above child's face. Pass if eyes follow 90° to midline. (Past midline; 180°)
5. Pass if child grasps rattle when it is touched to the backs or tips of fingers.
6. Pass if child continues to look where yarn disappeared or tries to see where it went. Yarn should be dropped quickly from sight from tester's hand without arm movement.
7. Pass if child picks up raisin with any part of thumb and a finger.
8. Pass if child picks up raisin with the ends of thumb and index finger using an over hand approach.

9. Pass any enclosed form. Fail continuous round motions.
10. Which line is longer? (Not bigger.) Turn paper upside down and repeat. (3/3 or 5/6)
11. Pass any crossing lines.
12. Have child copy first. If failed, demonstrate

When giving items 9, 11 and 12, do not name the forms. Do not demonstrate 9 and 11.

13. When scoring, each pair (2 arms, 2 legs, etc.) counts as one part.
14. Point to picture and have child name it. (No credit is given for sounds only.)

15. Tell child to: Give block to Mommie; put block on table; put block on floor. Pass 2 of 3. (Do not help child by pointing, moving head or eyes.)
16. Ask child: What do you do when you are cold? ..hungry? ..tired? Pass 2 of 3.
17. Tell child to: Put block <u>on</u> table; <u>under</u> table; <u>in front</u> of chair, <u>behind</u> chair. Pass 3 of 4. (Do not help child by pointing, moving head or eyes.)
18. Ask child: If fire is hot, ice is ?; Mother is a woman, Dad is a ?; a horse is big, a mouse is ?. Pass 2 of 3.
19. Ask child: What is a ball? ..lake? ..desk? ..house? ..banana? ..curtain? ..ceiling? ..hedge? ..pavement? Pass if defined in terms of use, shape, what it is made of or general category (such as banana is fruit, not just yellow). Pass 6 of 9.
20. Ask child: What is a spoon made of? ..a shoe made of? ..a door made of? (No other objects may be substituted.) Pass 3 of 3.
21. When placed on stomach, child lifts chest off table with support of forearms and/or hands.
22. When child is on back, grasp his hands and pull him to sitting. Pass if head does not hang back.
23. Child may use wall or rail only, not person. May not crawl.
24. Child must throw ball overhand 3 feet to within arm's reach of tester.
25. Child must perform standing broad jump over width of test sheet. (8-1/2 inches)
26. Tell child to walk forward, ⌀⌀⌀⌀→ heel within 1 inch of toe. Tester may demonstrate. Child must walk 4 consecutive steps, 2 out of 3 trials.
27. Bounce ball to child who should stand 3 feet away from tester. Child must catch ball with hands, not arms, 2 out of 3 trials.
28. Tell child to walk backward, ←⌀⌀⌀⌀ toe within 1 inch of heel. Tester may demonstrate. Child must walk 4 consecutive steps, 2 out of 3 trials.

<u>DATE AND BEHAVIORAL OBSERVATIONS</u> (how child feels at time of test, relation to tester, attention span, verbal behavior, self-confidence, etc,):

B

Fig. 15-50, cont'd **B,** Directions for Denver Developmental Screening Test. (From W.K. Frankenburg and J.B. Dobbs, University of Colorado Medical Center, 1969.)

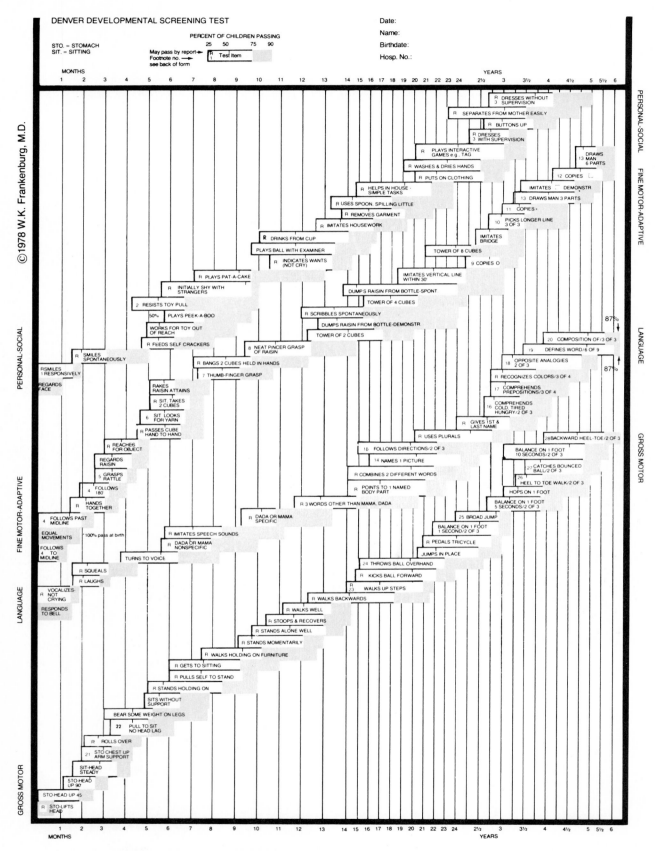

Fig. 15-51 Denver Developmental Screening Test Revised (DDST-R). (From Frankenburg WK, Sciarillo W, Burgess D: *J Pediatr* 99[6]:995, 1981.)

DENVER DEVELOPMENTAL SCREENING TOOLS

Denver Prescreening Developmental Questionnaire (PDQ)

Overview: This prescreening test is designed to identify children who require a more thorough screening with the DDST.

Use: Children 3 months to 6 years of age.

Limitations: Same as for the DDST.

Procedure: Uses 97 questions that focus on a child's current behavior. Ten questions must be answered for any one child. The questions are arranged chronologically according to the age at which 90% of the children pass the corresponding DDST item. Children with scores of 8 or below should be retested in approximately 1 month.

Denver Developmental Screening Test (DDST)

Overview: This test is composed of four major categories: personal/social, fine motor/adaptive, language, and gross motor.

Use: Children from ages 1 month through 6 years. The tool was developed for potential evaluation every month through 24 months, then every 6 months until age 6 years.

Limitations: Frankenburg and associates (*J Pediatr* 99(6):995, 1981) report that one weakness of the DDST is in terms of predictive validity with lower socioeconomic groups.

Procedure: The DDST takes approximately 30 minutes to administer. The examiner should use a regulated DDST kit and follow the procedure manual exactly.* According to the instructions, items are scored "P" for pass, "F" for fail, and "R" for refusal. *Fail* is used to designate any item not passed by the child being tested that is passed by 90% of all children of the same age. If it is determined that the child is not performing in his typical behavior, the DDST should be repeated at a later date.

Denver Developmental Screening Test Revised (DDST-R)

Overview: This test is composed of the same four categories (above) as the DDST.

Use: Same as for the DDST.

Limitations: Same as for the DDST.

Procedure: The DDST-R should take between 15 and 20 minutes to administer. Examiner should use a regulated DDST-R kit and follow the procedure manual exactly.* According to the instructions, only the items passed are scored. *Fail* is considered similar to the same designation in the DDST. Subsequent testing of the child requires administering only those items not previously scored with a "P" that are to the left of the child's age line.

*DDST and DDST-R kits and instruction manuals are available from LADOCA Publishing Foundation, E. Fifty-first and Lincoln St., Denver, CO 80216.

GOODENOUGH DRAW-A-PERSON TEST

Purpose: This screening test assesses mental or intellectual development in children from 3 to 10 years of age.

Instructions: The child is seated at a table and given a pencil with an eraser and a piece of paper. The examiner should tell the child to "draw the best picture of a man or a person that you can draw." No other instructions should be given. The child should then be left alone and given as much time as needed to draw the picture.

Scoring: Using the scoring criteria listed below, give one (1) point for each item in the drawing. Each point equals 3 months. The number of points are then converted to months and/or years. The final score in months or years is approximately equal to the child's mental age.

IQ: The child's IQ may be approximated by the following method: Divide the child's calculated mental age (determined by the Goodenough test) by his real chronologic age and then multiply that number by 100. This will give an approximate IQ.

Scoring criteria

1. Head present
2. Legs present
3. Arms present
4. Trunk present
5. Trunk longer than broad
6. Shoulder indicated
7. Both arms and legs attached to trunk
8. Legs and arms attached to trunk at proper level
9. Neck present
10. Outline of neck continuous with that of head or trunk or both
11. Eyes present
12. Nose present
13. Mouth present
14. Both nose and mouth in two dimensions; two lips shown
15. Nostrils indicated
16. Hair shown
17. Hair on more than circumference of head, nontransparent, better than scribble
18. Clothing present
19. Two articles of clothing, nontransparent
20. Entire clothing with sleeves and trousers shown, nontransparent
21. Four or more articles of clothing definitely indicated
22. Costume complete without incongruities
23. Fingers shown
24. Correct number of fingers
25. Fingers in two dimensions, length greater than breadth, angle subtended not greater than 180 degrees
26. Opposition of thumbs shown
27. Hands shown distinct from fingers and arms
28. Arm joints shown (elbow or shoulder or both)
29. Head in proportion
30. Arms in proportion
31. Legs in proportion
32. Feet in proportion
33. Arms and legs in two dimensions
34. Heel shown
35. Lines somewhat controlled
36. Lines well controlled
37. Head outline well controlled
38. Trunk outline well controlled
39. Outline of arms and legs well controlled
40. Outline of features well controlled
41. Ears present
42. Ears present in correct position
43. Eyebrows or lashes present
44. Pupil shown
45. Proportion of eyes correct
46. Glance directed to front in profile drawing
47. Both chin and forehead shown
48. Projection of chin shown
49. Profile with not more than one error
50. Correct profile

Data from Goodenough FI: *Management of intelligence by drawings,* New York, 1926, World Book.

TABLE 15-2   Normal developmental milestones

AGE	FINE MOTOR	GROSS MOTOR	SOCIAL/ADAPTIVE	LANGUAGE
1 month	Follows with eyes to midline	Turns head to side Keeps knees tucked under abdomen When pulled to sitting position, has gross head lag and rounded swayed back	Regards face	Responds to bell
2 months	Follows objects well; may not follow past midline (major developmental milestone)	Holds head in same plane as rest of body Can raise head and maintain position; looks downward	Smiles responsively	Vocalizes (not crying)
3 months	Follows past midline When in supine position puts hands together; will hold hands in front of face	Raises head to 45° angle Maintains posture Looks around with head May turn from prone to side position When pulled into sitting position, shows only slight head lag		Laughs
4 months	Grasps rattle Plays with hands together	Actively lifts head up and looks around Will roll from prone to supine position When pulled to sitting position, no longer has head lag When held in standing position, attempts to maintain some weight support		Squeals
5 months	Can reach and pick up object May play with toes	Able to push up from prone position and maintain weight on forearms Rolls from prone to supine and back to prone Maintains straight back when in sitting position	Smiles spontaneously	
6 months	Will hold spoon or rattle Will drop object and reach for second offered object	Begins to raise abdomen off table Sits, but posture still shaky May sit with legs apart; holds arms straight as prop between legs Supports almost full weight when pulled to standing position		

Data from Frankenburg WK, Sciarillo W, Burgess D: J Pediatr 99(6):995, 1981.   *Continued.*

TABLE 15-2   Normal developmental milestones—cont'd

AGE	FINE MOTOR	GROSS MOTOR	SOCIAL/ADAPTIVE	LANGUAGE
7 months	Can transfer object, one hand to other Grasps objects in each hand	Sits alone; still uses hands for support When held in standing position, bounces Puts feet to mouth		
8 months	Beginning thumb-finger grasping	Sits securely without support (major developmental milestone)	Feeds self crackers	Turns to voice
9 months	Continued development of thumb-finger grasp May bang objects together	Steady sitting; can lean forward and still maintain position Begins creeping (abdomen off floor) Can stand holding onto stabilizing object when placed in that position; still may not be able to pull self into standing position		
10 months	Practices picking up small objects Points with one finger Will offer toys to people but unable to let go of objects	Can pull self into standing position; unable to let self down again	Plays peek-a-boo	
11 months		Moves about room holding onto objects Preparing to walk independently; wide-base stance Stands securely, holding on with one hand		Imitates speech sound
12 months (1 year)	May hold cup and spoon and feed self fairly well with practice Can offer toys and release them	Able to twist and turn and maintain posture Able to sit from standing position May stand alone, at least momentarily		"Dada" or "mama" specific
14 months		Plays pat-a-cake		
15 months	Can put raisins into bottle Will take off shoes and pull toys	Walks alone well Able to seat self in chair		
16 months		Plays ball with examiner		

AGE	FINE MOTOR	GROSS MOTOR	SOCIAL/ADAPTIVE	LANGUAGE
18 months	Holds crayon Scribbles spontaneously (major developmental milestone)	May walk up and down stairs holding hand May show running ability		
20 months		Imitates housework		Three words other than "mama" or "dada"
24 months (2 years)	Able to turn doorknob Able to take off shoes and socks Able to build two-block tower Dumps raisins from bottle following demonstration	May walk up stairs by self, two feet on each step Able to walk backward Able to kick ball	Uses spoon	
28 months				Combines two words
30 months (2½ years)	Able to build four-block tower Scribbling techniques continue Feeding self with increased neatness Dumps raisins from bottle spontaneously	Able to jump from object Walking becomes more stable, wide-base gait decreases Throws ball overhanded		
36 months (3 years)	Can unbutton front buttons Copies vertical lines within 30° Copies 0 Able to build eight-block tower	Walks up stairs, alternating feet on steps Walks down stairs, two feet on each step Pedals tricycle Jumps in place Able to perform broad jump	Pulls on shoes	Follows two or three simple directions
48 months (4 years)	Able to copy + Picks longer line three out of three times	Walks down stairs, alternating feet on steps Able to button large front buttons Able to balance on one foot for approximately 5 seconds	Dresses with supervision	Gives first and last name
60 months (5 years)	Able to dress self with minimal assistance Able to draw three-part human figure Draws ☐ following demonstration Colors within lines	Hops on one foot Catches ball bounced to child two out of three times Able to demonstrate heel-toe walking	Dresses without supervision	Recognizes three colors

TABLE 15-3   Developmental lag warning signs

AGE	GENERAL	HEARING AND SPEECH	VISION	ARMS	LEGS
6 weeks	Tremors, asymmetry, or jerky spastic movements	Does not respond to loud noise by startle reflex High-pitched cry	Failure to follow or fix at 22- to 30.5-cm (9-inch to 12-inch) distance	Excessive head lag when pulled to sitting position	Immobility Continued limb extension
6 months	No smiling Jerky or spastic movements Does not seem to recognize parent	Failure to turn toward sound Does not laugh or squeal	Failure to fix or follow both near and distant objects	Failure to keep head steady when pulled to sitting position Persistent fisting Preference, one hand Fails to push up or roll over	Increased adductor tone Increased reflexes Clonus
10 months	Lack of imitation Does not reach for toy Not attempting to feed self or put things in own mouth	Does not babble Does not imitate speech sounds	Displays squint or nystagmus	Abnormal hand posture Failure to pass cube from one hand to other	Absence of weight bearing while held Failure to sit without support
18 months	Absence of constructive play Persistence of drooling Indicates wants only by crying	Lack of words, specifically "mama" or "dada"	Any apparent visual defect	No finger-thumb (pincer) grip Does not bang blocks together	Unable to stand bearing weight without support
2 years	Does not play peek-a-boo Not drinking from cup Failure to concentrate	Absence of words other than "mama" and "dada"	Failure to match toys	Does not attempt building with blocks Tremor or ataxia	Unable to walk without aid

Modified from Wood B, editor: A pediatric vade mecum, London, 1974, Lloyd-Luke (Medical Books).

• • •

In assessing the **infant (neonate to 12 months)** the examiner is primarily concerned with three factors:
- Reflex pattern and development
- Motor skills development
- Behavioral and socialization development

The infant develops greatly during the first year of life. In fact, there is more neurological maturation during the first year than in any other. The examiner must closely evaluate this development month by month. The infant should be assessed by the DDST, as well as according to the following clinical guidelines.

CLINICAL VARIATIONS: THE INFANT (NEONATE TO 12 MONTHS)

CHARACTERISTIC OR AREA EXAMINED	NORMAL FINDINGS	DEVIATIONS FROM NORMAL
1. Mental assessment	Appears quiet, content Eyes open Recognizes face of significant other Smiles responsively (after 2 months)	Fretful, tense Tremors or spastic movements
2. Speech	Cry loud and possibly angry Cooing after 3 months Babbles after 4 months One or two words (mama, dada) after 9 months	High pitched, shrill Penetrating cry
3. Cranial nerves: unable to directly test; observe child's functioning, involving at least partial intactness of following cranial nerves:		
a. CN III, IV, VI	Follows movement with eyes Matures from 1 month onward	Response not shown at time appropriate for age
b. CN V	Rooting reflex, sucking reflex	Asymmetry of response Asymmetry of face during response
c. CN VII	Wrinkles forehead, smiles after 2 months	Spastic or movement with tremor
d. CN VIII	Moro reflex to loud noise Turns head toward sound	
e. CN IX, X	Swallowing, gag reflex	
f. CN XII	Evaluated as infant sucks and swallows	
4. Proprioception, cerebellar function, and motor function	Observe infant for spontaneous activity, symmetry, and smoothness of movement Ease and passiveness during swallowing Fine and gross motor development as detailed in Chapter 14 in Table 14-1 (see also Table 15-2) Gradual, purposeful movement after age 2 months	Spasticity, tremors, jerky movements Frequent choking or difficulty with sucking Unable to achieve developmental milestones Any child in question should be evaluated by DDST

Continued.

CLINICAL VARIATIONS: THE INFANT (NEONATE TO 12 MONTHS)—cont'd

CHARACTERISTIC OR AREA EXAMINED	NORMAL FINDINGS	DEVIATIONS FROM NORMAL
5. Sensory function		
a. Light touch	Not normally tested	
b. Pain	Responds by withdrawal of all limbs and crying After 8 months may withdraw only limb tested	Withdrawal of limited limbs, asymmetrical withdrawal, no withdrawal
c. Vibratory	Not normally tested	
d. Discriminatory	Not normally tested	
6. Muscular function (muscle tone)		
a. General observation	Symmetry; limbs semiflexed and slightly abducted (see Fig. 14-43)	Frog position: hips in abduction (almost flat to table) with hips externally rotated Opisthotonos: infant prone, maintains back positions with neck hyperextended Hand-over-head position Any asymmetry or spasticity of movement
	Meaningful grasping after age 3 months	Persistence of fisted hand beyond 3 months
b. Evaluation by pulling infant to sitting position using wrists (pull-to-sit maneuver)	By 4 months head should remain in line with body and should no longer flop forward	Head flop beyond 4 months
c. Range of motion	Able to easily perform range of motion techniques as described in Chapter 14 in Table 14-1	Spastic muscular response Marked resistance to range-of-motion attempt Quick spastic response when limbs released
7. Reflex testing: deep tendon reflexes not normally tested; more important to evaluate infant responses, some of the most common of which are detailed in Table 15-1	Patellar reflex present at birth, followed by Achilles and brachial triceps reflex present by 6 months	If reflexes continue beyond expected disappearance age, examiner should become suspicious

• • •

As with the musculoskeletal examination, cleverness will determine the successfulness of data collection. The **toddler (1 to 3 years)** has outgrown much of the reflex assessment from the first year but is not yet able to cooperate as an adult. Children 2 years of age and older are said to have mature neurological systems in that much of the neurological response elicited by the examination will be similar to that of the adult. The problem is that the child's cognitive abilities are not mature enough to allow cooperation. For example, in testing sharp and dull sensory function, the child may not as yet have developed the concepts of sharp and dull. Likewise, the child may have already formed the concept of hurt and will not allow the examiner near with the percussion hammer. Therefore the examiner must still evaluate much of neurological function on the evidence of motor functioning and response. If the child grossly demonstrates motor, social, and language development appropriate for age by climbing, walking, reaching, babbling, smiling, and undressing techniques, a detailed neurological assessment is not always necessary.

CLINICAL VARIATIONS: THE TODDLER (1 TO 3 YEARS)

CHARACTERISTIC OR AREA EXAMINED	NORMAL FINDINGS	DEVIATIONS FROM NORMAL
1. Mental assessment	Happy, playful child Shows warm, caring relationship with parent; may demonstrate separation anxiety Recognizes and responds to name	Fretful, tense, frightened child Demonstrates no concern of relationship with parent
2. Speech	12 months: 1 to 3 words (nouns) 18 months: 10 to 20 words (nouns) 24 months: 200 to 300 words (adds verbs); two- to three-word sentences	No words by 18 months
	3 years: 900 words (all types); three- to four-word sentences	Very limited word usage by age 3 years
3. Cranial nerves: may be tested to a limited degree, depending on cooperation		
a. CN III, IV, VI	Follows toy with eyes (not valid if child turns head; may have parent immobilize head)	Asymmetry of response Asymmetry of face during response
b. CN V	Give child cookie or cracker to eat; note bilaterally strong chewing response Tickle child's forehead with cotton top; child responds by batting with hand	Absence of response may be caused by lack of cooperation and not actual defect; refer child if in doubt
c. CN VII	Note smile quality and bilaterally equal response Child may imitate frown or show teeth Taste may be evaluated, but examiner may lose child's cooperation; response to salt, sour, or bitter should be negative, batting away	Inability to elicit desired response may result from lack of cooperation
d. CN VIII	Responds to gross hearing evaluation (bell and whisper)	No response
e. CN IX, X	Gag reflex tested during mouth examination	
f. CN XI, XII	Not easily evaluated	

Continued.

CLINICAL VARIATIONS: THE TODDLER (1 TO 3 YEARS)—cont'd

CHARACTERISTIC OR AREA EXAMINED	NORMAL FINDINGS	DEVIATIONS FROM NORMAL
4. Proprioception, cerebellar, and motor function: observe child at play, bending over, reaching, grasping, returning to standing position	Strong coordinated movements One-year-old will show wide-base stance (Fig. 15-52); older child will demonstrate maturity of development (Fig. 15-53) (see "History and Clinical Strategies,", p. 483, for developmental normals)	Continued coordination difficulties beyond normal periods Unable to achieve developmental milestones Any children in question should be evaluated by DDST
5. Sensory function	Not routinely evaluated because almost impossible to separate actual sensory reaction from carefully watching and ready-to-reach toddler	
6. Muscular function	See Chapter 14 for assessment of muscular development of toddler; also see "History and Clinical Strategies," p. 474, associated with the pediatric client for normal developmental milestones	
7. Reflexes: not normally tested in healthy child during this time because of lack of cooperation	Response would be same as for adult	Response would be same as for adult

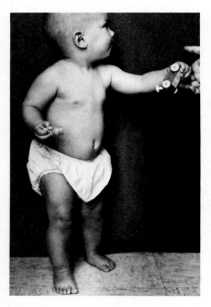

Fig. 15-52   Toddler's wide stance.

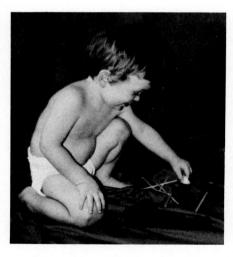

Fig. 15-53   Observing preschooler's coordinated movement.

• • •

Children beyond 3 years of age are normally assessed through the techniques of the adult neurological examination. As the child matures, the actual techniques of evaluation should become easier. The examiner may still need to "play games" with the preschool child to invite cooperation.

Because the actual techniques of the neurological examination are the same as for the adult, the following section was developed to discuss (1) areas to be evaluated, (2) assessment strategies, and (3) developmental variations.

CLINICAL VARIATIONS: THE CHILD (BEYOND 3 YEARS)

CHARACTERISTIC OR AREA EXAMINED	ASSESSMENT STRATEGIES	NORMAL FINDINGS
1. Mental	Questioning about happiness, school success, preferences during play periods Will participate in immediate recall of numbers	4-year-old repeats three-digit number 5-year-old repeats four-digit number 6-year-old repeats five-digit number
2. Speech	Converse with child; personally evaluate type of words used, speech patterns, or problems	4 years old: vocabulary 1500 words; uses plurals; four- to five-word sentences 5 years old: vocabulary approximately 2200 words; uses compound sentences, five to six words in length 6 years old: vocabulary approximately 3000 words; mature sentences over six words in length
3. Cranial nerves	Play games to test CN III to XII CN II not routinely tested until 6 or 7 years; then test as for adult CN III, IV, VI: instruct child to "freeze" neck, or have parent help immobilize CN V, VII: use imaginary bubble gum; have child chew and blow big beautiful bubbles; then bubble bursts; encourage child to play; may evaluate chewing, muscle function, blowing, frowning, eyes closed tight, smile, frown CN VIII: use whisper game CN IX, X: test during head and neck assessment CN XI: play game; have child show strength by pushing away examiner's hand with face and shoulders	

Continued.

CLINICAL VARIATIONS: THE CHILD (BEYOND 3 YEARS)—cont'd

CHARACTERISTIC OR AREA EXAMINED	ASSESSMENT STRATEGIES	NORMAL FINDINGS
	CN XII: famous "tongue dance" will usually aid evaluation of this cranial nerve; instruct child to stick out tongue and wiggle it back and forth	
4. Proprioception, cerebellar function, and motor function a. General screening b. Upper extremity testing c. Lower extremity testing (Also see following section, p. 570, for discussion of testing for neurological soft signs.)	Use variety of techniques from adult profile Even smaller children should be able to do variety of these techniques (Fig. 15-54) such as tasks presented on the Denver Developmental testing	Fine-motor coordination not fully developed until child reaches 4 to 6 years of with maturation; for example, during finger-nose touching, if child brings finger within 2.5 to 5 cm (1 or 2 inches) of end of nose, it is considered normal; *consistent* past pointing should arouse suspicion Developmental progression for one-foot standing: 4 years—5 seconds 6 years—5 seconds with arms folded across chest 7 years—5 seconds with eyes closed
5. Sensory function	After age 5 years child usually has enough trust to participate in sensory screening; helpful to show child cotton wisp, blunt end of paper clip, and tip of pin before starting; with child's eyes open, test each and discuss concepts of sharp, dull, and tickle; some authors suggest likening open pin to mosquito bite	

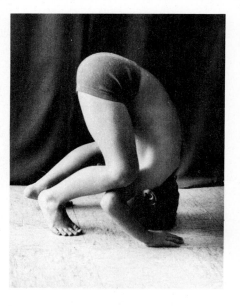

Fig. 15-54   Observing preschooler's coordinated movements of lower extremities.

CHARACTERISTIC OR AREA EXAMINED	ASSESSMENT STRATEGIES	NORMAL FINDINGS
	If child does not understand sharp, dull, and tickle, assessment will fail Two-point discrimination, graphesthesia, stereognosis, and kinesthetic evaluation should be done first with child's eyes open and in educational practice session before testing situation For graphesthesia, easy numbers to recognize: 0, 7, 3, 8, 1; for younger children, examiner may use 0, X, + To vary test further, examiner may make mark such as X twice and ask child if it is same or different; child must understand what same and different mean	
6. Muscular function	See musculoskeletal examination, Chapter 14, p. 440	Observe closely for any signs of muscular weakness as child matures Signs associated with muscular dystrophy: 1. Muscle atrophy or hypertrophy 2. Return to wide-base gait 3. Weakness when going up and down stairs 4. Difficulty arising from lying position; necessary to use arms to climb up and legs to push trunk into upright position
7. Reflexes	May be helpful to use reinforcement; if child shows all other healthy neurological signs, not always necessary to evaluate status of reflexes	

Screening Assessment of Neurological "Soft" Signs in the School-age Child

The term *soft signs,* although controversial, is used to describe vague and minimal dysfunctional signs, such as clumsiness, language disturbances, inconsistencies, motor overload, mirroring movements of extremities, or perceptual development difficulties.

These signs may be considered normal in the young child, but as the child matures, the signs should disap-pear. Their continued presence represents a develop-mental delay or lag in the sensory or motor system. The identification of soft signs indicates a failure of the child to perform age-specific activities.

Table 15-4 presents a series of evaluation techniques recommended by McMillan, Nieburg, and Oski. If the examiner elicits responses demonstrating difficulty in performing the task, the responses should be clustered and the child referred.

TABLE 15-4   Screening assessment of neurological "soft" signs

INSTRUCTIONAL TECHNIQUE	IMPORTANT OBSERVATIONS	VARIABLES AND CONSIDERATIONS
1. Evaluation of fine motor coordination: observe child during:		
a. Undressing, unbuttoning	Note child's general coordination	
b. Tying shoe		
c. Rapidly touching alternate fingers with thumb	Note if similar movement on opposite side	For items *c* to *e* and *h* and *i*, movement of other side noted as associated motor movements, adventitious overflow movements, or synkinesis
d. Rattling imaginary doorknob	Note if similar movement on other side	
e. Unscrewing imaginary light bulb	Note if similar movement on other side	May indicate difficulty with fine-motor coordination
f. Grasping pencil and writing	Note excessive pressure on pen-point; fingers placed directly over point, or placed greater than 2.5 cm (1 inch) up shaft	
g. Moving tongue rapidly		
h. Demonstrating hand grip	Note if similar movement on opposite side	
i. Inverting feet	Note if similar movement on opposite side	
j. Repeating several times "pa, ta, ka" or "kitty, kitty, kitty"	Accurate reproduction of these sounds indicates auditory coordination	
2. Evaluation of special sensory skills		
a. Dual simultaneous sensory tests (face-hand testing): first demonstrate technique, then instruct child to close eyes; examiner performs simultaneously:		
(1) Touch both cheeks	Failure to perceive hand stimulus when face simultaneously touched referred to as *rostral dominance*	About 80% of normal children able can perform this test by age 8 years without rostral dominance
(2) Touch both hands		
(3) Touch right cheek and right hand		
(4) Touch left cheek and right hand		
(5) Touch left cheek and left hand		
(6) Touch right cheek and left hand		

Data from McMillan J, Nieburg P, Oski F: The whole pediatrician catalog, *Philadelphia, 1977, WB Saunders.*

INSTRUCTIONAL TECHNIQUE	IMPORTANT OBSERVATIONS	VARIABLES AND CONSIDERATIONS
b. Finger localization test (finger agnosia test): touch two spots on one finger or two fingers simultaneously; child has eyes closed; ask "How many fingers am I touching, one or two?"	Evaluate number of correct responses with four trials for each hand Six out of eight possible correct responses passes	About 50% of all children pass test by age 6 years About 90% of all children pass by age 9 years This test reflects child's orientation in space, concept of body image, sensation of touch, and position sense

3. Evaluation of child's laterality and orientation in space
  a. Imitation of gestures: instruct child to use same hand as examiner and to imitate the following movements ("Do as I do."):
    (1) Extend little finger
    (2) Extend little and index fingers
 	
    (3) Extend index and middle fingers
    (4) Touch two thumbs and two index fingers together simultaneously
    (5) Form two interlocking rings—thumb and index finger of one hand, with thumb and index finger of other hand
    (6) Point index finger of one hand down toward cupped finger of opposite hand held below
	Note difficulty with fine finger movements, manipulation, or reproduction of correct gesture
	Note any marked right-left confusion regarding examiner's right and left hands
		This test helps to evaluate child's finger discrimination and awareness of body image, right, left, front, back, and up and down orientation
		Especially important after age 8 years if there continues to be marked right-left confusion

b. Following directions: ask child to:
    (1) Show me your left hand
    (2) Show me your right eye
    (3) Show me your left elbow
    (4) Touch your left knee with your left hand
    (5) Touch your right ear with your left hand
    (6) Touch your left elbow with your right hand
    (7) Touch your right cheek with your right hand
    (8) Point to my left ear
    (9) Point to my right eye
    (10) Point to my right hand
    (11) Point to my left knee
	Note any incorrect response
	Note any difficulty with following sequence of directions
		Items *1* through 7 mastered by approximately age 6 years
		
		Items *8* through *11* mastered by age 8 years

The Childbearing Woman

HISTORY AND CLINICAL STRATEGIES

- Common variations during pregnancy include:
  1. Side-waddling gait with broad-based support (from softening of pelvic joints and instability)
  2. Clumsy appearance with tendency to lose balance (from changes in the center of gravity from uterine weight)
- Supine hypotension syndrome may occur in third trimester. Symptoms include light-headedness, nausea and vomiting, fainting sensation, bradycardia, and hypotension. Back positions should not be maintained, since fetal distress can occur.

CLINICAL VARIATIONS: THE CHILDBEARING WOMAN

CHARACTERISTIC OR AREA EXAMINED	NORMAL FINDINGS	DEVIATIONS FROM NORMAL
1. Predelivery	Waddling, broad-based stride from softened pelvic joints and instability Loss of balance from center-of-gravity changes Light-headedness, fainting may occur (from vasodilation, hypoglycemia, hypotension)	Seizures (may be from toxemia) Increased seizures from preexisting condition (suggests inadequate medication) Pregnancy may alter or unveil multiple sclerosis, myasthenia gravis Carpal tunnel syndrome: burning, pain, tingling in hand, wrist, elbow (from edema and pressure on median nerve) Acroesthesia; hand numbness (from traction of brachial plexus)
2. Postdelivery	Balance and stride return to prepregnant state	

 The Older Adult

HISTORY AND CLINICAL STRATEGIES

- Following are significant symptoms that need careful attention (additional questions for symptom analysis).
  1. "Dizziness," "faintness," "spells," or "attacks"
     a. Describe the sensation: Does the room seem to be spinning around? Do you feel as though you are spinning around?
     b. Have you ever fallen down when having a dizzy spell, or lost consciousness?
     c. If you have lost consciousness, did anyone witness the episode and did they describe your behavior?
     d. Does the dizziness occur when you first sit up or stand up?
     e. Does it occur when you move your head from side to side or up and down?
     f. Does exertion cause you to feel faint? If so, describe the intensity and duration of the exertion.
     g. Are there any associated mood or mental changes?

h. Are there any associated symptoms (e.g., numbness or tingling of extremities—bilateral or unilateral, weakness or temporary loss of use of extremities, vision changes, facial expression changes, such as drooping of side of mouth, difficulty swallowing, difficulty speaking, or chest pain)?

i. Do your legs ever just "give way" so that you fall to the floor?

j. Have you (or your observers) noticed your skin color during the episode or during the recovery period (e.g., pallor, flushing)?

k. Describe the onset of the episode (sudden, slow, any warnings that the episode is going to occur).

l. Review all new and old prescribed and over-the-counter medications that the client is taking. (*Note*: Some hypotensives, phenothiazines, and antidepressants can cause dizziness). Review alcohol intake.

2. Weakness

a. Is it isolated to a specific body part or generalized (e.g., difficulty swallowing, lid drooping, unilateral or bilateral weakness in feet, ankles, hands, arms)?

b. Describe specific activities that alerted you to your weakness (e.g., lifting, stair climbing—how many stairs, rising from chair, walking on level ground, holding utensil such as a toothbrush in hand or manipulating it).

c. Does weakness occur at onset of activity or after activity has been sustained (how long or how much)?

d. What are associated symptoms (e.g., dizziness, "black-outs," numbness or tingling, pain, tics [fasciculations], tremors, shortness of breath)?

e. Associated stiffness of joints, spasms, or muscle tension (do these symptoms occur at night)?

f. Associated weight gain or loss?

g. Associated mood or mental changes?

h. Review all medications and alcoholic beverages being taken.

3. Headaches

a. Is this a problem that has occurred over a period of years, or is the pattern of headaches new to you?

b. Do you ever feel localized tenderness over your scalp, forehead, or face?

4. History of injuries, falls (inquire specifically about all recent accidents, minor "spills," or injuries). The client may not be aware that a pattern of increased stumbling, falls, or diminishing agility is emerging if injuries are not obvious or incapacitating.

5. Mental status changes (e.g., mood, thinking process, cognitive functions). (*Note*: A detailed history and observation assessment are covered in Chapter 2, pp. 38 and 39.)

6. Speech alterations (content or delivery) details for assessment are covered in Chapter 2, p. 43.

7. General considerations

a. Any history of weakness, falling, dizziness, pain, or disability should be explored in terms of loss of ability to carry out activities of daily living and concerns of safety. (The original older adult data base in Chapter 1, p. 26, offers detailed questions in these areas.)

b. All symptomatic clients should be asked if they live with someone or have access to someone (relative, neighbor, friend) who can be with them if they need immediate help (day and night).

c. The symptomatic client should be urged to discuss personal feelings about the symptoms (e.g., what is causing them, how serious it is, and any concerns related to living alone or lack of personal or immediate resources).

d. Careful exploration of the client's efforts to relieve symptoms or alleviate stress is important. Self-medication, self-imposed immobility, use of alcohol, social withdrawal, and denial are examples of new behaviors that might be uncovered with a careful history.

• The neurological screening examination can be used with the majority of elderly clients. The major variations in the aging client's responses to the examination follow:

1. Responses to the examiner's commands may be carried out more slowly.

2. The senses of smell and taste may be diminished.

3. Deep tendon reflexes may be slightly diminished (especially the ankle jerk); however, absence or exaggeration of any of the deep tendon reflexes should be reported as a problem.

4. The vibratory sensation in both feet and ankles may be diminished; however, full sensation should be reported at midcalf. (*Note*: Beginning practitioners should report this finding as a problem.)

• Neurological assessment of the elderly individual becomes complicated when the client is disabled by other problems. Diminished vision or hearing, arthritis, confusion or disorientation, or cardiorespiratory problems may be accompanied by fatigue, weakness, inattentiveness, or other symptoms that mask neurological deficits. Symptoms related to other illnesses may prevent the client from going through the motions of an examination. It might be helpful to conduct the examination over two or three sessions to avoid client fatigue. The beginning practitioner will have to seek advice from a preceptor regarding decisions about which functions are important for the client to complete if the client is greatly disabled.

- Following are some major physical signs for which the examiner should be alert:
  1. Facial asymmetry, drooping of the side of the mouth (flat nasolabial fold), asymmetrical wrinkling on forehead, drooling at side of mouth, or tongue fasciculation (while at rest in the mouth). If any are apparent, ask the client to swallow a sip of water. The observer should be alert for coughing, sputtering, dribbling, or fluid remaining in the mouth after the swallow.
  2. Weakness of extremities (unilateral or symmetrical response). Note the following:
     a. Extent of range of motion and strength to opposition
     b. Accompanying muscle atrophy
     c. Sensory responses to pain, touch, vibration, and temperature
     d. Reflexes (normal, present, absent, hyperactive, or diminished)
     e. Comparison of weakened side with other side in all areas of assessment
  3. Gait disturbances (see older adult section in Chapter 14, p. 508, for details to observe)
  4. Tremors. Some authors state that mild head tremors are normal for elderly individuals; however, the examiner should report all tremors for consultation.
     a. Anxiety or hyperthyroidism tremors are often fine, rapid, and irregular. Facial tics or twitching may be present. Tremors usually increase with action and decrease with relaxation. Excessive perspiration may be apparent.
     b. Parkinsonian tremors are slower and occur at rest. The "pill-rolling" pattern of thumb and opposing fingers may be evident. All body movements are slowed or diminished.
     c. Cerebellar tremors vary in rate and are usually intention tremors.
     d. Essential tremors (or those associated with aging) occur at a moderate rate and frequently involve the jaw, tongue, or entire head. The head may move up and down or laterally. The tremors disappear during relaxation and are usually not disabling; there is no accompanying rigidity. There may be a familial history of such tremors. The tremors may begin in middle age and continue at the same level of severity throughout the remainder of life.
     e. Metabolic tremors involve a flapping motion of the wrist, which suddenly drops and then returns to the original position. The client is usually very ill and manifests numerous other signs.

  5. Mental acuity alteration (see Chapter 2, pp. 47 and 48, for specific behaviors to assess).
  6. Labile emotional responses (specific behaviors listed in Chapter 2, pp. 36 and 37).

- *Stroke* is a word commonly used by professional and lay people to describe a sudden neurological deficit that results in a variety of signs, including paralysis or weakness of body parts. The cause of the problem is usually vascular, but the effects are neurological and are therefore described in this chapter. Strokes are often classified in terms of stages of appearance or severity:
  1. Transient ischemic attacks (TIAs) are neurological deficits with acute onset and limited duration (5 to 20 minutes). A variety of symptoms or signs might be manifested. Dizziness, confusion, unilateral weakness or numbness, and aphasia are some of the complaints. These episodes often leave few or no aftereffects and sometimes precede a stroke. The frequency and severity of these "spells" or "attacks" vary greatly among individuals.
  2. Reversible ischemic neurological deficit is similar to the transient attacks except that the signs and symptoms linger for several days before disappearing.
  3. Stroke-in-evolution is a slowly progressive focal deficit occurring and accumulating in a step-by-step or stuttering fashion over a period of days or weeks. Signs and symptoms become more apparent over this period of time.
  4. The onset of signs and symptoms of a completed stroke are abrupt and become stabilized (over a period of days or weeks or years).

RISK FACTORS ASSOCIATED WITH STROKES

- Family history of strokes or vascular disease
- Client history of hypertension
- Cardiac enlargement
- History of myocardial infarction or angina pectoris
- Congestive heart failure
- Diabetes mellitus
- History of peripheral vascular disease
- History of transient ischemic attacks

Study Questions

General

1. The cranial nerves are outside the brain and spinal cord. Therefore the cranial nerves are part of the:
   - ☐ a. Central nervous system
   - ☐ b. Peripheral nervous system

2. Every reflex arc pathway includes:
   - ☐ a. A receptor
   - ☐ b. An efferent fiber
   - ☐ c. An afferent fiber
   - ☐ d. A muscle or gland
   - ☐ e. A brain stem
   - ☐ f. All except c
   - ☐ g. All except a
   - ☐ h. All except e
   - ☐ i. All of the above

3. In assessing the client's proprioceptive or cerebellar function, which of the following tests *are* appropriate:
   - ☐ a. Instruct client to pat his leg as fast as he can with his hand
   - ☐ b. Instruct client to spread fingers as far as possible and to resist the examiner's attempt to squeeze them together
   - ☐ c. Instruct client to do a deep knee bend
   - ☐ d. Instruct client to take the heel of one foot and run it down the opposite shin
   - ☐ e. Instruct client to close his eyes; the examiner grasps the index finger of the client's hand and changes its position (e.g., up or down); the client then describes how the position was changed
   - ☐ f. None of the above
   - ☐ g. b, d, and e
   - ☐ h. b, c, and e
   - ☐ i. a, c, and d
   - ☐ j. a, b, and c

4. When performing a screening evaluation of sensory function, it is necessary to evaluate only the following areas:
   - ☐ a. Lateral aspect of upper thighs
   - ☐ b. Inner aspect of upper arms
   - ☐ c. Dorsal or palmar surface of hands
   - ☐ d. Bottom or dorsal surface of feet
   - ☐ e. Upper middle aspect of back
   - ☐ f. All of the above
   - ☐ g. a, b, and e
   - ☐ h. a and b
   - ☐ i. c, d, and e
   - ☐ j. c and d

5. Sensory function testing techniques include:
   - ☐ a. Pain sensation
   - ☐ b. Light touch sensation
   - ☐ c. Temperature identification
   - ☐ d. Vibration evaluation
   - ☐ e. Position sense
   - ☐ f. Stereognosis
   - ☐ g. All of the above
   - ☐ h. All except a
   - ☐ i. All except c
   - ☐ j. All except e
   - ☐ k. All except f

The Newborn

Match the terms in column A with their signs in column B.

Column A	Column B
6. ___ Symmetric retroflexion	a. clonus
7. ___ Movement toward stroking	b. Moro
8. ___ Dorsiflexion of foot	c. rooting

The Child

9. The examiner should expect a child to feed himself crackers or cookies by which of the following ages:
   - ☐ a. 4 months
   - ☐ b. 6 months
   - ☐ c. 8 months
   - ☐ d. 10 months
   - ☐ e. 12 months

10. Which of the following definitions best defines neurological "soft signs:"
   - ☐ a. Objective signs that are present because of an open portion of the spinal column
   - ☐ b. Objective findings of babies before mature development of neurological systems
   - ☐ c. Objective signs found in hyperactive children
   - ☐ d. Objective signs associated with vague complaints, such as clumsiness, motor overload, or mirroring of extremity movements
   - ☐ e. There is no such term

The Childbearing Woman

11. Softening of pelvic joints during pregnancy causes:
   - ☐ a. Stability
   - ☐ b. Waddling
   - ☐ c. Myasthenia gravis
   - ☐ d. Acroesthesia

The Older Adult

12. Neurological signs associated with the normal aging process might include:
   - ☐ a. Diminution or absence of ankle jerk response
   - ☐ b. Ptosis
   - ☐ c. Fasciculations of the tongue
   - ☐ d. All of the above
   - ☐ e. None of the above

13. Transient ischemic attacks:
   - ☐ a. May occur in the form of black-out spells
   - ☐ b. May affect speech ability
   - ☐ c. All of the above
   - ☐ d. None of the above

14. Risk factors associated with strokes might include:
   - ☐ a. A history of nervousness
   - ☐ b. A history of transient ischemic attacks
   - ☐ c. A history of hypothyroidism
   - ☐ d. All of the above
   - ☐ e. None of the above

SUGGESTED READINGS
General

Adams VM: *Principles of neurology,* ed 2, New York, 1981, McGraw-Hill.

Bates B: *A guide to physical examination,* ed 4, Philadelphia, 1987, JB Lippincott.

DeMeyer W: *Technique of neurological examination: a programmed text,* ed 3, New York, 1980, McGraw-Hill.

Essentials of the neurological examination, Philadelphia, 1974, SmithKline Corporation.

Malasanos L, Barkauskas V, Stoltenberg-Allen K: *Health assessment,* ed 4, St Louis, 1990, Mosby—Year Book.

Mandell EL: *Essentials of the neurological examination,* ed 2, Philadelphia, 1981, FA Davis.

Patient assessment: neurological examination. I. Programmed instruction, *Am J Nurs* 75:9, 1975.

Patient assessment: neurological examination. II. Programmed instruction, *Am J Nurs* 75:11, 1975.

Patient assessment: neurological examination. III. Programmed instruction, *Am J Nurs* 76:4, 1976.

Phipps WJ, Long BC, Woods NF, Cassmeyer VL: *Medical-surgical nursing: concepts and clinical practice,* ed 4, St Louis, 1991, Mosby—Year Book.

Prior JA, Silberstein JS, Stang JM: *Physical diagnosis: the history and examination of the patient,* ed 6, St Louis, 1981.

Seidel HM, Ball JW, Dains JE, Benedict GW: *Mosby's guide to physical examination,* ed 2, St Louis, 1991, Mosby—Year Book.

Thompson JM, McFarland GK, Hirsch JE, and others: *Mosby's manual of clinical nursing,* ed 2, St Louis, 1989, Mosby—Year Book.

Van Allen MW: *Pictorial manual of neurologic tests: a guide to the performance and interpretation of the neurologic examination,* ed 2, Chicago, Mosby—Year Book.

The newborn

Auvenshine MA, Enriquez MG: *Maternity nursing: dimensions of change,* Belmont, Calif, 1985, Wadsworth.

Bobak IM, Jensen MD: *Essentials of maternity nursing,* ed 3, St Louis, 1991, Mosby—Year Book.

Judd JM: Assessing the newborn from head to toe, *Nurs '85* 15(12):34, 1985.

Kiernan BS, Scoloveno MA: Assessment of the neonate, *Top Clin Nurs* 8(1):1, 1986.

The Organization of Obstetrical, Gynecological and Neonatal Nurses (NAACOG): *Physical assessment of the neonate,* OGN Nursing Practice Resource, Oct. 1986, The Association.

Pillitteri A: *Maternal-newborn nursing: care of the growing family,* ed 3, Boston, 1985, Little, Brown.

Scanlon JW, and others: *A system of newborn physical examination,* Baltimore, 1979, University Park Press.

Seidel HM, Ball JW, Dains JE, Benedict GW: *Mosby's guide to physical examination,* St Louis, 1991, Mosby—Year Book.

Whaley LF, Wong DL: *Nursing care of infants and children,* ed 4, St Louis, 1991, Mosby—Year Book.

The child

Barness L: *Manual of pediatric physical diagnosis,* ed 6, Chicago, 1990, Mosby—Year Book.

Frankenburg WK, Dick NP, Carland J: Development of preschool-aged children of different social and ethnic groups: implications for developmental screening, *J Pediatr* 87(7):125, 1975.

Frankenburg WK, and others: The newly abbreviated and revised Denver Developmental Screening Test, *J Pediatr* 99(6):995, 1981.

Goodenough FL: *Measurement of intelligence by drawings,* New York, 1926, World Book.

Hayes JS: The McCarthy scales of children's abilities: their usefulness in developmental assessment, *Pediatr Nurs* 7:35, 1981.

Hughes J: *Synopsis of pediatrics,* ed 6, St Louis, 1984, Mosby—Year Book.

Lowrey GH: *Growth and development of children,* ed 8, Chicago, 1986, Mosby—Year Book.

O'Pray M: Developmental screening tools: using them effectively, *Matern Child Nurs J* 5(2):126, 1980.

Pillitteri A: *Nursing care of the growing family: a child health text,* Boston, 1977, Little Brown.

Swaiman KF, Wright FS: *The practice of pediatric neurology,* ed 2, St Louis, 1982, Mosby—Year Book.

Whaley LF, Wong DL: *Essentials of pediatric nursing,* ed 3, St Louis, 1989, Mosby—Year Book.

The childbearing woman

Beischer NA, MacKay EV: *Obstetrics and the newborn: an illustrated textbook,* ed 2, Philadelphia, 1986, WB Saunders.

Pillitteri A: *Maternal-newborn nursing: care of the growing family,* ed 3, Boston, 1985, Little, Brown.

Pritchard JA, MacDonald PC: *Williams' obstetrics,* ed 17, New York, 1985, Appleton-Century-Crofts.

Whitley NA: *Manual of clinical obstetrics,* Philadelphia, 1985, JB Lippincott.

The older adult

Barry PP: Iatrogenic disorders in the elderly: preventive techniques, *Geriatrics* 41(9):42, 1986.

Carotenuto R, Bullock J: *Physical assessment of the gerontologic client,* Philadelphia, 1980, FA Davis.

Ebersole P, Hess P: *Toward healthy aging,* ed 3, St Louis, 1990, Mosby—Year Book.

Eliopoulos C: *Gerontological nursing,* ed 2, Philadelphia, 1987, JB Lippincott.

Granacher RP: The neurologic examination in geriatric psychiatry, *Psychosomatics* 22(6):485, 1981.

Steinberg FU, editor: *Care of the geriatric patient,* ed 6, St Louis, 1983, Mosby—Year Book.

CHAPTER 16

Physical examination integration format

This chapter discusses the integration of the total physical examination. Throughout, the description of the assessment techniques has been abbreviated. The examiner is referred to the individual chapters for a detailed description. The clinical information has been divided to show the following:

- The examination format
- The assessment techniques
- The systems involved in the assessment procedure
- Important strategies

At the end of this detailed description is a summary of variations and suggested approaches for the pediatric client.

Equipment for physical examination

Eye examination charts	Writing surface for examiner
Ophthalmoscope	Patient examination gown
Otoscope with pneumatic bulb	Vaginal speculum (for female clients)
Stethoscope	Pap smear materials
Tongue blades	Percussion hammer
Penlight	Tuning fork
4 × 4–inch gauze pads	Aromatic material
Examination gloves	Cotton balls
Cotton-tipped applicators	Sharp and dull testing instruments
Lubricant	
Drape sheet	Ruler
Gooseneck light	Goniometer
Examination table with stirrups	

DATA BASE HISTORY

Taking the data base history provides an opportunity for the examiner to get to know and develop a profile about the client. This profile should be synthesized and provide the examiner with a framework for approaching the client during the physical assessment.

- **Major concern of client.** The examiner must decide whether to examine the area of major concern first or whether to examine it during the normal sequence.
- **General approach to client.** The examiner will get to know the client during preparation of the rather lengthy data base. Although the examiner may decide to maintain a systematic and progressive physical examination approach, the client's personality and individual preferences should be incorporated. For example, if the client states that he becomes short of breath when he lies flat, the examiner may decide to keep the head of the examining table somewhat elevated and to keep the recumbent period to a minimum.
- **Major areas needing special attention.** Many times the examination simply confirms what the examiner already knows. Therefore the examiner should bring to the physical assessment session a "problem list" of areas needing special in-depth evaluation.

INTEGRATED PHYSICAL ASSESSMENT

- The physical examination of each client should begin as the examiner first meets the client. Assessment of objective data should continue throughout the subjective data base collection period.

During the initial introductory period, the examiner collects data by watching the client walk down the hall, come into the examination room, take off and hang up his coat, shake hands with the examiner, sit down on a chair in the office or examination room, and carry on all introductory conversation.

The examiner may identify areas with obvious difficulties or deviations. Areas requiring primary assessment follow:

1. Gait: difficulty walking, use of assisting devices
2. Stiffness, weakness
3. Difficulty standing, sitting, rising from sitting
4. Difficulty taking off coat or hanging it up
5. Obvious musculoskeletal deformities
6. General affect
7. Appearance of interest and involvement
8. Eye contact with examiner
9. Speech pattern or difficulties
10. Dress and posture
11. Overview of mental alertness, orientation, and thought process integrity
12. Tremors or motor difficulties
13. Obvious eye problem or blindness
14. Corrective lenses
15. Difficulty hearing
16. Obvious shortness of breath; posture that would facilitate breathing
17. Cyanosis, pale or flushed appearance
18. Language problem or foreign language speaker
19. Cultural orientation
20. Significant others accompanying client
21. Obesity or emaciation
22. Malnourishment

• After the initial assessment and data base collection, the client should be prepared for the physical assessment.

1. Instruct client to empty bladder (collect specimen if desired)
2. Instruct client to remove all clothing (including shoes, socks, bra, and underpants), put on gown, and sit on chair in examination room.

To perform the examination, the approach to body systems must be fragmented for two purposes: (1) to accommodate a regional physical assessment approach and (2) to coordinate client and examiner positions during the assessment process.

After the assessment the examiner must integrate the body systems data for the actual physical assessment write-up. The examiner should not feel compelled to follow the stated outline; the goal should be to develop an individualized routine.

• The examiner should perform a functional assessment where appropriate.

Text continues on p. 587.

CLINICAL GUIDELINES FOR PHYSICAL EXAMINATION INTEGRATION

PROCEDURE OR FORMAT/ASSESSMENT	BODY PART OR SYSTEMS INVOLVED	CLINICAL STRATEGIES (ADULT AND ELDERLY)
1. **Assess vital functions and other baseline measurements: client should be in gown and seated on end of examination table or in chair**		
Temperature	Cardiovascular	If deviation from normal discovered, reevaluate when associated system assessed
Blood pressure (both arms)	Thorax and lungs	
Radial pulse		
Respirations		
Height		
Weight		
Vision testing	Visual	
Snellen chart	Neurological—CN II	
External eye function	(optic nerve)	
Client is seated		
2. **Examine client's hands**		
Skin surface characteristics	Integumentary	Both examiner and client will be at ease if examiner starts with client's hands
Temperature and moisture of hands		
Characteristics of nails	Cardiovascular	
Clubbing	Respiratory	

PROCEDURE OR FORMAT/ASSESSMENT	BODY PART OR SYSTEMS INVOLVED	CLINICAL STRATEGIES (ADULT AND ELDERLY)
Skeletal characteristics and/or deformities of fingers and hands Range of motion and motor strength of fingers and hands Muscle wasting Asymmetry	Musculoskeletal	Fine motor neurological assessment may be included at this point; others find it more convenient to perform neurological assessment as a clustered procedure toward end of evaluation period
3. Examine client's arms from hands to shoulders Skin surface characteristics Muscle wasting Asymmetry	Integumentary Musculoskeletal	Examine each arm separately
Radial pulses: compare one arm to other	Cardiovascular	May have already been done during vital signs evaluation
Range of motion and motor strength of wrists, elbows, forearms, upper arm, shoulders	Musculoskeletal Neurological	Note that, again, neurological assessment has been delayed Use make/break techniques
Palpation of epitrochlear lymph nodes	Lymphatic	
4. Examine client's head and neck Facial characteristics and symmetry	Head and neck Neurological	Observe head and neck, gathering as much information as possible
Skin surface characteristics Symmetry and external characteristics of eyes and ears Hair characteristics: texture, distribution, quantity Palpation of hair and scalp	Integumentary	Do not touch until after thorough observation Palpate thoroughly; do not be intimidated by hair spray or dirty hair (may need to wash hands before progressing)
Palpation of facial bones Client opens and closes mouth for evaluation of temporomandibular joint Clenching teeth Palpation of sinus regions	Musculoskeletal Neurological—CN V (trigeminal nerve)	
Client clenches eyes tight, wrinkles forehead, smiles, sticks out tongue, and puffs out cheeks Eye and near-vision assessment External eye examination: eyebrows, eyelids, eyelashes, surface characteristics, lacrimal apparatus, corneal surface, anterior chamber, iris	Neurological—CN VII, XII (facial, hypoglossal nerves) Visual	Be straightforward Provide client with step-by-step instructions
Near-vision screening and eye function: pupillary response, accommodation, cover-uncover test	Neurological—CN II, III (optic, oculomotor nerves)	
Extraocular eye movements; vision field testing	Neurological—CN III, IV, VI, (oculomotor, trochlear, abducens nerves)	
Internal eye examination: red reflex, disc, cup margins, vessels, retinal surface, vitreous	Visual	Room must be darkened; should have small amount of secondary light Instruct client to focus on single object at distance

Continued.

CLINICAL GUIDELINES FOR PHYSICAL EXAMINATION INTEGRATION—cont'd

PROCEDURE OR FORMAT/ASSESSMENT	BODY PART OR SYSTEMS INVOLVED	CLINICAL STRATEGIES (ADULT AND ELDERLY)
Client is seated—cont'd		
Ear and hearing assessment	Ear and auditory	
External ear examination: alignment, surface characteristics, external canal		
Use ticking watch to evaluate hearing	Neurological—CN VIII (acoustic nerve)	Room must be quiet
Otoscope examination: characteristics of external canal, cerumen, eardrum (landmarks, deformities, inflammation)		Use largest speculum that will fit into canal; if necessary, review technique guidelines for using otoscope
Rinne and Weber tests	Auditory and neurological—CN VIII (acoustic nerve)	
Nasal examination: note structure, septum position; use nasal speculum to evaluate patency, turbinates, meatuses	Nose, mouth, and oropharynx	Even though uncomfortable, should be part of every thorough assessment
Evaluation of sense of smell	Neurological—CN I (olfactory nerve)	
Mouth examination: inspect gingivobuccal fornices, buccal mucosa, and gums	Nose, mouth, and oropharynx	
Inspection of teeth: number, color, surface characteristics		If client has dentures, they should be removed
Inspection and palpation of tongue: symmetry, movement, color, surface characteristics		
Inspection of floor of mouth: color, surface characteristics		
Inspection of hard and soft palates: color, surface characteristics		
Inspection of oropharynx: note mouth odor, anteroposterior pillars, uvula, tonsils, posterior pharynx		
Evaluation of gag reflex	Neurological—CN IX, X (glossopharyngeal, vagus nerves)	
Evaluation of range of motion of head and neck: instruct client to swing shoulders upward against examiner's resistance; head movement positions, neck flexion, extension, ear-to-shoulder flexion, chin-to-shoulder rotation	Musculoskeletal Neurological—CN XI (accessory nerve)	
Observation of symmetry and smoothness of neck and thyroid		Client's gown should be lowered slightly so that examiner may fully inspect neck
Palpation of carotid pulses	Cardiovascular	
Observation for jugular venous distention		
Palpation of trachea, thyroid (isthmus and lobes), lymph nodes (preauricular, postauricular, occipital, tonsillar, submaxillary, submental, superficial cervical chain, posterior cervical, deep cervical chain, and supraclavicular)	Lymphatic	Client may need drink of water to facilitate swallowing during thyroid evaluation

PROCEDURE OR FORMAT/ASSESSMENT	BODY PART OR SYSTEMS INVOLVED	CLINICAL STRATEGIES (ADULT AND ELDERLY)
Completion of assessment of cranial nerves: use cotton swab to evaluate light sensation to forehead, cheeks, chin (trigeminal nerve sensory tract)	Neurological—CN V (trigeminal nerve)	Client should be instructed to close eyes and identify where and when light touch felt
5. Assess posterior chest: examiner moves behind client; client seated; gown to waist for men; gown removed but pulled up to cover breasts for women		
Observation of posterior chest: symmetry of shoulders, muscular development, scapular placement, spine straightness, posture	Musculoskeletal	
Observation of skin: intactness, color, lesions	Integumentary	
Observation of respiratory movement: excursion, quality, depth, and rhythm of respirations	Thorax and lungs	
Palpation of posterior chest: evaluate muscles and bone structure, palpate excursion of chest expansion; palpate down vertebral column; note straightness	Musculoskeletal Thorax and lungs	
Palpation of posterior chest for fremitus		Palpate with base of fingers while client says "how now brown cow" or "ninety-nine"
Percussion of posterior chest for resonance, respiratory excursion	Thorax and lungs	During excursion evaluation, demonstrate to client how to take deep breath and hold it Measure amount of excursion with ruler
Percussion with fist along costovertebral angle for kidney tenderness	Genitourinary	
Inspection, bilateral palpation, and percussion along lateral axillary chest walls	Thorax and lungs	
Auscultation of posterior and axillary chest walls for breath sounds; note quality of sounds heard and presence of adventitious sounds	Thorax and lungs	Instruct client to breathe deeply by mouth
6. Assess anterior chest: move to front of client; client should lower gown to waist		
Inspection of skin color, intactness, presence of lesions, muscular symmetry, bilaterally similar bone structure	Integumentary Musculoskeletal	
Observation of chest wall for pulsations or heaving	Cardiovascular	
Observation of movement during respirations	Thorax and lungs	
Observation of client's ease with respirations, posture, pursing lips		
Female breasts: Note size, symmetry, contour, moles or nevi, breast or nipple deviation, dimpling, or lesions; evaluate range of motion of shoulders and regularity of breast tissue during various movements: a. Client's arms extended over head b. Client's arm behind head	Musculoskeletal Breast	It is helpful to explain to client basically what she will be expected to do and why before actual examination; may help to alleviate client anxiety as well as facilitate active participation

Continued.

CLINICAL GUIDELINES FOR PHYSICAL EXAMINATION INTEGRATION—cont'd

PROCEDURE OR FORMAT/ASSESSMENT	BODY PART OR SYSTEMS INVOLVED	CLINICAL STRATEGIES (ADULT AND ELDERLY)
Client is seated—cont'd		
c. Client's hands behind small of back d. Client's hands pushed tightly against each other at shoulder level		During examination, it may be helpful to discuss what is being observed; breast self-examination instruction should follow at some point to reiterate these and other aspects of breast examination
e. Client leaning forward slightly so that breasts hang away from chest wall; note symmetry and pull on suspensory ligaments		
Male breasts: Note size, symmetry, breast enlargement, nipple discharge, or lesions		
All clients: Palpation of anterior chest wall for stability, crepitations, muscular or skeletal tenderness	Musculoskeletal	
Palpation of precordium for thrills, heaves, pulsations	Cardiovascular	Evaluate chest while client is sitting upright and then leaning forward
Palpation of left chest wall to locate point of maximum impulse (PMI)		
Palpation of chest wall for fremitus, as with posterior chest	Thorax and lungs	
Percussion of anterior chest for resonance	Thorax and lungs	If examiner has difficulty percussing woman's anterior chest because of large breasts, percuss downward until breast tissue reached; then postpone further percussion until client lies down
For female clients: Palpation of breasts, including all four quadrants, tail of breast, and areolar area; note firmness, tissue qualities, lumps, areas of thickness, or tenderness	Breast	Client should be comfortably seated with arms resting at side
Palpation of nipples; note elasticity, tissue characteristics, discharge		As before, discuss what is being done so that client can incorporate similar techniques into breast self-examination
All clients: Palpation of lymph nodes associated with lymphatic drainage of breast, including supraclavicular and infraclavicular, central, lateral, axillary, pectoral, subscapular, scapular, brachial, intermediate, and internal mammary areas	Lymphatic	
For male clients: Palpation of breast; note swelling or presence of excessive tissue or lumps, nipple discharge, or lesions		
All clients: Auscultation of breath sounds of anterior chest from apex to base; note quality, rate, type, presence of adventitious sounds	Thorax and lungs	Instruct client to breathe deeply through mouth

PROCEDURE OR FORMAT/ASSESSMENT	BODY PART OR SYSTEMS INVOLVED	CLINICAL STRATEGIES (ADULT AND ELDERLY)
Auscultation of heart: aortic area, pulmonary area, Erb point, tricuspid area, apical area; note rate, rhythm, location, intensity, frequency, timing, and splitting of S_1, S_2, S_3, S_4 murmurs	Cardiovascular	Examiner must decide whether to start at apical area and work upward or start at aortic area and work downward; examiner should develop routine method of procedure If examining large-breasted woman, part of auscultatory evaluation may be deferred until client lying down
Client is assisted to lying or low Fowler position 7. **Assess anterior chest in recumbent position** Inspection of jugular venous pressure for height seen above sternal angle	Cardiovascular	Extend footrest for client's legs See "Clinical Tips and Strategies" (Chapter 9, p. 290) for cardiovascular examination techniques to measure jugular venous pressure
Female breast inspection: Symmetry, contour, venous pattern, skin color, areolar area (note size, shape, surface characteristics), nipples (note direction, size, shape, color, surface characteristics, possible crusting)	Breasts	Provide drape for legs and abdomen Place towel under back of side to be evaluated Instruct client to abduct arm overhead Explain procedures to client as performed
Female breast palpation: Note firmness, tissue qualities, lumps, areas of thickness, or tenderness; areolar and nipple area (note elasticity, tissue characteristics, discharge)		After breast palpation, may teach client to palpate own breasts
All clients: Palpation of anterior chest wall for cardiac movements or thrills, heaves, pulsations	Cardiovascular	
Auscultation of heart: aortic area, pulmonary area, Erb point, tricuspid area, apical area; note S_1, S_2, S_3, S_4 murmurs (location, rate, rhythm, intensity, frequency, timing, splitting); turn client slightly to left side; repeat assessment of these areas	Cardiovascular	
8. **Assess abdomen: provide chest drape for females; expose abdomen from pubis to epigastric region** Observation of skin characteristics from pubis to midchest region; note scars, lesions, vascularity, bulges, navel	Integumentary	Client should be comfortably positioned with pillow under head and knees slightly flexed to relax abdominal muscles
Observation of abdominal contour	Abdominal	
Observation of movement of abdomen, peristalsis, pulsations	Gastrointestinal Cardiovascular	

Continued.

CLINICAL GUIDELINES FOR PHYSICAL EXAMINATION INTEGRATION—cont'd

PROCEDURE OR FORMAT/ASSESSMENT	BODY PART OR SYSTEMS INVOLVED	CLINICAL STRATEGIES (ADULT AND ELDERLY)
Client is assisted to lying or low Fowler position—cont'd		
Auscultation of abdomen (all quadrants); note bowel sounds, bruits, venous hums	Gastrointestinal Cardiovascular	
Percussion of abdomen (all quadrants) and epigastric region for tone	Gastrointestinal	
Percussion of upper and lower liver borders and estimation of liver span		Liver percussion should occur at midclavicular line
Percussion of left midaxillary line for splenic dullness		
Light palpation of all four quadrants; note tenderness, guarding, masses		Allow client to become accustomed to examiner's hands
Deep palpation of all four quadrants; note tenderness, guarding, masses		Gently but firmly move palpation deeper and deeper until examiner convinced that abdomen sufficiently assessed
Deep palpation of right costal margin for liver border		Examiner must decide whether to use one-hand or two-hand approach
Deep palpation of left costal margin for splenic border		
Deep palpation of abdomen for right and left kidneys		
Deep palpation of midline epigastric area for aortic pulsation	Cardiovascular	Tenderness in epigastric area normal
Testing abdominal reflexes with pointed instrument	Neurological	
Client raises head for evaluation of flexion and strength of abdominal muscles	Musculoskeletal	Note use of arms or hands to assist; older client may have difficulty with this technique
Light palpation of inguinal region for lymph nodes, femoral pulses, and bulges that may be associated with hernia	Lymphatic Cardiovascular Abdominal	
9. **Assess lower limbs and hips: client is lying; abdomen and chest should be draped**		
Inspection of client's feet and legs for skin characteristics, vascular sufficiency, pulses; note deformities of toes, feet, nails, ankles, legs	Integumentary Cardiovascular, peripheral vascular Musculoskeletal	
Palpation of feet and lower legs; note temperature, pulses, tenderness, deformities	Cardiovascular Musculoskeletal	
Range of motion and motor strength of toes, feet, ankles, and knees	Musculoskeletal Neurological	Motor strength testing may be postponed until patient seated
Range of motion and motor strength of hips		
Palpation of hips for stability	Musculoskeletal	
10. **Assess genitalia, pelvic region, and rectum: client is lying and adequately draped**		
For males: Inspection and palpation of external genitalia, including pubic hair, penis and scrotum, testes, epididymides, and vas deferens; inspect sacrococcygeal and perianal areas and anus for surface characteristics (with client lying on left side with right hip and knee flexed)	Genitourinary	If mass in scrotal sac suspected, transilluminate

PROCEDURE OR FORMAT/ASSESSMENT	BODY PART OR SYSTEMS INVOLVED	CLINICAL STRATEGIES (ADULT AND ELDERLY)
Palpation of anus, rectum, and prostate gland with gloved finger		Lubricate finger and slowly insert; wait for sphincter to relax before advancing finger
Note characteristics of stool when gloved finger removed	Gastrointestinal	
For females (client should be lying in lithotomy position): inspection and palpation of external genitalia, including pubic hair, labia, clitoris, urethral and vaginal orifices, perineal and perianal area and anus for surface characteristics	Genitourinary	
Insertion of vaginal speculum and inspection of surface characteristics of vagina and cervix		
Collection of Pap smear and culture specimen		
Bimanual palpation to assess form, size, and characteristics of vagina, cervix, uterus, adnexa		Lubricate first two fingers of gloved hand to be inserted internally; other hand should be positioned on abdomen directly above internal hand
Vaginal-rectal examination to assess rectovaginal septum and pouch, surface characteristics, broad ligament tenderness		When examination completed, client should be offered tissue for drying of genital area
Rectal examination to assess anal sphincter tone, surface characteristics (anal culture may be obtained)		
Note characteristics of stool when gloved finger removed	Gastrointestinal	
Client is seated		
11. **Assess neurological system: assist client to sitting position; should have gown on and be draped across lap**		
Observation of client moving from lying to sitting position; note use of muscles, ease of movement, and coordination	Neurological Musculoskeletal	
Testing sensory function of neurological system by using light and deep (dull and sharp) sensation on forehead, paranasal sinus area, hands, lower arms, feet, lower legs	Neurological (sensory function)— CN V (trigeminal nerve)	Client's eyes should be closed; instruct client to either point to or verbally report area that has been touched Alternate light, dull, and pinprick sensations Test bilaterally
Bilateral testing and comparison of vibratory sensations of ankle, wrist, sternum		
Testing two-point discrimination of palms, thighs, back	Cortical, discriminatory, sensory functions of neurological system	
Testing stereognosis or graphesthesia		
Testing fine-motor functioning and coordination of upper extremities by instructing client to perform at least two of following: a. Alternating pronation and supination of forearm	Proprioception and cerebellar function of neurological system	Perform technique bilaterally and compare responses

Continued.

CLINICAL GUIDELINES FOR PHYSICAL EXAMINATION INTEGRATION—cont'd

PROCEDURE OR FORMAT/ASSESSMENT	BODY PART OR SYSTEMS INVOLVED	CLINICAL STRATEGIES (ADULT AND ELDERLY)
Client is seated—cont'd		
b. Touching nose with alternating index fingers		
c. Rapidly alternating finger movements to thumb		
d. Rapid movement of index finger between nose and examiner's finger		
Testing and bilaterally comparing fine-motor functioning and coordination of lower extremities by instructing client to run heel down tibia of opposite leg		
Alternately crossing legs over knee	Musculoskeletal	
Testing and bilaterally comparing deep tendon reflexes, including:	Reflex status of neurological system	If client shows any neurological problems, evaluate by Babinski and ankle clonus tests
a. Biceps tendon		
b. Triceps tendon		
c. Brachioradial tendon		
d. Patellar tendon		
e. Achilles tendon		
Client is standing		
12. **Palpate scrotum and inguinal region (male)**		
13. **Assess neurological and musculoskeletal system**		
Palpation of scrotum and inguinal regions for characteristics and hernias	Genitourinary	Instruct client to bear down or cough during hernia evaluation
Assessment of client's gait: observe and palpate straightness of client's spine as client stands and bends forward to touch toes	Musculoskeletal Neurological	Elderly clients may not be able to do this
With client's waist stabilized, evaluation by hyperextension, lateral bending, rotation of upper trunk		
Assessment of proprioception and cerebellar and motor functions by using at least two of following:		Client's age and general ability may help define which technique to use
a. Romberg test (eyes closed)		Protect client from falling by remaining close and ready to catch him if necessary
b. Walking straight heel-to-toe formation		Elderly clients may not be able to do this
c. Standing on one foot and then other (eyes closed)		
d. Hopping in place on one foot and then other		
e. Knee bends		

INTEGRATION OF THE NEONATAL AND PEDIATRIC EXAMINATION

The procedure for integrating the pediatric examination will depend entirely on the age and cooperation of the child. By the time the child reaches school age, he should be able to participate fully in a cooperative manner. It is the younger child who will present the challenge. The following format changes should facilitate a thorough assessment.

NEONATAL AND PEDIATRIC EXAMINATION

AGE AND PREPARATION/ASSESSMENT PROCEDURE	BODY PART OR SYSTEMS INVOLVED
1. **Newborn to 6 months: undressed, lying on examination table**	
Obtain history, highlighting developmental or problem areas	
Check vital signs: temperature, pulse, respiration	
Record weight, length, chest and head circumference	
Observe child lying on examination table; note color, general health, body symmetry, gross motor movement, alertness, gross and fine motor development, language development, social adaptive development, skin characteristics, and response to sound and vision stimulation	Cardiovascular, neurological, musculoskeletal, integumentary, visual, auditory
Examine and manipulate hands, arms, shoulders, feet, legs; note range of motion and tone	Musculoskeletal, neurological
Examine skin over extremities, chest, abdomen, and back	Integumentary, cardiovascular
Auscultate thorax, lungs, heart, abdomen	Thorax, lungs, cardiovascular, gastrointestinal
Palpate and examine external characteristics of head, neck, face, axillary region	Lymphatic, head, neck, visual, auditory, oral, nasal
Palpate thorax, abdomen, and umbilical area	Thorax, abdomen
Observe and palpate external genitalia, inguinal area, and hip stability	Genital, musculoskeletal
Examine eyes with ophthalmoscope	Visual
Examine mouth, teeth (development), tongue, posterior pharynx, nose	Oral, nasal
Examine ears with otoscope	Auditory
2. **Six months to 2 years: child in diaper, sitting on parent's lap; examiner's chair should be in front of parent's chair, and examiner's knees should touch parent's; during supine examination, child may lie on parent's and examiner's lap**	
Obtain history highlighting developmental or problem areas	
Perform developmental, social, vision, speech, hearing, and fine and gross motor assessment during play and initial "get acquainted" period	Neurological, visual, speech, auditory, musculoskeletal
Record weight, length, and chest and head circumference (until 18 months)	

Continued.

NEONATAL AND PEDIATRIC EXAMINATION—cont'd

AGE AND PREPARATION/ASSESSMENT PROCEDURE	BODY PART OR SYSTEMS INVOLVED
Check vital signs, including blood pressure in children over 18 months of age; may be postponed until later if child becomes agitated	
Auscultate lungs and heart	Thorax, cardiovascular
Examine skin over extremities, chest, abdomen, and back	Integumentary, cardiovascular
Examine and manipulate hands, arms, shoulders, feet, legs; note range of motion and tone	Neurological, musculoskeletal
Palpate and examine external characteristics of head, neck, face, axillary region	Lymphatic, head, neck, visual, auditory, oral, nasal
Auscultate abdomen with child in supine position on parent's and examiner's lap	Gastrointestinal
Palpate thorax, abdomen, and umbilical area	Thorax and abdomen
Observe and palpate external genitalia, inguinal area, and hip stability	Genital, musculoskeletal
Examine eyes with ophthalmoscope	Visual
Examine mouth, teeth (development), tongue, posterior pharynx, nose	Oral, nasal
Examine ears with otoscope	Auditory
3. **Two to 4 years: undressed to underpants; may be examined either on parent's lap or examination table; much of assessment may be informal as examiner observes and plays with child**	
Same as for child from 6 months to 2 years; refer to individual chapter for detailed discussion of strategies	
4. **Four to 6 years: undressed to underpants, sitting on examination table; assessment should move toward adult format; child's developmental immaturity may necessitate that examiner alter various examination techniques to facilitate child's participation and correct response.**	
Same as for child from 6 months to 2 years	
5. **Over 6 years old: in gown on examination table**	
Same as for adult client	

GUIDELINES FOR EXAMINATION OF CHILDBEARING WOMEN

Printed formats are available for examiners who concentrate on prenatal, postpartum, and neonatal assessment. Sample forms available from Problem Oriented Pregnancy Risk Assessment System (POPRAS) are shown in Fig. 16-1, *A* and *B* (pp. 590-591). Consistent examination is especially important during pregnancy, delivery, and the neonatal period.

PHYSICAL EXAMINATION WRITE-UP

The data base and the information collected during the physical assessment must be organized and documented. The components of the documentation are (1) subjective data base, (2) physical assessment, (3) risk profile, and (4) problem list. Before the actual documentation the examiner must decide whether to record the data on plain paper or on a predesigned form. Each has advantages and disadvantages.

Advantages

Plain paper

Documentation space is not a problem.

Specific data for individual client may be emphasized as necessary.

Predeveloped form

Departmental continuity is maintained.

Data will be easy to locate by other examiners.

It is a reminder for completeness.

Disadvantages

The examiner must be organized; if not, rambling and insignificant data may be a problem.

All examiners in the agency may not use the same format.

Individual situations may be difficult to emphasize.

Examiner may not have adequate space for documentation.

If form was developed before examiner's input, it may not include all data the examiner wants to collect

Separate forms necessary for pediatric and geriatric clients.

Once the style of documentation is determined, the examiner must synthesize the client's historical and physical data and record information in the following areas. The examiner is urged to record *what* is observed, heard, percussed, or palpated and to avoid vague and nondescriptive terms, such as *normal, negative, good,* or *poor.*

DOCUMENTATION FORMAT
Subjective Data Base
- Biographical data
- Reason for visit
- Present health status
- Current health data: immunizations, allergies, last examination
- Past health status: childhood illnesses, serious or chronic illnesses, serious accidents or injuries, hospitalizations, operations, emotional health, obstetrical health
- Family history
- Review of physiological systems: general, nutritional, integumentary, head, eyes, ears, nose, mouth, neck, breast, cardiovascular, respiratory, hematolymphatic, gastrointestinal, urinary, genital, musculoskeletal, central nervous system, endocrine, and allergic and immunological
- Psychosocial history: general status, response to illness, significant others, occupational history, educational level, activities of daily living, habits, financial status
- Health maintenance efforts: maintenance of self health, health care patterns
- Environmental health: general assessment, employment, home, neighborhood, community

Physical Assessment
- Vital Statistics
  - Age
  - Race
  - Nutritional status
  - Height
  - Weight
  - Temperature
  - Pulse
  - Blood pressure (both arms, lying and sitting)
  - Communication skills
- General Statement of Appearance
- Integumentary
  - Color
  - Integrity
  - Texture
  - Presence or absence of lesions, edema, unusual odors

  Distribution and texture of hair
- Head and Neck
  - Size, symmetry, and contour of head and face
  - Edema or puffiness
  - Palpation of lymph nodes
  - Palpation of thyroid
  - Palpation of sinuses
- Nose
  - Position
  - Nasal patency
  - Presence of polyp(s)
  - Appearance of turbinates
  - Position of septum
- Mouth and Pharynx
  - Condition and alignment of teeth
  - Color and characteristics of tongue, mucosa, pharynx, gums
  - Position and appearance of tonsils and palate
  - Symmetry and movement of tongue and uvula
  - Taste and gag reflex
- Ears and Auditory System
  - Position and alignment of auricles
  - Surface characteristics of external ear and canal
  - Characteristics of temporomandibular joint
  - Rinne and Weber tests
- Eyes and Visual System
  - Visual acuity and visual fields
  - Appearance of surface characteristics of eyes
  - Extraocular movements
  - Corneal light reflex
  - Characteristics of cornea
  - Consensual response to light
  - Findings from ophthalmoscopic examination
- Thorax and Lungs
  - Chest wall configuration and anteroposterior diameter
  - Respiratory rate and depth
  - Palpation to evaluate symmetry and tactile fremitus
  - Percussion to evaluate tones and diaphragm excursion
  - Auscultation to identify breath sound characteristics and adventitious sounds
  - Auscultation of other sounds
- Cardiovascular
  - Location and characteristics of the apical impulse
  - Auscultation of S_1 and S_2 to note location, pitch, intensity, timing, splitting, systole, and diastole
  - Presence and characteristics of extra sounds, such as murmurs, clicks, snaps, S_3, and S_4
  - Jugular vein distention
  - Peripheral pulses: quality of pulses, bilaterally equal
  - Allen's test

A

PAST PREGNANCIES

INTAKE DATE & INITIALS:

OB INDEX

Age	Term	Premi	Ab-Ectop	Living

BIRTH CONTROL PILLS IN PAST YEAR ☐ Yes ☐ No

MENSES Onset/Int/Dur

CYCLES ☐ Regular ☐ Irregular

LMP: ☐ Normal ☐ Abnormal   PMP:

EDC:

POSITIVE PREGNANCY TEST

Date:

Preg-nancy No.	Termi-nation Date Mo.	Yr.	EARLY LOSS < 20 wks Spon	Ec-top	In-duced*	GA wks	Birth Wt	Sex	Living Y/N**	Spon Vtx	Br	For-ceps	CPD	Fetal Dis-tress	Abn Pres	Re-peat	Other/Unk	ASSOCIATED PROBLEMS
1																		
2																		
3																		
4																		
5																		
6																		
7																		
8																		

≥ 20 wks LIVE OR STILLBORN — VAGINAL — C-SECTION

*D&C S(Suction) Sa(Saline) P(Prostaglandin) H(Hysterotomy) O(Other) U(Unknown) **S(Stillbirth) N(Neonatal) I(Infant) C(Childhood)

Prob. No.	±	Risk Value	HISTORICAL PROBLEMS	HEALTH STATUS INDICATORS
1		5	☐ **AGE < 17** ☐ **AGE ≥ 35**	**YEARS OF EDUCATION** Mother _____ Father _____
2		5	**MULTIPARITY** (5 or more ≥ 20 weeks)	**DIET (Ex, G, P, Undet)** Calories _____ Protein _____ Iron _____
3		5	**INDUCED ABORTION**	**INSURANCE** ☐ Public ☐ Private ☐ None
4		10	**HABITUAL ABORTION** (3 or more)	Carrier _____ # _____ # _____
5		10	**PREMATURE** (< 37 weeks) ☐ **LGA**	Carrier _____ # _____ # _____
				ALLERGIES
6		10	**SGA** (Small for Gestational Age)	**COMMENTS**
7		5	**BIRTH WEIGHT > 4000 gms or 9 lbs**	SPECIAL COMMENTS FOR DATA ENTRY
8		10	**PERINATAL DEATH** ☐ Stillborn ☐ Neonatal	
9		5	**POST NEONATAL PROBLEM** ☐ Sudden Infant Death ☐ Neurologic Handicap ☐ Mental Retardation	
10		10	**NEONATAL JAUNDICE** ☐ Rh ☐ ABO ☐ Physiologic ☐ Unknown ☐ Other:	
11		5	**GENETIC DISEASE** ☐ Chromosomal ☐ CNS ☐ Inborn Errors of Metabolism ☐ Other: ☐ Structural Congenital Anomalies	
12		5	**HISTORY OF INFERTILITY** ☐ Primary ☐ Secondary ☐ Treated ☐ Untreated	
13		10	**UTERINE-CERVICAL ABNORMALITY** ☐ Uterine Anomaly ☐ Corrected ☐ Incomp Cx ☐ Cerclage Removed ☐ Yes ☐ No	
14		5	**PREVIOUS UTERINE SURGERY C-Section:** ☐ Classical ☐ Low Trans ☐ Low Vert ☐ Unknown ☐ Hysterotomy ☐ Myomectomy	
15		5	**HEMORRHAGE** ☐ Previa ☐ Abruptio ☐ Other 3rd Trimester ☐ Post Partum ☐ Transfusion	
16		5	**PREGNANCY-INDUCED HYPERTENSION** ☐ Required Hosp ☐ Required Early Delivery ☐ Developed Eclampsia	
17		10	**CHRONIC HYPERTENSION** (BP ≥ 140/90 non-pregnant) ☐ On Drug Therapy:	
18		10	**HEART DISEASE** ☐ Rheumatic ☐ Congenital ☐ Arteriosclerotic ☐ Other ☐ Surgical Correction ☐ Hx of CHF or Arrhythmia ☐ No limitation of physical activity ☐ Slight limitation ☐ Marked limitation ☐ Unable to carry on any physical activ. w/out discomfort	
19		5	**PULMONARY DISEASE** ☐ Asthma ☐ Chronic Bronchitis ☐ Tuberculosis ☐ Other	
20		5	**GENITOURINARY INFECTIONS** ☐ Asymptomatic Bacteruria ☐ Cystitis ☐ Pyelonephritis ☐ Gonorrhea ☐ Syphilis ☐ Genital Herpes	
21		10	**RENAL DISEASE** ☐ Glomerulo ☐ Chronic Pyelo ☐ Diabetic ☐ Collagen-vas ☐ Calculi ☐ Other:	
22		10	**DIABETES** ☐ A ☐ B ☐ C ☐ D ☐ F-R ☐ Insulin, Pre-preg Dosage:	
23		10	**THYROID DISEASE** ☐ Hypo ☐ Thyroiditis ☐ Hyper: treated with ☐ Drugs ☐ Surgery ☐ I-131	
24		10	**OTHER MEDICAL** ☐ Phlebitis ☐ Embolus ☐ Collagen-vas ☐ On Drug Therapy: ☐ Hematologic:	
25		10	**EPILEPSY** ☐ On Therapy: ☐ Phenobarb ☐ Dilantin ☐ Mysoline ☐ Other:	
26		5	**PSYCHIATRIC** ☐ Hospitalized ☐ On Drug Therapy:	
27		5	**PREVIOUS OPERATIONS** ☐ Diag D&C ☐ Laparoscopy ☐ Appendectomy ☐ Cholecystectomy ☐ Other:	
28		10	**EXCESSIVE USE** ☐ Alcohol ☐ Tobacco ☐ Marijuana ☐ Narcotics:	
29		5	**MATERNAL ONLY** ☐ Hypertension ☐ Multiple Births ☐ Diabetes ☐ Hemoglobinopathy ☐ DES ☐ Other:	
30		5	**MAT. OR PATERNAL** ☐ Mental Retardation ☐ Congen Anom ☐ Congen Hearing Loss ☐ Allergies ☐ Other:	

Row categories (left margin): PREVIOUS INFANTS (5–11), GYN (12–14), PREG. COMPLICATIONS (15–16), MEDICAL-SURGICAL (17–27), HABITS (28), FAMILY HISTORY (29–30)

Patient Address _____ City _____ State _____ Zip _____ Birth Date _____

Home Phone _____ Preferred Language _____ Marital Status **M W D SEP S**

Contact Phone _____ Race-Ethnicity **W B H I A O** Spouse's Name _____

Last Name _____ First Name _____ Middle Initial _____

Pat Hosp # _____

Referred By _____ Hospital of Delivery _____

Fam File Name _____ Pat Clinic # _____

COPYRIGHT © POPRAS, 1975, 1977, 1978, 1981

1 PRENATAL HISTORY

Maiden Name _____ Mother's Maiden Name _____

Clinic/Physician _____ Referral Clinic _____

Fig. 16-1   A, Sample form for prenatal history. **B,** Sample form for prenatal screening. (From Problem Oriented Pregnancy Risk Assessment System [POPRAS], Los Angeles.)

B

DATE:	PHYSICAL EXAM								LAB DATA BASE		

PHYSICAL EXAM

Normal	Yes No	Normal	Yes No	Normal	Yes No	Normal	Yes No
SKIN		LUNGS		ABDOMEN		VAGINA	
HEENT		BREASTS		EXTREMITIES		CERVIX	
MOUTH		NIPPLES		NEUROLOGIC		UTERUS	
THYROID		HEART		PERINEUM		ADNEXA	
				VULVA		RECTAL	

UTERINE SIZE/DATES: ____ / ____ □ Comparable □ Smaller □ Larger

PELVIS □ Adequate □ Borderline □ Inadequate □ Clinical □ X-ray

ABNORMAL FINDINGS

LAB DATA BASE

Date	TYPE □ A □ B □ O □ AB	Date	HCT ____ HGB ____
	Rh □ Neg □ Pos □ Du+		**HGB ELECT** (circle 2)
	ANTIBODY SCREEN □ Neg □ Pos		A₁ A₁ A₂ F / S S C
	VDRL □ Neg □ Pos		**PPD** □ Neg □ Pos:
	FTA □ Neg □ Pos		**CHEST X-RAY** □ Neg □ Pos:
	RUBELLA □ Neg Titer:		**PAP** □ Neg □ Infl □ Pos
	URINE CULTURE:		**DYSPLASIA** □ Mild □ Mod □ Sev
	U **PROTEIN** □ Neg □ Tr □ 1+ □ 2+ □ 3+		**G-C CULTURE** □ Neg □ Pos:
	R I N **SUGAR** □ Neg □ Pos		**FATHER'S Rh** □ Pos □ Neg □ Homozyg □ Heterozyg
	E **MICRO** □ Neg □ Pos		
	BLOOD SUGAR	FASTING 1 HR	PP 2 HR PG

MEDICATIONS

COMMENTS

SPECIAL COMMENTS FOR DATA ENTRY

DEVELOPING PROBLEMS

Prob. No.	±	Date Positive	R	Risk Val.			
31				5	**ANATOM-ICAL**	**PRE-PREG WT** □ < 100 lb □ > 200 lb	
32				10		**SIZE-DATE DISCREPANCY**	
33				5		**SMALL PELVIS**	
34				5	**POSITIVE LAB**	**Rh NEG** □ Not Sensitized	
35				10		□ Sensitized	
36				5		**G-U TESTS** □ Abn Pap □ Pos GC □ Asymp Bacteruria	
37				5		**POS** □ SEROLOGY □ PPD	
38				5		**ANEMIA** □ Mild < 11 gms or 27-33% □ Severe < 9 gms or < 27%	
39				5		**ABNORMAL HBG** □ SS □ AS □ Thalassemia □ Other:	
40				10	**EARLY PREG-NANCY**	**THREATENED AB** □ Hosp □ Drug Therapy:	
41				■		**EARLY TERMINATION** (< 20 wks) □ Spontaneous □ Induced □ Ectopic	
42				5		**HYPEREMESIS GRAVIDARUM** □ Hosp □ Drug Therapy:	
43				10		**INCOMPETENT CERVIX** □ Cerclage, Date: □ Drug Therapy:	
44				10	**INFECTION**	**TORCH** □ Toxoplasmosis □ Syphilis □ Rubella □ Cytomegalovirus □ Herpes	
45				5		**FLU SYNDROME** □ High Fever □ Gastroenteritis □ Hosp	
46				5		**GENITAL-URINARY** □ Vaginitis □ Asymp Bacteruria □ Cystitis □ GC □ Genital Herpes	
47				10		**PYELONEPHRITIS**	
48				10	**MEDICAL-SURGICAL**	**DIABETES** (in this pregnancy) □ A □ B □ C □ D □ F-R Rx: □ Diet □ Insulin	
49				10		**THROMBOPHLEBITIS** □ Hosp □ Anticoagulant □ Embolus	
50				10		**CARDIOPULMONARY** □ Asthmatic Attack □ Bronchitis □ Pneumonia □ Active TB □ Tachycardia □ Arrhythmia □ CHF	
51				10		**OTHER MEDICAL** □ Hepatitis □ Late Anemia □ Other:	
52				5		**SURGICAL** □ Adnexal □ Appendectomy □ Other:	
53				5	**PSYCHO-SOCIAL**	□ Marital □ Coping & Support □ Unresolved Grief □ Family □ Sexual □ Financial □ Relocation □ Prior OB Experience □ Other:	
54				5	**ANATOM-ICAL ABNORMAL-ITIES**	**MATERNAL WEIGHT GAIN** □ < ½ lb/wk □ > 2 lb/wk	
55				10		**UTERINE SIZE** □ Suspected IUGR □ Suspected LGA □ Polyhydramnios □ Mult Preg □ Myomata	
56				5		**FETAL POSITION** □ Breech □ Transverse Lie □ Oblique	
57				5	**ABNORMAL-ITIES OF FUNCTION**	**BLOOD PRESSURE** □ Preg-Induced Hypertension Mild □ 1 = BP ≥ 140/90 or ↑ 30 mm systolic or ↑ 15 mm diastolic □ 2 = Proteinuria 1+ or 2+ □ 3 = Persistent Edema	
58				10		□ Superimposed Severe □ BP ≥ 160/110 or □ Proteinuria > 2+ both after 26 wks GA	
59				10		**BLEEDING > 20 WKS** □ Cervical □ Previa □ Low-lying □ Undetermined	
60				5		**LABOR, HOSPITALIZED FOR** □ Suspected Premature Labor □ False Labor > 37 wks □ Pharmacologic Rx:	
61				10		**POST-TERM > 42 WKS** (over 42 weeks from LMP or estimated from early physical exam)	
62				■		**ANTEPARTUM FETAL DEATH**	
63						**PROTOCOL** □□□ □□□	

First Total		↑ PRENATAL SCORE	Sig/Date ____
36 Wk Total			Sig/Date ____

Last Name ____ First Name ____ Middle Initial ____

Pat Hosp # _____

Clinic/Physician _____ # ____

Patient Clinic # _____

2 **PRENATAL SCREENING**

- Breasts
  Bilaterally equal
  Symmetry
  Presence of masses, tenderness, discharge, dimpling
  Presence of scars
  Lymphatic assessment
- Abdomen
  Contour, visible aortic pulsations
  Auscultation of all four quadrants to identify bowel sounds
  Palpation of all four quadrants to identify organs, tenderness, masses
  Costovertebral angle tenderness
  Hernia
  Findings from rectal examination
- Genital: Female
  Characteristics of external genitalia
  Speculum examinations: note discharge, pain, surface characteristics of vagina, cervix, adnexa
  Bimanual examination: note tenderness, masses, size of uterus and ovaries
  Rectal examination
- Genital: Male
  Characteristics of external genitalia
  Palpation of penis and scrotum to note tenderness, discharge, lesions
  Investigation of inguinal hernia to note swelling or tenderness
  Prostate evaluation
  Rectal examination
- Musculoskeletal
  Gait
  Alignment of extremities and spine, symmetry of body
  Joint evaluation
  Muscle development, symmetry, and strength
  Range of motion
  Drawer test
  McMurray's test
- Neurological
  Mental status, thought process, cognitive assessment
  Gait
  Cranial nerves assessment
  Fine and gross motor function
  Sensory evaluation
  Reflexes

Risk Profile

The risk profile should include those items from the client's history and physical assessment that might indicate risk to the overall health state. They are potential problems. Examples that may be considered a risk for some clients are detailed in the data base in Chapter 1.

Problem List

The problem list should be a synthesis of those items that are currently identified as stressors for the client. The stressors may be physiological, sociological, psychological, or a combination of them. The problems are those items that reduce the client's overall level of health. Once the problems are listed and assigned a priority, it can be decided which are within the examiner's scope of practice to handle and which must be referred.

It is important for the examiner to cluster subjective and objective data to describe problems. The following unrelated examples demonstrate a holistic approach to problem identification.

Weight gain: 18 pounds in past year; exercise limited to game of tennis twice a month; expresses desire to diet but needs direction

Shortness of breath when walking up more than one flight of stairs; moderate edema below midcalf bilaterally; fine rales in lower bases bilaterally

Limited range of motion in right shoulder, which interferes with activities of daily living; dressing, preparing meals

Cataracts bilaterally, which interfere with reading and driving at night

BP 180/120 (right arm) lying, 172/112 (right arm) sitting; retinal A-V ratio appears to be 2/4; arteriolar narrowing

Periodic slight urinary incontinence since birth of child 3 years ago; cystocele noted during vaginal examination.

Complaints of LLQ discomfort for 6 months; cyclic with menses; increased discomfort at ovulation time and just before menses; thickening in left adnexa area; increased tenderness with palpation of left adnexa area; menses regular; pinpoint tenderness on deep palpation in LLQ

Smokes one pack of cigarettes a day for past 15 years; deep, nonproductive cough for past 5 years, becoming worse; increased breathing difficulty when climbing more than one flight of stairs; decreased breath sounds on right; bilateral rales or rhonchi in base of lungs; slight clearing with cough

Death of spouse 2 months ago; since then increased periods of depression, 10-pound weight loss, decreased desire to maintain own health state

Study Questions

1. The examiner usually decides to concentrate on this area first:
   - ☐ a. The major concern of the client
   - ☐ b. The head examination, with intent to finish at the feet
   - ☐ c. Review of systems
   - ☐ d. Snellen screening

2. An examiner moves behind the client to assess the:
   - ☐ a. Peripheral circulation
   - ☐ b. Posterior chest
   - ☐ c. Spleen and gallbladder
   - ☐ d. Epigastric region

3. What position is used for conducting a pelvic examination:
   - ☐ a. Prone
   - ☐ b. Knee-chest
   - ☐ c. Lithotomy
   - ☐ d. Trendelenburg

4. Adult examination procedures are usually done when a child reaches the age of:
   - ☐ a. 2 years
   - ☐ b. 4 years
   - ☐ c. 6 years
   - ☐ d. 8 years

5. Which of the following is one benefit of using printed forms for childbearing women:
   - ☐ a. Patients can complete their own forms
   - ☐ b. All major areas of assessment are addressed
   - ☐ c. New examiners can perform examinations without supervision
   - ☐ d. The examiner can spend more time with the client

6. Which item relates to subjective data:
   - ☐ a. Hernia
   - ☐ b. Vital signs
   - ☐ c. Condition of teeth
   - ☐ d. Reason for visit

Mark each statement as either "T" for true or "F" for false.

7. ＿＿ Subjective and objective data are used to describe problems.

8. ＿＿ Objective and subjective data are gathered at the same time.

9. ＿＿ The precordium is palpated for thrills, heaves, and pulsations.

10. ＿＿ Deep palpation is used to determine the liver border.

11. ＿＿ Examination procedure depends on the age of the child.

12. ＿＿ Variation is expected during an examination of systems.

SUGGESTED READINGS

Cohen J: The adult health screen in general practice, *Aust Fam Phys* 17(7):584, 1988.

Finch CE, Schneider EL: *Handbook of the biology of aging,* ed 2, New York, 1985, Van Nostrand Reinhold.

Malasanos L, Barkauskas V, Stoltenberg-Allen K: *Health assessment,* ed 4, St Louis, 1990, Mosby–Year Book.

Oboler SK, and others: The periodic physical examination in asymptomatic adults, *Ann Intern Med* 110:214, 1989.

Pritchard JA, MacDonald PC: *Williams' obstetrics,* ed 17, New York, 1985, Appleton-Century-Crofts.

Problem Oriented Pregnancy Risk Assessment System (POPRAS), 5910 West 77th Place, Los Angeles, CA 90045.

Seidel HM, Ball JW, Dains JE, Benedict GW: *Mosby's guide to physical examination,* ed 2, St Louis, 1991, Mosby–Year Book.

Whaley LF, Wong DL: *Nursing care of infants and children,* ed 4, St Louis, 1991, Mosby–Year Book.

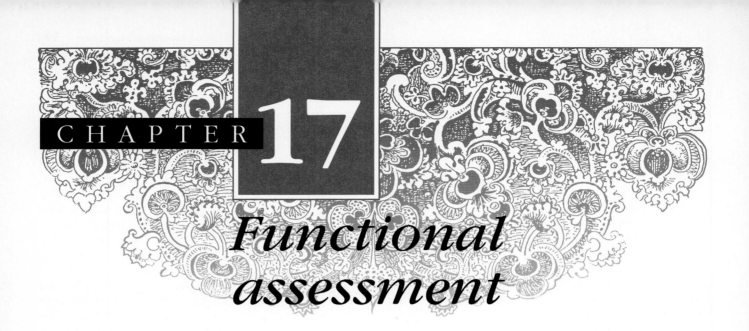

CHAPTER 17

Functional assessment

VOCABULARY

cognitive functioning Appraisal of an individual's perception of his intellectual awareness, his potential for growth, and his recognition by others for his mental skills and contributions.

emotional functioning Appraisal of an individual's access to his own feelings, his satisfaction with his feelings, his ability to express his feelings effectively, and his capacity to resolve or deal with stressors.

environment Composition of physical facilities, resources, and people that affect an individual's capacity to exist to his satisfaction.

functional assessment Appraisal of an individual's perception of his capacity to maneuver within a defined environment.

general well-being assessment Appraisal of an individual's view of his worth and his capability for maintaining and/or enhancing his quality of life.

physical functioning Appraisal of an individual's perception of his ability to control and manipulate his physical en-

vironment, as well as his judgment of the ability of his inner resources to control and use his body effectively.

psychosocial functioning Appraisal of an individual's capacity to attain and maintain satisfactory intimate and social relationships with others.

spiritual state An individual's version of his effectiveness in developing and sustaining a belief and value system that assists him in self-acceptance and in his relationship to others and to a Higher Being.

PRINCIPLES AND CONCEPTS

Functional assessment explores how an individual is able to manipulate, accommodate, and find comfort within a given environment. It is an inquiry about how a person perceives himself and all that surrounds him. Successful living can be affected by physical, emotional, or spiritual incapacities, but one's perception of what is happening can overturn or exaggerate an unfortunate circumstance. All of the questions in this functional assessment are posed to elicit *the client's version* of how satisfactorily he conducts his life. The realms of general well-being, and emotional, psychosocial, physical, cognitive, and spiritual functioning are covered in this format. Functional assessment can be used with clients who are very ill, dying, undergoing rehabilitation, or in

"perfect health." It can be used with very young adults or the very old. People in all of these circumstances share the need to have control over their environment to the extent that they feel effective as human beings and sufficiently in touch with others for loving and understanding.

The purpose of functional assessment is to clarify an individual's status in his world as he perceives it. The outcome of the ensuing analysis, planning, intervention and evaluation may lead to restoration of full functioning, maintenance of present level, or improving some aspects of functioning while other segments deteriorate. An individual with a terminal disease can strengthen his capacity for fulfillment with family relationships and self-acceptance even though his physical functioning will not improve. A person in "perfect health" may report insufficient energy to enjoy his family after a working day. Further investigation of nutritional and sleep habits, stress at work, family relationships, and self-expectations may lead to a solution that would further enhance his state of well-being.

Functional assessment complements the traditional body systems assessment. The traditional assessment in this text is tempered with questions about interference with activities of daily living, but it is generally aimed at a search for symptoms and medical disorders. This search is a legitimate and necessary reason for performing an assessment; however, the identification of medical disorders or symptoms does not really convey to the examiner a client's capacity to negotiate his environment. The format of this chapter deliberately excludes a body systems approach; instead, it focuses on the client's perceptions of his capabilities in leading a successful and satisfying life within the context of his present circumstances.

Functional assessment has existed for many years. Although a variety of tools have been developed to assess a client's level of functioning, they have addressed specific groups of clients or have served narrow purposes. For instance, geriatric practitioners and researchers have devised a number of assessment instruments to measure the physical, cognitive, and psychosocial skills of the elderly. These early tools were used to appraise candidates for institutional placement and level of care. The ability to dress, bathe, toilet, ambulate, transfer self (in and out of bed or chair), feed self, and remain continent were classified in self-care categories defined as "independent" or "dependent." These levels of functioning helped to standardize corresponding levels of care, as well as facility and staffing design, and served as research data as large groups of individuals were assessed.

In recent years, numerous assessment tools have been used in psychiatric and rehabilitative settings to provide a data base of an individual's level of functioning and to follow that person's progress while being treated. Experience gained from using these tools to assess large groups of people has resulted in more flexible interventions and in altering hostile environments that impede or fail to support the client's progress. Nevertheless, there has been growing recognition for the need to incorporate functional assessment into the general health assessment performed by nurses.

Environmental Assessment

In the context of this assessment, the environment includes all of the physical facilities, resources, and people that affect an individual's capacity to exist to his satisfaction. One's environment may be narrowed to a hospital bed, including all of the institutional resources, or it may encompass a home and a community with its variety of resources.

Environmental assessment has been traditionally incorporated into family and community nursing textbooks and practices. Many of these assessments, usually of the home, family, and community, are very detailed and have served as an entry into the family realm for students learning about families and for practitioners providing home care.

Halbert Dunn (Pender), a contemporary theorist in the area of high level wellness, proposed a health grid (Fig. 17-1, p. 596), indicating that an individual's level of health (a functional state) can be enhanced or deterred by his environment. If an individual is impaired, his functional status is improved if he lives in a favorable environment. For example, if an arthritic client reports that she is unable to manipulate eating utensils or tie her shoelaces because of stiff, painful fingers, an environmental assessment may lead to the acquisition of special utensils and Velcro fasteners. If a resident in an extended care facility indicates that he has a need for privacy, examination of the facilities may lead to identification of a quiet place where he can seek refuge when needed. If an individual cannot be restored to full function (or peak wellness), his environment must be examined and possibly altered to support the impairment—hence the advent of ramps, the development of support networks, or the instigation of a toileting program to support the needs of an incontinent individual. The environmental assessment in this text has been designed to match the areas of concern in the functional assessment.

COGNITIVE OBJECTIVES

At the end of this chapter the learner will demonstrate knowledge of functional assessment by the ability to do the following:
- Define the following terms and give examples of each:
  1. Cognitive functioning
  2. Emotional functioning
  3. Environment
  4. Functional assessment
  5. General well-being assessment
  6. Physical functioning
  7. Psychosocial functioning
  8. Spiritual state
- Describe the connection between one's capacity to function and the effect that one's environment has on that capacity by giving examples of the interplay between human functioning and environment.

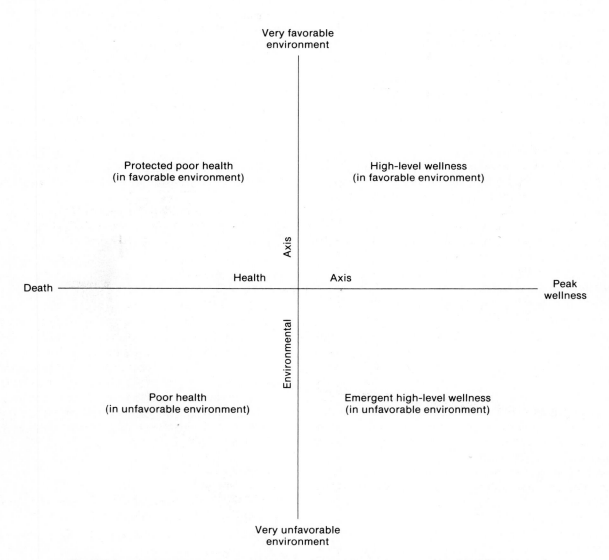

Fig. 17-1   Health grid: its axes and quadrants. (From U.S. Department of Health, Education and Welfare, Public Health Service, National Office of Vital Statistics.)

- Offer a rationale for complementing the traditional body system assessment with a functional assessment.
- Identify at least four reasons why the nurse is professionally suited to perform a comprehensive functional assessment.
- Appreciate the flexibility of functional assessment in terms of using portions of it according to the status of the client.

CLINICAL OUTLINE

At the end of this chapter the learner will perform a systematic functional assessment, demonstrating the ability to do the following:

- Assess the client's state of general well-being by posing specific questions about:
  1. Self-perception
  2. Stability
  3. Self-actualization
  4. Health maintenance
- Assess the client's emotional functioning by posing specific questions about:
  1. Mood expression
  2. Coping capacity
- Assess the client's psychosocial functioning by posing specific questions.
- Assess the client's physical functioning by posing specific questions about:
  1. Performance
  2. Sensory functions
  3. Body image
  4. Rest, activity, energy expenditure
- Assess the client's cognitive functioning by posing specific questions.
- Assess the client's spiritual state by posing specific questions.
- Assess the environmental state of the client by posing specific questions in the areas of:
  1. General well-being
  2. Emotional functioning
  3. Psychosocial functioning
  4. Physical functioning
  5. Cognitive functioning
  6. Spiritual state
- Compile the findings of both the functional and environmental assessments and examine the relationships between the two in preparation for further analysis and intervention.

FUNCTIONAL ASSESSMENT AND THE ROLE OF THE NURSE

Although a number of allied health professionals have special skills to perform detailed assessment of specific aspects of a client's ability to function, the nurse, for the following reasons, is perhaps in the best position to perform a comprehensive functional assessment.

- Typically, the nurse has the greatest amount of contact with the client. This contact allows her to question and observe through numerous interactions with the client, enabling her to note changes in functioning over a period of time.
- The nurse provides holistic health care, which holds that the client can be separated neither into parts nor from his environment.
- The character of interaction between nurse and client promotes wide-ranging discussions spanning the many dimensions of health.
- The interaction between nurse and client promotes trust so that the less obvious functional implications (e.g., ones in the psychosocial and spiritual realms) come to the surface.
- Because of her central role in client care, the nurse interacts with other health professionals involved with the client's care, as well as with family members and other individuals, such as friends and co-workers who are important to the client's general well-being. Interaction with these individuals can be useful, not only because of their importance to the client, but also because they can help evaluate the reliability of the information provided by the client.
- Finally, the nurse is often in the best position to evaluate the practicality of the client's environment, including the support systems represented by other individuals heavily involved in the client's life circumstances.

A TWO-PART TOOL FOR PERFORMING A GENERAL FUNCTIONAL ASSESSMENT

The purpose of the following assessment is to provide the examiner with the means (1) to screen for the client's functional impairments and (2) to describe the corresponding environmental effects on the client's functions. After performing the functional assessment part of the tool, the examiner performs the environmental assessment to correlate the client's functional needs with the resources that need to be present in his environment.

Functional Assessment

The functional assessment is incorporated into a tool that permits the client to respond "not applicable," "yes," "sometimes," or "no" to any of the questions. The questions are worded so that *yes* indicates full satisfaction with functioning, and *sometimes* or *no* indicates a problem in that area. This format permits the examiner to be alert for all of the *sometimes* and *nos* when evaluating the total set of responses. Values (numbers) are assigned to each of the responses. Each *no* is worth two points, each *sometimes* is worth one point, and *yes* and *NA* (not applicable) are worth zero points. Therefore the higher the score for each section, the higher the indication of

functional deficits will be. This author cannot offer a standard for evaluating the totals (or percentages), since this tool has not been researched to provide reliable norms for deficits. However, the quantification of the results would be helpful if the same client would use this tool over a period of time. The decline of totals (or the increase) would indicate improvement (or regression) in a particular functional area. Following is a table of functional categories and their potential deficit totals. (It is helpful to review the vocabulary section of this chapter before beginning the assessment to assist in clarifying the intention [purpose] for each question.)

Text continues on p. 604.

FUNCTIONAL CATEGORY	POTENTIAL TOTAL POINTS FOR DEFICITS
General well-being	
Self-perception	12
Stability	10
Self-actualization	10
Health maintenance	22
	TOTAL 54
Emotional functioning	
Mood/expression	14
Coping capacity	18
	TOTAL 32
Psychosocial functioning	TOTAL 16
Physical functioning	
Performance	142
Sensory functions	32
Body image	6
Rest, activity, energy expenditure	14
	TOTAL 194
Cognitive functioning	TOTAL 16
Spiritual state	TOTAL 12

FUNCTIONAL ASSESSMENT	(Points)	NA* (0)	Yes (0)	Sometimes (1)	No (2)	

General well-being

1. Self-perception
   Do you feel as though you generally like yourself?
   Do you like to spend some time by yourself?
   Do you believe you function effectively (in terms of problem solving, participating in events or decisions)
     In the work setting?
     With your family?
     With your friends?
     In other situations?

POSSIBLE SUBTOTAL 12

2. Stability
   Is your personal life as stable as you want it to be? Areas of concern are
     Budgeting for necessities
     Satisfaction with employment
     Seeking advice/comfort from significant others
   Do you believe that you have control over the important parts of your life?
   Do you believe that your life has purpose?

POSSIBLE SUBTOTAL 10

3. Self-actualization
   Do you generally feel optimistic about your life?
   Are you able to accomplish the goals that you set for yourself?
   Do you enjoy creative expression (e.g., recreation, exercise, music, the arts, writing)
   Do you feel you live in the present (vs. the past or future)?
   Do you enjoy changes in your life?

POSSIBLE SUBTOTAL 10

4. Health maintenance
   Do you believe that your level of health is average or above average?
   Do you feel confident that you can take care of the problem when you are sick?
   Do you generally feel well?
   Do you feel comfortable seeking professional help when you need it?
     Physician
     Nurse
     Clinic
     Dentist
     Counselor
     Other
   Do you trust your health care provider?
   Do you believe that you take good care of yourself?

POSSIBLE SUBTOTAL 22

General well-being   POSSIBLE TOTAL 54

*NA, *Not applicable.*

Continued.

FUNCTIONAL ASSESSMENT	(Points)	NA (0)	Yes (0)	Sometimes (1)	No (2)	

Emotional functioning

1. Mood/expression

When you feel sad, blue, or depressed, is it self-contained (i.e., short-lived and controllable)?

When you feel nervous, is it self-contained (i.e., controllable)?

Do you feel a sense of belonging with other people?

Do you believe that other people are generally kind and compassionate?

Are you able to control your anger so that you can function effectively?

Are you able to express your anger when you want to?

Are you able to accomplish important tasks to your satisfaction?

POSSIBLE SUBTOTAL 14

2. Coping capacity

When stressors descend on you, are you able to handle them to your satisfaction?

Is it easy to seek out friends for advice/comfort?

Is it easy to go to your family (or significant other) with problems/distress?

When you are distressed, does your health remain stable?

Do you have an outlet for relieving your tension (e.g., relaxation methods, reading, sports, crying, talking, keeping a journal)?

Is your alcohol consumption at a limited, moderate (or controllable) level?

Are you able to maintain a satisfactory feeling of contentment without medications or drugs?

Are you able to control your nerves without medications or drugs?

Are you able to feel enthusiastic, energetic, and confident without medications or drugs?

POSSIBLE SUBTOTAL 18

Emotional functioning   POSSIBLE TOTAL 32

Psychosocial functioning

1. Are you satisfied with the amount of time that you spend with other people?
2. Do you feel that your close friends understand you?
3. Do you feel that your family (or significant others) understand you?
4. Do you feel that you really care about your friends?
5. Do you feel that you really care about your family (or significant others)?
6. Are you satisfied with the loving and affection that you share with others?
7. Are you satisfied with your level of sexual expression and fulfillment?
8. If you needed emergency assistance, do you feel that you could count on someone to respond?

Psychosocial functioning   POSSIBLE TOTAL 16

FUNCTIONAL ASSESSMENT	(Points)	NA* (0)	Yes (0)	Sometimes (1)	No (2)	

Physical functioning

1. Performance
   a. Are you able to provide self-care?
      (1) *Dressing, undressing, and clothing*
         Keeping clothes in good repair (mending)
         Having access to clothes
         Getting into and out of underwear (bra, girdle, underpants,
            pantyhose, stockings, garter belt, undershirt)
         Putting on and removing pants
         Getting arms in sleeves
         Managing zippers, buttons, snaps (especially in the back),
            and ties
         Putting on socks, shoes, tying laces
         Applying prostheses (e.g., glasses, hearing aid, brace)
      (2) *Grooming and hygiene*
         Washing, drying, brushing hair
         Brushing teeth
         Cleaning and putting in dentures
         Shaving
         Nail care (feet and hands)
         Applying makeup
         Preparing bath water and testing the temperature
         Getting into and out of the tub or shower
         Reaching and cleaning all body parts

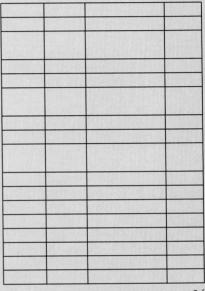

POSSIBLE SELF-CARE TOTAL 34

   b. Are you able to move about successfully?
      Sitting up, rising from bed
      Transferring from bed to chair
      Lowering to or rising from chair
      Walking (short distances)
      Walking (long distances)
      Opening doors
      Climbing stairs
      Descending stairs
      Lifting
      Reaching items in cupboards

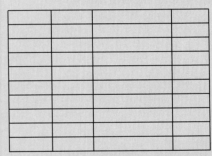

POSSIBLE MOBILITY TOTAL 20

   c. Are your elimination habits under control and comfortable?
      Controlling urination
      Controlling bowel movements
      Assuming sitting position on toilet
      Lowering onto and rising from toilet
      Wiping and cleansing self

POSSIBLE ELIMINATION TOTAL 10

Continued.

FUNCTIONAL ASSESSMENT	(Points)	NA (0)	Yes (0)	Sometimes (1)	No (2)

Physical functioning—cont'd

1. Performance—cont'd

d. Are you able to accomplish eating to your satisfaction
   (use nutritional section from traditional assessment for
   details about appetite, food consumption, and weight patterns)
   Handling knife, fork, spoon
   Cutting foods (meat)
   Getting food to mouth
   Chewing
   Swallowing
   Preparing food (opening cans, packages, using stove)
   Access to dishes, pots, utensils
   Access to market
   Carrying packages

POSSIBLE EATING TOTAL **18**

e. Are you able to communicate to your satisfaction?
   Speaking clearly
   Dialing telephone
   Answering door
   Immediate access to neighbors; calling for help

POSSIBLE COMMUNICATION TOTAL **8**

f. Are you satisfied with your housekeeping capabilities?
   Making bed
   Sweeping, mopping floors
   Dusting
   Cleaning dishes
   Cleaning tub, bathroom
   Picking up clutter (to client's satisfaction)
   Taking out trash, garbage
   Using basement (stairs, cleaning)
   Using laundry facilities (in home or near residence; washtub,
      clothes line)
   Performing yard care (garden, bushes, grass)
   Performing other home maintenance concerns (e.g., access to
      fuse box, storm windows, furnace filters, painting)

POSSIBLE HOME CARE TOTAL **22**

g. Are you able to manage your medications?
   Scheduling numerous dosages
   Remembering to take medications
   Being able to see, understand labels, directions
   Keeping medications in one area and safe from others
   Getting prescriptions filled
   Being able to afford prescriptions

POSSIBLE MEDICATION TOTAL **12**

h. Are you able to leave your residence and get into the commu-
   nity?
   Walking
   Using stairs, curbs
   Being in traffic, crowds
   Using the bus
   Driving (self or service from others)
   Feeling safe on the streets

POSSIBLE COMMUNITY ACCESS TOTAL **12**

FUNCTIONAL ASSESSMENT	(Points)	NA (0)	Yes (0)	Sometimes (1)	No (2)

Physical functioning—cont'd

1. Performance—cont'd
   i. Other functional concerns
      Caring for spouse/relative/companion/children successfully
      Managing finances (access to your money, making payments, cashing/writing checks)
      Care of pet(s)

POSSIBLE OTHER PHYSICAL CONCERNS TOTAL 6

POSSIBLE PERFORMANCE TOTAL 142

2. Sensory functions
   a. Are you able to maintain your balance?
   b. Are you able to see clearly?
      Near vision
      Far vision
   c. Can you tolerate glare?
      During daytime
      During nighttime
   d. Are you able to hear
      Speech tones
      Television
      Telephone
      Someone at door
   e. Are you able to tolerate
      Excessive noise
      Background noise
   f. Is your sense of smell intact (consider enjoyment of food and detection of offensive or dangerous odors)?
   g. Are you free of pain?
   h. If you have pain, are you able to reduce it (to toleration) or get rid of it?
   i. Are you comfortable with the degree of cold temperature to which you are exposed?
   j. Are you comfortable with the degree of heat that your body feels or to which your body is exposed?

POSSIBLE SENSORY FUNCTIONS TOTAL 32

3. Body image
   a. Do you like the way your body looks?
   b. Do you like the way your body functions?
   c. Do you feel that you can count on your body to function when necessary?

POSSIBLE BODY IMAGE TOTAL 6

4. Rest, activity, energy expenditure
   a. Do you awaken in the morning feeling rested?
   b. Can you fall asleep easily?
   c. Can you stay asleep to your satisfaction?
   d. Do you have the energy to get through
      your day?
      your evening?
   e. Are you able to relax?
   f. Are you able to find time for recreation?

POSSIBLE REST, ACTIVITY, ENERGY EXPENDITURE TOTAL 14

Physical functioning POSSIBLE TOTAL 194

Continued.

FUNCTIONAL ASSESSMENT	(Points)	NA (0)	Yes (0)	Sometimes (1)	No (2)	

Cognitive functioning

1. Do you generally feel alert and clearheaded?
2. Do you look forward to (or plan on) learning something new?
3. Do you believe your intellect (or knowledge) is satisfactorily used (or recognized)?
   At work
   With friends
   With family (or significant others)
4. Are you able to maintain/control your mental capacity (thinking, perceiving, problem solving) in spite of
   Medication
   Stress
   Other

Cognitive functioning   POSSIBLE TOTAL 16

Spiritual state

1. Are you satisfied with
   Your spiritual state (your personal philosophy and value system)
   Your relationship to a Higher Being
   Your relationship with other people
   Your religious practices
2. Do your spiritual or religious convictions provide you with the comfort you need in your present circumstances?
3. Are you comfortable seeking spiritual guidance if you need it?

Spiritual state   POSSIBLE TOTAL 12

Environmental Assessment

The environmental assessment allows the client the opportunity to respond to each question with "not applicable," "yes," "sometimes," or "no." The questions in this format are also worded so that the *sometimes* or *no* responses indicate a deficit in the environment. Numbers (values) were not added to this section because this tool is less complicated and it is easier to identify the negative responses for further action or evaluation.

The categories of concern are exactly the same and in the same order as in the functional assessment tool so that the responses of the client can be compared and contrasted between the two tools.

ENVIRONMENTAL ASSESSMENT	NA*	Yes	Sometimes	No	

General well-being

1. Self-perception
   Do you have access to privacy?
   Do you have access to others for understanding, feedback, problem-solving?
      Employers, peers at work?
      Family, significant others?
      In other situations?
2. Stability
   Do you have financial stability (adequate income for necessities)?
   Do you have secure living arrangements (shelter, safety, heat, food)?
   Do you have secure employment?
   Do you have dependable access to people important to your survival (physical, emotional)?

*NA, *Not applicable.*

ENVIRONMENTAL ASSESSMENT	NA	Yes	Sometimes	No	

General well-being—cont'd

3. Self-actualization
   Do you have financial comfort (income for enrichment)?
   Do you have recreational facilities available (sports, fitness, libraries, parks, cultural resources)?
4. Health maintenance
   Do you have access to health care services (hospital, ambulance services, dental care, counseling or support services)?
   Do you have insurance or financial freedom to seek care?
   Do you have automobile or vehicle services (or reasonable walking distance to services)?
   Do you have access to responsive and competent health care providers?
   Do you have exposure to clean air?
   Do you have adequate police, fire protection?

Emotional functioning

1. Mood/expression
   Do you have family or significant others who offer support, caring?
   Do you have responsive, competent professional support?
2. Coping capacity
   Do you have limited (or manageable) stressors (Fig. 17-2, pp. 607-608)?
   Do you have family or significant others who offer support, caring?
   Do you have responsive, competent professional support?

Psychosocial functioning

Do you have adequate support systems available (according to client's definition)?
   Friends?
   Family?
   Significant other(s)?
   Pets?
   Emergency network?

Physical functioning

1. Performance
   Home (or living space)
      Do you have adequate space for the number of people residing there (includes sleeping, space for belongings, eating, cooking utensils and facilities, furniture, laundry, privacy)?
      Do you have reasonable walking distance between living areas (from bedroom to kitchen to bathroom to sitting area to outdoors)?
      Do you have manageable number of stairs between living areas (from bedroom to kitchen to sitting area to outdoors to basement)?
      Do you have adequate temperature regulation?
      Do you have indoor plumbing?
      Do you have effective prosthetic devices (wheelchair, walker, crutches, glasses, hearing aid, dentures, other)?
      Do you have adequate facilities for prosthetic devices (e.g., if wheelchair is in use, adequate space in doorways, maneuvering in rooms, ramps, toilet usage, reaching high places)?
      Do you have availability of others in facility to assist with physical performance?
      Do you have a telephone?
      Do you have a call button (or bell)?

Continued.

ENVIRONMENTAL ASSESSMENT	NA	Yes	Sometimes	No	

Physical functioning—cont'd

1. Performance—cont'd

    Home—cont'd

    Do you have other safety needs?

    Railings in bathtub, bathroom, hallway, stairways

    Adequate lighting (stairways, nightlight, absence of glare)

    Nonslippery floors, rugs

    Freedom from clutter

    Smoke alarm

    Ability to secure safety (lock doors, maintain belongings, food, medications)

    Community

    Do you have access to

    Automobile (self-use or services from others)

    Busline

    Other public vehicles

    Are nearby roads, sidewalks paved and maintained?

    Are the following available?

    Market

    Laundry

    Pharmacy

    Trash disposal

    Legal services

    Repair services

    Veterinarian

    Public health services

    Is your community sufficiently quiet?

2. Sensory functions

    Do you have professional resources to assess and intervene with impairments? (NOTE: Temperature regulation, vision, and hearing are covered in assessment on previous page.)

3. Body image

    Do you have professional resources to assess and intervene with impairments?

    Do you have sufficient support from family or significant others in coping with impairments?

4. Rest, activity, energy expenditure

    Do you have access to privacy (freedom from noise and distractions)?

    Do you have freedom from noise during sleeping times?

    Do you have vacation time from employment?

    Do you have support from family or significant others for relaxation time?

    Do you have professional resources to assess and intervene with unresolvable fatigue or sleep deprivation?

Cognitive functioning

    Do you have professional resources to assess and intervene with identified impairment?

    Do you have support from significant others and health care providers for identified impairment?

    Do you have community resources for enrichment (schools, continuing education, libraries, special services for identified impairment)?

Spiritual state

    Do you have spiritual guidance (or comfort) available?

    Do you have family members (or significant others) who support (or do not interfere with) your beliefs?

Please check those life changes that you have experienced personally during the past *two years*.

Life event	Scale of impact	
Death of spouse (or significant other)	100	_____
Divorce (or termination of long-term relationship)	73	_____
Marital separation	65	_____
Jail term	63	_____
Death of close family member	63	_____
Personal injury or illness	53	_____
Marriage (or commitment to permanent relationship)	50	_____
Fired at work	47	_____
Marital or relationship reconciliation	45	_____
Retirement	45	_____
Change in health of family member	44	_____
Pregnancy	40	_____
Sex difficulties	39	_____
Gain of new family member	39	_____
Business readjustment	39	_____
Change in financial state	38	_____
Death of close friend	37	_____
Change to different line of work	36	_____
Change in number of arguments with spouse	35	_____
Mortgage over $20,000	31	_____
Foreclosure of mortgage or loan	30	_____
Change in responsibilities at work	29	_____
Son or daughter leaving home	29	_____
Trouble with in-laws	29	_____
Outstanding personal achievement	28	_____
Spouse begins or stops work	26	_____

Fig. 17-2 Life-change index. (Modified from Holmes T, Rahe E: *J Psychosom Res* 11:213, 1967. Copyright © 1967, Pergamon Press.)

Continued.

Fig. 17-2, cont'd   Life-change index.

Life event	Scale of impact	
Begin or end school	26	_____
Change in living conditions	25	_____
Revision of personal habits	24	_____
Trouble with boss	23	_____
Change in work hours or conditions	20	_____
Change in residence	20	_____
Change in schools	20	_____
Change in recreation	19	_____
Change in church activities	19	_____
Change in social activities	18	_____
Mortgage or loan less than $20,000	17	_____
Change in sleeping habits	16	_____
Change in number of family get-togethers	15	_____
Change in eating habits	15	_____
Vacation	13	_____
Christmas (if approaching)	12	_____
Minor violations of the law	11	_____
TOTAL		========

SCORING THE LIFE-CHANGE INDEX

Score range	Interpretation
0-150	No significant problems, low or tolerable life change
150-199	Mild life change (approximately 33% chance of illness)
200-299	Moderate life change (approximately 50% chance of illness)
300 or over	Major life change (approximately 80% chance of illness)

CLINICAL TIPS AND STRATEGIES

- **The entire assessment is subjective, i.e., the client's version of his own lifestyle and capabilities:** It may be helpful to complement this tool with portions of the traditional (objective) assessment to increase the reliability of the findings if the client's version is questionable. Examples of useful objective assessments follow:
  1. Mental status observations
  2. Musculoskeletal observations
  3. Neurological observations
  4. Vision and hearing screening
  5. Nutritional assessment
- **If the client does seem to be unreliable or dis-** oriented, it may be helpful to pose some of the questions to a family member/significant other to increase the reliability of the responses: This questioning would be particularly useful in the physical functioning category. It is doubtful that anyone but the client could describe his sense of well-being or his spiritual state.
- **Regardless of the client's reliability in judging his own capabilities, his version is important and legitimate:** He must live, function, and deal with his environment and himself according to his perceptions.
- **It is also helpful to complement the functional assessment with the traditional assessment:** The traditional assessment (and ensuing medical diagno-

sis) often provides an explainable cause for functional impairments, as well as a prognosis in terms of a predictable time frame for improvement or resolution of the problem.

- **As you study these functional and environmental formats, you will note that they are extremely useful for assessing individuals with obvious physical impairments to generate baseline data for evaluating how successfully they maneuver in their world:** These tools can also be modified or used, in part, to assess a client's capacity to maintain a high level of wellness. The general well-being section poses questions about how the client perceives himself in his present developmental phase and life circumstance. The subset of questions in the physical performance section can be eliminated if an individual is physically fit. The emotional and psychosocial sections may alert an examiner to a client's emotional crisis or stress-laden life circumstance. The spiritual questions have been particularly useful to this author in talking with chronically or terminally ill individuals.

These tools are intended to be flexible and to conform to the examiner's *purpose* for initiating an assessment, as well as the needs and circumstances of the client.

FUNCTIONAL ASSESSMENT AND THE NURSING PROCESS

Inasmuch as assessment is the initial phase of the five-step nursing process, the data derived from the functional assessment is used to formulate appropriate nursing diagnoses. Although nursing diagnosis is beyond the scope of this text, the examiner is urged to think about the rich opportunities for diagnoses suggested by the kind of data developed from a comprehensive functional assessment. Many NANDA-approved nursing diagnoses are strikingly appropriate to the kind of findings generated by a functional assessment, as the following sampling attests:

Activity intolerance
Impaired adjustment
Ineffective family coping: disabling
Diversional activity deficit
Altered family processes
Altered health maintenance
Impaired home maintenance management
Functional incontinence
Knowledge deficit (specify)
Impaired physical mobility
Altered role performance
Bathing/hygiene self-care deficit
Dressing/grooming self-care deficit
Feeding self-care deficit
Toileting self-care deficit
Body-image disturbance
Sensory/perceptual alterations: visual, auditory, kinesthetic, gustatory, tactile, olfactory

Sexual dysfunction
Impaired skin integrity
Social isolation
Spiritual distress (distress of the human spirit)
Unilateral neglect

In addition, the results of the functional assessment enable the nurse to plan, implement, and evaluate nursing care, completing the nursing process.

In a general sense, the functional assessment will continue to fulfill its traditional role in determining the level of care clients require. However, today's nurse must be prepared to use the general functional assessment to match functional needs to therapeutic environments in an infinite number of situations, extending far beyond the traditional issue of nursing home placement. Such recommendations may include visits by home health care nurses, specialized rehabilitation programs, counseling, self-care, and countless specific alterations in lifestyle and environmental modifications. All these living situations and treatment modalities can be properly recommended only when they are based on the results of a comprehensive functional assessment.

FUNCTIONAL ASSESSMENT AS AN ONGOING ACTIVITY

It was noted earlier that the numerical totals of the functional assessment become more meaningful as evaluative indices when the examiner has gained a sense of judgment based on assessing a large number of clients. However, the numerical totals have immediate significance when they are used to measure an individual client's progress or regression based on repeated administrations of the assessment. Indeed, the assessment should be administered periodically to evaluate the effectiveness of the nursing care as part of the nursing process.

The level of a client's functioning usually evolves rather than remains static. The assessment is a means of measuring that evolution. But even an obvious impairment, such as an amputation, which implies obvious physical limitations, may conceal hidden functional disabilities. These functional disabilities may not be fully grasped by the client, so they may require ongoing investigation by the examiner through an interactive discovery process shared with the client. In many cases, the social and emotional implications of a physical impairment may be more devastating to the client (resulting in a more profound loss of functional ability) than the loss of physical functioning in areas such as mobility. The functional status of the client should be constantly monitored through reassessment so that the nurse, by remaining alert to these functional changes, can review and revise the goals of nursing care to conform to the shifting level of human functioning.

SUGGESTED READINGS

Balaban DJ and others: Weights for scoring the quality of well-being instrument among rheumatoid arthritics, *Med Care* 24:11, 973, 1986.

Dean P: Expanding our sights to include social networks, *Nurs Health Care,* 545, December 1986.

Duke University Center for the Study of Aging and Human Development: *Multidimensional functional assessment: the OARS methodology,* Durham, NC, 1978, Duke University.

Friedman MM: *Family nursing: theory and assessment,* New York, 1981, Appleton-Century-Crofts.

Granick S: Psychologic assessment technology for geriatric practice, *J Am Geriatr Soc* 31:12, 728, 1986.

Gross-Andrew S, Zimmer A: Incentives for families caring for disabled elderly: research and demonstration project to strengthen the natural support system, *J Gerontol Soc Work* 1:119, 1978.

Guccione AA, Felson DT, Anderson JJ: Defining arthritis and measuring functional status in elders: methodological issues in the study of disease and physical disability, *Am J Public Health* 80(8):945, 1990.

Harris BA and others: Validity of self-report measures of functional disability, *Top Geriatr Rehabilitation* 1:3, 31, 1986.

Henderson V: *The nature of nursing,* New York, 1966, MacMillan.

Hill L, Smith N: *Self-care nursing,* ed 2, Norwalk, Conn, 1990, Appleton & Lange.

Jette AM: Functional disability and rehabilitation of the aged, *Top Geriatr Rehabilitation* 1:3, 1986.

Kahn RL: Productive behavior: assessment, determinants and effects, *J Am Geriatr Soc* 31:12, 750, 1983.

Katz S: Assessing self-maintenance: activities of daily living, mobility and instrumental activities of daily living, *J Am Geriatr Soc* 31:12, 721, 1983.

Katz S and others: Studies of illness in the aged. The index of ADL: a standardized measure of biological and psychological function, *JAMA* 185:914, 1963.

Kim MJ, McFarland GK, McLane AM: *Pocket guide to nursing diagnoses,* ed 3, St Louis, 1989, Mosby—Year Book.

Lawton MP: The impact of the environment on aging and behavior. In Birren J, Schaie E, Warners K, editors: *Handbook of the psychology of aging,* New York, 1977, Van Nostrand Reinhold.

Llewellyn TH and others: Describing health states: methodologic issues in obtaining values for health states, *Med Care* 22:6, 543, 1984.

Pender NJ: *Health promotion in nursing practice,* Norwalk, Conn, 1982, Appleton-Century-Crofts.

Stanhope M, Lancaster J: *Community health nursing: process and practice for promoting health,* ed 2, St Louis, 1988, Mosby—Year Book.

Thompson JM, McFarland GK, Hirsch JE, and others: *Mosby's manual of clinical nursing,* ed 2, St Louis, 1989, Mosby—Year Book.

Travis SS: Personalizing self-care, *Geriatr Nurs* 11(2):72, 1990.

Williams FT: Comprehensive functional assessment: an overview, *J Am Geriatr Soc* 31:11, 637, 1983.

Zielstorff RD and others: Functional assessment in an automated medical record system for coordination of long-term care, *Top Geriatr Rehabilitation* 1:3, 43, 1986.

Answers

Chapter 1

1. T
2. T
3. T
4. F
5. T
6. T
7. T
8. F
9. T
10. T

Chapter 2

1. Any of the following are correct, in any order:
   Client's initial response to examiner
   Body appearance
   Body movements
   Gait
   Facial expression
   Vocal tones
   Speech
   Apparel
   Grooming
   Odors
   General mannerisms

2. c
3. d
4. e
5. a
6. b
7. d
8. b
9. c
10. b
11. b
12. a

Chapter 3

1. e
2. b
3. d
4. d
5. c
6. d
7. g
8. h
9. c
10. f
11. g
12. j
13. a
14. i
15. l
16. d
17. k
18. b
19. h
20. e
21. f
22. e
23. g
24. d
25. a
26. b
27. c
28. f
29. e
30. b
31. a
32. d
33. c
34. e
35. a
36. b
37. c
38. d
39. a
40. d
41. c
42. e
43. b
44. b
45. c
46. d
47. c
48. e

Chapter 4

1. d
2. c
3. a
4. e
5. c
6. b
7. b
8. d
9. b
10. a
11. i
12. c
13. g
14. e

Chapter 5

1. f
2. b
3. b
4. a
5. i
6. c
7. f
8. c
9. b
10. a
11. c
12. a
13. c
14. b
15. c
16. e
17. c
18. d
19. d
20. f
21. c
22. f

Chapter 6

1. c
2. c
3. i
4. c
5. i
6. d
7. b
8. h
9. d
10. b
11. d
12. T
13. F
14. T
15. F

Chapter 7

1. b
2. g
3. j
4. c
5. b
6. g
7. f
8. g
9. b
10. j
11. i
12. e
13. h
14. a
15. j
16. a
17. e
18. e
19. a
20. d
21. d
22. e
23. c
24. c
25. e
26. c
27. b
28. a

Chapter 8

1. F
2. T
3. T
4. F
5. F
6. F
7. d
8. j
9. d
10. c
11. a
12. b
13. d
14. d
15. d
16. i
17. f
18. c

Chapter 9

1. i
2. g
3. i
4. f
5. f
6. g
7. h
8. b
9. a
10. Amplitude
11. Contour
12. Amplitude pattern
13. a. Superior vena cava
    b. Inferior vena cava
    c. Right atrium
    d. Tricuspid valve
    e. Right ventricle
    f. Pulmonary valve
    g. Pulmonary artery
    h. Pulmonary vein
    i. Aorta
    j. Left atrium
    k. Aortic valve
    l. Mitral valve
    m. Left ventricle
14. Mitral; tricuspid; systole
15. Aortic, pulmonary; diastole
16. a
17. b
18. b
19. a
20. a
21. b
22. a
23. a
24. c
25. c
26. e
27. d
28. b
29. a
30. h
31. a
32. b

Chapter 10

1. b
2. c
3. i
4. j
5. d
6. c
7. i
8. a
9. c
10. a

Chapter 11

1. Student can compare own drawing of major abdominal organs with textbook illustration.
2. Any five of the following are correct:
   Client supine with arms on chest or at sides
   Small pillow under head
   Knees slightly flexed
   Warm room
   Client's breasts and pubis draped
   Examiner's hands warm
   Short fingernails
   Warm stethoscope
   Client breathing slowly through mouth
   Examiner explaining procedure
3. g
4. g
5. c
6. a
7. b
8. d
9. e
10. c
11. c
12. b
13. d
14. g
15. c or e

Chapter 12

1. n
2. g
3. o
4. b
5. h
6. f
7. c
8. l
9. k
10. d
11. j
12. i
13. m
14. a
15. e
16. b
17. b
18. c
19. a
20. b
21. c
22. d
23. d
24. c
25. i
26. i

Chapter 13

1. l
2. f
3. c
4. k
5. h
6. a
7. e
8. i
9. b
10. g
11. d
12. j
13. d
14. g
15. b
16. h
17. k
18. c
19. m
20. f
21. a
22. l
23. i
24. e
25. j
26. j
27. f
28. b
29. g
30. h
31. g
32. b
33. d
34. T
35. F
36. T
37. T
38. F
39. c
40. b
41. a
42. c
43. b
44. c
45. a
46. g
47. c
48. h

Chapter 14

1. T
2. T
3. T
4. F
5. T
6. T
7. F
8. F
9. T
10. F
11. a
12. a
13. j
14. c
15. a
16. b
17. h
18. a
19. b
20. c
21. d
22. h
23. c
24. f
25. e

Chapter 15

1. b
2. h
3. i
4. j
5. g
6. b
7. c
8. a
9. c
10. d
11. b
12. a
13. c
14. b

Chapter 16

1. a
2. b
3. c
4. c
5. b
6. d
7. T
8. T
9. T
10. T
11. T
12. T

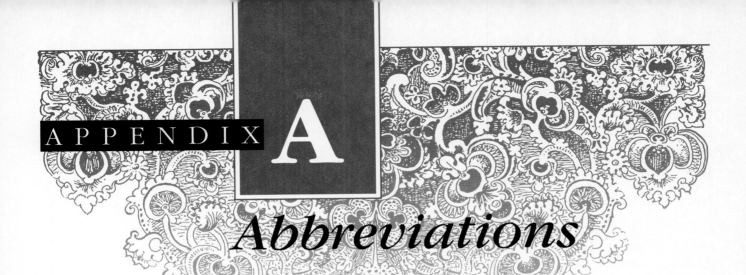

APPENDIX A

Abbreviations

A & P	Anterior and posterior; auscultation and percussion
A & W	Alive and well
abd	Abdomen; abdominal
a̅c̅	Before meals
ADL	Activities of daily living
AJ	Ankle jerk
AK	Above knee
ANS	Autonomic nervous system
AP	Anteroposterior
bid	Twice a day
BK	Below knee
BP	Blood pressure
BPH	Benign prostatic hypertrophy
BS	Bowel sounds; breath sounds
c̅	With
CC	Chief complaint
CHD	Childhood disease; congenital heart disease; coronary heart disease
CHF	Congestive heart failure
CNS	Central nervous system
c/o	Complains of
COPD	Chronic obstructive pulmonary disease
CV	Cardiovascular
CVA	Costovertebral angle; cerebrovascular accident
CVP	Central venous pressure
Cx	Cervix
D & C	Dilation and curettage
D/C	Discontinued
DM	Diabetes mellitus
DOB	Date of birth
DOE	Dyspnea on exertion
DTRs	Deep tendon reflexes

DUB	Dysfunctional uterine bleeding
Dx	Diagnosis
ECG, EKG	Electrocardiogram; electrocardiograph
EENT	Eye, ear, nose, and throat
ENT	Ear, nose, and throat
EOM	Extraocular movement
FB	Foreign body
FH	Family history
FROM	Full range of motion
FTT	Failure to thrive
Fx	Fracture
GB	Gallbladder
GE	Gastroesophageal
GI	Gastrointestinal
GU	Genitourinary
GYN	Gynecologic
HA	Headache
HCG	Human chorionic gonadotropin
HEENT	Head, eyes, ears, nose, and throat
HOPI	History of present illness
HPI	History of present illness
Hx	History
ICS	Intercostal space
IOP	Intraocular pressure
IUD	Intrauterine device
IV	Intravenous
JVP	Jugular venous pressure
KJ	Knee jerk
KUB	Kidneys, ureters, and bladder

lat	Lateral
LCM	Left costal margin
LE	Lower extremities
LLL	Left lower lobe (lung)
LLQ	Left lower quadrant (abdomen)
LMD	Local medical doctor
LMP	Last menstrual period
LOC	Loss of consciousness; level of consciousness
LS	Lumbosacral; lumbar spine
LSB	Left sternal border
LUL	Left upper lobe (lung)
LUQ	Left upper quadrant (abdomen)
M	Murmur
MAL	Midaxillary line
MCL	Midclavicular line
MGF	Maternal grandfather
MGM	Maternal grandmother
MSL	Midsternal line
MVA	Motor vehicle accident
N & T	Nose and throat
N & V	Nausea and vomiting
NA	No answer; not applicable
NKA	No known allergies
NPO	Nothing by mouth
NSR	Normal sinus rhythm
OD	Oculus dexter; right eye
OM	Otitis media
OS	Oculus sinister; left eye
OTC	Over the counter
OU	Oculus uterque; both eyes
p̄	After
P & A	Percussion and auscultation
p̄c	After meals
PE	Physical examination
PERRLA	Pupils equal, round, react to light and accommodation
PGF	Paternal grandfather
PGM	Paternal grandmother
PI	Present illness

PID	Pelvic inflammatory disease
PMH	Past medical history
PMI	Point of maximum impulse; point of maximum intensity
PMS	Premenstrual syndrome
prn	As necessary
Pt	Patient
PVC	Premature ventricular contraction
q	Every
qd	Every day
qh	Every hour
qod	Every other day
RCM	Right costal margin
REM	Rapid eye movement
RLL	Right lower lobe (lung)
RLQ	Right lower quadrant (abdomen)
RML	Right middle lobe (lung)
ROM	Range of motion
ROS	Review of systems
RSB	Right sternal border
RUL	Right upper lobe (lung)
RUQ	Right upper quadrant (abdomen)
s̄	Without
SCM	Sternocleidomastoid
SQ	Subcutaneous
Sx	Symptoms
T & A	Tonsillectomy and adenoidectomy
TM	Tympanic membrane
TPR	Temperature, pulse, and respiration
UE	Upper extremities
URI	Upper respiratory infection
UTI	Urinary tract infection
WD	Well developed
WN	Well nourished
x	Times; by (size)

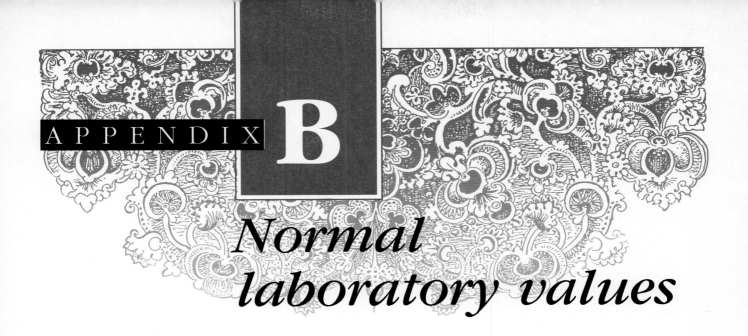

Normal laboratory values

ABBREVIATIONS USED IN TABLES

<	= less than	mg	= milligram	ng	= nanogram
>	= greater than	ml	= milliliter	pg	= picogram
dl	= 100 ml	mM	= millimole	μEq	= microequivalent
g	= gram	mm Hg	= millimeters of mercury	μg	= microgram
IU	= International Unit	mIU	= milliInternational Unit	μIU	= microInternational Unit
kg	= kilogram	mOsm	= milliosmole	μl	= microliter
mEq	= milliequivalent	mμ	= millimicron	μU	= microunit

TABLE B-1   Whole blood, serum, and plasma chemistry

		TYPICAL REFERENCE INTERVALS		
COMPONENT	SYSTEM	CONVENTIONAL UNITS	FACTOR*	RECOMMENDED SI UNITS†
Acetoacetic acid				
Qualitative	Serum	Negative	—	Negative
Quantitative	Serum	0.2-1.0 mg/dl	98	19.6-98.0 μmol/L
Acetone				
Qualitative	Serum	Negative	—	Negative
Quantitative	Serum	0.3-2.0 mg/dl	172	51.6-344.0 μmol/L
Albumin				
Quantitative	Serum	3.2-4.5 g/dl (salt fraction-ation)	10	32-45 g/L
		3.2-5.6 g/dl (electropho-resis)		32-56 g/L
		3.8-5.0 g/dl (dye binding)		38-50 g/L
Alcohol, ethyl	Serum or whole blood	Negative—but presented as mg/dl	0.22	Negative—but presented as mmol/L

From Henry JB: Todd-Sanford-Davidsohn clinical diagnosis and management by laboratory methods, *ed 17, Philadelphia, 1984, WB Saunders.*
*Factor, *Number factor (note that units are not presented).*   *Continued.*
†Value in SI units, *Value in conventional units × factor.*

TABLE B-1 Whole blood, serum, and plasma chemistry—cont'd

COMPONENT	SYSTEM	TYPICAL REFERENCE INTERVALS		
		CONVENTIONAL UNITS	FACTOR	RECOMMENDED SI UNITS
Aldolase	Serum			
Adults		3-8 Sibley-Lehninger U/dl at 37° C	7.4	22-59 mU/L at 37° C
Children		Approximately 2 times adult levels		Approximately 2 times adult levels
Newborn		Approximately 4 times adult levels		Approximately 4 times adult levels
Alpha-amino acid nitrogen	Serum	3.6-7.0 mg/dl	0.714	2.6-5.0 mmol/L
δ-Aminolevulinic acid	Serum	0.01-0.03 mg/dl	76.3	0.76-2.29 μmol/L
Ammonia	Plasma	20-120 μg/dl (diffusion)	0.554	11.1-67.0 μmol/L
		40-80 μg/dl (enzymatic method)		22.2-44.3 μmol/L
		12-48 μg/dl (resin method)		6.7-26.6 μmol/L
Amylase	Serum	60-160 Somogyi units/dl	1.85	111-296 U/L
Arginosuccinic lyase	Serum	0-4 U/dl	10	0-40 U/L
Arsenic*	Whole blood	<7 μg/dl	0.13	<0.91 μmol/L
Ascorbic acid (vitamin C)	Plasma	0.6-1.6 mg/dl	56.8	34-91 μmol/L
	Whole blood	0.7-2.0 mg/dl		40-114 μmol/L
Barbiturates	Serum, plasma, or whole blood	Negative	—	Negative
Base excess	Whole blood			
Male		−3.3 to +1.2 mEq/L	1	−3.3 to +1.2 mmol/L
Female		−2.4 to +2.3 mEq/L		−2.4 to +2.3 mmol/L
Base, total	Serum	145-160 mEq/L	1	145-160 mmol/L
Bicarbonate	Plasma	21-28 mM	1	21-28 mmol/L
Bile acids	Serum	0.3-3.0 mg/dl	10	3.0-30.0 mg/L
Bilirubin	Serum			
Direct (conjugated)		Up to 0.3 mg/dl	17.1	Up to 5.1 μmol/L
Indirect (unconjugated)		0.1-1.0 mg/dl		1.7-17.1 μmol/L
Total		0.1-1.2 mg/dl		1.7-20.5 μmol/L
Newborn's total		1-12 mg/dl		17.1-205.0 μmol/L
Blood gases				
pH	Whole blood	7.38-7.44 (arterial)	1	7.38-7.44
		7.36-7.41 (venous)		7.36-7.41
Pco_2	Whole blood	35-40 mm Hg (arterial)	0.133	4.66-5.32 kPa
		40-45 mm Hg (venous)		5.32-5.99 kPa
Po_2	Whole blood	95-100 mm Hg (arterial)	0.133	12.64-13.30 kPa
Bromide	Serum	0-5 mg/dl	0.125	0-0.63 mmol/L
BSP (Bromsulphalein) (5 mg/kg)	Serum	Less than 6% retention 45 min after injection	0.01	Fraction retention <0.06 at 45 min after dye injection
Calcium				
Ionized	Serum	4-4.8 mg/dl	0.25	1.0-1.2 mmol/L
		2.0-2.4 mEq/L	0.5	
		30%-58% of total	0.01	0.30-0.58 of total
Total	Serum	9.2-11.0 mg/dl	0.25	2.3-2.8 mmol/L
		4.6-5.5 mEq/L	0.5	23-28 mmol/L

*Usually not measured in blood (preferred specimen in urine, hair, or nails except in acute cases where gastric contents are used).

TABLE B-1 Whole blood, serum, and plasma chemistry—cont'd

COMPONENT	SYSTEM	TYPICAL REFERENCE INTERVALS		
		CONVENTIONAL UNITS	FACTOR	RECOMMENDED SI UNITS
Carbon dioxide (CO_2 content)	Whole blood (arterial)	19-24 mM	1	19-24 mmol/L
	Plasma or serum (arterial)	21-28 mM		21-28 mmol/L
Carbon dioxide	Whole blood (venous)	22-26 mM	1	22-26 mmol/L
	Plasma or serum (venous)	24-30 mM		24-30 mmol/L
CO_2 combining power	Plasma or serum (venous)	24-30 mM	1	24-30 mmol/L
CO_2 partial pressure (Pco_2)	Whole blood (arterial)	35-40 mm Hg	0.133	4.66-5.32 kPa
	Whole blood (venous)	40-45 mm Hg		5.32-5.99 kPa
Carbonic acid (H_2CO_3)	Whole blood (arterial)	1.05-1.45 mM	1	1.05-1.45 mmol/L
	Whole blood (venous)	1.15-1.50 mM		1.15-1.50 mmol/L
	Plasma (venous)	1.02-1.38 mM		1.02-1.38 mmol/L
Carboxyhemoglobin (carbon monoxide hemoglobin)	Whole blood			Fraction hemoglobin saturated
	Suburban non-smokers	<1.5% saturation of hemoglobin	0.01	<0.015
	Smokers	1.5-5.0% saturation		0.015-0.050
	Heavy smokers	5.0-9.0% saturation		0.050-0.090
Carotene, beta	Serum	40-200 μ/dl	0.0186	0.74-3.72 μmol/L
Ceruloplasmin	Serum	23-50 mg/dl	10	230-500 mg/L
Chloride	Serum	95-103 mEq/L	1	95-103 mmol/L
Cholesterol				
Total	Serum	150-250 mg/dl (varies with diet, sex, and age)	0.026	3.90-6.50 mmol/L
Esters	Serum	65%-75% of total cholesterol	0.01	Fraction of total cholesterol 0.65-0.75
Cholinesterase (pseudocholinesterase)	Erythrocytes	0.65-1.3 pH units	1	0.65-1.3 units
	Plasma	0.5-1.3 pH units		0.5-1.3 units
		8-18 IU/L at 37° C	1	8-18 U/L at 37° C
Citrate	Serum or plasma	1.7-3.0 mg/dl	52	88-156 μmol/L
Copper	Serum, plasma			
	Male	70-140 μg/dl	0.157	11.0-22.0 μmol/L
	Female	80-155 μg/dl		12.6-24.3 μmol/L
Cortisol	Plasma			
	8 AM-10 AM	5-23 μg/dl	27.6	138-635 nmol/L
	4 PM-6 PM	3-13 μg/dl		83-359 nmol/L
Creatine as creatinine	Serum or plasma			
	Male	0.1-0.4 mg/dl	76.3	7.6-30.5 μmol/L
	Female	0.2-0.7 mg/dl	76.3	15.3-53.4 μmol/L
Creatine kinase (CK)	Serum			
	Male	55-170 U/L at 37° C	1	55-170 U/L at 37° C
	Female	30-135 U/L at 37° C	1	30-135 U/L at 37° C
Creatinine	Serum or plasma	0.6-1.2 mg/dl (adult)	88.4	53-106 μmol/L
		0.3-0.6 mg/dl (children <2 yr)		27-54 μmol/L

Continued.

TABLE B-1 Whole blood, serum, and plasma chemistry—cont'd

COMPONENT	SYSTEM	TYPICAL REFERENCE INTERVALS		
		CONVENTIONAL UNITS	FACTOR	RECOMMENDED SI UNITS
Creatinine clearance (endogenous)	Serum or plasma and urine			
Male		107-139 ml/min	0.0167	1.78-2.32 ml/sec
Female		87-107 ml/min		1.45-1.79 ml/sec
Cryoglobulins	Serum	Negative	—	Negative
Electrophoresis, protein	Serum	Percent		Fraction of total protein
Albumin		52%-65% of total protein	0.01	0.52-0.65
Alpha-1		2.5%-5.0% of total protein	0.01	0.025-0.05
Alpha-2		7.0%-13.0% of total protein	0.01	0.07-0.13
Beta		8.0%-14.0% of total protein	0.01	0.08-0.14
Gamma		12.0%-22.0% of total protein	0.01	0.12-0.22
		Concentration		
Albumin		3.2-5.6 g/dl	10	32.56 g/L
Alpha-1		0.1-0.4 g/dl		1-4 g/L
Alpha-2		0.4-1.2 g/dl		4-12 g/L
Beta		0.5-1.1 g/dl		5-11 g/L
Gamma		0.5-1.6 g/dl		5-16 g/L
Fats, neutral (see Triglycerides)				
Fatty acids				
Total (free and esterified)	Serum	9-15 mM	1	9-15 mmol/L
Free (nonesterified)	Plasma	300-480 μEq/L	1	300-480 μmol/L
Ferritin	Serum			
Male		15-200 ng/ml		15-200 μg/L
Female		12-150 ng/ml		15-150 μg/L
Fibrinogen	Plasma	200-400 mg/dl	0.01	2.00-4.00 g/L
Fluoride	Whole blood	<0.05 mg/dl	0.53	<0.027 mmol/L
Folate	Serum	5-25 ng/ml (bioassay)	2.27	11-56 nmol/L
		>2.3 ng/ml (radioassay)		>5.2 nmol/L
	Erythrocytes	166-640 ng/ml (bioassay)		376-1452 nmol/L
		>140 ng/ml (radioassay)		>318 nmol/L
Galactose	Whole blood			
Adults		None	—	None
Children		<20 mg/dl	0.055	<1.1 mmol/L
Gamma globulin	Serum	0.5-1.6 g/dl	10	5-16 g/L
Globulins, total	Serum	2.3-3.5 g/dl	10	23-35 g/L
Globulins, fasting	Serum or plasma	70-110 mg/dl	0.055	3.85-6.05 mmol/L
	Whole blood	60-100 mg/dl		3.30-5.50 mmol/L
Glucose tolerance				
Oral	Serum or plasma			
Fasting		70-110 mg/dl	0.055	3.85-6.05 mmol/L
30 min		30-60 mg/dl above fasting		1.65-3.30 mmol/L above fasting
60 min		20-50 mg/dl above fasting		1.10-2.75 mmol/L above fasting
120 min		5-15 mg/dl above fasting		0.28-0.83 mmol/L above fasting
180 min		Fasting level or below		Fasting level or below

TABLE B-1 Whole blood, serum, and plasma chemistry—cont'd

COMPONENT	SYSTEM	TYPICAL REFERENCE INTERVALS		
		CONVENTIONAL UNITS	FACTOR	RECOMMENDED SI UNITS
Intravenous	Serum or plasma			
Fasting		70-110 mg/dl		3.85-6.05 mmol/L
5 min		Maximum of 250 mg/dl		Maximum of 13.75 mmol/L
60 min		Significant decrease		Significant decrease
120 min		Below 120 mg/dl		Below 6.60 mmol/L
180 min		Fasting level		Fasting level
Glucose 6-phosphate dehydrogenase (G6PD)	Erythrocytes	250-500 units/10^6 cells	1	250-500 μunits/cells
		1200-2000 mIU/ml packed erythrocytes		1200-2000 U/L packed erythrocytes
γ-Glutamyl transferase	Serum	5-40 IU/L	1	5-40 U/L at 37° C
Glutathione	Whole blood	24-37 mg/dl	0.032	0.77-1.18 mmol/L
Growth hormone	Serum	<10 ng/ml	1	<10 μg/L
Guanase	Serum	<3 nM/ml/min	1	<3 U/L at 37° C
Haptoglobin	Serum	60-270 mg/dl	0.01	0.6-2.7 g/L
Hemoglobin	Serum or plasma			
Qualitative		Negative	—	Negative
Quantitative		0.5-5.0 mg/dl	10	5-50 mg/L
	Whole blood			
Female		12.0-16.0 g/dl	10	1.86-2.48 mmol/L
Male		13.5-18.0 g/dl		2.09-2.79 mmol/L
α-Hydroxybutyrate dehydrogenase	Serum	140-350 U/ml	1	140-350 kU/L
17-Hydroxycorticosteroids	Plasma			
Male		7-19 μg/dl	10	70-190 μg/L
Female		9-21 μg/dl		9-21 μg/L
After 24 USP units of ACTH IM		35-55 μg/dl		350-550 μg/L
Immunoglobulins	Serum			
IgG		800-1801 mg/dl	0.01	8.0-18.0 g/L
IgA		113-563 mg/dl		1.1-5.6 g/L
IgM		54-222 mg/dl		0.54-2.2 g/L
IgD		0.5-3.0 mg/dl	10	5.0-30 mg/L
IgE		0.01-0.04 mg/dl		0.1-0.4 mg/L
Insulin	Plasma			
Bioassay		11-240 μIU/ml	0.0417	0.46-10.00 μg/L
Radioimmunoassay		4-24 μIU/ml		0.17-1.00 μg/L
Insulin tolerance (0.1 unit/kg)	Serum			
Fasting		Glucose of 70-110 mg/dl	0.055	Glucose of 3.85-6.05 mmol/L
30 min		Fall to 50% of fasting level	0.01	Fall to 0.5 of fasting level
90 min		Fasting level		Fasting level
Iodine				
Butanol-extraction (BEI)	Serum	3.5-6.5 μg/dl	0.079	0.28-0.51 μmol/L
Protein bound (PBI)	Serum	4.0-8.0 μg/dl		0.32-0.63 μmol/L
Iron, total	Serum	60-150 μg/dl	0.179	11-27 μmol/L
Iron binding capacity	Serum	250-400 μg/dl	0.179	54-64 μmol/L
Iron saturation	Serum	20%-55%	0.01	Fraction of total iron binding capacity: 0.20-0.55
Isocitric dehydrogenase	Serum	50-240 units/ml at 25° C (Wolfson-WIlliams Ashman units)	0.0167	0.83-4.18 U/L at 25° C

Continued.

TABLE B-1 Whole blood, serum, and plasma chemistry—cont'd

| COMPONENT | SYSTEM | TYPICAL REFERENCE INTERVALS | | |
		CONVENTIONAL UNITS	FACTOR	RECOMMENDED SI UNITS
Ketone bodies	Serum	Negative	—	Negative
17-Ketosteroids	Plasma	25-125 μg/dl	0.01	0.25-1.25 mg/L
Lactic acid (as lactate)	Whole blood			
	Venous	5-20 mg/dl	0.111	0.6-2.2 mmol/L
	Arterial	3-7 mg/dl		0.3-0.8 mmol/L
Lactate dehydrogenase (LDH)	Serum	(Lactate→pyruvate) 80-120 units at 30° C	0.48	38-62 U/L at 30° C
		(Pyruvate→lactate) 185-640 units at 30° C	0.48	90-310 U/L at 30° C
		(Lactate→pyruvate) 100-190 U/L at 37° C	1	100-190 U/L at 37° C
Lactate dehydrogenase isoenzymes	Serum			Fraction of total LDH
LDH$_1$ (anode)		17%-27%	0.01	0.17-0.27
LDH$_2$		27%-37%		0.27-0.37
LDH$_3$		18%-25%		0.18-0.25
LDH$_4$		3%-8%		0.03-0.08
LDH$_5$ (cathode)		0%-5%		0.00-0.05
Lactate dehydrogenase (heat stable)	Serum	30%-60% of total	0.01	Fraction of total LDH: 0.30-0.60
Lactose tolerance	Serum	Serum glucose changes similar to glucose tolerance test	—	Serum glucose changes similar to glucose tolerance test
Lead	Whole blood	0-50 μg/dl	0.048	0-2.4 μmol/L
Leucine aminopeptidase (LAP)	Serum			
	Male	80-200 U/ml (Goldbarg-Rutenberg)	0.24	19.2-48.0 U/L
	Female	75-185 U/ml (Goldbarg-Rutenberg)		18.0-44.4 U/L
Lipase	Serum	0-1.5 U/ml (Cherry-Crandall)	278	0-417 U/L
		14-280 mIU/ml	1	14-280 U/L
Lipids, total	Serum	400-800 mg/dl	0.01	4.00-8.00 g/L
Cholesterol		150-250 mg/dl	0.026	3.9-6.5 mmol/L
Triglycerides		10-190 mg/dl	0.109	1.09-20.71 mmol/L
Phospholipids		150-380 mg/dl	0.01	1.50-380 g/L
Fatty acids (free)		9.0-15.0 mM/L	1	9.0-15.0 mmol/L
		300-480 μEq/L	0.01	300-480 μmol/L
Phospholipid phosphorus		8.0-11.0 mg/dl	0.323	2.58-3.55 mmol/L
Lithium	Serum	Negative	—	Negative
Therapeutic interval		0.5-1.4 mEq/L	1	0.5-1.4 mmol/L
Long-acting thyroid-stimulating hormone (LATS)	Serum	None	—	None

TABLE B-1   Whole blood, serum, and plasma chemistry—cont'd

		TYPICAL REFERENCE INTERVALS		
COMPONENT	**SYSTEM**	**CONVENTIONAL UNITS**	**FACTOR**	**RECOMMENDED SI UNITS**
Leutinizing hormone (LH)	Serum			
	Male	6-30 mIU/ml	0.23	1.4-6.9 mg/L
	Female	Midcycle peak: 3 times baseline value		Midcycle peak: 3 times baseline value
		Premenopausal <30 mIU/ml		Premenopausal <5 times baseline value
		Postmenopausal >35 mIU/ml		Postmenopausal >5 times baseline value
Macroglobulins, total	Serum	70-430 mg/dl	0.01	0.7-4.3 g/L
Magnesium	Serum	1.3-2.1 mEq/L	0.5	0.7-1.1 mmol/L
		1.8-3.0 mg/dl	0.41	0.7-1.1 mmol/L
Methemoglobin	Whole blood	0-0.24 g/dl	10	0.0-2.4 g/L
		<1% of total hemoglobin	0.01	Fraction of total hemoglobin <0.01
Mucoprotein	Serum	80-200 mg/dl	0.01	0.8-2.0 g/L
Muramidase	Serum	4-13 mg/L		4-13 mg/L
Nonprotein nitrogen (NPN)	Serum or plasma	20-35 mg/dl	0.714	14.3-25.0 mmol/L
	Whole blood	25-50 mg/dl		17.9-35.7 mmol/L
5'Nucleotidase	Serum	0-1.6 units at 37° C	1	0-1.6 units at 37° C
Ornithine carbamyl transferase	Serum	8-20 mIU/ml at 37° C	1	8-20 U/L at 37° C
Osmolality	Serum	280-295 mOsm/kg	1	280-295 mmol/L
Oxygen				
Pressure (P_{O_2})	Whole blood (arterial)	95-100 mm Hg	0.133	12.64-13.30 kPa
Content	Whole blood (arterial)	15-23 volume %	0.01	Volume fraction: 0.15-0.23
Saturation	Whole blood (arterial)	94%-100%		0.94-1.00
pH	Whole blood (arterial)	7.38-7.44	1	7.38-7.44
	Whole blood (venous)	7.36-7.41		7.36-7.41
	Serum or plasma (venous)	7.35-7.45		7.35-7.45
Phenylalanine	Serum			
	Adults	<3.0 mg/dl	0.061	<0.18 mmol/L
	Newborns (term)	1.2-3.5 mg/dl		0.07-0.21 mmol/L
Phosphatase				
Acid phosphatase	Serum	0.13-0.63 U/L at 37° C (paranitrophenylphosphate)	16.67	2.2-10.5 U/L at 37° C
Alkaline phosphatase	Serum	20-90 IU/L at 30° C (paranitrophenylphosphate in AMP buffer)	1	20-90 U/L at 30° C
Phospholipid phosphorus	Serum	8-11 mg/dl	0.323	2.6-3.6 mmol/L
Phospholipids	Serum	150-380 mg/dl	0.01	1.50-3.80 g/L
Phosphorus, inorganic	Serum			
	Adults	2.3-4.7 mg/dl	0.323	0.78-1.52 mmol/L
	Children	4.0-7.0 mg/dl		1.29-2.26 mmol/L

Continued.

TABLE B-1 Whole blood, serum, and plasma chemistry—cont'd

		TYPICAL REFERENCE INTERVALS		
COMPONENT	SYSTEM	CONVENTIONAL UNITS	FACTOR	RECOMMENDED SI UNITS
Potassium	Plasma	3.8-5.0 mEq/L	1	3.8-5.0 mmol/L
Prolactin	Serum			
Female		1-25 ng/ml	1	1-25 µg/L
Male		1-20 ng/ml		1-20 µg/L
Proteins	Serum			
Total		6.0-7.8 g/dl	10	60-78 g/L
Albumin		3.2-4.5 g/dl		32-45 g/L
Globulin		2.3-3.5 g/dl		23-35 g/L
Protein fractionation		See electrophoresis		See electrophoresis
Protoporphyrin	Erythrocytes	15-50 µg/dl	0.018	0.27-0.90 µmol/L
Pyruvate	Whole blood	0.3-0.9 mg/dl	114	34-103 µmol/L
Salicylates	Serum	Negative	—	Negative
Therapeutic interval		15-30 mg/dl	0.072	1.44-1.80 mmol/L
		150-300 µg/ml	0.0072	1.08-2.16 mmol/L
Sodium	Plasma	136-142 mEq/L	1	136-142 mmol/L
Sulfate, inorganic	Serum	0.2-1.3 mEq/L	0.5	0.10-0.65 mmol/L
		0.9-6.0 mg/dl as SO_4	0.104	0.09-0.62 mmol/L as SO_4
Sulfhemoglobin	Whole blood	Negative	—	Negative
Sulfonamides	Serum or whole blood	Negative	—	Negative
Testosterone	Serum or plasma			
Male		300-1200 ng/dl	0.035	10.0-42.0 nmol/L
Female		30-95 ng/dl		1.1-3.3 nmol/L
Thiocyanate	Serum	Negative	—	Negative
Thyroid hormone tests	Serum			
a) Expressed as thyroxine				
T_4 by column		5.0-11.0 µg/dl	13.0	65-143 nmol/L
T_4 by competitive binding—Murphy-Pattee		6.0-11.8 µg/dl		78-153 nmol/L
T_4 RIA		5.5-12.5 µg/dl	13.0	72-163 nmol/L
Free T_4		0.9-2.3 ng/dl		12-30 pmol/L
b) Expressed as iodine				
T_4 by column		3.2-7.2 µg/dl	79.0	253-569 nmol/L
T_4 by competitive binding—Murphy-Pattee		3.9-7.7 µg/dl		308-608 nmol/L
Free T_4		0.6-1.5 ng/dl	79.0	47-119 pmol/L
T_3 resin uptake		25-38 relative % uptake	0.01	Relative uptake fraction 0.25-0.38

TABLE B-1 Whole blood, serum, and plasma chemistry—cont'd

COMPONENT	SYSTEM	TYPICAL REFERENCE INTERVALS		
		CONVENTIONAL UNITS	FACTOR	RECOMMENDED SI UNITS
Thyroxine-binding globulin (TBG)	Serum	10-26 µg/dl	10	100-260 µg/L
TSH	Serum	<10 µU/ml	1	$<10^{-3}$IU/L
Transferases				
Aspartate amino transferase (AST or SGOT)	Serum	10-40 U/ml (Karmen) at 25° C	0.48	8-29 U/L at 30° C
		16-60 U/ml (Karmen) at 30° C		8-33 U/L at 37° C
Alanine amino transferase (ALT or SGPT)	Serum	10-30 U/ml (Karmen) at 25° C	0.48	4-24 U/L at 30° C
		8-50 U/ml (Karmen) at 30° C		4-36 U/L at 37° C
Gamma glutamyl transferase (GGT)		5-40 IU/L at 37° C	1	5.40 U/L at 37° C
Triglycerides	Serum	10-190 mg/dl	0.011	0.11-2.09 mmol/L
Urea nitrogen	Serum	8-23 mg/dl	0.357	2.9-8.2 mmol/L
Urea clearance	Serum and urine			
Maximum clearance		64-99 ml/min	0.0167	1.07-1.65 ml/sec
Standard clearance		41-65 ml/min, or more than 75% of normal clearance		0.68-1.09 ml/sec or more than 0.75 of normal clearance
Uric acid	Serum			
Male		4.0-8.5 mg/dl	0.059	0.24-0.5 mmol/L
Female		2.7-7.3 mg/dl		0.16-0.43 mmol/L
Vitamin A	Serum	15-60 µg/dl	0.035	0.53-2.10 µmol/L
Vitamin A tolerance	Serum			
Fasting 3 hr or 6 hr after 5000 units		15-60 µg/dl	0.035	0.53-2.10 µmol/L
Vitamin A/kg 24 hrs		200-600 µg/dl Fasting values or slightly above	—	7.00-21.00 µmol/L Fasting values or slightly above
Vitamin B$_{12}$	Serum	160-950 pg/ml	0.74	118-703 pmol/L
Unsaturated vitamin B$_{12}$ binding capacity	Serum	1000-2000 pg/ml	0.74	740-1480 pmol/L
Vitamin C	Plasma	0.6-1.6 mg/dl	56.8	34-91 µmol/L
Xylose absorption	Serum			
Normal		25-40 mg/dl between 1 and 2 hr	0.067	1.68-2.68 mmol/L between 1 and 2 hr
In malabsorption		Maximum approximately 10 mg/dl		Maximum approximately 0.67 mmol/L
Dose: Adult		25 g D-xylose	0.067	0.167 mol D-xylose
Children		0.5 g/kg D-xylose		3.33 mmol/kg D-xylose
Zinc	Serum	50-150 µg/dl	0.153	7.65-22.95 µmol/L

TABLE B-2 Urine

COMPONENT	TYPE OF URINE SPECIMEN	TYPICAL REFERENCE INTERVALS		
		CONVENTIONAL UNITS	FACTOR	RECOMMENDED SI UNITS
Acetoacetic acid	Random	Negative	—	Negative
Acetone	Random	Negative	—	Negative
Addis count	12 hr collection	WBC and epithelial cells		
		1,800,00/12 hr	1	$1.8 \times 10^6/12$ hr
		RBC 500,000/12 hr	1	$0.5 \times 10^6/12$ hr
		Hyaline casts: 0-5000/12 hr	1	$5.0 \times 10^3/12$ hr
Albumin				
Qualitative	Random	Negative	—	Negative
Quantitative	24 hr	15-150 mg/24 hr	1	0.015-0.150 g/24 hr
Aldosterone	24 hr	2-26 μg/24 hr	2.77	5.5-72.0 nmol/24 hr
Alkapton bodies	Random	Negative	—	Negative
Alpha-amino acid nitrogen	24 hr	100-290 mg/24 hr	0.0714	7.14-20.71 mmol/24 hr
δ-Aminolevulinic acid	Random			
Adult		0.1-0.6 mg/dl	76.3	7.6-45.8 μmol/L
Children		<0.5 mg/dl		<38.1 μmol/L
	24 hr	1.5-7.5 mg/24 hr	7.63	11.15-57.2 μmol/24 hr
Ammonia nitrogen	24 hr	20-70 mEq/24 hr		
		500-1200 mg/24 hr	0.071	35.5-85.2 mmol/24 hr
Amylase	2 hr	35-260 Somogyi units/hr	0.185	6.5-48.1 U/hr
Arsenic	24 hr	<50 mg/L	0.013	<0.65 μmol/L
Ascorbic acid	Random	1-7 mg/dl	0.057	0.06-0.40 mmol/L
	24 hr	>50 mg/24 hr	0.0057	>0.29 mmol/24 hr
Bence Jones protein	Random	Negative	—	Negative
Beryllium	24 hr	<0.05 μg/24 hr	111	<5.55 nmol/24 hr
Bilirubin, qualitative	Random	Negative	—	Negative
Blood, occult	Random	Negative	—	Negzative
Borate	24 hr	<2 mg/L	16	<32 μmol/L
Calcium				
Qualitative (Sulkowitch)	Random	1+ turbidity	1	1+ turbidity
Quantitative	24 hr			
Average diet		100-240 mg/24 hr	0.025	2.50-6.25 mmol/24 hr
Low calcium diet		<150 mg/24 hr		<3.75 mmol/24 hr
High calcium diet		240-300 mg/24 hr		6.25-7.50 mmol/24 hr
Catecholamines	Random	0-14 μg/dl	10	0-140 μg/L
	24 hr	<100 μg/24 hr (varies with activity)	1	<100 μg/24 hr
Epinephrine		<10 ng/24 hr	5.46	<55 nmol/24 hr
Norepinephrine		<100 ng/24 hr	5.91	<590 nmol/24 hr
Total free catecholamines		4-126 μg/24 hr	1	4-126 μg/24 hr
Total metanephrines		0.1-1.6 mg/24 hr	1	0.1-1.6 mg/24 hr
Chloride	24 hr	140-250 mEq/24 hr	1	140-250 mmol/24 hr
Concentration test (Fishberg)	Random—after fluid restriction			
Specific gravity		>1.025	1	>1.025

TABLE B-2 Urine—cont'd

| COMPONENT | TYPE OF URINE SPECIMEN | TYPICAL REFERENCE INTERVALS | | |
		CONVENTIONAL UNITS	FACTOR*	RECOMMENDED SI UNITS†
Osmolality		>850 mOsm/L	1	>850 mmol/L
Copper	24 hr	0-50 µg/24 hr	0.016	0-0.48 µmol/24 hr
Coproporphyrin	Random			
Adult		3-20 µg/dl	0.015	0.045-0.30 µmol/L
	24 hr			
Adult		50-160 µg/24 hr	0.0015	0.075-0.24 µmol/24 hr
Children		0-80 µg/24 hr	0.0015	0.00-0.12 µmol/24 hr
Creatine	24 hr			
Male		0-40 mg/24 hr	0.0076	0-0.30 mmol/24 hr
Female		0-100 mg/24 hr		0-0.76 mmol/24 hr
		Higher in children and during pregnancy	—	Higher in children and during pregnancy
Creatinine	24 hr			
Male		20-26 mg/kg/24 hr	0.0088	0.18-0.23 mmol/kg/24 hr
		1.0-2.0 g/24 hr	8.8	8.8-17.6 mmol/24 hr
Female		14-22 mg/kg/24 hr	0.0088	0.12-0.19 mmol/kg/24 hr
		0.8-1.8 g/24 hr	8.8	7.0-15.8 mmol/24 hr
Cystine, qualitative	Random	Negative	—	Negative
Cystine and cysteine	24 hr	10-100 mg/24 hr	0.0083	0.08-0.83 mmol/24 hr
Diacetic acid	Random	Negative	—	Negative
Epinephrine	24 hr	0-20 µg/24 hr	0.0055	0.00-0.11 µmol/24 hr
Estrogens				
Total	24 hr			
Male		5-18 µg/24 hr	1	5-18 µg/24 hr
Female				
Ovulation		28-100 µg/24 hr		28-80 µg/24 hr
Luteal peak		22-80 µg/24 hr		22-105 µg/24 hr
At menses		4-25 µg/24 hr		4-25 µg/24 hr
Pregnancy		Up to 45,000 µg/24 hr		Up to 45,000 µg/24 hr
Postmenopausal		Up to 10 µg/24 hr		Up to 10 µg/24 hr
Fractionated	24 hr, nonpregnant, midcycle			
Estrone (E¹)	—	2.25 µg/24 hr	3.7	7-93 nmol/24 hr
Estradiol (E²)	—	0-10 µg/24 hr	3.7	0-37 nmol/24 hr
Estriol (E³)	—	2-30 µg/24 hr	3.5	7-105 nmol/24 hr
Fat, qualitative	Random	Negative	—	Negative
FIGLU (N-formiminoglutamic acid)	24 hr	<3 mg/24 hr	5.7	<17.0 µmol/24 hr
	After 15 g of L-histidine	4 mg/8 hr	5.7	23.0 µmol/8 hr
Fluoride	24 hr	<1 mg/24 hr	0.053	0.053 mmol/24 hr
Follicle-stimulating hormone (FSH)	24 hr			
Adult		6-50 Mouse uterine units (MUU)/24 hr	1	4-25 mIU/ml
Prepubertal		<10 MUU/24 hr	1	4-30 mIU/ml
Postmenopausal		>50 MUU/24 hr	1	40-50 mIU/ml
Midcycle		2× baseline		
Fructose	24 hr	30-65 mg/24 hr	0.0056	0.17-0.36 mmol/24 hr

Continued.

TABLE B-2 Urine—cont'd

| COMPONENT | TYPE OF URINE SPECIMEN | TYPICAL REFERENCE INTERVALS | | |
		CONVENTIONAL UNITS	FACTOR*	RECOMMENDED SI UNITS†
Glucose				
Qualitative	Random	Negative	—	Negative
Quantitative	24 hr			
Copper-reducing substances 0.5-1.5 g/24 hr			0.5-1.5 g/24 hr	1
Total sugars		Average 250 mg/24 hr	1	Average 250 mg/24 hr
Glucose		Average 130 mg/24 hr	0.0056	Average 0.73 mmol/24 hr
Gonadotropins, pituitary (FSH and LH)	24 hr	10-50 MUU/24 hr	1	10-50 IU/24 hr
Etiocholanolone	24 hr			
Male		1.4-5.0 mg/24 hr	3.44	4.8-17.2 μmol/24 hr
Female		0.8-4.0 mg/24 hr		2.8-13.8 μmol/24 hr
Dehydroepiandrosterone	24 hr			
Male		0.2-2.0 mg/24 hr	3.46	0.7-6.9 μmol/24 hr
Female		0.2-1.8 mg/24 hr		0.7-6.2 μmol/24 hr
11-Ketoandrosterone	24 hr			
Male		0.2-1.0 mg/24 hr	3.28	0.7-3.3 μmol/24 hr
Female		0.2-0.8 mg/24 hr		0.7-2.6 μmol/24 hr
11-Ketoetiocholanolone	24 hr			
Male		0.2-1.0 mg/24 hr	3.28	0.7-3.3 μmol/24 hr
Female		0.2-0.8 mg/24 hr		0.7-2.6 μmol/24 hr
11-Hydroxyandrosterone	24 hr			
Male		0.1-0.8 mg/24 hr	3.26	0.3-2.6 μmol/24 hr
Female		0.0-0.5 mg/24 hr		0.0-1.6 μmol/24 hr
11-Hydroxyetiocholanolone	24 hr			
Male		0.2-0.6 mg/24 hr	3.26	0.7-2.0 μmol/24 hr
Female		0.1-1.1 mg/24 hr		0.3-3.6 μmol/24 hr
Lactose	24 hr	14-40 mg/24 hr	2.9	41-116 μmol/24 hr
Lead	24 hr	<100 μg/24 hr	0.0048	<0.48 μmol/24 hr
Magnesium	24 hr	6.0-8.5 mEq/24 hr	0.5	3.0-4.3 mmol/24 hr
Melanin, qualitative	Random	Negative	—	Negative
3-Methoxy-4-hydroxymandelic acid (VMA)	24 hr			
Adults		1.5-7.5 mg/24 hr	5.05	7.6-37.9 μmol/24 hr
Infants		83 μg/kg/24 hr	0.0051	0.4 μmol/kg/24 hr
Mucin	24 hr	100-150 mg/24 hr	1	100-150 mg/24 hr
Muramidase (lysozyme)	24 hr	1.3-36 mg/24 hr		1.3-36 mg/24 hr
Myoglobin				
Qualitative	Random	Negative	—	Negative
Quantitative	24 hr	<4 mg/L	1	<4 mg/L
Osmolality	Random	500-800 mOsm/kg water	1	500-800 mmol/kg
Pentoses	24 hr	2-5 mg/kg/24 hr	1	2-5 mg/kg/24 hr

TABLE B-2   Urine—cont'd

| COMPONENT | TYPE OF URINE SPECIMEN | TYPICAL REFERENCE INTERVALS | | |
		CONVENTIONAL UNITS	FACTOR*	RECOMMENDED SI UNITS†
pH	Random	4.6-8.0	1	4.6-8.0
Phenolsulfon-	6 mg			Fraction dye excreted
phthalein (PSP)	PSP IV			
	15 min	20%-50% dye excreted	0.01	0.2-0.5
	30 min	16%-24% dye excreted		0.16-0.24
	60 min	9%-17% dye excreted		0.09-0.17
	120 min	3%-10% dye excreted		0.03-0.10
Phenylpyruvic acid, qualitative	Random	Negative	—	Negative
Phosphorus	Random	0.9-1.3 g/24 hr	32	29-42 mmol/24 hr
Porphobilinogen				
Qualitative	Random	Negative	—	Negative
Quantitative	24 hr	0-1.0 mg/24 hr	4.42	0-4.4 μmol/24 hr
Potassium	24 hr	40-80 mEq/24 hr	1	40-80 mmol/24 hr
Pregnancy tests	Concentrated morning specimen	Positive in normal pregnancies or with tumors producing chorionic gonadotropin	—	Positive in normal pregnancies or with tumors producing chorionic gonadotropin
Pregnanediol	24 hr			
Male		0-1.5 mg/24 hr	3.12	0-4.7 μmol/24 hr
Female		1-8 mg/24 hr		3-25 μmol/24 hr
Peak		1 week after ovulation	—	1 week after ovulation
Pregnancy		<50 mg/24 hr		156 μmol/24 hr
Children		Negative	—	Negative
Pregnanetriol	24 hr			
Male		0.4-2.4 mg/24 hr	2.97	1.2-7.1 μmol/24 hr
Female		0.5-2.0 mg/24 hr		1.5-5.9 μmol/24 hr
Children		Up to 1 mg/24 hr		Up to 3 μmol/24 hr
Protein, qualitative	Random	Negative	—	Negative
	24 hr	40-150 mg/24 hr	1	40-150 mg/24 hr
Reducing substances, total	24 hr	0.5-1.5 mg/24 hr	1	0.5-1.5 mg/24 hr
Sodium	24 hr	75-200 mEq/24 hr	1	75-200 mmol/24 hr
Solids, total	24 hr	55-70 g/24 hr	1	55-70 g/24 hr
		Decreases with age to 30 g/24 hr	—	Decreases with age to 30 g/24 hr
Specific gravity	Random			Relative density (U 20° C/ water 20° C)
		1.016-1.022 (normal fluid intake)	1	1.016-1.022 (normal fluid intake)
		1.001-1.035 (range)		1.001-1.034 (range)
Sugars (excluding glucose)	Random	Negative	—	Negative
Titratable acidity	24 hr	20-50 mEq/24 hr	1	20-50 mmol/24 hr

Continued.

TABLE B-2   Urine—cont'd

| COMPONENT | TYPE OF URINE SPECIMEN | TYPICAL REFERENCE INTERVALS | | |
		CONVENTIONAL UNITS	FACTOR	RECOMMENDED SI UNITS
Urea nitrogen	24 hr	6-17 g/24 hr	0.0357	0.21-0.60 mol/24 hr
Uric acid	24 hr	250-750 mg/24 hr	0.0059	1.48-4.43 mmol/24 hr
Urobilinogen	2 hr	0.3-1.0 Ehrlich units	—	
	24 hr	0.05-2.5 mg/24 hr or	1.69	0.09-4.23 μmol/24 hr
		0.5-4.0 Ehrlich units/24 hr	—	
Uropepsin	Random	15-45 units/hr (Anson)	7.37	111-332 U/hr
	24 hr	1500-5000 units/24 hr (Anson)		11-37 kU/hr
Uroporphyrins				
Qualitative	Random	Negative	—	Negative
Quantitative	24 hr	10-30 μg/24 hr	0.0012	0.012-0.37 μmol/24 hr
Vanillylmandelic acid (VMA)	24 hr	1.5-7.5 mg/24 hr	5.05	7.6-37.9 μmol/24 hr
Volume, total	24 hr	600-1600 ml/24 hr	0.001	0.6-1.6 L/24 hr
Zinc	24 hr	0.15-1.2 mg/24 hr	15.3	2.3-18.4 μmol/24 hr

TABLE B-3   Synovial fluid

| COMPONENT | TYPICAL REFERENCE INTERVALS | | |
	CONVENTIONAL UNITS	FACTOR	RECOMMENDED SI UNITS
Blood-serum-synovial fluid glucose difference	<10 mg/dl	0.055	<0.55 mmol/L
Differential cell count	Granulocytes <25% of nucleated cells	0.01	Granulocyte number fraction: <25% of nucleated cells
Fibrin clot	Absent	—	Absent
Mucin clot	Abundant	—	Abundant
Nucleated cell count	<200 cells/μl	10^6	$<2 \times 10^8$ cells/L
Viscosity	High	—	High
Volume	<3.5 ml	0.001	<0.0035 L

TABLE B-4   Seminal fluid

| COMPONENT | TYPICAL REFERENCE INTERVALS | | |
	CONVENTIONAL UNITS	FACTOR	RECOMMENDED SI UNITS
Liquefaction	Within 20 min	1	Within 20 min
Sperm morphology	>70% normal mature spermatozoa	0.01	Number fraction: >0.7 normal, mature spermatozoa
Sperm motility	>60%	0.01	Number fraction: >0.6
pH	>7.0 (average 7.7)	1	>7.0 (average 7.7)
Sperm count	60-150 million/ml	10^5	$60\text{-}150 \times 10^9$/L
Volume	1.5-5.0 ml	0.001	0.0015-0.005 L

TABLE B-5   Gastric fluid

COMPONENT	TYPICAL REFERENCE INTERVALS		
	CONVENTIONAL UNITS	FACTOR	RECOMMENDED SI UNITS
Fasting residual volume	20-100 ml	0.001	0.02-0.10 L
pH	<2.0	1	<2.0
Basal acid output (BAO)	0-6 mEq/hr	1	0-6 mmol/hr
Maximum acid ouput (MAO) (after histamine stimulation)	5-40 mEq/hr	1	5-40 mmol/hr
BAO/MAO ratio	<0.4	1	<0.4

TABLE B-6   Hematology

COMPONENT	TYPICAL REFERENCE INTERVALS		
	CONVENTIONAL UNITS	FACTOR	RECOMMENDED SI UNITS
Red cell volume			
Male	20-36 ml/kg body weight	0.001	0.020-0.036 L/kg body weight
Female	19-31 ml/kg body weight	—	0.019-0.031 L/kg body weight
Plasma volume			
Male	25-42 ml/kg body weight		0.040-0.050 L/kg body weight
Female	28-45 ml/kg body weight	—	0.040-0.050 L/kg body weight
Coagulation and hemostatic tests			
Bleeding time			
Mielke template	2-8 minutes		2-8 min
Simplate	3-8 minutes		3-8 min
Antithrombin III			
Immunologic	21-30 mg/dl		210-310 mg/L
Functional	80%-120%		0.8-1.2
Clot reaction	40%-94% of serum extruded in 1 hr at 37° C		
Euglobulin clot lysis time	Clot lyses between 2 and 4 hr at 37° C		
Factor assays (procoagulant)	0.5-1.5 U/ml		0.5-1.5
Factor VIII antigen (Factor VIIIR: Ag; Laurell)	0.5-1.5 U/ml		0.5-1.5
Ristocetin cofactor (Factor VIIIR: RCoF)	0.5-1.5 U/ml		0.5-1.5
Factor XIII (screening test)	Clot insoluble in 5M urea at 24 hr		
Fibrinogen	200-400 mg/dl		2-4 g/dl
Fibrinogen split products	10 µg/ml		10 mg/L
Partial thromboplastin time (PTT)	Depends upon phospholipid reagent used, typically 60-80 sec		
Activated PTT	Depends upon activator and phospholipid reagents used, typically 20-35 sec		
Plasminogen			
Immunologic	10-20 mg/dl		100-200 mg/L
Functional	2.2-4.2 CTA U/ml*		
Prothrombin time	Depends upon thromboplastin reagent used, typically 9.5-12 sec		
Thrombin time	Depends upon concentration of thrombin reagent used, typically 20-29 sec		
Whole blood clot lysis time	None in 24 hr		
Complete blood count (CBC)			
Hematocrit			
Male	40%-54%	0.01	Volume fraction: 0.40-0.54
Female	38%-47%		0.38%-0.47%
Hemoglobin			
Male	13.5-18.0 g/dl	0.155	2.09-2.79 mmol/L
Female	12.0-16.0 g/dl		1.86-2.48 mmol/L

*CTA, *Committee on Thrombotic Agents.*

Continued.

TABLE B-6 Hematology—cont'd

COMPONENT	TYPICAL REFERENCE INTERVALS			
	CONVENTIONAL UNITS		FACTOR	RECOMMENDED SI UNITS
Red cell count				
Male	$4.6\text{-}6.2 \times 10^6/\mu l$		10^6	$4.6\text{-}6.2 \times 10^{12}/L$
Female	$4.2\text{-}5.4 \times 10^6/\mu l$			$4.2\text{-}5.4 \times 10^{12}/L$
White cell count	$4.5\text{-}11.0 \times 10^3/\mu l$		10^6	$4.5\text{-}11.0 \times 10^9/L$
Erythrocyte indices				
Mean corpuscular volume (MCV)	80-96 cu microns		1	80-96 fl
Mean corpuscular hemoglobin (MCH)	27-31 pg		1	27-31 pg
Mean corpuscular hemoglobin concentration (MCHC)	32%-36%		0.01	Concentration fraction: 0.32-0.36

White blood cell differential (adult):

COMPONENT	*Mean percent*	*Range of absolute counts*	FACTOR	*Mean number fraction**	*Range of absolute count*
Segmented neutrophils	56%	$1800\text{-}7000/\mu l$	10^6	0.56	$1.8\text{-}7.8 \times 10^9/L$
Bands	3%	$0\text{-}700/\mu l$	10^6	0.03	$0\text{-}0.70 \times 10^9/L$
Eosinophils	2.7%	$0\text{-}450/\mu l$	10^6	0.027	$0\text{-}0.45 \times 10^9/L$
Basophils	0.3%	$0\text{-}200/\mu l$	10^6	0.003	$0\text{-}0.20 \times 10^9/L$
Lymphocytes	34%	$1000\text{-}48000/\mu l$	10^6	0.34	$1.0\text{-}4.8 \times 10^9/L$
Monocytes	4%	$0\text{-}800/\mu l$	10^6	0.04	$0\text{-}0.80 \times 10^9/L$

COMPONENT	CONVENTIONAL UNITS	FACTOR	RECOMMENDED SI UNITS
Hemoglobin A_2	1.5%-3.5% of total hemoglobin	0.01	Mass fraction: 0.015-0.035 of total hemoglobin
Hemoglobin F	<2%	0.01	Mass fraction: <0.02

Osmotic fragility:

% NaCl	*% Lysis* Fresh	*% Lysis* 24 hr at 37°C	FACTOR	NaCl mmol/L	*Lysed fraction* Fresh	*Lysed fraction* 24 hr at 37°C
0.2	—	95-100	% NaCl—171	34.2	—	0.95-1.00
0.3	97-100	85-100	% Lysis—0.01	51.3	0.97-1.00	0.85-1.00
0.35	90-99	75-100		59.8	9.90-0.99	0.75-1.00
0.4	50-95	65-100		68.4	0.50-0.95	0.65-1.00
0.45	5-45	55-95		77.0	0.05-0.45	0.55-0.95
0.5	0-6	40-85		85.5	0-0.06	0.40-0.85
0.55	0	15-70		94.1	0	0.15-0.70
0.6	—	0-40		102.6	—	0-0.40
0.65	—	0-10		111.2	—	0-0.10
0.7	—	0-5		119.7	—	0-0.05
0.75	—	0		128.3	—	0

COMPONENT	CONVENTIONAL UNITS	FACTOR	RECOMMENDED SI UNITS
Platelet count	$150,000\text{-}400,000/\mu l$	10^6	$0.15\text{-}0.4 \times 10^{12}/L$
Reticulocyte count	0.5%-1.5%	0.01	Number fraction: 0.005-0.015
	25,000-75,000 cells/μl	10^6	$25\text{-}75 \times 10^9/L$
Sedimentation rate (ESR) (Westergren)			
Men under 50 yrs	<50 mm/hr	1	<15 mm/hr
Men over 50 yrs	<20 mm/hr		<20 mm/hr
Women under 50 yrs	<20 mm/hr		<20 mm/hr
Women over 50 yrs	<30 mm/hr		<30 mm/hr
Viscosity	1.4-1.8 times water	1	1.4-1.8 times water
Zeta sedimentation ratio	41%-54%	0.01	Fraction: 0.41-0.54

*All percentages are multiplied by 0.01 to give fraction.

TABLE B-7   Amniotic fluid

| COMPONENT | TYPICAL REFERENCE INTERVALS | | |
	CONVENTIONAL UNITS	FACTOR	RECOMMENDED SI UNITS
Appearance			
Early gestation	Clear	—	Clear
Term	Clear or slightly opalescent	—	Clear or slightly opalescent
Albumin			
Early gestation	0.39 g/dl	10	3.9 g/dl
Term	0.19 g/dl		1.9 g/dl
Bilirubin			
Early gestation	<0.075 mg/dl	17.1	<1.28 μmol/L
Term	<0.025 mg/dl		<0.43 μmol/L
Chloride			
Early gestation	Approximately equal to serum chloride	—	Approximately equal to serum chloride
Term	Generally 1-3 mEq/L lower than serum chloride	1	Generally 1-3 mmol/L lower than serum chloride
Creatinine			
Early gestation	0.8-1.1 mg/dl	88.4	70.7-97.2 μmol/L
Term	1.8-4.0 mg/dl (generally >2 mg/dl)		159.1-353.6 μmol/L (generally >176.8 μmol/L)
Estriol			
Early gestation	<10 μg/dl	0.035	<0.35 μmol/L
Term	>60 μg/dl		>2.1 μmol/L
Lecithin/sphingomyelin		1	
Early (immature)	<1:1	1	<1:1
Term (mature)	>2:1	1	>2:1
Osmolality			
Early gestation	Approximately equal to serum osmolality	1	Approximately equal to serum osmolality
Term	230-270 mOsm/L	1	<230-270 mmol/L
Pco_2			
Early gestation	33-55 mm Hg	0.133	4.39-7.32 kPa
Term	42-55 mm Hg (increases toward term)		5.59-7.32 kPa (increases toward term)
pH			
Early gestation	7.12-7.38	1	7.12-7.38
Term	6.91-7.43 (decreases toward term)		6.91-7.43
Protein, total			
Early gestation	0.60 ± 0.24 g/dl	10	6.0 ± 2.4 g/L
Term	0.26 ± 0.19 g/dl		2.6 ± 1.9 g/L
Sodium			
Early gestation	Approximately equal to serum sodium	—	Approximately equal to serum sodium
Term	7-10 mEq/L lower than serum sodium	1	7-10 mmol/L lower than serum sodium
Staining, cytologic			
Oil red O			Stained fraction
Early gestation	<10%	0.01	<0.1
Term	>50%		>0.5
Nile blue sulfate			Stained fraction
Early gestation	0	0.01	0
Term	>20%		>0.2

Continued.

TABLE B-7 Amniotic fluid—cont'd

COMPONENT	TYPICAL REFERENCE INTERVALS		
	CONVENTIONAL UNITS	FACTOR	RECOMMENDED SI UNITS
Urea			
Early gestation	18.0 ± 5.9 mg/dl	0.166	2.99 ± 0.98 mmol/L
Term	30.3 ± 11.4 mg/dl		5.03 ± 1.89 mmol/L
Uric acid			
Early gestation	3.72 ± 0.96 mg/dl	0.059	0.22 ± 0.06 mmol/L
Term	9.90 ± 2.23 mg/dl		0.58 ± 0.13 mmol/L
Volume			
Early gestation	450-1200 ml	0.001	0.45-1.2 L
Term	500-1400 ml (increases toward term)		0.5-1.4 L (increases toward term)

TABLE B-8 Cerebrospinal fluid

COMPONENT	TYPICAL REFERENCE INTERVALS		
	CONVENTIONAL UNITS	FACTOR	RECOMMENDED SI UNITS
Albumin	10-30 mg/dl	10	100-300 mg/L
Calcium	2.1-2.7 mEq/L	0.5	1.05-1.35 mmol/L
Cell count	0-5 cells/µl	10^6	$0-5 \times 10^6$/L
Chloride			
Adult	118-132 mEq/L	1	118-132 mmol/L
Glucose	50-80 mg/dl	0.055	2.75-4.40 mmol/L
Lactate dehydrogenase (LDH)	Approximately 10% of serum level	—	Activity fraction: approximately 0.1 of serum level
Protein			
Total CSF	15-45 mg/dl	10	150-450 mg/L
Ventricular fluid	5-15 mg/dl		50-150 mg/L
Protein electrophoresis			Fraction
Prealbumin	2%-7%	0.01	0.02-0.07
Albumin	56%-76%		0.56-0.76
Alpha-1 globulin	2%-7%		0.02-0.07
Alpha-2 globulin	4%-12%		0.04-0.12
Beta globulin	8%-18%		0.08-0.18
Gamma globulin	3%-12%		0.03-0.12
Xanthochromia	Negative	—	Negative

TABLE B-9 Miscellaneous

COMPONENT	SPECIMEN	TYPICAL REFERENCE INTERVALS		
		CONVENTIONAL UNITS	FACTOR	RECOMMENDED SI UNITS
Bile, qualitative	Random stool	Negative in adults	—	Negative in adults
		Positive in children	—	Positive in children
Chloride	Sweat	4-60 mEq/L	1	4-60 mmol/L
Clearances	Serum and urine (timed)			
Creatinine, endogenous		115 + 20 ml/min	0.0167	1.92 + 0.33 ml/sec
Diodrast		600-720 ml/min		10.02-12.02 ml/sec
Inulin		100-150 ml/min		1.67-2.51 ml/sec
PAH		600-750 ml/min		10.02-12.53 ml/sec
Diagnex blue (tubeless gastric analysis)	Urine	Free acid present	—	Free acid present
Fat	Stool, 72 hr			
Total fat		<5 g/24 hr	0.01	<5 g/24 hr
				Mass fraction
		10%-25% of dry matter	0.01	0.1-0.24 of dry matter
Neutral fat		1%-5% of dry matter	0.01	0.01-0.05 of dry matter
Free fatty acids		5%-13% of dry matter	0.01	0.05-0.13 of dry matter
Combined fatty acids		5%-15% of dry matter	0.01	0.05-0.15 of dry matter
Nitrogen, total	Stool, 24 hr			Mass fraction
		10% of intake	0.01	0.1 of intake
		1-2 g/24 hr	0.071	0.071-0.142 mol/24 hr
Sodium	Sweat	10-80 mEq/L	1	10-80 mmol/L
Trypsin activity	Random, fresh stool	Positive (2+ to 4+)	—	Positive (2+ to 4+)
Thyroid ^{31}L uptake		7.5%-25% in 6 hr	0.01	Fraction uptake: 0.075-0.25 in 6 hr
Urobilinogen				
Qualitative	Random stool	Positive	—	Positive
Quantitative	Stool, 24 hr	40-200 mg/24 hr	0.00169	0.068-0.34 mmol/24 hr
		80-280 Ehrlich units/ 24 hr		

Index